# HEPATOBILIARY AND PANCREATIC SURGERY

*Seventh Edition*

**A Companion to Specialist Surgical Practice**

**Seventh Edition**

Series Editors
**O. James Garden**
**Simon Paterson-Brown**

# HEPATOBILIARY AND PANCREATIC SURGERY

Edited by

**Rowan W. Parks, MB BCh BAO, FRCSI, FRCS(Ed), FFST(RCSEd), FCSSL(Hon), FCPSP(Hon), FAIS(Hon)**
Professor of Surgical Sciences, Clinical Surgery, The University of Edinburgh;
Honorary Consultant HPB Surgeon, Royal Infirmary of Edinburgh,
Edinburgh, UK

**Stephen J. Wigmore, BSc(Hons), MBBS, MD, FRCSEd, FRCS(Gen Surg), FRCPE, FRSE**
Regius Professor of Clinical Surgery, The University of Edinburgh;
Honorary Consultant HPB Surgeon, Royal Infirmary of Edinburgh,
Edinburgh, UK

For additional online content visit eBooks+

ELSEVIER

First edition 1997
Second edition 2001
Third edition 2005
Fourth edition 2009
Fifth edition 2014
Sixth edition 2019
Seventh edition 2024

---

**Notices**

Practitioners and researchers must always rely on their own experience and knowledge in evaluating and using any information, methods, compounds or experiments described herein. Because of rapid advances in the medical sciences, in particular, independent verification of diagnoses and drug dosages should be made. To the fullest extent of the law, no responsibility is assumed by Elsevier, authors, editors or contrib-utors for any injury and/or damage to persons or property as a matter of products liability, negligence or otherwise, or from any use or operation of any methods, products, instructions, or ideas contained in the material herein.

---

ISBN: 978-0-7020-8457-7

Content Strategist: Alexandra Mortimer
Content Project Manager: Arindam Banerjee
Design: Ryan Cook
Art Buyer: Muthukumaran Thangaraj
Marketing Manager: Deborah Watkins

Printed in India

Last digit is the print number:  9  8  7  6  5  4  3  2  1

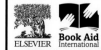

Working together
to grow libraries in
developing countries

www.elsevier.com • www.bookaid.org

# Contents

# Series Editors' preface

The *Companion to Specialist Surgical Practice* series has now reached its Seventh Edition and continues to remain popular for both surgeons in training as well as consultant surgeons in independent practice. The strength of this series has always been founded on contemporary, evidence-based information on the subspecialist areas relevant to their general surgical practice and this Seventh Edition has followed this plan.

This Edition continues to keep abreast of increasing subspecialisation in general surgery. The ongoing developments in minimal access and increasingly robotic surgery are discussed, along with the desire of some subspecialities, such as breast and vascular surgery, to separate away from 'general surgery' in some countries. However, all volumes also underline the importance for all surgeons of being aware of current developments in their surgical field. The importance of evidence-based practice and in particular the management of emergency conditions remains throughout, and authors have provided recommendations and highlighted key resources within each chapter. The ebook version of the textbook has also enabled improved access to the reference abstracts and links to video content relevant to many of the chapters.

As in all the previous editions, we are greatly indebted to the volume editors, and contributors, who have all put so much hard work into delivering such a high quality piece of work. We remain grateful for the support and encouragement of the team at Elsevier and we trust that our original vision of delivering an up-to-date, affordable text has been met and that readers, whether in training or independent practice, will find this Seventh Edition an invaluable resource.

We are grateful to Kathryn Rigby and Jonathan Michaels who wrote the guidelines on Evidence-based Practice in Surgery for previous editions of the series. These have been well received and have been retained again for this new edition in order to help guide readers in their assessment of the various levels of evidence discussed in each chapter.

**O. James Garden**, CBE, BSc, MBChB, MD, DSc(Hon), FRCS (Glas), FRCS(Ed), FRCP(Ed), FRACS(Hon), FRCSC (Hon), FACS(Hon), FCSHK(Hon), FRCSI(Hon), FRCS(Engl)(Hon), FRSE, MAMSE, FFST(RCSEd)
Professor Emeritus, Clinical Surgery, University of Edinburgh, UK.

**Simon Paterson-Brown**, MBBS, MPhil, MS, FRCS(Ed), FRCS (Engl), FCSHK, FFST(RCSEd)
Honorary Senior Lecturer, Clinical Surgery, University of Edinburgh, UK.

# Editors' preface

The Seventh Edition of *Hepatobiliary and Pancreatic Surgery* builds on the strong foundation of previous editions and the groundwork provided by our colleague Professor James Garden, who was involved in the first five editions. Over the past 25 years, this volume and indeed, the entire *Companion to Specialist Surgical Practice* series, has become well established with a remarkable reputation. It is a privilege to be able to build on this legacy.

Each new edition brings the opportunity to update and refresh the content and format of the book. For this Seventh Edition, two new chapters on Perioperative Care in HPB Surgery and HPB Cancer Biology have been added and many of the existing chapters have been delivered by new contributors.

The aim has been to secure further leading international experts to ensure contemporary, evidence-based content on the various aspects of benign and malignant liver, biliary and pancreatic disease. All chapters have been brought up to date with new content highlighting current guidelines and practice, with high-quality images and figures to enhance the resources available to the reader.

## ACKNOWLEDGEMENTS

We wish to acknowledge the wonderful contribution of our friend and colleague Dr Cornelius de Jong known to all as 'Kees' who sadly passed away during the production of this edition. We are grateful to colleagues at Elsevier, particularly Alexandra Mortimer and Arindam Banerjee, for their guidance and encouragement during this project and for trying to keep progress on schedule. We would also wish to acknowledge the tremendous support and tolerance of our wives, Janet and Lynne, and wider families, in allowing us to deliver this volume.

*Rowan W. Parks*
*Stephen J. Wigmore*
*Edinburgh*

# Evidence-based practice in surgery

Critical appraisal for developing evidence-based practice can be obtained from a number of sources, the most reliable being randomised controlled clinical trials, systematic literature reviews, meta-analyses and observational studies. For practical purposes three grades of evidence can be used, analogous to the levels of 'proof' required in a court of law:

1. **Beyond all reasonable doubt**. Such evidence is likely to have arisen from high-quality randomised controlled trials, systematic reviews or high-quality synthesised evidence such as decision analysis, cost-effectiveness analysis or large observational datasets. The studies need to be directly applicable to the population of concern and have clear results. The grade is analogous to burden of proof within a criminal court and may be thought of as corresponding to the usual standard of 'proof' within the medical literature (i.e. $P < 0.05$).

2. **On the balance of probabilities**. In many cases a high-quality review of literature may fail to reach firm conclusions due to conflicting or inconclusive results, trials of poor methodological quality or the lack of evidence in the population to which the guidelines apply. In such cases it may still be possible to make a statement as to the best treatment on the 'balance of probabilities'. This is analogous to the decision in a civil court where all the available evidence will be weighed up and the verdict will depend upon the balance of probabilities.

3. **Not proven**. Insufficient evidence upon which to base a decision, or contradictory evidence.

Depending on the information available, three grades of recommendation can be used:

Strong recommendation, which should be followed unless there are compelling reasons to act otherwise.

a. A recommendation based on evidence of effectiveness, but where there may be other factors to take into account in decision-making, for example the user of the guidelines may be expected to take into account patient preferences, local facilities, local audit results or available resources.

b. A recommendation made where there is no adequate evidence as to the most effective practice, although there may be reasons for making a recommendation in order to minimise cost or reduce the chance of error through a locally agreed protocol.

Evidence where a conclusion can be reached '**beyond all reasonable doubt**' and therefore where a strong recommendation can be given.

This will normally be based on evidence levels:
- Ia. Meta-analysis of randomised controlled trials
- Ib. Evidence from at least one randomised controlled trial
- IIa. Evidence from at least one controlled study without randomisation
- IIb. Evidence from at least one other type of quasi-experimental study.

Evidence where a conclusion might be reached '**on the balance of probabilities**' and where there may be other factors involved which influence the recommendation given. This will normally be based on less conclusive evidence than that represented by the double tick icons:
- III. Evidence from non-experimental descriptive studies, such as comparative studies and case–control studies
- IV. Evidence from expert committee reports or opinions or clinical experience of respected authorities, or both.

Evidence that is associated with either a **strong recommendation** or **expert opinion** is highlighted in the text in panels such as those shown above, and is distinguished by either a double or single tick icon, respectively. The references associated with double-tick evidence are listed as Key References at the end of each chapter, along with a short summary of the paper's conclusions where applicable. The full reference list for each chapter is available in the ebook.

The reader is referred to Chapter 1, 'Evaluation of surgical evidence' in the volume *Core Topics in General and Emergency Surgery* of this series, for a more detailed description of this topic.

# Contributors

**Ian Beckingham, DM, FRCS**
Consultant Hepatobiliary Surgeon
Department of Surgery
Queens Medical Centre
Nottingham, United Kingdom

**M.G. Besselink, MD, MSc, PhD**
Professor of Surgery
Department of Surgery
Amsterdam UMC
Amsterdam, The Netherlands

**Garrison Carlos, MD, BS**
General Surgery Resident
Stanford University
Stanford, California, United States

**John Casey, PhD, MB ChB**
Consultant Transplant Surgeon and Honorary Reader
Edinburgh Transplant Centre
Royal Infirmary of Edinburgh
Edinburgh, United Kingdom

**Ashley Clift, MA, MBBS, DPhil, AFHEA**
Clinical Research Fellow
Cancer Research UK Oxford Centre
University of Oxford
Oxford, United Kingdom

**Jordan M. Cloyd, MD**
Assistant Professor of Surgery
Ward Family Professor of Surgical Oncology
The Ohio State University Wexner Medical Center
James Comprehensive Cancer Center
Columbus, Ohio, United States

**Elizabeth M.E. Cole, BMBS, BSc(Hons), FRCA**
Specialty Trainee in Anaesthesia
Royal Infirmary of Edinburgh
Edinburgh, United Kingdom

**Kevin C. Conlon, MB, MCh, FRCSI, FRCSEd, FRCSGlas, FACS, MBA, MA, FTCD**
Professor and Academic Head
Department of Surgery
Trinity College Dublin;
Consultant HPB Surgeon
Department of HPB Surgery
St Vincents University Hospital;
Consultant Surgeon
Tallaght University Hospital
Tallaght, Dublin, Ireland

**Michael I. D'Angelica, MD, FACS**
Enid Haupt Chair in Surgery
Memorial Sloan Kettering Cancer Center;
Professor of Surgery
Weil Cornell School of Medicine
New York, United States

**Cornelius H.C. Dejong, MD, PhD, FRCSEd**
Professor of HPB Surgery
Maastricht University Medical Center+
Maastricht, The Netherlands

**Marcel den Dulk, MD, PhD, FRCS**
Hepato-pancreato-biliary Surgeon
Maastricht Universiy Medical Center+
Maastricht, The Netherlands

**C.H.J. van Eijck, MD, PhD**
Professor of Surgery
Department of Surgery
Erasmus MC
Rotterdam, The Netherlands

**T.R. Jeff Evans, MBBS, MD, FRCP, FRCPE, FRCPGlasg**
Professor of Translational Cancer Research
University of Glasgow;
Honorary Consultant in Medical Oncology
Beatson West of Scotland Cancer Centre;
Lead
Glasgow Experimental Cancer Medicine Centre
Clinical Lead
NHS Research Scotland Cancer Research Network;
Editor-in-Chief
British Journal of Cancer;
School of Cancer Sciences
University of Glasgow
Glasgow, United Kingdom

**Cecilia G. Ethun, MD, MS**
Assistant Professor of Surgery
Division of Surgical Oncology
Harold C. Simmons Comprehensive Cancer Center
Dallas, Texas, United States

**Stephen W. Fenwick, BMedSci, BM, BS, MD, FRCS**
Consultant Hepatobiliary Surgeon
Department of Hepatobiliary Surgery
Royal Liverpool University Hospital
Liverpool, United Kingdom

**Andrea Frilling, MD, PhD, FACS, FRCS, FEBS**
Chair in Endocrine Surgery
Professor of Surgery
Department of Surgery and Cancer
Imperial College London
London, United Kingdom

**Steven Gallinger, MD, MSc, FRCSC**
Professor
Department of General Surgery
University Health Network
Toronto, Ontario, Canada

**Rachel V. Guest, MBBS, BSc(Hons), PhD, FRCSEd**
Senior Lecturer and Honorary Consultant HPB Surgeon
Department of Clinical Surgery
University of Edinburgh
Edinburgh, United Kingdom

**Andrew J. Healey, MBChB, MDRes, FRCSEd**
Consultant Surgeon and Honorary Clinical Senior
    Lecturer
General and HPB Surgery
Royal Infirmary of Edinburgh
Edinburgh, United Kingdom

**Michael Hughes, MBChB, BMedSci, MD, FRCS**
Consultant Hepatobiliary Surgeon and Honorary Senior
    Lecturer
Royal Infirmary of Edinburgh
Edinburgh, United Kingdom

**William R. Jarnagin, MD, FACS**
Chief, Hepatopancreatobiliary Service
Leslie H. Blumgart Chair in Surgical Oncology
Memorial Sloan-Kettering Cancer Center;
Professor of Surgery
Weill Medical College of Cornell University
New York, United States

**Chris J.C. Johnston, PhD, MRCP, FRCS**
Consultant Transplant Surgeon
Edinburgh Transplant Centre
Royal Infirmary of Edinburgh;
Honorary Clinical Senior Lecturer
Clinical Surgery
University of Edinburgh
Edinburgh, United Kingdom

**Geoffrey W. Krampitz, MD, PhD**
General Surgeon
Sharp Rees-Stealy Medical Group
Sharp Healthcare
San Diego, California, United States

**Kristoffer Lassen, MD, Dr. Med.**
GI/HPB Surgery
Oslo University Hospital
Oslo, Norway;
Professor
Institute of Clinical Medicine
Arctic University of Norway
Tromsø, Norway

**Caitlin A. McIntyre, MD**
Fellow, Complex General Surgical Oncology
Department of Surgery
Memorial Sloan Kettering Cancer Center
New York, United States

**Carol-Anne Moulton, MD, PhD**
Associate Professor
Department of General Surgery
University Health Network
Toronto, Ontario, Canada

**Gabriel C. Oniscu, MD, FRCS(Ed), FRCS(Glas), KOSM**
Professor of Transplantation Surgery
Head of Transplant Division
Department of Clinical Science, Intervention and
    Technology
Karolinska Institutet
Stockholm, Sweden

**Timothy M. Pawlik, MD, PhD, MPH, MTS, MBA, FACS**
Professor and Chair
Department of Surgery
The Ohio State University Medical Center;
The Urban Meyer III and Shelley Meyer Chair for Cancer
    Research
Wexner Medical Center at The Ohio State University
Columbus, Ohio, United States

**Chaya Shwaartz, MD**
Assistant Professor of Surgery
Abdominal Transplant & HPB Surgical Oncology
Department of General Surgery
University Health Network
Toronto, Ontario, Canada

**Ajith K. Siriwardena, MD FCS**
Professor of Hepatobiliary Surgery
Regional Hepato-Pancreato-Biliary Unit
Manchester Royal Infirmary
Manchester, United Kingdom

**Benjamin M. Stutchfield, FRCS**
Clinical Lecturer
Department of Surgery
Royal Infirmary Edinburgh
Edinburgh, United Kingdom

**Andrew Sutherland, MB ChB, BSc(Hons), DPhil(Oxon), FRCS(Ed)**
Consultant Transplant Surgeon
Honorary Senior Lecturer
University of Edinburgh
Edinburgh, United Kingdom;
Clinical Lead Scottish Pancreas Transplant Unit
National Research Scotland Clinician

**Vikram Tewatia, MD, MCh**
Assistant Professor of Surgery
Trinity College Dublin
Dublin, Ireland

**Benjamin N.J. Thomson, MBBS, DMedSc, FRACS, FACS**
Director of Surgical Services
The Royal Melbourne Hospital
Parkville, Victoria, Australia;
Chief Surgical Advisor
Victorian Department of Health
Honorary Clinical Professor
The University of Melbourne
Melbourne, Australia

**Helen M.E. Usher, BSc, MBChB, MRCP, FRCA**
Consultant Anaesthetist
Royal Infirmary of Edinburgh
Edinburgh, United Kingdom

**H.C. van Santvoort, MD, PhD**
Department of Surgery
University Medical Center Utrecht
Utrecht, The Netherlands

**C.L. van Veldhuisen, MD, PhD Candidate**
Pancreatitis Werkgroep Nederland
Department of Gastroenterology and Department of
   Surgery
Amsterdam UMC
Amsterdam, The Netherlands

**Brendan Visser, MD**
Professor of Surgery
Hepatobiliary and Pancreatic Surgery
HPB Fellowship Program Director
Medical Director
Cancer Center GI Clinical Care Program
Stanford University School of Medicine
Stanford, California, United States

**Stephen J. Wigmore, BSc(Hons), MBBS, MD, FRCSEd, FRCS(Gen Surg), FRCPE, FRSE**
Regius Professor of Clinical Surgery
The University of Edinburgh;
Honorary Consultant HPB Surgeon
Royal Infirmary of Edinburgh
Edinburgh, United Kingdom

**Vincent S. Yip, MBChB, MD, FRCS**
Consultant HPB and General Surgery
Barts and the London HPB Centre
Royal London Hospital
London, United Kingdom

# Hepatic, biliary and pancreatic anatomy

Vincent S. Yip | Stephen W. Fenwick

This chapter will provide a basic anatomical foundation for performing liver, biliary and pancreatic surgery. Anatomical features that are clinically unimportant have been omitted. It is self-evident that surgeons operating in this area must have a full working knowledge of the anatomy of the liver, biliary system and pancreas. Furthermore, with ongoing advances in modern imaging techniques, surgeons must be able to translate their understanding of anatomy from the screen to the patient. Surgeons must also be aware that whilst there is a normal or *prevailing pattern* of anatomy, variations, which are termed *anomalies*, are frequent.

## LIVER

### OVERVIEW OF HEPATIC ANATOMY AND TERMINOLOGY

The most significant advances in the understanding of the surgical anatomy of the liver were made by the late French surgeon and anatomist Claude Couinaud during his studies with vasculo-biliary casts of the liver during the 1950s.[1] This work demonstrated that the liver appeared to consist of eight distinct functional segments, with each segment having its own dual vascular inflow, biliary drainage and lymphatic drainage (Fig. 1.1). Although more recent studies have questioned the validity of some aspects of this system, it remains the most relevant for the hepatic surgeon. It is clearly important to have uniformity and clarity of anatomical nomenclature pertaining to liver resectional surgery. Previously this was somewhat chaotic, with multiple terms being used for the same structure or operation, or some individual terms being used for more than one structure or operation. As a result, a terminology committee was formed by the International Hepato-Pancreato-Biliary Association (IHPBA), and the proposed system, which is primarily based on hepatic artery and bile duct ramifications, will be used throughout this chapter.[2]

### DIVISIONS OF THE LIVER BASED ON THE HEPATIC ARTERY

The proper hepatic artery arises as a branch of the common hepatic artery. The primary (first-order) division of the proper hepatic artery is into the right and left hepatic arteries (Fig. 1.2). These branches supply arterial inflow to the right and left hemilivers (Fig. 1.3). The plane between the two distinct zones of vascular supply is called a watershed. The border or watershed of the first-order division is called the *midplane of the liver*. It intersects the gallbladder fossa and

the fossa for the inferior vena cava (IVC) (Fig. 1.4). The right hemiliver usually has a larger volume than the left hemiliver (60:40), although this is variable.

The second-order divisions (Figs. 1.2 and 1.4) of the hepatic artery supply four distinct zones of the liver. Each is referred to as a *section*. The right liver is divided into two sections, the *right anterior section* and the *right posterior section*. These sections are supplied by the right anterior sectional hepatic artery and the right posterior sectional hepatic artery (Fig. 1.2). The plane between these sections is the *right intersectional plane*, which does not have any surface markings to indicate its position. The left liver is also divided into two sections, the *left medial section* and the *left lateral section* (Fig. 1.4), which are supplied by the left medial sectional hepatic artery and the left lateral sectional hepatic artery (Fig. 1.2). The plane between these sections is referred to as the *left intersectional plane*, which is marked on the surface of the liver by the umbilical fissure and the line of attachment of the falciform ligament. The third-order divisions of the hepatic artery divide the right and left hemilivers into *segments* (Sg) 2–8 (Figs. 1.2 and 1.5). Each of the segments has its own feeding segmental artery. The left lateral section is divided into Sg2 and Sg3. The ramification of vessels within the left medial section does not permit subdivision of this section into segments, each with its own arterial blood supply. Therefore, the left medial section and Sg4 are synonymous. However, Sg4 is arbitrarily divided into superior (4a) and inferior (4b) parts without an exact anatomical plane of separation. The right anterior section is divided into two segments, Sg5 and Sg8. The right posterior section is divided into Sg6 and Sg7. The planes between segments are referred to as intersegmental planes. The ramifications of the bile ducts are identical to that described for the arteries, as are the zones of the liver drained by the respective ducts.

Segment 1 (caudate lobe) is a distinct portion of the liver, separate from the right and left hemilivers (Fig. 1.6). It is appropriately referred to as a lobe since it is demarcated by visible fissures. It consists of three parts: the bulbous left part (Spigelian lobe), which wraps around the left side of the vena cava and is readily visible through the lesser omentum; the paracaval portion, which lies anterior to the vena cava; and the caudate process, on the right. The caudate process merges indistinctly with the right hemiliver. The caudate lobe is situated posterior to the hilum and the portal veins (PVs). Lying anterior and superior to the paracaval portion are the hepatic veins, which limit the upper extent of the caudate lobe[1,3] (Fig. 1.6). The caudate lobe receives vascular supply from both right and left hepatic arteries and PVs. Caudate bile ducts drain into both right and left

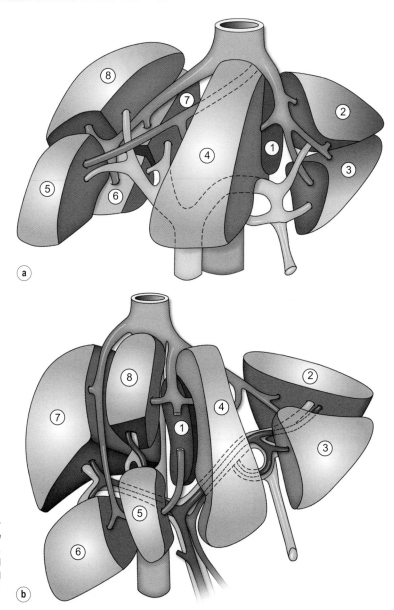

**Figure 1.1** Functional division of the liver into eight segments as described by Couinaud: **(a)** as observed in the anatomical position in the patient; **(b)** as observed ex vivo. (Adapted from Poston GJ, D'Angelica M, editors. Surgical management of hepatobiliary and pancreatic disorders. 2nd ed. 2010. Informa Healthcare, Taylor and Francis Group. Chapter 1, Figure 1.7.)

hepatic ducts.[1] The caudate lobe is drained by several short caudate veins that enter the IVC directly from the caudate lobe. Their number and size are variable, and they must be ligated when mobilising the caudate lobe from the vena cava. Commonly, these veins enter the IVC on either side of the midplane of the vessel, an anatomical feature that allows the creation of a tunnel behind the liver on the surface of the IVC without encountering the caudate veins. A 'hanging manoeuvre' can be performed by lifting up on a tape placed through this tunnel (see below).

## RESECTIONAL TERMINOLOGY

The terminology of hepatic resections is based upon the terminology of hepatic anatomy. Resection of one side of the liver is called a hepatectomy or hemihepatectomy (Fig. 1.3). Resection of the right side of the liver is a right hepatectomy or hemihepatectomy and resection of the left side of the liver is a left hemihepatectomy or hepatectomy. Resection of a liver section is referred to as a sectionectomy (Fig. 1.4).

Resection of the liver to the left side of the umbilical fissure is a left lateral sectionectomy. The other sectionectomies are named accordingly, e.g. right anterior sectionectomy. Resection of the right hemiliver plus Sg4 is referred to as a right trisectionectomy (Fig. 1.4). Similarly, resection of the left hemiliver plus the right anterior section is referred to as a left trisectionectomy.

Resection of one of the numbered segments is referred to as a segmentectomy (Fig. 1.5).

## SURGICAL ANATOMY FOR LIVER RESECTIONS

### HEPATIC ARTERIES AND LIVER RESECTIONS

In the prevailing anatomical pattern, the coeliac artery terminates to divide into left gastric, splenic and common hepatic arteries. The common hepatic artery runs for 2–3 cm anteriorly and to the right to ramify into gastroduodenal and proper hepatic arteries. The proper hepatic artery enters the hepatoduodenal ligament and normally runs for 2–3 cm along the left side of the common bile duct (CBD) and terminates by dividing into the right and left hepatic arteries, the right immediately passing behind the common hepatic duct (CHD). The four sectional arteries arise from the right and left arteries 1–2 cm from the liver (Fig. 1.7). While this is the commonest pattern, variations from this pattern are also very common. Thus it is imperative that the surgeon does not make assumptions regarding hepatic arteries based on size or position, but instead on complete dissection, trial clamping and intraoperative imaging. 'Replaced' and 'aberrant' arteries are surgically important anomalies. 'Replaced' means that the artery supplying a particular volume of liver is in an unusual location and also that it is the sole supply to that volume of liver. 'Aberrant' means the structure is in an unusual location.

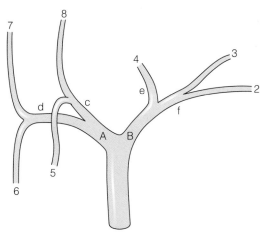

**Figure 1.2**  Ramification of the hepatic artery in the liver. The prevailing pattern is shown. The first-order division of the proper hepatic artery is into the right (A) and left (B) hepatic arteries, which supply right and left hemilivers (see Fig. 1.3), respectively. The second-order division of the hepatic arteries supplies the four sections (see Fig. 1.4). The third-order division supplies the segments (see Fig. 1.5). The caudate lobe is supplied by branches from (A) and (B). Bile duct anatomy and nomenclature is similar to that of the hepatic artery. (© Washington University in St Louis.)

While the definition of 'aberrant' does not state whether the structure provides sole supply, it is usually considered to be synonymous with 'replaced' in respect to these arteries. 'Accessory' refers to an artery that is additional, i.e. is present in addition to the normal structure and as a result is *not* the sole supply to a volume. Consequently, ligation of an accessory artery does not result in ischaemia.

In about 25% of individuals, part or all of the liver is supplied by a replaced (or aberrant) artery. The *replaced right hepatic artery* arises from the superior mesenteric artery (SMA). It runs from left to right behind the lower end of the CBD to emerge and course on its right posterior border. It may supply a segment, section or the entire right hemiliver. Rarely, this artery supplies the entire liver and then it is called a *replaced hepatic artery* (Fig. 1.8). The *replaced left hepatic artery* arises from the left gastric artery and courses in the lesser omentum in conjunction with vagal branches to the liver (hepatic nerve). As with the right artery, it may supply a segment, section (usually the left lateral section), hemiliver or very rarely the whole liver. Sometimes left hepatic arteries arising from the left gastric artery are actually accessory rather than replaced and exist in conjunction with normally situated left hepatic arteries. Knowledge of these particular arterial variations is of importance not only in hepatobiliary surgery, including transplantation, but also in gastric surgery and pancreatic surgery. Transection of the left gastric artery at its origin during gastrectomy may cause ischaemic necrosis of the left hemiliver if a replaced left artery is present. The same may occur on the right side as a result of injury to a replaced right artery. Also, and of particular importance, these vessels must be preserved and perfused during donor hepatectomy for transplantation.

Replaced arteries may confer an advantage during surgery. For instance, when a replaced left artery supplies the left lateral section, it is possible to resect the entire proper hepatic artery when performing a right trisectionectomy for hilar cholangiocarcinoma. The replaced right artery is sometimes invaded by pancreatic head tumours and is in danger of injury during pancreatico-duodenectomy. This is only a brief description of replaced arteries and there are

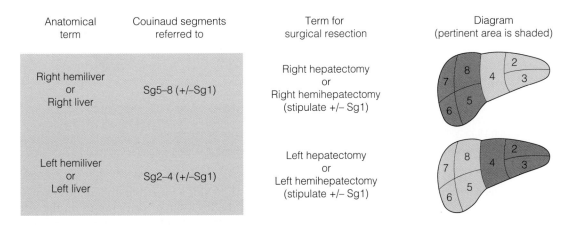

| Anatomical term | Couinaud segments referred to | Term for surgical resection | Diagram (pertinent area is shaded) |
|---|---|---|---|
| Right hemiliver or Right liver | Sg5–8 (+/–Sg1) | Right hepatectomy or Right hemihepatectomy (stipulate +/– Sg1) | |
| Left hemiliver or Left liver | Sg2–4 (+/–Sg1) | Left hepatectomy or Left hemihepatectomy (stipulate +/– Sg1) | |

Border or watershed: The border or watershed of the first-order division which separates the two hemilivers is a plane which intersects the gallbladder fossa and the fossa for the IVC and is called the midplane of the liver.

**Figure 1.3**  Nomenclature for first-order division anatomy (hemilivers or livers) and resections. IVC, inferior vena cava; Sg, segment. (© Washington University in St Louis.)

Second-order division
(second-order division based on bile ducts and hepatic artery)

| Anatomical term | Couinaud segments referred to | Term for surgical resection | Diagram (pertinent area is shaded) |
|---|---|---|---|
| Right anterior section | Sg 5,8 | Add (-ectomy) to any of the anatomical terms as in Right anterior sectionectomy | 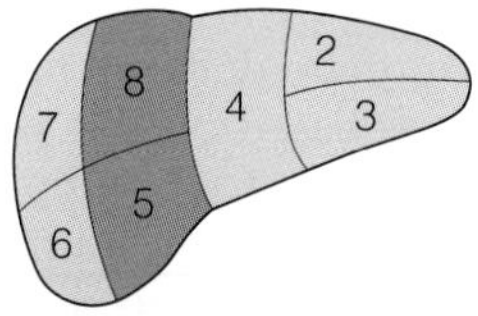 |
| Right posterior section | Sg 6,7 | Right posterior sectionectomy | 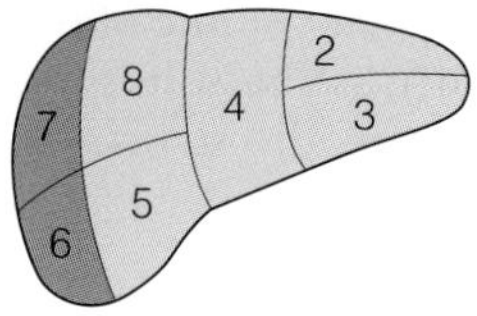 |
| Left medial section | Sg 4 | Left medial sectionectomy or Resection segment 4 (also see third order) or Segmentectomy 4 (also see third order) | 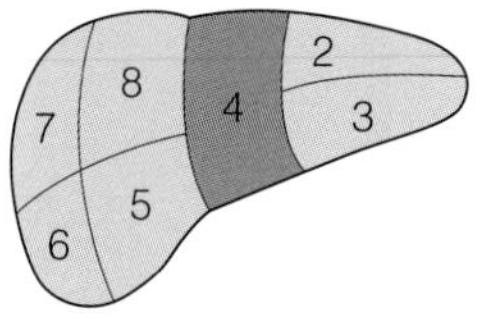 |
| Left lateral section | Sg 2,3 | Left lateral sectionectomy or Bisegmentectomy 2,3 (also see third order) | 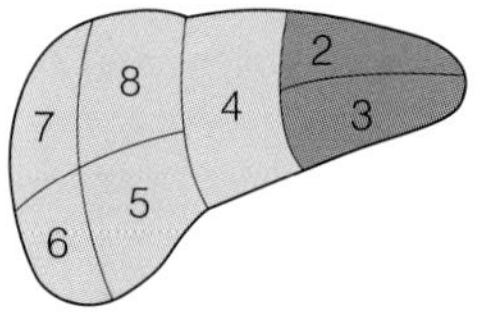 |

Other sectional liver resections

| | Sg 4–8 (+/–Sg1) | Right trisectionectomy (preferred term) or Extended right hepatectomy or Extended right hemihepatectomy (stipulate +/– Sg1) | 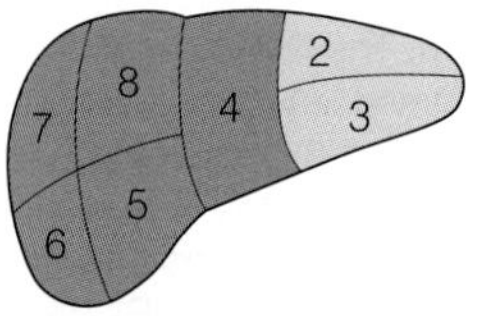 |
|---|---|---|---|
| | Sg 2,3,4,5,8 (+/–Sg1) | Left trisectionectomy (preferred term) or Extended left hepatectomy or Extended left hemihepatectomy (stipulate +/– Sg1) | 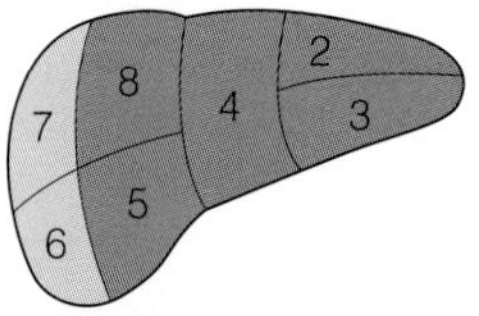 |

Border or watershed: The borders or watersheds of the sections are planes referred to as the right and left intersectional planes. The left intersectional plane passes through the umbilical fissure and the attachment of the falciform ligament. There is no surface marking of the right intersectional plane.

**Figure 1.4**   Nomenclature for second-order division anatomy (sections) and resections including extended resections. (© Washington University in St Louis.)

many variations of replaced arteries, especially on the right, depending on the relationship of the artery to the pancreatic head and neck, the bile duct and the PV.[4]

In performing hepatectomies by the standard technique of isolating individual structures instead of pedicles, it is critical to correctly identify the particular artery(ies) supplying the volume of liver to be resected. One important anatomical point is that an artery located to the right side of the bile duct always supplies the right side of the liver, but arteries found on the left side of the bile duct may supply either side of the liver. Therefore, when using the individual vessel ligation method, it is important to be aware of the position of the CHD. A trial occlusion of an artery with an atraumatic clamp should always be performed in order to be sure that there is a good pulse to the future remnant liver.

Third-order division

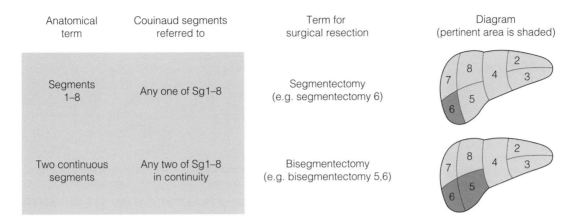

| Anatomical term | Couinaud segments referred to | Term for surgical resection | Diagram (pertinent area is shaded) |
|---|---|---|---|
| Segments 1–8 | Any one of Sg1–8 | Segmentectomy (e.g. segmentectomy 6) | |
| Two continuous segments | Any two of Sg1–8 in continuity | Bisegmentectomy (e.g. bisegmentectomy 5,6) | |

Border or watershed: The borders or watersheds of the segments are planes referred to as intersegmental planes.

**Figure 1.5**  Nomenclature for third-order division anatomy (segments) and resections. (© Washington University in St Louis.)

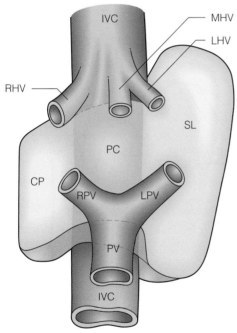

**Figure 1.6**  Schematic representation of the anatomy of the caudate lobe. The caudate lobe consists of three parts: the caudate process (*CP*), on the right, the paracaval portion anterior to the vena cava (*PC*) and the bulbous left part (Spigelian lobe, *SL*). *IVC*, inferior vena cava; *PV*, portal vein; *RHV, MHV, LHV*, right hepatic, middle hepatic and left hepatic vein, respectively. (© Washington University in St Louis.)

## BILE DUCTS AND LIVER RESECTIONS

### Prevailing pattern and important variations of bile ducts draining the right hemiliver

Normally only a short portion of the right hepatic duct, approximately 1 cm, is in an extrahepatic position. The prevailing pattern of bile duct drainage from the right liver is shown in Fig. 1.9a. The segmental ducts from Sg6 and Sg7 (called *B6, B7*) unite to form the *right posterior sectional bile duct* and the segmental ducts from Sg5 and Sg8 (*B5, B8*) unite to form the *right anterior sectional bile duct* (Fig. 1.9a). The sectional

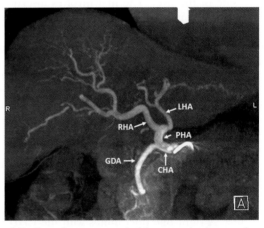

**Figure 1.7**  Cone beam computed tomography image of conventional hepatic arterial anatomy. *CHA*, common hepatic artery; *GDA*, gastroduodenal artery; *LHA*, left hepatic artery; *PHA*, proper hepatic artery; *RHA*, right hepatic artery.

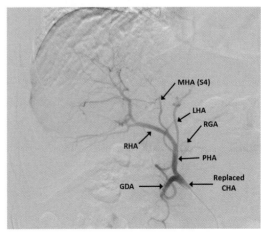

**Figure 1.8**  Superior mesenteric arteriogram showing replaced common hepatic artery. *CHA*, common hepatic artery; *GDA*, gastroduodenal artery; *PHA*, proper hepatic artery; *RGA*, right gastric artery; *RHA, LHA, MHA,* right hepatic, middle hepatic and left hepatic artery, respectively.

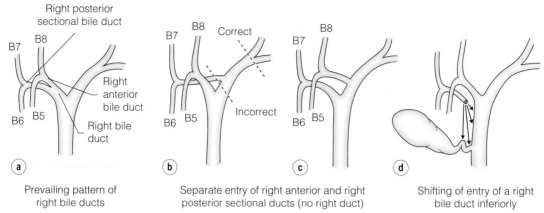

**Figure 1.9**  Prevailing pattern **(a)** and important variations **(b–d)** of bile ducts draining the right hemiliver (see text). (© Washington University in St Louis.)

ducts unite to form the *right hepatic duct*, which unites with the left hepatic duct at the *confluence* to form the *CHD*.

There are two important sets of biliary anomalies on the right side of the liver. The first involves insertion of a right sectional duct into the left bile duct. This is a common anomaly. The right posterior sectional duct inserts into the left hepatic duct in 20% of individuals (Fig. 1.9b) and the right anterior bile duct does so in 6% (Fig. 1.9c). In these situations there is no right hepatic duct. A right sectional bile duct inserting into the left hepatic duct is in danger of injury during left hepatectomy if the left duct is divided at its termination. Therefore, when performing left hepatectomy, the left hepatic duct should be divided close to the umbilical fissure to avoid injury to a right sectional duct.

The second important anomaly is insertion of a right bile duct into the biliary tree at a lower level than the prevailing site of confluence. Low union may affect the right hepatic duct, a sectional right duct, a segmental duct or a subsegmental duct. A right bile duct unites with the CHD below the prevailing site of confluence in about 2% of individuals. Sometimes the duct unites with the cystic duct and then with the CHD. The latter anomaly places the aberrant duct at great risk of injury during laparoscopic cholecystectomy.

Very rarely the right hepatic duct terminates in the gallbladder. This may be congenital or acquired. In the latter case, a gallstone has effaced a cystic duct which united with the right hepatic duct, giving the appearance that it joins the gallbladder. An extremely rare anomaly is the absent CHD. In these cases, the right and left hepatic duct enters the gallbladder and the duct emerging from the gallbladder runs downward to join with the duodenum.[5] In the presence of these anomalies, which would be extremely difficult to detect, a complete cholecystectomy will result in ductal injury. These ducts should not be confused with ducts of Luschka (see below).

The right *posterior* sectional duct normally hooks over the origin of the right *anterior* sectional PV ('Hjortsjo's crook'),[6] where it is in danger of being injured if the right anterior sectional pedicle is clamped too close to its origin (Fig. 1.10).

### Prevailing pattern and important variations of bile ducts draining the left hemiliver

The prevailing pattern of bile duct drainage from the left liver is shown in Fig. 1.11a. It is present in only 30% of

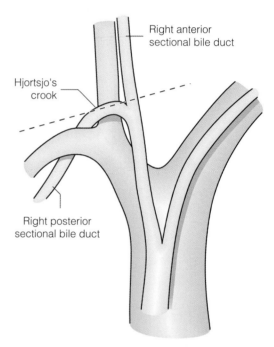

**Figure 1.10**  Hjortsjo's crook. Note that the right posterior sectional bile duct (RPSBD) crosses the origin of the right anterior sectional portal vein. (© Washington University in St Louis.)

individuals, i.e. variations (anomalies) are present in the majority of individuals. In the prevailing pattern, the segmental ducts from Sg2 and Sg3 (*B2, B3*) unite to form the *left lateral sectional bile duct*. This duct passes behind the umbilical portion of the PV and unites with the duct from Sg4 (**B4**; also called the left medial sectional duct since section and segment are synonymous for this volume of liver). The site of union of these ducts to form the left hepatic duct lies about one-third of the distance between the umbilical fissure and the midplane of the liver. The left hepatic duct continues from this point for 2–3 cm along the base of Sg4 to its confluence with the right hepatic duct. Note that it is in an extrahepatic position and that it has a much longer extrahepatic course than the right bile duct. The extrahepatic position of the left hepatic duct is a key anatomical feature, which makes this section of duct the prime site for high biliary–enteric anastomoses.

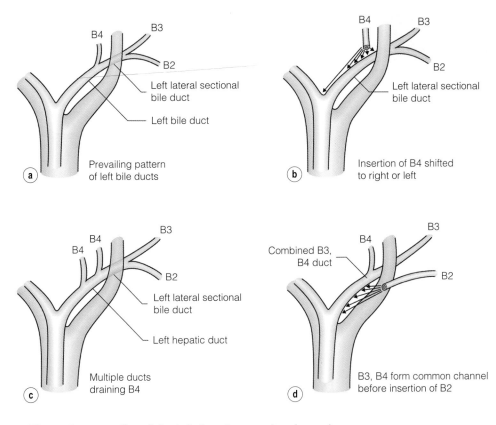

**Figure 1.11** Prevailing pattern **(a)** and important variations **(b–d)** of bile ducts draining the left hemiliver. (© Washington University in St Louis.)

The main anomalies of the left ductal system involve variations in the site of insertion of B4 (Fig. 1.11b), multiple ducts coming from B4 (Fig. 1.11c) and primary union of B3 and B4 with subsequent union of B2 (Fig. 1.11d). B4 may join the left lateral sectional duct to the left or right of its point of union in the prevailing pattern (Fig. 1.11b); in the former case, the insertion of B4 is at the umbilical fissure and in the latter the insertion may occur at any place to the right of the prevailing location up to the point where the left hepatic duct normally unites with the right hepatic duct. In the latter instance, which according to Couinaud is present in 8% of individuals, there is no left hepatic duct. Instead there is a confluence of three ducts, the left lateral sectional duct, B4 and the right hepatic duct, to form the CHD. These variations are important in split liver transplantation and in diagnosis and repair of biliary injuries.

The bile duct to Sg3 has been used to perform biliary bypass and can be isolated by following the superior surface of the ligamentum teres down to isolate the portal pedicle to Sg3. The technique is less commonly used now that internal endoscopic stenting has been developed.

**Prevailing pattern of bile ducts draining the caudate lobe (Sg1)**

Normally, two to three caudate ducts enter the biliary tree. Their orifices are usually located posteriorly on the left duct, right duct or right posterior sectional duct.

## PORTAL VEINS AND LIVER RESECTIONS

On the right side of the liver, the PV divisions correspond to those of the hepatic artery and bile duct, and they supply the same hepatic volumes. Therefore, there is a right PV that supplies the entire right hemiliver (Fig. 1.12). It divides into two sectional and four segmental veins, as do

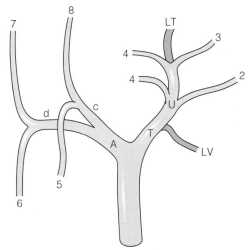

**Figure 1.12** Ramification of the portal vein in the liver. The portal vein divides into right (*A*) and left (*T*) branches. The branches in the right liver correspond to those of the hepatic artery and bile duct (Fig. 1.2). The branching pattern on the left is unique. The left portal vein has transverse (*T*) and umbilical portions (*U*). The transition point between the two parts is marked by the attachment of the ligamentum venosum (*LV*). All major branches come off the umbilical portion (see text). The vein ends blindly in the ligamentum teres (*LT*). (© Washington University in St Louis.)

the arteries and bile ducts. On the left side of the liver, however, the left PV is quite unusual because of the fact that its structure was adapted to function in utero as a conduit between the umbilical vein and the ductus venosus, whilst postnatally the direction of flow is reversed. The left PV consists of a *horizontal or transverse portion*, which is located under Sg4, and a *vertical part or umbilical portion*, which

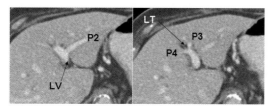

**Figure 1.13** Ramification of the left portal vein as seen on computed tomography. Note the branches to segments 2–4 and the ligamentum teres *(LT)*. The arrow pointing to the ligamentum venosum *(LV)* and the groove between the left lateral section and the caudate lobe. This is also the site of origin of the ligamentum venosum where the transverse portion of the left portal vein becomes the umbilical portion of the vein, proving conclusively that the branch to Sg2 is not part of a terminal division of the transverse portion of the vein as might be concluded from case studies.[7] (© Washington University in St Louis.)

is situated in the umbilical fissure (Fig. 1.13). Unlike the right PV, neither portion of the left PV actually enters the liver, but rather they lie directly on its surface. Often the umbilical portion is hidden by a bridge of tissue passing between left medial and lateral sections. This bridge of liver tissue may be as thick as 2 cm or be only a fibrous band. The junction of the transverse and umbilical portions of the left PV is marked by the attachment of a stout cord— the ligamentum venosum. This structure, the remnant of the fetal ductus venosus, runs in the groove between the left lateral section and the caudate lobe and attaches to the left hepatic vein/IVC junction.

**Ramification of the left portal vein**

The transverse portion of the left PV sends only a few small branches to Sg4. Large branches from the PV to the left liver arise exclusively beyond the attachment of the ligamentum venosum, i.e. from the umbilical part of the vein.[7] These branches come off both sides of the vein—those arising from the right side pass into Sg4 and those from the left supply Sg2 and Sg3. There is usually only one branch to Sg2 and Sg3, but often there is more than one branch to Sg4. The left PV terminates in the ligamentum teres at the free edge of the left liver. Note that the umbilical portion of the PV has a unique pattern of ramification. The pattern is similar to an air-conditioning duct that sends branches at right angles from both of its sides to supply rooms (segments), tapering as it does so, finally to end blindly (in the ligamentum teres). Other vascular and biliary structures normally ramify by dividing into two other structures at their termination and not by sending out branches along their length.

Although the divisions of the PV are unusual, for the embryonic reasons described above, it is uncommon to have variations from this pattern. Probably the most common variation is absence of the right PV. In these cases, the right posterior and right anterior sectional PVs originate independently from the main PV. Under these circumstances, the anterior sectional vein is usually quite high in the porta hepatis and may not be obvious. An unsuspecting surgeon may divide the posterior sectional vein thinking that it is the right PV and become confused when the anterior sectional vein is subsequently revealed during hepatic transection.

The PV branches to Sg4 may be isolated in the umbilical fissure on the right side of the umbilical portion of the left

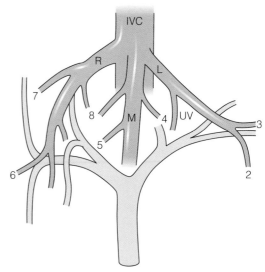

**Figure 1.14** Hepatic veins. There are normally three hepatic veins: right *(R)*, middle *(M)* and left *(L)*. Note the segments drained. The umbilical vein *(UV)* normally drains part of Sg4 into the left hepatic vein. The latter is proof that the terminal portion of the left vein lies in the intersectional plane of the left liver. *IVC,* inferior vena cava. (© Washington University in St Louis.)

PV. The veins here are associated with the bile ducts and the arteries passing to Sg4, i.e. they enter sheaths as they go into the liver substance. Isolation in this location may provide extra margin when resecting a tumour in Sg4 that impinges upon the umbilical fissure. Normally the branches to Sg4 are isolated after dividing the parenchyma of the liver of Sg4 close to the umbilical fissure, an approach that is used to avoid injury to the umbilical portion of the left PV. Injury to this vein could, of course, deprive Sg2 and Sg3 of PV supply as well as Sg4. For instance, if this occurs when performing a right trisectionectomy, the only portion of the liver to be retained would be devascularised of PV flow. However, isolation of these structures within the umbilical fissure does provide an extra margin of clearance on tumours and can be done safely if care is taken to ascertain the position of the PV. Likewise, it is possible to isolate the PV branches going into Sg2 and Sg3 in the umbilical fissure and to extend a margin when resecting a tumour in the left lateral section. For the same reasons given above, caution must be taken when doing this in order not to injure the umbilical portion of the PV. In order to access the PV in this location, it is usually necessary to divide the bridge of liver tissue between the left medial and lateral sections. This is done by passing a blunt instrument behind the bridge before dividing it, usually with cautery. Note that arteries and bile ducts passing to the left lateral section are in danger of being injured as one isolates the most posterior–superior portion of the bridge. To facilitate passage of an instrument behind the bridge, the peritoneum at the base of the bridge may be opened in a preliminary step. The instrument being passed behind the bridge should never be forced.

**HEPATIC VEINS AND LIVER RESECTION (FIG. 1.14)**

There are normally three large hepatic veins. These run in the midplane of the liver (middle hepatic vein), the right intersectional plane (right hepatic vein) and the left intersectional plane (left hepatic vein). The left hepatic vein actually begins in the plane between Sg2 and Sg3 and travels in that plane for most of its length. It becomes quite a large vein even in that location. It leaves the plane between Sg2 and Sg3 and enters the left intersectional plane about 1 cm from where it terminates by uniting with the middle hepatic vein to form a common channel that enters the IVC. It receives the umbilical vein from Sg4 in its short course in the left intersectional plane. Note that this is the same plane in which the umbilical portion of the left PV lies. It is important not to confuse the 'umbilical portion of the left PV' with the 'umbilical vein'. The latter is a tributary of the left hepatic vein that normally drains the most leftward part of Sg4.[8,9] The left and middle hepatic veins usually fuse at a distance of about 1–2 cm from the IVC, so that when viewed from within the IVC there are only two hepatic vein openings. Rarely, hepatic veins join the IVC above the diaphragm.

In about 10% of individuals there is more than one large right hepatic vein. In addition to the right superior hepatic vein (normally called the right hepatic vein), which enters the IVC just below the level of the diaphragm, there is a right inferior hepatic vein that enters the IVC 5–6 cm below this level. If this inferior hepatic vein is present, resections of Sg7 and Sg8 may be performed, including resection of the right superior vein, without compromising the venous drainage of Sg5 and Sg6.

The caudate lobe is drained by its own veins—several short veins that enter the IVC directly from the caudate lobe. When performing a classical right hepatectomy, caudate veins are divided in the preliminary stage of the dissection. As dissection moves up the anterior surface of the vena cava to isolate the right hepatic vein, a bridge of tissue lateral to the IVC referred to as the hepato-caval ligament is encountered.[10] It connects the posterior portion of the right liver to the caudate lobe behind the IVC. This bridge of tissue usually consists of fibrous tissue, but occasionally is a bridge of liver parenchyma. It limits exposure of the right side of the IVC at a point just below the right hepatic vein and must be divided in order to isolate the right vein extrahepatically. This must be done with care as the ligament may contain a large vein and forceful dissection of the ligament may also result in injury to the right lateral side of the IVC. Isolation of the right hepatic vein is also aided by clearing the areolar tissue between the right and middle hepatic veins down to the level of the IVC when exposing these veins from above.

Another approach to right hepatectomy is to leave division of the caudate and right hepatic veins until after the liver is transected. In this case, an instrument may be passed up along the anterior surface of the vena cava from below to emerge between the right and middle hepatic veins. Once an umbilical tape is passed, the liver may be hung to facilitate transection ('hanging manoeuvre').[11]

The left and middle veins can also be isolated prior to division of the liver. There are several ways to achieve this anatomically. One method is to divide all the caudate veins as well as the right hepatic vein. This exposes the entire anterior surface of the retrohepatic vena cava and leaves the liver attached to the vena cava only by the middle and left hepatic veins, which are then easily isolated. This is suitable when performing a right hepatectomy or extended right hepatectomy, especially when the caudate lobe is also to be resected. The advantage of having control of these veins during operations on the right liver is that total vascular occlusion

is possible without occlusion of the IVC and haemodynamically the effect is not much different from occlusion of the main portal pedicle alone (Pringle manoeuvre).

In performing a left hepatectomy, the right hepatic vein is conserved and a different anatomical approach to isolation of the left and middle hepatic veins is required. They may be isolated from the left side by dividing the ligamentum venosum, where it attaches to the left hepatic vein, then dividing the peritoneum at the superior tip of the caudate lobe and gently passing an instrument on the anterior surface of the vena cava to emerge between the middle and right veins and/or between the left and middle veins. Again, care needs to be applied when performing this manoeuvre in order to avoid injury to the structures.

Isolation of the vena cava above and below the hepatic veins is also a technique that should be in the armamentarium of every surgeon performing major hepatic resection. It is not usually necessary when performing standard liver resections, but surgeons should be familiar with the anatomical technique of doing so. Isolation of the vena cava superior to the hepatic veins is done by dividing the left triangular ligament and the lesser omentum, being careful to first look for a replaced left hepatic artery. The peritoneum on the superior border of the caudate lobe is then divided and a finger is passed behind the vena cava to come out just inferior to the crus of the diaphragm. The crus of the diaphragm makes an easily identified column on the right side. This column passes across the right side of the vena cava and dissection of the space inferior to this column and behind the vena cava facilitates passage of the finger from the left side to the right side in the space behind the vena cava. Isolation of the vena cava below the liver is more straightforward, but one should be aware of the position of the adrenal vein and in some cases, it is necessary to isolate the adrenal vein if bleeding is persisting after occlusion of the vena cava above and below the liver.

Finally, the surgeon should be aware that during transection of the liver large veins will be encountered in certain planes of transection. For instance, in its passage along the midplane the middle hepatic vein usually receives two large tributaries, one from Sg5 inferiorly and the other from Sg8 superiorly. Both are routinely encountered in performing right hepatectomy. The venous drainage of the right side of the liver is highly variable and additional large veins, including one from Sg6, may also enter the middle hepatic vein.

### Liver capsule, attachments and the plate system

The liver is encased in a thin fibrous capsule, called Glisson's capsule, which covers the entire organ except for a large bare area posteriorly where the organ is in contact with the IVC and with the diaphragm to the right of the IVC. The bare area stretches superiorly to include the termination of the three hepatic veins and ends in a point, which is also where the attachment of the falciform ligament ends. The limit of the bare area, where the peritoneum passes between the body wall and the liver, is called the coronary ligament. It is one of three structures that connect the liver to the abdominal wall 'dorsally', the other two being the right and left triangular ligaments. The liver also has another bare area, best thought of as a bare crease, where the hepatoduodenal ligament and the lesser omentum attach on the 'ventral' surface. It is through this crease that the

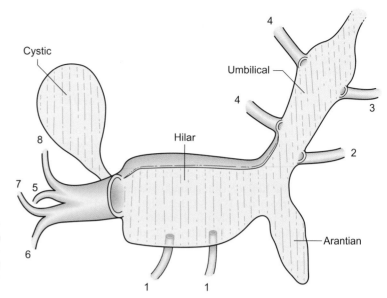

**Figure 1.15** The plate/sheath system of the liver. (Adapted from Strasberg SM, Linehan DC, Hawkins WG. Isolation of right main and right sectional portal pedicles for liver resection without hepatotomy or inflow occlusion. J Am Coll Surg 2008;206:390–6. With permission of the Journal of the American College of Surgeons.)

portal structures enter the liver at the hilum. The other ligamentous structures of interest to surgeons are the ligamentum teres, falciform ligament and the ligamentum venosum. The ligamentum teres (teres = 'round') is the obliterated left umbilical vein and runs in the free edge of the falciform ligament from the umbilicus to the termination of the umbilical portion of the left PV. The falciform (falciform = 'scythe shaped') is the filmy fold that runs between the anterior abdominal wall above the umbilicus and attaches to the anterior surface of the liver between the left medial and left lateral sections.

There are four fibrous plates on the surface of the liver (hilar, cystic, umbilical and Arantian) (Fig 1.15). These fibrous plates are condensations of Glisson's capsule. The hilar plate is the most important plate in liver surgery. Incising the junction between the base of Sg4 and the hilar plate is referred to as 'lowering the hilar plate' and is an important step in the surgical exposure of the extrahepatic bile ducts, particularly the left hepatic duct.

The sheath of the right portal pedicle extends off the hilar plate like a sleeve into the liver surrounding the portal structures, i.e. PV, hepatic artery and bile duct. The combined structure is referred to as a 'portal pedicle'. As the right portal pedicle enters the liver, it divides into a right anterior and right posterior portal pedicle supplying the respective sections, and then segmental pedicles supplying the four segments. On the left side, only the segmental structures are sheathed. There is no sheathed main portal pedicle because the main PV, proper hepatic artery and CHD are not close enough to the liver to be enclosed in a sheath.

The cystic plate is the ovoid fibrous sheet on which the gallbladder lies (Fig. 1.15). When a cholecystectomy is performed, this plate is normally left behind. In its posterior extent, the cystic plate narrows to become a stout cord that attaches to the anterior surface of the sheath of the right portal pedicle. The latter is a point of anatomical importance for the surgeon wishing to expose the anterior surface of the right portal pedicle, since this cord must be divided to do so.[12] With severe chronic inflammation, the cystic plate may become shortened and thickened so that the distance

between the top of the cystic plate and the right portal pedicle is likewise much shorter than usual. This places the structures in the right pedicle in danger during cholecystectomy when dissection is performed 'top down' as a primary strategy. The other plates are the umbilical and Arantian, which underlie the umbilical portion of the left PV and the ligamentum venosum, respectively (Fig. 1.15). The other sheaths carry segmental bilovascular pedicles of the left liver and caudate lobe.

In performing a right hepatectomy, there are two methods of managing the right-sided portal vessels and bile ducts. The first is to isolate the hepatic artery, PV and bile duct individually and either control them or ligate them extrahepatically, and the second is to isolate the entire portal pedicle and staple the pedicle. Isolation of the right portal pedicle can be performed by making hepatotomies above the right portal pedicle in Sg4 and in the gallbladder fossa after removing the gallbladder. A finger is passed through the hepatotomy to isolate the right portal pedicle. This technique usually requires inflow occlusion. It can also be done without inflow occlusion by lowering the hilar plate and coming around the right portal pedicle directly on its surface (Fig. 1.16).[13] It is advisable to divide caudate veins in the area below the vena caval ligament before performing pedicle isolation, since haemorrhage from these veins can be considerable if they are injured during isolation of the right portal pedicle.

## LIVER VOLUME AND REGENERATION

The normal adult human liver is approximately 2% of total body mass. This represents a relative surplus of functioning liver tissue. A key factor that must be considered when planning a liver resection is the likely volume of the future remnant liver. For patients with healthy liver parenchyma, this can be as low as 25% of original hepatic volume. Resecting beyond this risks the development of post hepatectomy liver failure. When a proposed liver resection risks leaving a small future remnant, or where there is concern regarding the quality of the liver parenchyma, it is possible to induce relative regeneration in the future remnant liver, largely through hyperplasia. This is most often achieved

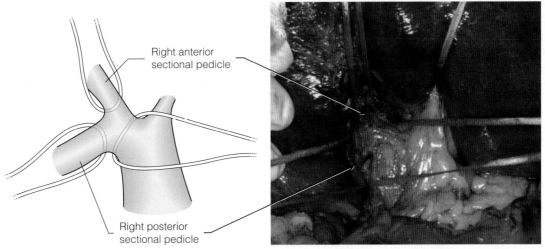

Right anterior
sectional pedicle

Right posterior
sectional pedicle

**Figure 1.16**    Isolation of right portal pedicle and sectional pedicles by the technique of dissection on the surface of pedicles. No inflow occlusion or separate hepatotomies are used (see reference 13). The umbilical tape in the upper right of the photograph is around the bridge of liver tissue over the umbilical fissure. (Reproduced from Strasberg SM, Linehan DC, Hawkins WG. Isolation of right main and right sectional portal pedicles for liver resection without hepatotomy or inflow occlusion. J Am Coll Surg 2008;206:390–6. With permission of the Journal of the American College of Surgeons.)

by means of partial vascular occlusion to the part of the liver to be resected, commonly through ligation or embolisation of the respective branch of the PV. This principle can be adapted to enable a two-stage procedure, which is usually indicated when a patient requires a right hemihepatectomy along with multiple resections from the left hemiliver. The first stage involves the clearance of all disease from the left hemiliver and ligation of the right PV. The patient is then given 4–6 weeks during which the left hemiliver regenerates, following which a right hepatectomy can be safely performed. A more recent evolution of the principle of the two-stage resection is the ALPPS procedure (Associating Liver Partition and Portal vein ligation for Staged hepatectomy). This involves the addition of a parenchymal separation of the future remnant liver during the first-stage operation.[14] The ALPPS procedure remains controversial, as although it produces rapid hypertrophy of the future liver remnant permitting the second-stage resection to be performed within 1 week, there is increased morbidity and mortality when compared with traditional two-stage hepatectomy.

## GALLBLADDER AND EXTRAHEPATIC BILE DUCTS

### GALLBLADDER

The gallbladder lies on the cystic plate. The cystohepatic triangle is an important anatomical space bordered by the cystic duct/gallbladder wall inferiorly, the CHD medially and the inferior surface of the liver superiorly. The eponymous term 'Calot's triangle' is often used interchangeably to describe the cystohepatic triangle, although the original description by Calot was of a space bounded by the cystic duct, cystic artery and CHD. The cystohepatic triangle contains the cystic artery and cystic lymph node and a portion of the right hepatic artery, as well as fat and fibrous tissue. Clearance of this triangle along with isolation of the cystic duct and elevation of the base of the

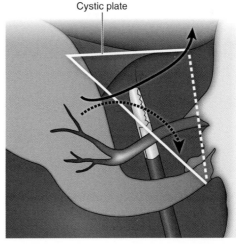

Cystic plate

**Figure 1.17**    The critical view of safety. The cystohepatic triangle has been dissected free of fat and fibrous tissue. Gallbladder, right side of the common hepatic duct (not displayed) and the liver form the border of the cystohepatic triangle. The cystic artery is within the cystohepatic triangle, and is branched into anterior and posterior branches. The *solid and dotted arrows* indicate the direction of dissection during cholecystectomy. The *dotted arrow* indicates leaving areolar tissue on the cystic plate; whereas the *solid arrow* indicates leaving the areolar tissue with the gallbladder during dissection.

gallbladder off the lower portion of the cystic plate gives the 'critical view of safety' that has been described for identification of the cystic structures during laparoscopic cholecystectomy[15] (Fig. 1.17). A large number of curiosities of the gallbladder, e.g. the Phrygian cap, have been described. The following are anomalies of importance to the biliary surgeon.

### AGENESIS OF THE GALLBLADDER

Agenesis occurs in approximately 1 in 8000 patients. It can be difficult to recognise but when it is suspected, axial imaging may confirm. If doubt remains, laparoscopy is definitive.

## DOUBLE GALLBLADDER

This is also a very rare anomaly but can be the cause of persistent symptoms after cholecystectomy. The gallbladder may also be bifid which typically does not cause symptoms, or have an hourglass constriction which may cause symptoms due to obstruction of the upper segment.

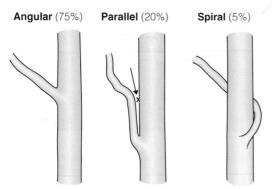

**Figure 1.18**  The three types of cystic duct/common hepatic duct confluence. The parallel union confluence is shown in the middle. Dissection of this type of cystic duct *(arrow)* may lead to injury to the side of the common hepatic duct during laparoscopic cholecystectomy. This is often a cautery injury. (Adapted from Warrren KW, McDonald WM, Kune GA. Bile duct strictures: new concepts in the management of an old problem. In: Irvine WT, editor. Modern trends in surgery. London: Butterworth; 1966. With permission from Elsevier.)

## CYSTIC DUCT

This structure is normally 1–2 cm in length and 2–3 mm in diameter. It joins the CHD at an acute angle to form the CBD. The cystic duct normally joins the CHD approximately 4 cm above the duodenum. However, the cystic duct may enter at any level from the biliary confluence down to the ampulla. The cystic duct may also join directly into the right hepatic duct, either when the right duct is in its normal position or in an aberrant location.

There are three patterns of confluence of the cystic duct and CHD (Fig. 1.18). In 20% of patients there is a parallel union and the surgeon approaching the CHD by dissecting the cystic duct is at risk of injuring the side of the former structure (Fig. 1.18). When making a choledochotomy in this situation, the incision should be started on the lateral side of the midplane of the bile duct in order to avoid entering a septum between the two fused ducts. When performing cholecystectomy, the cystic duct should be occluded in such a way that there is a visible section of cystic duct between the clip and the CBD.

Although a gallbladder with two cystic ducts has been described, the author has not seen convincing proof that this anomaly actually exists. If it does, it must be an anomaly of extreme rarity.

## CYSTIC ARTERY

The cystic artery is about 1 mm in diameter and normally arises from the right hepatic artery in the cystohepatic triangle (Fig. 1.19a). Typically the cystic artery runs for 1–2 cm

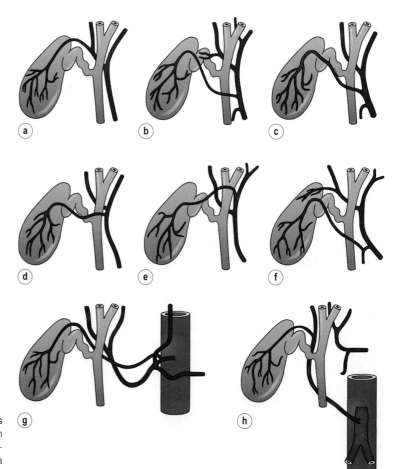

**Figure 1.19**  The eight **(a–h)** common anatomical variations of the cystic artery to the gallbladder. (Adapted from Poston GJ, Blumgart LH, editors. Surgical management of hepatobiliary and pancreatic disorders. 2nd ed. 2010. Ch. 2, p. 10. Boca Raton: CRC Press.)

to meet the gallbladder superior to the insertion of the cystic duct. The artery ramifies into an anterior and posterior branch at the point of contact with the gallbladder and these branches continue to divide on their respective surfaces. Sometimes the cystic artery divides into branches before the gallbladder is reached. In this situation, the anterior branch may be mistaken as the cystic artery proper and the posterior branch will not be discovered until later in the dissection, when it may be divided inadvertently. The artery may ramify into several branches before reaching the gallbladder, giving the impression that there is no cystic artery. The anterior and posterior branches may arise independently from the right hepatic artery, giving rise to two distinct cystic arteries. It is important to bear in mind other anatomical variations which are of significance during cholecystectomy including (Fig. 1.19):

1. A cystic artery that arises from the hepatic artery proper and runs anterior to the CHD (Fig. 1.19c).
2. A cystic artery that arises from the right hepatic artery on the left side of the CHD (Fig. 1.19d) or from the left hepatic artery (Fig. 1.19e) and runs anterior to the CHD, while the right hepatic artery runs behind it. Such cystic arteries tend to tether the gallbladder and make dissection of the cystohepatic triangle more difficult.
3. A cystic artery that arises from the gastroduodenal artery (GDA) (Fig. 1.19f) or an aberrant right hepatic artery coming off the SMA (Fig. 1.19h). In this case the cystic artery and not the cystic duct tends to be in the free edge of the fold leading from the hepatoduodenal ligament to the gallbladder. This should be suspected whenever the 'cystic duct' looks smaller than the 'cystic artery'.

Multiple small **cystic veins** drain into intrahepatic PV branches by passing into the liver around or through the cystic plate. Sometimes there are cystic veins in the cystohepatic triangle that run parallel to the cystic artery and enter the main PV.

The **cystic plate** has been described above. Small bile ducts may penetrate the cystic plate to enter the gallbladder. These 'ducts of Luschka' are very small, usually submillimetre accessory ducts. However, when divided during cholecystectomy, postoperative bilomas may occur if they are not visualised and occluded. Bilomas and haemorrhage may also be caused by penetration of the cystic plate during dissection. In about 10% of patients there is a large peripheral bile duct immediately deep to the plate, disruption of which will cause copious bile drainage. The origin of the middle hepatic vein is also in this location, and if it is injured massive haemorrhage may ensue. There is areolar tissue between the muscularis of the gallbladder and the cystic plate. At the top of the gallbladder, the layer is very thin. This areolar layer thickens if retrograde dissection from the top of the gallbladder in a medial direction is performed. If areolar tissue is left on the cystic plate, the surgeon will arrive on the posterior surface of the cystic artery and cystic duct (Fig. 1.17, *dotted arrow*). Conversely, if dissection is performed on the cystic plate leaving the areolar tissue on the gallbladder, the surgeon will arrive at the right portal pedicle (Fig. 1.17, *solid arrow*). If this is not anticipated, structures in the right portal pedicle may be injured. This dissection method is significantly more challenging in the presence of an inflamed gallbladder or

Mirizzi syndrome, when the areolar tissue between the gallbladder and cystic plate is fused together.

## EXTRAHEPATIC BILE DUCTS

The CHD is a structure formed by union of the right and left hepatic ducts. The union normally occurs at the right extremity of the base of Sg4, anterior and superior to the PV bifurcation. The CHD travels in the right edge of the hepatoduodenal ligament for 2–3 cm, where it joins the cystic duct to form the CBD. The latter has a supraduodenal course of 3–4 cm and then passes behind the duodenum to run in or occasionally behind the pancreas to enter the second portion of the duodenum. Details of its lower section and relation to the pancreatic duct are described in the final section of this chapter. The external diameter of the CBD varies from 5 to 13 mm when distended to physiological pressures. However, the duct diameter at surgery, i.e. in fasting patients with low duct pressures, may be as small as 3 mm. Radiologically, the internal duct diameter is measured on fasting patients. Under these conditions, the upper limit is normally 8 mm. Size should never be used as a sole criterion for identifying a bile duct. Caution is required in situations where a structure seems larger than expected. Although the cystic duct may be enlarged due to passage of stones, the surgeon should take extra precaution before dividing a 'cystic duct' that is greater than 2 mm in diameter because the CBD can be 3 mm in diameter and aberrant ducts may be smaller.

### ANOMALIES OF EXTRAHEPATIC BILE DUCTS

As already noted, there are biliary anomalies of the right and left ductal systems that can affect the outcome of hepatic surgery. The same is true for biliary surgery. The most important clinical anomaly is low insertion of right hepatic ducts referred to above. Because of its low location, it may be mistaken as the cystic duct and be injured during cholecystectomy. This is even more likely to occur when the cystic duct unites with an aberrant duct as opposed to joining the CHD. Left hepatic ducts can also join the CHD at a low level. They are less prone to injury since dissection during cholecystectomy is on the right side of the biliary tree.

### EXTRAHEPATIC ARTERIES

The course of these arteries has been described above. Anomalies of the hepatic artery are important in gallbladder surgery. Normally the right hepatic artery passes posterior to the bile duct (80%) (Fig. 1.19a) and gives off the cystic artery in the cystohepatic triangle. However, in 20% of cases, the right hepatic artery runs anterior to the bile duct (Fig. 1.19b–f). The right hepatic artery may lie very close to the gallbladder and chronic inflammation can draw the right hepatic artery directly on to the gallbladder, where it lies in an inverse U-loop and is prone to injury. In the 'classical injury' in laparoscopic cholecystectomy when the CBD is mistaken for the cystic duct, an associated right hepatic artery injury is very common.

### BLOOD SUPPLY OF BILE DUCTS

Many studies, dating back to the 19th century, have examined the blood supply of the extrahepatic bile ducts in

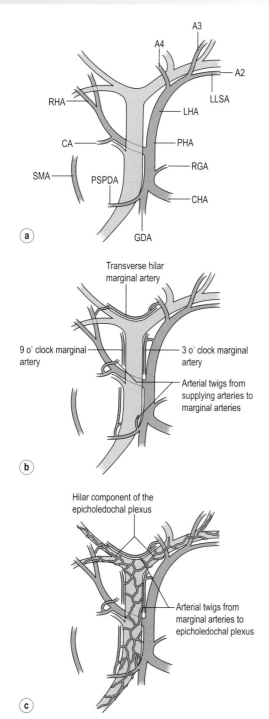

**Figure 1.20**  **(a)** The supplying arteries. All arteries shown can all give branches to the marginal arteries or in some cases directly supply the epicholedochal plexus. (*A2, A3, A4*, arteries to Sg2, 3 and 4; *CA*, cystic artery; *CHA*, common hepatic artery; *GDA*, gastroduodenal artery; *LHA*, left hepatic artery; *LLSA*, left lateral sectional artery; *PHA*, proper hepatic artery; *PSPDA*, posterior superior pancreaticoduodenal artery, the most important and constant artery; *RHA*, right hepatic artery). Replaced arteries arising from the superior mesenteric artery may also supply the bile ducts. **(b)** Marginal arteries. Marginal arteries are disposed at 3 and 9 o'clock (and occasionally at 12 o'clock) on the common bile duct/common hepatic duct. The hilar marginal artery runs across the top of the confluence of the right and left hepatic ducts. **(c)** Epicholedochal plexus. The epicholedochal plexus is supplied by the marginal arteries. (Adapted from Strasberg SM, Helton WS. An analytical review of vasculobiliary injury in laparoscopic and open cholecystectomy. HPB 2011;13(1):1–14. With permission from John Wiley & Sons.)

cadaveric specimens. A key observation made by Rappaport is that the bile ducts are supplied by the hepatic artery only,[16] unlike the liver, which has a dual blood supply from the hepatic artery and the PV. The arterial blood supply can be thought of as having three anatomical elements. The first consists of afferent vessels from the hepatic artery and its branches (Fig. 1.20a). The second element is longitudinal arteries that run parallel to the long axis of the bile duct and that receive blood from the afferent vessels (Fig. 1.20b). The third element is an arterial plexus encasing the bile ducts that receives blood from the marginal arteries (Fig. 1.20c). Tiny branches of the plexus pierce the bile duct wall to supply the capillaries of the bile duct.

The afferent vessels are branches of the hepatic arteries and less commonly of the SMA or other upper abdominal arteries. The most constant and important artery supplying the bile duct is the posterior superior pancreaticoduodenal artery, usually the first branch of the GDA. Arterial branches pass to the duct as the artery winds around the lower end of the duct. These branches supply much of the retroduodenal and intrapancreatic bile duct, but also ascend the bile duct to supply the supraduodenal bile duct. The lowest portion of the duct near the ampulla is also supplied by the anterior superior pancreatic artery from the inferior pancreatico-duodenal artery. Other vessels that commonly send afferents to the supraduodenal duct are the proper hepatic artery, cystic artery and artery to Sg4. Furthermore, body wall collaterals such as phrenic arteries can at times supply the bile ducts (as well as the liver) since bile duct infarction is much more common when there is occlusion of the common hepatic artery after a transplant than it is in an in-situ liver. The notion that the extrahepatic bile duct is supplied by arteries that join it only at the bottom and top of its course is incorrect. Supplying arteries from the cystic artery, right and left hepatic arteries and proper hepatic artery may also supply it.

The afferent vessels usually supply the longitudinal or 'marginal' arteries that run parallel to the long axis of the bile ducts (also called 'marginal anastomotic loop').[17] These vessels are disposed at 3 and 9 or, less commonly, at 12 o'clock on the CBD/CHD, or run across the top of the confluence and the right and left bile ducts. This 'hilar marginal artery' has been called the 'caudate arcade' or 'communicating arcade'. This artery is of great importance in maintaining blood supply to the liver when one hepatic artery (right or left) is occluded.[18]

The third element of this system is the 'epicholedochal plexus', a fine arterial plexus that lies on and surrounds the entire CBD and the left and right bile ducts. The latter is the hilar component of the epicholedochal plexus. The vessels of the plexus tend to run along the long axis of the ducts so that on the common duct many of the vessels are vertical, while those around the confluence and the right and left ducts are disposed horizontally. In the portion of the biliary tree that lies adjacent to the hilar plate or which has entered the fibrous sheaths, the epicholedochal plexus lies between the sheath and the wall of the bile duct. Dissection in this plane has the potential to devascularise bile ducts.[19]

Transection of the bile duct may result in ischaemia of the duct. For instance, if the duct is transected at the level

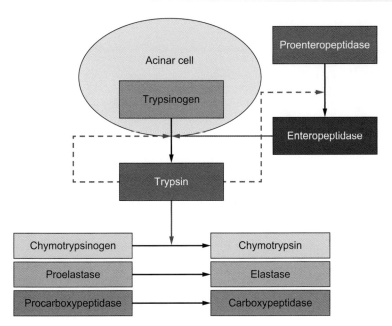

**Figure 1.21** Pancreatic zymogen activation cascade. Trypsinogen is secreted from the acinar cells. Upon reaching the duodenum, trypsinogen is cleaved and activated by enteropeptidase to become trypsin, which then activates chymotrypsinogen, proelastase and procarboxypeptidase. The formation of trypsin also allows the cleavage of more trypsinogen and the precursor of enteropeptidase.

of the duodenum, ischaemia of a portion of the bile duct above this level may occur since blood flow originating from the superior pancreatico-duodenal artery and passing up along the marginal artery is cut off. Similarly, in a high transection at the level of the confluence, the lower cut end of the duct may become ischaemic. This problem is thought to be an important contributory cause to the frequent failure of choledocho-choledochotomy as a form of biliary reconstruction. To avoid this problem, the bile duct is trimmed back to within 1 cm of the confluence and an hepatico-jejunostomy is fashioned.

## PANCREAS

### EMBRYOLOGICAL DEVELOPMENT OF THE PANCREAS

The thickening of the endoderm on the dorsal side of the gut tube opposite the hepatic bulge marks the development of the dorsal pancreas. The bulging of the dorsal pancreas into the mesenchyme becomes paired with the growth of the ventral foregut endoderm, which becomes the ventral pancreas. During the clockwise rotation of the gut tube, the ventral and dorsal buds come together and subsequently fuse. Pancreatic progenitor cells undergo further differentiation and commit to the major pancreatic lineages depending on either endocrine or exocrine pathways. Acinar cells are produced and proliferate around the epithelial tip, whilst islets of Langerhans are derived at a later stage, and continue to develop beyond the first week of the postnatal period.

### ANATOMICAL STRUCTURE AND FUNCTIONS OF THE PANCREAS

The pancreas is a retroperitoneal organ lying obliquely across the upper abdomen so that the tail is superior to the head. It is approximately 22 cm in length. The head of the pancreas is discoid in shape and terminates inferiorly

and medially in the hook-like uncinate process. The neck, body and tail are shaped like a flattened cylinder, sometimes somewhat triangular in cross-section with a flat anterior and pointed posterior surface. These divisions of the organ are somewhat arbitrary, but the neck of the pancreas sits anterior to the superior mesenteric and PV. The consistency of pancreatic gland is normally soft.

The pancreas has two key functions: endocrine and exocrine. For the exocrine function, pancreatic juice is secreted from acinar cells to intralobular ducts, which in turn drain into the main pancreatic duct and then to the duodenum. The enzyme produced from the acinar cell is secreted as an inactive form, called zymogen, which is then cleaved and activated by enteropeptidase upon reaching the duodenum (Fig. 1.21).

The endocrine function of the pancreas is contributed by four types of pancreatic islet cells, namely α-(alpha-)cells (secreting glucagon), β-(beta-)cells (insulin), δ-(delta-)cells (somatostatin) and γ-(gamma-)cells (pancreatic polypeptide). Insulin acts to decrease blood glucose level, whereas glucagon balances it out. These hormones are secreted by the islet cells directly into the bloodstream, and function independently from the exocrine role of the pancreas.

### PANCREATIC DUCTS

The prevailing anatomical pattern of the pancreatic duct is the result of union of the ventral main duct (Wirsung) with the dorsal accessory duct (Santorini), along with partial regression of the dorsal duct in the head. The 'genu' of the duct (genu = knee) is the bend in the duct where the ventral duct joins the dorsal duct. In the prevailing pattern, both ducts communicate with the duodenum, the dorsal duct entering at the minor papilla approximately 2 cm above and 5 mm anterior to the major papilla. Other ductal patterns are possible that involve various degrees of dominance or regression of portions of the ducts in the head of the pancreas. For instance, the ducts may not unite, resulting in separate drainage from the ventral and dorsal pancreas (pancreas divisum), the dorsal duct may lose its connection

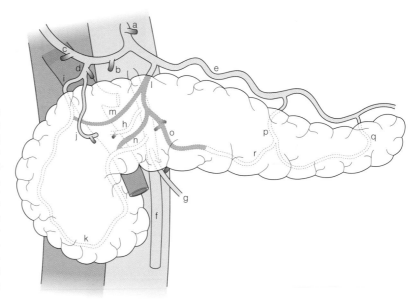

**Figure 1.22** Arterial blood supply to the pancreas. The dorsal pancreatic artery is shown shaded. Alternative origins of the artery are shown as black stumps. Key: *a*, coeliac artery; *b*, common hepatic artery; *c*, right hepatic artery; *d*, gastroduodenal artery; *e*, splenic artery; *f*, superior mesenteric artery; *g*, middle colic artery; *h*, right hepatic artery (aberrant); *i*, superior pancreatico-duodenal artery; *j*, right gastroepiploic artery; *k*, inferior pancreatico-duodenal artery; *l*, dorsal pancreatic artery (DPA); *m*, right anastomotic branch of DPA to superior part of pancreatico-duodenal arcade; *o*, left anastomotic branch of DPA becomes transverse pancreatic artery; *p*, pancreatica magna artery; *q*, caudal pancreatic artery; *r*, transverse pancreatic artery. (© Washington University in St Louis.)

to the duodenum; or the dorsal duct in the head may lose its connection to the rest of the ductal system and drain only a small section of the head into the duodenum. Alternatively, the ventral duct may regress and the dorsal duct drain more or all of the pancreas through the minor ampulla. The uncinate process is served by its own duct, which joins the main pancreatic duct 1–2 cm from its entry into the duodenum.

The pancreatic duct (and pancreas) are often referred to as proximal (head) and distal (tail). These may be confusing terms—as may the terms proximal and distal bile duct. The bile duct nearest to the ampulla is commonly referred to as 'distal', but the pancreatic duct in this region as 'proximal'. An alternative is to refer to the pancreatic portion or lower bile duct and the upper extrahepatic or hilar bile duct. For the pancreas, the duct may be referred to as the 'pancreatic head duct', 'pancreatic body duct', etc.

The ventral duct usually joins the CBD to form a common channel several millimetres from the ampulla of Vater, usually within the wall of the duodenum. The bile duct traverses the duodenal wall obliquely and the pancreatic duct at a right angle. Each duct and the common channel have their own sphincters. The common channel may be longer or absent, with both ducts entering the duodenum separately, the pancreatic duct more inferiorly. In performing a sphincteroplasty, it is advisable to open the common opening superiorly (10–12 o'clock position in the mobilised duodenum) to avoid the orifice of the pancreatic duct (4 o'clock). The ampulla is normally at the midpoint of the second part of the duodenum. It is rarely higher but can be as low as the midpoint of the third part of the duodenum. When the dorsal duct has its own communication with the duodenum, it is found at the 'minor papilla', about 2 cm proximal and 1 cm anterior to the major papilla.

## BLOOD SUPPLY OF THE PANCREAS

The arterial supply of the pancreas consists of two vascular systems, one supplying the head and uncinate, and the other the body and tail. The neck is a watershed area between these two vascular systems.[20] The head and uncinate process are supplied by the pancreatico-duodenal arcade, which

consists of two to several loops of vessels that arise from the superior pancreatico-duodenal (branch of the GDA) and inferior pancreatico-duodenal (branch of the SMA) arteries. The arcades run on the anterior and posterior surface of the pancreas next to the duodenum, the anterior arcade lying somewhat closer to the duodenum. The second system arises from the splenic artery, which gives rise to three arteries into the dorsal surface of the gland (Fig. 1.22). The dorsal pancreatic artery is the most medial of the three and the most important. It anastomoses with the pancreatico-duodenal arcade in the neck of the pancreas. It is the most aberrant artery in the upper abdomen and may arise from vessels that are routinely occluded during pancreatico-duodenectomy, which may account in part for fistula formation after this procedure.

This unique arterial arcade between the inferior pancreatico-duodenal and the GDA at the head of the pancreas provides an additional surgical option in achieving resectability for pancreatic body tumours encasing the coeliac axis. By resecting the coeliac axis in these rare circumstances, the liver will then rely on the backflow arterial supply from the GDA to the hepatic artery proper. The GDA will also provide the only arterial supply to the stomach via the gastroepiploic artery, since the left gastric and splenic arteries would have been sacrificed during the coeliac axis resection. This procedure is known as the 'Appleby' procedure, which was first described by Lyon Appleby in 1953.[21]

Venous drainage generally follows the arterial supply (Fig. 1.23). The veins of the body and tail of the pancreas drain into the splenic vein, which lies partly embedded in the posterior surface of the gland. These veins are short and fragile. The right gastroepiploic and anteroinferior pancreatico-duodenal veins provide drainage for the head and uncinate process. These two tributaries form the gastrocolic trunk, which in turn drains into the superior mesenteric vein (SMV) on the right lateral side, and then to the PV above the porto-splenic confluence. The gastrocolic trunk is a key tributary that is ligated during pancreatico-duodenectomy. A nearly constant posterosuperior pancreatico-duodenal vein enters the right lateral side of the PV at the level of

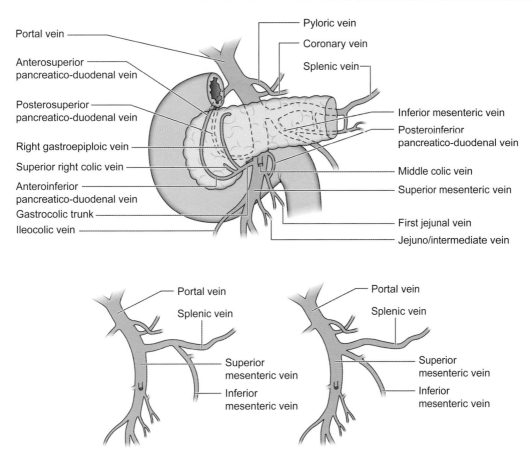

**Figure 1.23**  Venous drainage of the pancreas. Variations in the relation of the portal, splenic, superior mesenteric and inferior mesenteric veins are shown at the bottom. (Adapted from Vickers SM, Arnoletti JP, Brunicardi FC, Andersen DK. Pancreas anatomy and physiology. In: Mulholland MW, Lillemoe KD, Doherty GM, editors. Greenfield's surgery: scientific principles and practice. 4th edition. Philadelphia: Lippincott Williams & Wilkins; 2006. Copyright © 2006 Lippincott Williams & Wilkins.)

the duodenum. During the isolation of all venous tributaries prior to performing a SMV/PV resection, it is important to be mindful of the insertion of the coronary vein, which provides drainage for the left gastric vein immediately above the porto-splenic confluence. The inferior mesenteric vein (IMV) normally drains into the splenic vein. However, the IMV can occasionally drain directly to the SMV, and can be damaged during surgical dissection.

## LYMPHATICS OF THE PANCREAS

For surgical purposes, the lymphatic drainage of the pancreas is best considered with respect to resection of the pancreatic head and resection of the pancreatic body and tail. Nomenclature for nodal stations is currently based on the classification of the Japanese Pancreas Society as recommended by the International Study Group on Pancreatic Surgery (ISGPS).[22]

There is a ring of nodes around the pancreas that drain the adjacent sections of the gland and are denoted by various lymph node stations (Ln), depending on their location.[23] The lymphatics of the head and uncinate process drain into lymph nodes in the pancreatico-duodenal groove anteriorly (Ln17) and posteriorly (Ln13), and infrapyloric nodes inferiorly (Ln6). These in turn drain into nodes adjacent to the CBD (Ln12) and hepatic artery superiorly (Ln8), and into nodes along the SMA (Ln14), coeliac axis (Ln9) and aorta (axial nodes). Understanding these lymph node stations is

important as current practice is a standard lymphadenectomy for pancreatico-duodenectomy, which does not include coeliac (Ln9), splenic (Ln11) and left gastric (Ln7) nodes.

The lymphatics of the body and tail are shown in Fig. 1.24. These are lymph nodes around the splenic hilum (Ln10), splenic artery (Ln11) and inferior border of body/tail of pancreas (Ln18). Resection of Ln9 is only indicated in tumours involving the body of the pancreas.

## ANATOMICAL RELATIONS AND LIGAMENTS OF THE PANCREAS

The pancreas is a deeply seated organ that, unlike the liver and most of the biliary tree, is not obvious when opening the abdomen. The anatomical relations of the pancreas are very important in pancreatic surgery. The structures emphasised in the following section are those that are commonly invaded by tumours.

The pancreas lies in the pararenal space anterior to the anterior renal fascia and behind the peritoneum. Posteriorly, the pancreas is related, from right to left, to the right kidney and perinephric fat, IVC and right gonadal vein, aorta, left renal vein (slightly inferior), retropancreatic fat, left adrenal gland and the superior pole of the left kidney. All of the former structures lie in the perirenal space and behind the anterior renal fascia. In the case of oncological resections, the plane of dissection should be behind the anterior renal fascia in order to maximise the chance of obtaining

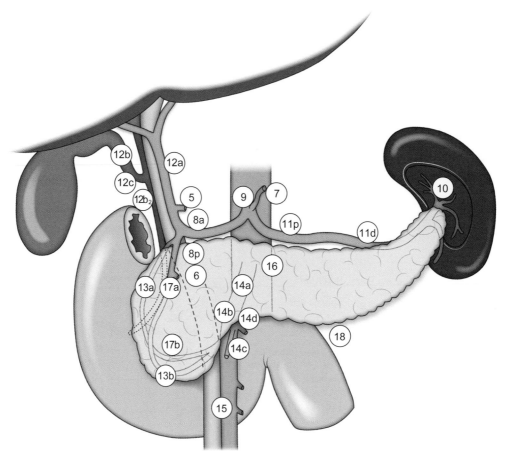

**Figure 1.24** Japan Pancreas Society nomenclature of peripancreatic lymph nodes. (Adapted from Japan Pancreas Society. Classification of pancreatic carcinoma. 2nd English edition. Tokyo: Kanehara & Co. Ltd; 2003.)

negative margins as described for the radical antegrade modular pancreatosplenectomy (RAMPS) procedure.[24]

The SMV and PV are posterior relations to the neck of the pancreas, and *splenic vein* to the body and tail. The SMA is a posterior relation of the junction of the neck and body of the gland lying posterior and medial to the SMV. The SMA and SMV are both related to the uncinate process and give branches into and receive tributaries from the uncinate process, respectively. Often the uncinate veins enter a large tributary of the SMV, the first jejunal vein, which also abuts the uncinate process. These short arteries and veins are of importance surgically as they are divided when the head of the pancreas is resected. The *coeliac artery* rises vertically superior to the SMA close to the superior edge of the pancreas, where it gives off the common hepatic artery and the *splenic artery*. The former runs anteriorly and to the left in approximation to the superior border of the pancreas. At the point where the artery passes in front of the PV, it divides into the *gastroduodenal artery*, which passes anterior to the neck of the pancreas, sometimes buried within it. It terminates in the right gastroepiploic artery that rises in a fold of tissue toward the pylorus, a fold that also contains the right gastroepiploic vein and subpyloric nodes. The splenic artery snakes along the superior border of the pancreas to leave it 2–3 cm from the termination of the pancreas.

The head of the pancreas is wrapped in the first three parts of the duodenum and the tail ends in relation to the splenic hilum. There is variability in the proximity of the tail of the pancreas to the spleen. In some cases, the pancreas terminates 2 cm from the splenic substance and in others it abuts it. The anterior surface of the body and tail of the pancreas is covered by peritoneum, which is the posterior wall of the lesser sac, and then by the posterior wall of the stomach anterior to this. The transverse mesocolon is related to the inferior border of the pancreas, and the right and left extremities of the transverse colon are related to the head and tail of the gland. The IMV is related to the inferior border of the neck of the pancreas and may pass behind it to enter the splenic vein or turn medially to enter the SMV.

The pancreas is normally accessed surgically by entering the lesser sac either by division of the greater omentum below the gastroepiploic arcade or by releasing the greater omentum from its attachment to the transverse colon. When the lesser sac is entered, the anterior surface of the neck, body and tail are often visible, but may be obscured by congenital filmy adhesions to the posterior wall of the stomach. To expose the head of the pancreas, it is necessary to mobilise the right side of the transverse colon and hepatic flexure inferiorly and to divide the right gastroepiploic vein. The latter crosses the inferior border of the pancreas to join with the middle colic vein to form the gastrocolic trunk, which then enters the SMV. For complete exposure, e.g. for a Frey procedure, the right gastroepiploic artery is also divided and it and the subpyloric nodes are swept upwards off the pancreas. To access the SMV at the inferior border of the pancreas, the peritoneum at the inferior border of the neck is divided and the dissection is carried inferiorly and laterally to open a groove between the uncinate process and the mesentery. Division of the right gastroepiploic vein at the inferior border of the pancreas greatly facilitates this manoeuvre. Normally no veins enter the SMV or PV from the posterior surface of the neck of the pancreas. Consequently, the neck of the pancreas can be separated from the anterior surface of the SMV/PV in this avascular plane. The peritoneum at the inferior border of the neck, body and tail of the pancreas is avascular, and there are few vascular connections between the back of the body and tail of the pancreas and retroperitoneal tissues. As a result, the pancreas may be readily dissected free from the retroperitoneum. The splenic vein is partly embedded in the back of the pancreas from the point that it reaches the gland on the left to about 1 cm from its termination at its confluence with the SMV.

## INNERVATION OF THE PANCREAS

The pancreas is a highly innervated visceral organ. Pancreatic nerves are sensitive to both chemical and mechanical stimuli. These nerves transmit nociceptive and visceral afferent signals to the coeliac plexus, which is the largest of the three plexuses of the sympathetic system. Normally, the preganglionic efferent fibres exit the spinal cord to form the sympathetic chain. Instead of synapsing at the sympathetic chain, the greater, lesser and least splanchnic nerves pass through the sympathetic chain to form the coeliac ganglia, and provide the major preganglionic contribution to the coeliac plexus. The parasympathetic supply of the pancreas is provided by the left and right vagal trunks, which do not connect at the coeliac ganglia. This coeliac plexus most commonly consolidates around the origin of the coeliac axis and SMA.[25]

An understanding of this pancreatic innervation has led to the development of various non-surgical and surgical techniques for treating pain in chronic pancreatitis. These include the coeliac plexus block most commonly performed under endoscopic guidance[26] and selective pancreatic denervation by splanchnicectomy and ganglionectomy.[27,28]

### Key points

- A prevailing pattern of hepatic, biliary and pancreatic anatomy exists, but variations (anomalies) are frequent.
- All HPB operations should be conducted with the strong suspicion that an anatomical anomaly may be present.

 References available at http://ebooks.health.elsevier.com/

### KEY REFERENCES

[2]  Terminology Committee of the IHPBA. The brisbane 2000 terminology of liver anatomy and resections. HPB 2000;2:333–9.
    *The Scientific Committee of the IHPBA created a Terminology Committee to deal with the confusion in nomenclature of hepatic anatomy and liver resections. The resulting terminology is presented in this paper. This use of agreed anatomical and surgical terms permits a meaningful and consistent approach to liver resection terminology in all clinical and academic writing.*

[14]  Schnitzbauer AA, Lang SA, Goessmann H, et al. Right portal vein ligation combined with in situ splitting induces rapid left lateral liver lobe hypertrophy enabling 2-staged extended right hepatic resection in small-for-size settings. Ann Surg 2012;255:405–14. PMID: 22330038.
    *First report of a novel two-stage hepatic resection performing surgical exploration, portal vein ligation and in-situ splitting, resulting in marked and rapid hypertrophy of functional liver tissue enabling curative resection of marginally resectable liver tumours or metastases.*

[15]  Strasberg SM, Brunt LM. Rationale and use of the critical view of safety in laparoscopic cholecystectomy. J Am Coll Surg 2010;211:132–8. PMID: 20610259.
    *This paper describes the use of the critical view of safety (CVS) method of identification of the cystic duct and cystic artery during laparoscopic cholecystectomy, in order to minimise the risk of common bile duct injury.*

[22]  Tol JA, Gouma DJ, Bassi C, et al. Definition of a standard lymphadenectomy in surgery for pancreatic ductal adenocarcinoma: a consensus statement by the International Study Group on Pancreatic Surgery (ISGPS). Surgery 2014;156(3):591–600. PMID: 25061003.
    *This paper describes the lymph node stations surrounding the pancreas and provides the definitions required for standard lymphadenectomy in surgery for ductal adenocarcinoma located in different parts of the pancreas.*

# 2 Liver function and failure

Benjamin M. Stutchfield | Stephen J. Wigmore

## OVERVIEW OF LIVER FUNCTIONS AND EVOLUTION

The liver is the largest solid organ in the human body. It has a unique structure with a dual blood supply, being approximately one-third from the hepatic artery and two-thirds from the portal venous system. Within the liver substance, blood flows through sinusoids between plates of hepatocytes into central veins, which in turn join the hepatic veins draining into the vena cava. The liver is a major site of protein synthesis exporting plasma proteins to maintain oncotic pressure and coagulation factors. Acute-phase proteins that act as antiproteases, opsonins and metal ion carriers are synthesised by the liver in response to injury or infection. Numerous immune cells populate the liver and the resident tissue macrophages, the Kupffer cells, form an important component of the innate immune system. Nutrients are extracted from portal blood by the liver and processed, and the liver acts as an important reservoir for glycogen. Waste products are either modified in the liver for excretion by the kidneys or are excreted into bile. Many drugs are taken up by the liver and metabolised, giving either active metabolites or inactive metabolites for excretion. In humans, as in many vertebrates, the liver's capacity for metabolism and clearance far exceeds what is required for day-to-day life. It is possible that this ability offers a significant advantage in terms of survival from poisoning, starvation or trauma.

## SYMPTOMS OF LIVER FAILURE: ACUTE AND CHRONIC

In the acute setting, liver failure can present with a number of symptoms, but it is important to note that not all of these may be present at the same time. Typically, a patient with acute liver failure after surgery, transplantation or due to acute poisoning will be confused or cognitively impaired as a result of encephalopathy, which may progress to loss of consciousness and a need to protect the airway by intubation and mechanical ventilation. Patients are often not immediately jaundiced, but jaundice may develop over the course of several days. Patients may be hypoglycaemic, and the requirement for intravenous infusion of dextrose is a sinister development and an indicator of severe acute liver failure. Coagulopathy may develop, with evidence of bruising or bleeding from line sites or surgical scars. Severe acute liver failure can be assessed using the King's College Hospital criteria, which were designed to predict mortality in paracetamol- and non-paracetamol-dependent acute liver failure.[1] Later, this scoring system was adopted in the UK to determine criteria indicating likely benefit from liver transplantation. In the surgical patient, the development of acute liver failure is usually more gradual and less dramatic; a useful scoring system for liver dysfunction in the acute setting has been reported by Schindl et al.[2] (Box 2.1).

## COMMON CAUSES OF ACUTE LIVER FAILURE: HEPATIC INSUFFICIENCY FOLLOWING LIVER RESECTION

Liver resection has the potential to cure patients with cancers that have originated in the liver itself (primary liver cancer) or that have originated elsewhere and have subsequently spread to the liver (metastatic liver cancer). Equally, it is a preferred therapy in patients with benign liver tumours that have the potential of malignant transformation (uncertain benign primary liver tumours). Resection of up to 70% of the liver is feasible, because the liver has a remarkable capacity to regenerate. Within 6–8 weeks following 60–70% hepatectomy, the liver has regained nearly all of its original size and weight.

The most common cause of liver metastases is from primary colorectal cancer, and it is estimated that in the West there is a yearly incidence of 300 new cases of colorectal liver metastases per million population. The current estimate is that this should lead to approximately 100–150 patients per million eligible for liver resection for this indication. To this should be added the patients with primary benign and malignant liver tumours, and hence about 150–200 liver resections should probably be performed per million population each year.

Ever since the first liver resection by Langenbuch in 1887, this procedure has remained a major undertaking and even in the recent past, liver resection was still a dangerous surgical procedure with a high mortality of 20–30% in the 1970s. This was mainly due to excessive intraoperative bleeding; however, over the subsequent decades, the procedure has become increasingly safer due to improvements in surgical and anaesthetic techniques. At present, mortality rates are reported to be well below 5%. Currently, the single most important cause of lethal outcome following hepatic resection is liver failure. For this reason, many researchers and clinicians have attempted to design methods to identify patients at risk of liver failure (and hence mortality) following liver surgery. However, the development of such a method has been hampered by several factors, as outlined below.

The critical point determining lethal outcome following liver resection has been a failure of the residual liver to function properly. Focus in this research area has been to determine a single liver function test that identifies patients with impaired liver function. This has proven exceedingly difficult, and such a test is not available for a number of reasons.

First, as outlined above, the liver has a remarkable capacity to regenerate very rapidly, which emphasises that there is tremendous overcapacity of several liver functions. In this context, it is known that it is entirely safe to resect 50% of an otherwise healthy liver, because the residual half liver will simply take over all vital liver functions such as clearing bacteria, urea synthesis and synthesis of crucial proteins. It has been estimated that a crucial liver function, such as urea synthesis, has an overcapacity of 300%, which implies that a static preoperative liver function test will be unable to assess this particular function. An alternative and innovative strategy would be to give a challenge to the liver and measure the ability of the liver to respond or cope—a dynamic test.

The critical minimum residual liver volume for healthy liver parenchyma has been estimated to be approximately 25% after resection.[2]

The second crucial problem has been that there is only a poor correlation between volume and function. However, it is still unclear why some patients with smaller hepatic remnants do not develop liver failure whilst some with greater residual volumes do. These observations suggest, however, that peri- and intraoperative events superimposed on the innate hepatic capacity to withstand injury play a role. Hepatic insufficiency in this situation may arise either if not enough liver volume is left after partial hepatectomy or if the residual volume does not function properly. A functional limitation may arise, for example, in patients who have received chemotherapy in order to reduce the number and size of metastases prior to surgical treatment by liver resection. One of the factors contributing to defective defence may be preoperative fasting,[3] but equally, prior chemotherapy and pre-existent steatosis may play a role.

A third important aspect is that during liver surgery, deliberate hypotension and temporary hepatic blood inflow occlusion (Pringle manoeuvre) are used by many surgeons to reduce blood loss during hepatic surgery (15 minutes ischaemia, 5 minutes reperfusion [15/5 Pringle]). Other surgeons do not use this manoeuvre, assuming that it causes oxidative stress and ischaemia/reperfusion (I/R) injury.[4,5] There is little doubt that this procedure does cause oxidative stress and I/R injury; however, the consequence of this is variable. In a situation where defence mechanisms against oxidative stress are deficient, it may adversely affect liver function. In this situation, hepatic steatosis may constitute an additional predisposing factor to damage by I/R.

Ischaemia/reperfusion is the basis of ischaemic preconditioning, a process in which temporary clamping and release of the liver blood flow has been shown to be beneficial in terms of increasing resistance to subsequent injury.[6]

In this situation, it is assumed that defence mechanisms against oxidative stress are adequate and are indeed enhanced by short-term I/R injury.[7]

The above three factors explain why it has been exceedingly difficult to design a proper liver function test that reliably singles out those patients at risk of liver failure following liver resection. The term 'liver function' is a rather crude denominator for a range of functions that includes ammonia detoxification, urea synthesis, protein synthesis and breakdown, bile synthesis and secretion, gluconeogenesis and detoxification of drugs, bacteria and bacterial toxins.

## CHRONIC LIVER FAILURE

The clinical signs of chronic liver failure are often insidious and can also be related to the type of disease. Cirrhosis is associated with a failure of hepatic function and the consequences of increased hepatic vascular resistance. Metabolic impairment is manifest by jaundice, coagulopathy, impaired ammonia clearance and encephalopathy, hypoalbuminaemia and oedema. The presence of increased vascular resistance is associated with the development of splenomegaly, ascites and gastro-oesophageal or abdominal wall varices. The slow progression of many chronic liver diseases, over years, implies a gradual, almost incremental, loss of liver cell mass or function. There are many causes of liver failure, including hepatitis B and C virus, autoimmune diseases such as primary biliary cirrhosis, primary sclerosing cholangitis and autoimmune hepatitis, alcoholic liver disease, Wilson's disease, $\alpha_1$-antitrypsin deficiency and others. All are associated with chronic or repeated cell injury and attempts at repair. The fibrosis and scarring associated with this regeneration and repair lead to the clinical condition termed cirrhosis, with a typically small shrunken irregular liver and an increased risk of cancer.

The Child–Pugh score for chronic liver disease[8] has served as a useful means of categorising patients based on the severity of their liver disease. It employs five clinical measures of liver disease and each measure is scored 1–3, with 3 indicating the most severe derangement (Table 2.1). In the setting of liver transplantation, the Model for End-stage Liver Disease (MELD) or MELD-Na (MELD including sodium) score or in

**Table 2.1**   Child–Pugh score for chronic liver disease

| Measure | 1 point | 2 points | 3 points | Units |
|---|---|---|---|---|
| Bilirubin (total) | < 34 (< 2) | 34–50 (2,3) | > 50 (> 3) | μmol/L (mg/dL) |
| Serum albumin | > 35 | 28–35 | < 28 | g/L |
| INR | < 1.7 | 1.71–2.20 | > 2.20 | No unit |
| Ascites | None | Suppressed with medication | Refractory | No unit |
| Hepatic encephalopathy | None | Grade I–II (or suppressed with medication) | Grade III–IV (or refractory) | No unit |

Child–Pugh A = 5–6 points; Child–Pugh B = 7–9 points; Child–Pugh C = 10–15 points. 1-year survival: A = 100%; B = 80%; C = 45%.

the United Kingdom UKELD score has partly replaced Child–Pugh scoring in the assessment of severity of liver disease.

## METABOLIC LIVER FUNCTION

The liver plays a central role in fat, carbohydrate and protein metabolism, as well as in acid–base homeostasis. In the context of liver failure, disturbances of fat metabolism are probably not crucially important. With respect to carbohydrate metabolism, it is well known that the liver plays a central role in the conversion of lactate to glucose. Part of this lactate is formed due to anaerobic metabolism of, amongst others, glucose in skeletal muscle. This metabolic route of glucose to lactate (muscle) and then back to glucose (liver) is very important for glycaemic homeostasis and is called the Cori cycle. Liver failure will be manifested by lactic acidosis and hypoglycaemia.

Next to its role in carbohydrate metabolism, the liver plays a central function in nitrogen homeostasis. Hepatic synthesis and breakdown of proteins and amino acids, and detoxification and clearance of the nitrogenous waste products from other organs are of central importance. For example, the gut uses the amino acid glutamine as a fuel for enterocytes, which results in the production of waste end-products of intestinal metabolism, such as ammonia. This ammonia is then transported via the portal vein to the liver, where it is detoxified with the formation of urea.

## WHY DO PATIENTS DIE FROM LIVER FAILURE?

The failing liver can trigger a range of events resulting in multi-organ failure, sepsis and death. When three or more organs are involved, the chance of death approaches 80%.[9] Bacterial infection and hepatic encephalopathy are the leading causes of death in this group who experience progressive systemic failure.

Risk of bacterial infection is increased considerably following partial hepatectomy.[2] Immune function is compromised as the liver's phagocytic and synthetic capacity is impaired by its reduced size. The shear force generated by increased portal venous blood flow per unit area, as well as ischaemic injury at the time of surgery, can further impair immune capacity.[10] Management of sepsis in these patients necessitates intensive care, multi-organ support and broad-spectrum antibiotics subsequently guided by culture results.

Hepatic encephalopathy is a reversible neuropsychiatric syndrome, with a multifactorial cause. It is characterised by cerebral oedema, raised intracranial pressure, with risk of brain herniation and death.[11] A range of factors may contribute to this phenomenon, including rising concentration of ammonia, glutamine and lactate. Ammonia has a range of effects on brain function, affecting neurotransmission as well as impairing mitochondrial function and key cellular transport systems. There is a direct correlation between arterial ammonia concentration and the presence of brain herniation.[12] Brain glutamine concentration is elevated in acute liver failure, which may influence the development of hepatic encephalopathy through toxic metabolites, modulation of hepatic blood flow or by amplifying the toxic effects of ammonia.[13] Lactate can result in significant swelling of astrocytes in culture[14] and raised brain lactate concentration is seen in a wide range of experimental models of acute liver failure.

Therapeutic approaches in hepatic encephalopathy aim to address these areas with strategies to lower ammonia levels, protect systems by inducing mild hypothermia, reduce blood–brain ammonia transfer, decrease brain lactate synthesis and reduce inflammation. However, in the face of overwhelming liver failure, attempts to modulate these mechanisms of hepatic encephalopathy have been shown at best to prolong life by hours to a few days. In some selected patients, this may provide a 'bridge to liver transplantation'; however, patients undergoing surgery for metastatic disease are ineligible for transplantation and therefore their only hope lies in the intrinsic ability of the liver to regenerate.

## ASSESSMENT OF THE LIVER

### MEASURING LIVER VOLUME

Advances in imaging techniques have permitted the development of in vivo imaging of the liver. Three-dimensional models of the liver can be constructed from computed tomography (CT) or other cross-sectional imaging modalities, such as magnetic resonance imaging (MRI). The volume of the liver can then be calculated based on known separation of image slices combined with planar mapping of cross-sectional areas. In addition, such three-dimensional computer models can be simulated to map the effects of surgery by performing virtual hepatic resection, and studies have demonstrated that there is a good correlation between computer modelling and actual resection weight of surgical liver specimens (Figs. 2.1–2.3).[2,15] Some centres use 3D printers to create a replica of the patient's liver. This enables the relationship between the tumour and the vascular/biliary anatomy of the liver to be better understood, aiding complex liver resections.[16]

### BLOOD TESTS OF LIVER FUNCTION

Liver function tests refer to the transaminases, alkaline phosphatase, γ-glutamyl transferase and bilirubin. They are

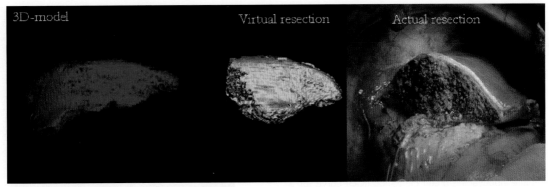

**Figure 2.1** Three-dimensional (3D) reconstruction of the liver preoperatively *(red)* showing tumours. Computer prediction of residual liver volume based on virtual hepatectomy of 3D model *(yellow)* and actual photograph of resection showing residual liver segments. (Reproduced from Schindl MJ, Redhead DN, Fearon KC, et al. The value of residual liver volume as a predictor of hepatic dysfunction and infection after major liver resection. Gut 2005;54:289–96. With permission from the BMJ Publishing Group Ltd.)

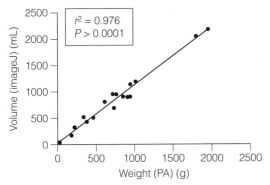

**Figure 2.2** Correlation between volume of resection calculated with ImageJ and actual measured weights of the resection specimens (*n* = 15, Pearson's test). (Reproduced with permission from Dello SA, van Dam RM, Slangen JJ, et al. Liver volumetry plug and play: do it yourself with ImageJ. World J Surg 2007;31:2215–21.)

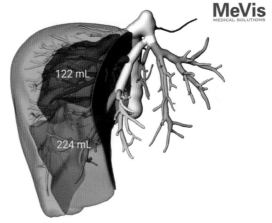

**Figure 2.3** Mapping the territory of the right hepatic lobe drained by the middle hepatic vein. The numbers represent the volumes of the territories at risk if segment 5 and 8 tributaries of the middle hepatic vein were not reconstructed in a potential right lobe living-donor liver transplant. (Image courtesy of © 2023 MeVis Medical Solutions AG, Bremen, Germany.)

not truly measures of function but do give an indication of processes going on within the liver. Aspartate aminotransferase and alanine aminotransferase are hepatocyte enzymes that are released in conditions in which hepatocytes are damaged or killed, such as ischaemic injury, hepatitis, severe sepsis and in response to cancer. Liver-specific alkaline phosphatase is expressed predominantly in the biliary epithelium and is elevated in conditions such as cholangitis or biliary obstruction. γ-Glutamyl transferase is expressed by both hepatocytes and biliary epithelium; it is often elevated in patients with cancer but can also be induced by high alcohol consumption.

Biochemical markers of true liver function vary depending on whether acute or chronic liver failure or injury is being considered (Table 2.2).

**Table 2.2 Blood tests useful to assess function in acute and chronic liver injury**

|  | Acute | Chronic |
|---|---|---|
| Albumin | – | +++ |
| Prothrombin time | +++ | +++ |
| Bilirubin | + | +++ |
| Lactate | ++ | – |
| Glucose requirement | ++ | – |
| Ammonia | + | + |

## TESTS OF LIVER FUNCTION MEASURING SUBSTANCE CLEARANCE

The ability to accurately predict postoperative outcome based on preoperative liver function would be a valuable addition to preoperative assessment. The tests currently in common use include the indocyanine green (ICG) clearance test, hepatobiliary scintigraphy with radioisotope clearance, lidocaine clearance test, aminopyrine breath test and the galactose elimination test. These tests aim to provide an indicator of dynamic liver function, in that they can provide real-time assessment of liver function in response to a challenge. However, none of these tests challenge the liver to demonstrate its full functional capacity. Serum bilirubin and clotting factors provide a static indirect estimation of liver metabolism and synthetic function, but are influenced by a range of other factors that limit their relevance and suitability to predict postoperative outcome. The most commonly used test for liver function prior to liver resections is the ICG clearance test.

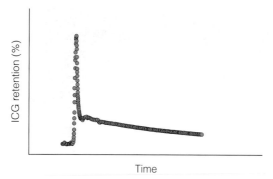

**Figure 2.4** Typical indocyanine green clearance (ICG) curve for a subject with healthy liver function.

## INDOCYANINE GREEN

ICG is a compound that is used widely to measure liver function. It is rapidly cleared from blood, specifically by hepatocytes, and is excreted into bile without enterohepatic circulation. Hepatocytes are highly effective at clearing ICG such that hepatic blood flow is the limiting factor in patients with otherwise normal liver parenchyma. In more severe liver disease, both hepatic blood flow and hepatocyte function may be compromised, thereby impairing the clearance of ICG. ICG clearance can be measured as 'disappearance' from the blood or can also be measured as accumulation in bile. Liver dysfunction is suggested by a slower rate of clearance from the blood and is usually expressed as percentage retention at 5 or 15 minutes after injection. Continuous measurement of ICG clearance can also be performed, offering potentially improved accuracy, by measurement of the area under the clearance curve (Fig. 2.4). In some centres, ICG clearance is routinely performed during preoperative work-up, with cut-off values set for which patients are 'safe' to proceed to resection. However, there is no evidence to suggest that outcomes are improved in centres that use this test compared with centres that do not. In chronic liver disease, the discriminative ability of ICG clearance is greatest in those with intermediate to severe liver failure. Addition of this test to the MELD score can improve prognostic accuracy for patients with intermediate to severe liver dysfunction.[17] However, given the relationship with hepatic blood flow, caution should be exercised when interpreting ICG clearance in the context of abnormally high cardiac output.

## HEPATOBILIARY SCINTIGRAPHY AND SINGLE-PHOTON EMISSION COMPUTED TOMOGRAPHY

Using a radiolabelled tracer that is eliminated exclusively by the liver, such as [$^{99m}$Tc]mebrofenin (technetium is a gamma-emitting radioisotope), blood clearance and hepatic uptake can be measured using a gamma camera to provide an indication of hepatic function (Fig. 2.5). Hepatobiliary scintigraphy may improve predictive value compared to future liver remnant volume, especially in patients with uncertain quality of liver parenchyma.[18] Combining nuclear medicine techniques with CT (single-photon emission computed tomography [SPECT]) enables the generation of a 3D image of liver function which can be related to liver volume. Using this technique, segmental liver function and liver functional volume can be calculated.

In 2010, de Graaf et al.[19] demonstrated that by combining CT with [$^{99m}$Tc]mebrofenin SPECT, the function of the

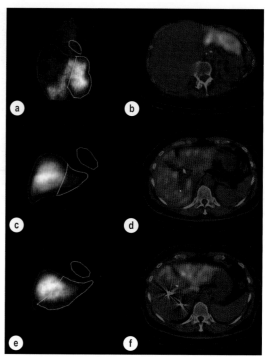

**Figure 2.5** Hepatobiliary scintigraphy before major liver surgery in a patient with a large hepatocellular carcinoma of the right liver **(a, b)** and a patient with a Klatskin type IIIa tumour before **(c, d)** and 3 weeks after portal vein embolisation (PVE) **(e, f)**. Panels a and b show a large afunctional right-sided hepatic mass with sufficient future liver remnant function in segments 2–3. Panels c and d show relatively small liver segments 2–3 with insufficient future liver remnant function (1%/min/m$^2$). Volume and function of segments 2–3 increased significantly after PVE (panels e and f) with sufficient future liver remnant function (2.7%/min/m$^2$) for safe resection (extended right hemihepatectomy). (Images courtesy of R. Bennink, Amsterdam Medical Centre, Netherlands.)

proposed future liver remnant can be accurately obtained. This group, based at the Amsterdam Medical Centre, subsequently demonstrated that routine implementation of this technique for patients requiring major liver resection significantly reduced postoperative liver failure and failure-related mortality.[20] The authors reported that a better understanding of preoperative liver function improved patient selection and led to an increased use of portal vein embolisation (PVE) to optimise the future liver remnant.

✓✓ Combining CT with nuclear medicine techniques enables regional liver function to be calculated and can be used to assess preoperative function.[19,20]

## LIDOCAINE

Lidocaine, also known as monoethylglycinexylidide (MEG-X), is a local anaesthetic that is taken up by the liver and undergoes biotransformation by a cytochrome P450 enzyme, CYP1A2. The rate of disappearance of lidocaine from plasma correlates with liver function; however, measurement of lidocaine is more complex than that of ICG.

## AMINOPYRINE BREATH TEST

The aminopyrine breath test was the first breath test proposed for the assessment of liver function in patients with liver disease. The test uses $^{13}C_2$-aminopyrine, which is a stable, non-radioactive, isotopically labelled compound eliminated almost exclusively by the liver. Following oral intake, the compound is taken up by the gut and then transported to the liver, where it is metabolised by microsomal cytochrome P450 function. This metabolism liberates $13CO_2$, which can be measured non-invasively in exhaled air. This test is not readily available at the bedside and requires fairly sophisticated apparatus to measure stable isotopic enrichment in the exhaled air. Induction of microsomal metabolism by various drugs may constitute a problem.

## UREA SYNTHESIS

Recently, the feasibility of measuring urea synthesis using stable isotopes and relating this to liver volume in patients undergoing liver resection was explored.[21] As liver failure is almost always accompanied by hyperammonaemia, it was hypothesised that this is related to a presumed failure of hepatic urea synthesis. Using stable isotopically $^{13}C$-labelled urea, urea synthesis was measured before and after major hepatic resection, and liver volumes before and after resection were determined using CT.

✓✓ Major hepatic resection did not affect total body ureagenesis, because the synthesis of urea per gram of residual liver increased 2.6-fold.[21] Therefore, it is unlikely that urea synthesis is a limiting factor in the initial aetiology of liver failure and this test is not likely to contribute to predicting liver failure following liver resection.

## GLUTATHIONE SYNTHESIS

Unfortunately, most of the above tests focus on very specific functions or pathways. None of them assesses the main hepatic protection system against many diverse forms of stress and intoxications: the intracellular content and synthesis of glutathione (GSH). It is generally accepted that GSH plays a key role in the protection of the liver against many forms of stress, ischaemia and toxic compounds such as paracetamol. Unfortunately, there is currently no adequate test to assess hepatic GSH synthesis and metabolism in vivo in humans, even though such a test would be of great clinical importance. We have previously explored the feasibility of measuring GSH synthesis in vivo during liver surgery in humans using stable isotopically labelled $^2H_2$-glycine, a component of GSH (γ-glutamyl-cysteinyl-glycine), but this approach was not suitable because part of the deuterium label of glycine was lost (unpublished data). It is possible to measure toxic metabolites of paracetamol (acetaminophen) which are managed by the GSH pathway, such as 5-oxoproline, but these are usually only detectable at extremes of liver injury.[22] Future research will have to focus on designing a test that is both dynamic and focuses on the GSH system, making it possible to determine liver function correlated to liver volume, and assess an individual's risk of developing liver failure following hepatic resection.

## MEASURING LIVER BLOOD FLOW

Blood flow in the splanchnic area, particularly the gut and liver, can be measured in a number of ways. These can basically be either invasive (i.e. intraoperative) or non-invasive. During open abdominal surgery, blood flow can be measured in the portal vein and hepatic artery. Portal vein blood flow measurements provide predominantly information on the flow across the intestines. By summing up the blood flow in the hepatic artery and portal vein, total hepatic blood flow can be calculated. Theoretically, this could also be achieved by measuring hepatic venous outflow, but this is impractical in humans because of the short common outflow tract of the three hepatic veins. Non-invasive MRI-based techniques are being developed that may offer improved accuracy of measurement of liver blood flow and provide the potential for repeat measurements.[23] The ratio of portal vein to hepatic artery blood flow changes with increasing resistance of the liver and may indicate the development of fibrosis or cirrhosis. Methodology for assessing the importance of blood flow as a predictor of liver parenchymal condition has not been fully evaluated, but may provide a means of determining regenerative capacity and safety of surgery in some patients.

Such measurements of hepatic and portal arterial blood flow can be obtained using 6–8 mm and 12–14 mm handle ultrasonic flow probes (Transonic Systems, Kimal PLC, Uxbridge, UK). Essentially, the vessels have to be dissected free for this flow measurement and the three-quarters circular probe is applied to the vessel. These probes are believed to provide the most accurate technique for assessing flow in relatively small vessels. However, there is considerable variability in measurement related to Doppler ultrasound signal strength and coupling with the vessel wall. Also, there are likely to be changes in diameter of the artery, in particular related to its handling during surgery. However, the advantage is that repeated measurements can be obtained and the surgeon can operate this application without help from a radiologist. Furthermore, post-resection blood flow measurements can be taken before closure of the abdomen, typically 1–2 hours after the first measurement. This gives an impression of blood flow across the residual liver following major resection.

During liver surgery, organ blood flow can also be measured by means of colour Doppler ultrasound scanning (e.g. Aloka Prosound SSD 5000; Aloka Co. Ltd, Tokyo, Japan). A 5-MHz probe is used to trace the vessels and calculate the cross-sectional area. Then, time-averaged mean velocities of the bloodstream are measured at the point where the cross-sectional area of the portal vein and hepatic artery have been measured. For accurate velocity measurements, care must be taken to keep the angle between the ultrasonic beam direction and blood flow direction below 60°. If an accessory hepatic artery is present, flow in both arteries should obviously be measured.[24,25] In our experience, this method gives roughly the same values as the ultrasonic flow measurement described above. Theoretically, it is possible to perform such flow measurements preoperatively or postoperatively using a percutaneous approach, although the measurement in the hepatic artery requires a skilled ultrasonographer.

In recent years, technical improvements in hardware and software applications for MRI have made it possible to measure blood flow in the portal vein and hepatic artery non-invasively. By linking this method of flow measurement to hepatic volumetry, blood flow per volume unit of liver can be calculated.[26,27] It has been suggested that MRI may provide a more accurate and reliable assessment of portal vein and hepatic artery blood flow than ultrasonography, particularly given the wide interobserver variability seen with the latter technique.[23] Although limited to the preoperative period, MRI flow studies may provide complementary information to intraoperative ultrasonography.

A further technique that is emerging is the use of near-infrared spectroscopy. This technique measures absorption of near-infrared wavelength light and from this can be calculated tissue oxygenation, since haemoglobin oxygenation status alters absorption of this wavelength light. This technique is more useful for estimating tissue oxygenation and perfusion at a sinusoidal level, but could potentially be combined with other measures to estimate liver blood flow.[28]

## EFFECT OF MAJOR LIVER RESECTION ON HEPATIC BLOOD FLOW

Direct measurement of hepatic artery and portal vein blood flow before and after liver resection reveals interesting results. When expressed as absolute values, portal blood flow does not change significantly whereas hepatic artery blood flow generally falls. Typically, portal vein flow is approximately 840 mL/min and post-resection 805 mL/min, whereas hepatic artery flow pre-resection is approximately 450 mL/min and post-resection 270 mL/min. When these flows are expressed in relation to the preoperative and residual postoperative liver volume, it can be seen that the portal blood flow increases from a mean of 0.55 mL/min per gram of liver to 1.09 mL/min per gram of liver, and the hepatic artery flow remains relatively constant (Fig. 2.6).

In experimental research, pressure measurements can also be obtained using radial artery invasive monitoring to estimate hepatic artery pressure and direct portal vein pressure measurement, using a small needle coupled to a pressure transducer similar to that used for measuring central venous pressure. The combination of flow and pressure measurement then allows calculation of hepatic sinusoidal resistance (Fig. 2.6).

## ASSESSMENT OF INNATE IMMUNITY

The liver forms an important part of the innate immune system by producing acute-phase proteins and other opsonins,

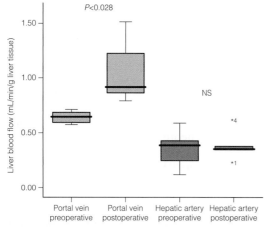

**Figure 2.6**   Directly measured blood flow intraoperatively in six patients during major hepatic resection. Measurements were taken from the main portal vein and the main hepatic artery simultaneously using multichannel Transonics ultrasound flow probes. During the liver resection one branch of each of the portal vein and hepatic artery is ligated. The post-resection blood flow measurement has been taken just before closure of the abdomen, typically 1–2 hours after the first measurement. Results are expressed per gram of liver tissue.

proteins that bind to bacteria facilitating their phagocytosis. In addition, 85% of the reticuloendothelial system is located in the liver (Kupffer cells) and clearly surgical resection will involve a reduction of this cell mass.

It is not unreasonable to expect that major liver resection might result in some impairment of innate immunity. Our group has previously demonstrated that major liver resection is associated with increased frequency of infection as well as increased likelihood of objective evidence of liver function impairment.[2]

In a separate study, our group has also shown that major liver resection is associated with a temporary defect in the ability of the reticuloendothelial system to clear albumin microspheres that were used as a surrogate for bacteria.[29] In a separate but related study, we showed that patients with advanced cirrhosis have a similar defect of innate immunity as patients who have undergone major liver resection and that this defect is more or less immediately corrected by liver transplantation.[30]

✔ Loss of approximately 50% of liver volume, such as that might occur during a right hepatectomy, is associated with impairment of reticuloendothelial cell clearance equivalent to that of non-surgical patients with Child C chronic liver disease.[29,30]

The liver also synthesises and exports many acute-phase proteins involved in innate immunity or homeostasis. C-reactive protein, for example, binds to phosphoryl choline moieties of encapsulated bacteria and acts as an opsonin, promoting phagocytosis. Mannan-binding lectin, complement fragments and $\alpha_1$-acid glycoprotein (orosomucoid) can also act as opsonins. Transferrin and caeruloplasmin are important in the binding and carriage of free metal ions and $\alpha_1$-antitrypsin and $\alpha_1$-antichymotrypsin act as antiproteases. Liver failure or liver surgery may be associated with a reduction in synthesis of some of these acute-phase proteins (mannan-binding lectin, haptoglobin, $\alpha$-fetuin and fibronectin), whereas the concentrations of others may be increased despite a reduction in functional liver tissue (C-reactive protein, liver fatty acid-binding protein; unpublished data). The exact significance of these changes is unclear but may contribute to a global impairment in innate immunity in the injured liver.

## LIVER REGENERATION

The liver is unique in that it is the only organ in the adult that is capable of regenerating or renewing itself to restore the ratio between pre-injury liver volume and body weight. Knowledge of the capacity for the liver to regenerate is presumed to be ancient and is the basis for the punishment meted out by Zeus to Prometheus, who according to Greek mythology was chained to a rock and had his liver eaten daily by an eagle, only for it to regenerate overnight. This continued for several years until the eagle was finally killed by Hercules, who also released Prometheus. While the speed of liver regeneration is exaggerated in this myth, it is true that it is an extremely rapid process. In the context of surgery, liver regeneration happens very rapidly, with most of the cell division required for regeneration occurring within 72 hours of injury in mice. Full liver function and volume are usually restored within 6–12 weeks in humans. In chronic injury or in the presence of fibrosis, liver regeneration can be chaotic with repeated insults causing scarring, and nodular regeneration with disordered architecture leading to cirrhosis.

## MOLECULAR SIGNALS FOR HEPATIC REGENERATION

At a cellular level, liver regeneration depends on the coexistence of three key factors: changes in the microenvironment of the liver cell supporting growth, the ability of differentiated hepatocytes to proliferate and inhibition of processes, linking injury to programmed cell death.

Stimuli for liver regeneration stimulate transcription factors that turn on a variety of genes expressing growth factors. Although not direct growth factors, the hormones insulin and adrenaline potentiate the effects of growth factors on hepatocyte regeneration. All elements of the liver are required to regenerate; however, the coordination of these processes is complex. Removal of the stimulus for regeneration by growth to pre-injury capacity and transforming growth factor-β act as brakes that slow regeneration of liver elements (Fig. 2.7). Barriers to hepatic regeneration include cirrhosis and fibrosis and ongoing liver injury such as might occur with biliary obstruction or sepsis.

## CELL POPULATIONS INVOLVED IN LIVER REGENERATION

Histology of normal liver regeneration following resection or acute injury shows the presence of high mitotic rates in mature hepatocytes. Normally, these cells are mitotically quiescent but can move into S phase extremely rapidly. For example, following 70% hepatectomy in rat, approximately 30–40% of hepatocytes are seen to be undergoing mitosis within 48 hours of surgery and the liver will regain its normal size within 10 days. The situation is more complex in chronically injured liver (e.g. cirrhotic liver); here, the hepatocytes are less able to undergo mitosis and are frequently in cell cycle arrest. Furthermore, the accumulation of excess

scar tissue deposited in cirrhosis contributes to the inability of the liver to respond to injury and regenerate effectively. In this setting, a second population of cells becomes activated and may contribute to parenchymal regeneration. These intrahepatic cells are located in the canal of Hering (the most distal branch of the biliary tree); termed hepatic progenitor cells (HPCs), they are bipotential and are capable of giving rise to both biliary and hepatocyte populations under the influence of macrophage-derived factors.[31] This response is seen in chronic or severe injury and sometimes appears as a ductular reaction. It is also worth noting that there is an increasing recognition that intrahepatic stem cells are a likely source of a significant proportion of liver cancers. The role of circulating extrahepatic cells in liver regeneration has received interest recently and the potential bone marrow (BM) origin of hepatocytes has been suggested. However, if this phenomenon occurs at all, it is extremely rare. The BM does, however, supply macrophages and myofibroblasts that are involved in the liver's scarring response to injury. The relationship between BM-derived cells and the response to injury is complex, with different macrophage subtypes shown to either promote fibrosis or repair. However, administration of BM-derived macrophages to the fibrotic liver via the portal vein has been shown to reduce fibrosis and improve markers of regeneration in preclinical models.[32] The use of BM populations to stimulate liver regeneration in both animal models and clinical studies is likely to be an area of future development (see later).

## CONSEQUENCES OF SURGERY

Unfortunately, at present it is unclear what the key mechanisms of liver failure are, and why the liver usually regenerates but sometimes progresses into liver failure. It is believed that I/R injury plays an important role in the sequence of events leading to liver failure. Hepatic resections are major

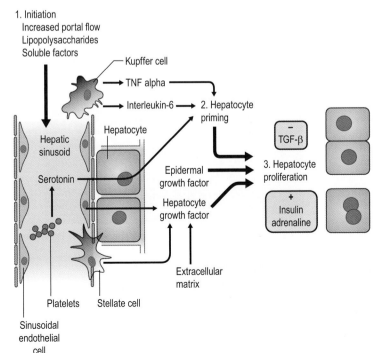

**Figure 2.7** Schematic of some of the factors known to regulate liver regeneration.

surgical procedures, often leading to significant blood loss. In order to reduce blood loss, central venous pressure is reduced during liver surgery and hepatobiliary surgeons frequently occlude hepatic blood inflow temporarily (Pringle manoeuvre). Obviously, all these factors may contribute to an I/R injury in the liver. A key component of I/R injury is the generation of oxygen free radicals. The latter can induce ischaemic necrosis and caspase-dependent apoptosis, and may contribute to failure of vital metabolic synthetic pathways. However, it remains to be investigated which one of these plays a key role during liver failure. In this context, it has been proposed that the balance between hepatocyte regeneration and apoptosis can be tipped towards either side by hepatic defence mechanisms against oxygen free radical damage. Also, oxygen free radicals play a role in determining whether apoptosis or ischaemic necrosis occurs in the liver. Apparently, the equilibrium between oxygen free radicals and their scavengers plays a pivotal role in determining whether regeneration or decay occurs. GSH is the principal oxygen free radical scavenger in the liver and the principal defence mechanism against I/R damage. Hepatic GSH levels decrease following I/R damage, inflammation and nutritional deprivation. It seems conceivable that a reduction in liver volume following surgery contributes to insufficient hepatic free radical scavenging capacity as a consequence of reduced GSH synthesis. I/R injury may aggravate this situation.

## SMALL-FOR-SIZE SYNDROME

The original descriptions of small-for-size syndrome described a condition arising in split liver transplantation characterised by the development of ascites, portal hypertension and liver dysfunction in an otherwise healthy transplanted portion of liver. The underlying cause for this syndrome is believed to relate to blood flow and the failure of a small liver volume to cope with often very high blood flows in patients with previous chronic liver disease undergoing transplantation. The validity of this hypothesis was supported by the observation that partial diversion of portal blood flow into the graft using a portocaval shunt could limit or prevent the development of small-for-size syndrome. Subsequently, other manoeuvres have also been affected, such as ligation or embolisation of the splenic artery, which works in the same way by reducing portal vein flow.

In patients undergoing even very major liver resection, it is rare to develop small-for-size syndrome. Some patients do, however, develop ascites, jaundice and chronic liver dysfunction, and it is more likely that this syndrome is more dependent on a failure to regenerate than on excessive blood flow.

## HEPATIC STEATOSIS

Fat infiltration of the liver is an increasing problem with increased prevalence of obesity and the metabolic syndrome (obesity and type 2 diabetes). Macroscopically the liver may appear enlarged, pale or yellow-coloured with rounded edges. Microscopically the liver can have microsteatosis (small fat droplets within every hepatocyte) or macrosteatosis (regional infiltration of hepatocytes with large fat droplets) (Fig. 2.8).

### ASSESSMENT OF STEATOSIS

Assessment of hepatic steatosis is notoriously difficult. Experienced surgeons can estimate liver fat by judging the size, whether the edges of the liver are rounded or sharp, and its general appearance. Even using colour as an estimate is prone to error, as can be seen in Fig. 2.9.

The gold standard for hepatic fat assessment is histology. Trucut or wedge biopsies can be assessed by a pathologist and a reliable estimate of the percentage fat content produced. In addition, useful information including the distribution—macrosteatosis or microsteatosis—and the presence of fibrosis or inflammation can be provided. New MRI techniques are, however, challenging the accuracy of pathological assessment of steatosis and offer the potential advantage of being non-invasive.[33]

## CHEMOTHERAPY-INDUCED LIVER CHANGES

Increased usage of neoadjuvant chemotherapy, particularly oxaliplatin and irinotecan, has resulted in liver changes. These range from a soft, fragile pale liver to steatosis, steatohepatitis and sinusoidal dilatation. Surgery should be deferred until 6 weeks after chemotherapy and studies, although conflicting, suggest that tolerance of major liver resection may be reduced and complications more frequent in individuals who have received chemotherapy. A study by Mehta et al.[34] showed that oxaliplatin-based chemotherapy was associated with increased blood loss and prolonged hospital stay.

## PORTAL VEIN EMBOLISATION

Morbidity and mortality after hepatectomy have constituted a limitation on the number of patients eligible for resection, and currently only 8% of patients with colorectal liver

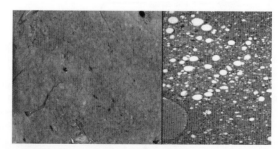

**Figure 2.8** Macroscopic and microscopic images of steatotic liver.

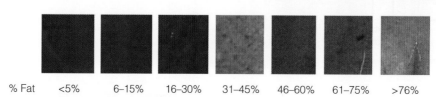

| % Fat | <5% | 6–15% | 16–30% | 31–45% | 46–60% | 61–75% | >76% |

**Figure 2.9** Physical appearance of livers with varying fat content confirmed by histology to demonstrate the poor correlation between colour and objective measurement of fat content.

metastases are candidates for curative hepatic resection. Liver function is correlated with liver volume, and consequently hepatic insufficiency in this situation may arise because not enough functional liver volume is left after surgical removal of part of the liver. As noted above, removal of part of the liver induces the residual liver regenerating to the point where the preoperative liver weight to body weight ratio is regained. This notion led to the belief that if it were possible to increase preoperatively the volume of the future residual liver, it would be possible to perform more extensive liver resections and more patients would be eligible for hepatic resection. It has long been recognised that interruption of one part of the liver portal blood flow usually leads to hypertrophy of normally vascularised liver. This has been observed in patients with Klatskin tumours, which have a tendency to invade the portal vein, causing ipsilateral atrophy and contralateral hypertrophy. This concept has subsequently been harnessed by manoeuvres such as PVE. Embolising the right portal vein prior to surgical resection leads to hypertrophy of the left liver lobe and facilitates the subsequent safe extensive resection of the right liver (extended right hepatectomy) 6 weeks later (Fig. 2.10). This phenomenon has been harnessed to maximise the residual functional liver volume of patients who are predicted to have a small remnant liver

volume. This approach is fully based on the concept that, in the normal liver, volume is correlated with function and hence liver failure occurs when residual liver volume is too small. A completely different and novel approach would be to improve liver function per volume unit of liver. Recent evidence from studies using mebrofenin suggests that functional improvement of the future liver remnant following PVE may precede changes in liver volume.[35] This important observation suggests that surgery earlier after PVE may be possible. Limitations to PVE-induced hypertrophy include pre-existing hepatic fibrosis or cirrhosis and technical or anatomical inability to completely obstruct a major portal vein branch. Despite the often marked increase in future liver remnant volume following PVE, sufficient future liver remnant volume may still not be reached. Other techniques can be used, however, in an attempt to further enhance future liver remnant growth.

### TECHNIQUE

The most common technique of PVE is to puncture a branch of the vein using a percutaneous approach. A venogram is obtained to demonstrate all of the relevant branches. The branch to be embolised is subsequently cannulated and coils and embolic material delivered to obstruct portal flow. A check angiogram can be performed to demonstrate success of the technique. Usually either a left or right main branch is occluded. To obtain hypertrophy of segments 2 and 3 in large right-sided tumours, it is not sufficient to embolise just the right portal vein and it is recommended that the branches supplying segment 4 should also be embolised. Patients usually tolerate PVE remarkably well, presumably because of the dual blood supply of the liver, and complications are uncommon. Significant hypertrophy can be achieved, as can be seen in Fig. 2.11.

### COMBINED PORTAL VEIN AND HEPATIC VEIN EMBOLISATION

In cases where portal vein embolization alone has either been ineffective in generating sufficient future liver

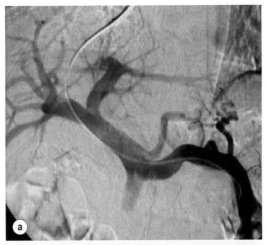
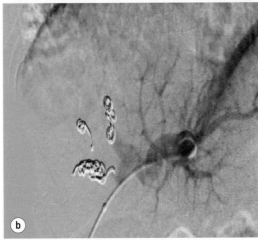

**Figure 2.10** Portal venograms showing the main left and right branches prior to embolisation **(a)** and after embolisation of the right portal vein **(b)**.

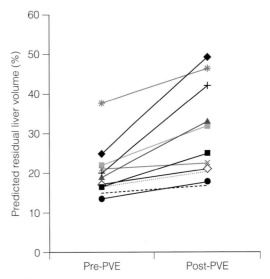

**Figure 2.11** Calculated residual liver volumes before and after portal vein embolisation (PVE) in patients scheduled to undergo major liver resection.

remnant growth or where PVE is predicted to be insufficient, the hepatic veins draining the part of the liver to be resected can also be embolized (hepatic vein embolisation [HVE]). This combination of PVE and HVE aims to completely deprive the future liver remnant of blood flow and can lead to more rapid and pronounced future liver remnant growth.[36] This technique is also known as liver venous deprivation. A recent case-controlled study showed that future liver remnant growth was significantly greater with the combined PVE/HVE technique (60% increase versus 30% with PVE alone).[37]

While PVE is performed by a transhepatic percutaneous approach, HVE is performed via either a transjugular or transhepatic approach.[38] A vascular plug, glue or coils are used to occlude the hepatic vein. Histology of the occluded portion of liver has demonstrated hepatocyte atrophy and necrosis.[37]

## ASSOCIATING LIVER PARTITION AND PORTAL VEIN LIGATION FOR STAGED HEPATECTOMY (ALPPS PROCEDURE)

This technique, first described in 2011, aims to enable surgery with curative intent in patients who would otherwise be unsuitable for liver resection due to insufficient future liver remnant volume and in whom PVE is not possible or did not achieve sufficient hypertrophy.[39] The technique involves two distinct stages. The first stage involves division of the liver along the line of proposed resection (between segment 2/3 and segment 4) and ligation of the portal blood supply to liver segments 4–8. Segments 4–8 retain both arterial blood supply and biliary drainage, thereby enabling these de-portalised liver segments to provide auxiliary support to the future liver remnant (segments 2/3) while they undergo a process of hypertrophy and hyperplasia. Tumours within segments 2/3 can also be removed at this stage. On completion of the first stage, the future liver remnant enlarges rapidly over several weeks. This initial growth is at least in part related to the change in haemodynamics, with greater blood flow through the future liver remnant. Increase in size should not necessarily therefore be interpreted as improved liver function.[40] When the future liver remnant (segment 2/3) has enlarged sufficiently (1–2 weeks), the right side (segments 4–8 + 1) is then removed. Early attempts were plagued by complications, including bleeding and liver failure with high mortality rates. However, there are patients who may benefit from this approach. It has become clear that identifying the most appropriate candidates, ensuring sufficient enlargement and function of the future liver remnant and further refinement of the technique are crucial to successful outcomes. It remains to be seen whether the percutaneous approach of combined PVE/HVE can lead to similar growth rates and an improved safety profile when compared with the ALPPS procedure.

## SUPPORTING THE FAILING LIVER

### N-ACETYL CYSTEINE

GSH depletion is a major problem in patients with paracetamol (acetaminophen) toxicity. N-acetyl cysteine has been used for many years as a treatment for early paracetamol poisoning. It is thought to act by replenishing GSH stores and by providing alternative thiol groups to which damaging reactive oxygen species can bind. The realisation that reactive oxygen species can be generated by conditions other than paracetamol poisoning such as sepsis and I/R has led to N-acetyl cysteine being used in a more general way to support patients with early evidence of liver dysfunction or failure.

## NUTRITIONAL SUPPORT IN LIVER FAILURE

The role of nutritional support in acute liver failure is uncertain, largely because of a lack of evidence in the literature. Enteral nutrition is known to preserve gut barrier function and thus might be considered to be beneficial in the context of liver failure. In addition, the provision of energy might be considered beneficial in the context of glycogen storage failure, and to fuel the regeneration of liver tissue and recover function. The limited ability of the failing liver to handle nitrogen and synthesise urea (potentially exacerbating encephalopathy) would argue against excessive provision of proteins unless these were in a form where they did not contribute to the circulating ammonia load.

## EXTRACORPOREAL LIVER SUPPORT

For the vast majority of patients who take toxic doses of paracetamol, suffer alcohol-induced liver injury or develop liver dysfunction following liver resection, the regenerative capacity of the liver is sufficient to prevent irretrievable liver failure and death. However, when this regenerative capacity is overwhelmed, treatment strategies to temporarily or permanently replace the failing liver are required. The ability to provide short-term extracorporeal liver support, either during the wait for transplantation or to facilitate liver regeneration and avoid transplantation, is an attractive option. A range of devices have been developed, either focusing on the detoxification functions of liver (artificial liver support) or also incorporating bioreactors intended to perform synthetic liver functions (bioartificial liver support). Assessment of efficacy has been hampered by the limited number of randomised controlled trials and small sample size, but a recent meta-analysis does suggest overall survival benefit in acute liver failure.[41]

### ARTIFICIAL LIVER SUPPORT

Artificial systems include the Molecular Adsorbent Recirculating System (MARS) device, Prometheus and the BioLogic-DT (now called the Liver Dialysis Device, currently being redesigned). The greatest experience has been with the MARS device, which deploys an albumin dialysis circuit to remove both water-soluble and protein-bound toxins.[42] Thus, a low Fischer ratio can be corrected by recirculating albumin dialysis.[43] Because the system preferentially removes AAAs, compared with BCAAs, the Fischer ratio significantly increases, predominantly by the removal of AAAs in a small series of patients.[43–46] MARS has been shown to be useful in fulminant hepatic failure, by attenuating the increase in intracranial pressure, which plays a major role in this situation. There may also be an effect on survival and an improvement of hepatic encephalopathy in patients with acute or chronic liver failure.[43,46] Equally, the system has been tested on artificial neuronal networks showing a normalisation of abnormal signals if the medium (plasma derived from rats with liver failure) was pre-treated with MARS. The role of MARS in a more chronic situation of mild hepatic encephalopathy, when correction of an abnormal Fischer ratio would likely be more important if this were a major pathogenetic factor, is still largely unknown and deserves further study.[47] It has been suggested that the role of MARS and bioartificial liver support systems should be limited to carefully designed clinical trials.[48] It is currently uncertain how hepatic excretory assistance devices, such as MARS, compare with bioartificial liver assistance devices, which in addition to their excretory functions aim to provide biosynthetic capacity.[49]

## BIOARTIFICIAL LIVER SYSTEMS

Bioartificial systems incorporate a bioreactor containing either human hepatoblastoma cell lines (e.g. the HepatAssist device) or porcine hepatocytes (e.g. the ELAD—Extracorporeal Liver Assist Device), through which the patient's blood is perfused. An additional filter component may be included to aid detoxification and improve bioreactor survival.

One of the major problems with these systems is what type of cells to use, and a variety of different approaches have been taken. Animal hepatocytes perform many of the same functions as human hepatocytes, although some of the proteins produced are obviously different. Human immortalised cell lines are an attractive proposition and some of the more differentiated cell lines can replicate many of the normal hepatocyte functions. Regardless, the true functionality of these cells in the clinical setting is uncertain. The design of bioartificial liver systems is challenging and the large surface area of hepatocytes needed to be effective is difficult. Engineering scaffolds of membranes or tubules has been the most popular approach. In normal liver, hepatocytes are polarised and have an epithelial surface. However, it is still to be determined how to recreate this polarity and its absolute importance has yet to be defined. Hepatocytes proliferate and function better in association with non-parenchymal cells; however, the creation of co-cultures in reactors produces its own problems. Cells must maintain viability or be able to be replenished to provide liver support over a prolonged period of time. In addition, very sick patients require a short time period to set up the support system, and the reactor must be easy to use by critical care nurses, safe from contamination and not overly expensive. For all of these reasons, bioartificial liver systems remain a tantalising prospect that has yet to break through into routine clinical practice.

## LIVER TRANSPLANTATION

Irreversible acute or chronic liver failure is amenable to treatment by liver transplantation. It is extremely uncommon for patients who have undergone liver resection to subsequently require or proceed to liver transplantation. Although rare, the limited evidence available suggests that this is a good indication for liver transplantation with the ability to rescue patients with acutely deteriorating liver function.[50] While liver transplantation is routinely performed for hepatocellular carcinoma and in some centres selected patients with cholangiocarcinoma or colorectal liver metastasis, a patient undergoing partial hepatectomy will not have undergone the required assessment process for transplantation. In unselected cancer patients, outcomes are typically poor following transplantation, owing to aggressive recurrence in the context of immunosuppression. A number of patients with bile duct injury have progressed to transplantation, usually in a chronic setting following the development of biliary stricture, cholangitis and secondary biliary cirrhosis. Similarly, a number of patients who have undergone a 'cancer resection' for what turned out to be a benign biliary stricture, perhaps due to primary sclerosing cholangitis, fail to regenerate their livers and may progress to transplantation.

## CELL THERAPY IN LIVER DISEASE

A number of key principles have operated as key drivers for the development of cell therapies for clinical treatment of liver failure. Firstly, it is recognised that the injured liver usually provides a rich environment stimulating tissue regeneration and the liver can normally 'heal' itself. Secondly, in animal models there is evidence that stem cells or nonparenchymal cells can support regeneration of hepatocytes. Thirdly, it is recognised that the difference between liver failure and compensated liver function in terms of cellular functional equivalents is probably very small. Finally, it would be preferable to support the liver by techniques that are within the body rather than using extracorporeal devices. This desire has stimulated research into therapeutic application of cell or stem cell transplantation.

The dual goals of stem cell therapy in the context of acute liver failure or injury are to promote rapid recovery of hepatocyte function and to allow regeneration of liver tissue without excessive scarring. Direct administration of hepatocytes or stem cell-derived hepatocytes to the injured liver has been met with little success in preclinical studies. However, BM-derived cells to enhance endogenous processes may support the regenerating liver, enabling effective regeneration.[51] A first in human study of autologous macrophage therapy has recently been completed in patients with chronic liver disease, demonstrating safety and feasibility of the approach.[52]

## HAEMOPOIETIC STEM CELL THERAPY FOR LIVER DISEASE IN HUMANS

There are several reports in the scientific literature of BM stem cell therapy in patients with advanced liver disease. It was first reported that BM stem cells could increase the liver's ability to regenerate in patients who were undergoing hepatic resection for various liver cancers sited in the right lobe. Here the patients underwent embolisation of the right branch of the portal vein prior to surgery to stimulate compensatory hypertrophy of the left lobe. Autologous CD133-positive BM stem cells were injected into the blood vessels that supply the left liver lobe shortly after the surgery and accelerated regeneration of the non-embolised section of the liver was seen compared with control patients.[53] The second report used BM stem cells in patients with liver cirrhosis.[54] CD34-positive stem cells were isolated from the patients' own blood following granulocyte colony-stimulating factor (GCSF)-induced haematopoietic stem cell mobilisation and were re-injected into the blood supply to the liver—preliminary results appeared to show improvement in liver function in three out of five of the patients. In the third study, patients with liver cirrhosis had mononuclear cells isolated from their own BM during general anaesthesia.[55] These cells were re-injected into the patient's bloodstream and again the patient's liver function appeared to improve. Although these studies are very encouraging, they are preliminary, of small numbers and non-randomised. Furthermore, in none of these studies were the cells marked to enable identification either by radiological tracking or in subsequent biopsies of the liver tissue. Therefore, a number of important questions are unanswered. It is not certain that these cells definitely settled in the liver over a period of time, whether some of the cells engrafted other organs in the body and by what mechanisms the cells were having their positive effects within the recipient livers. The potential benefits of this approach have yet to be seen in randomized controlled trials.

## FUTURE DEVELOPMENTS

The ability to exert greater control in modulating liver volume and function in the surgical patient would be a major advantage. Preoperative functional enhancement might expand the group of patients who would be amenable to surgery, while postoperative intervention might be useful in liver resection, transplantation and acute liver failure as a means of rescuing a failing liver. The potential to use autologous stem cells derived from BM to stimulate liver regeneration is enormous if its positive effects are seen in larger randomised studies.

## Key points

- Conventional measures of liver function are poor and take no account of liver volume.
- Liver resection leaving a residual liver volume of < 25% is associated with a high risk of liver dysfunction and infection.
- In patients with chronic liver disease, smaller resections can be dangerous.
- The combination of liver dysfunction and sepsis can be fatal.
- Preoperative portal vein embolisation and newer regenerative strategies may improve the safety of liver surgery.

 References available at http://ebooks.health.elsevier.com/

## KEY REFERENCES

[2] Schindl MJ, Redhead DN, Fearon KC, et al. The value of residual liver volume as a predictor of hepatic dysfunction and infection after major liver resection. Gut 2005;54:289–96. PMID: 15647196.
  *The first paper providing strong evidence of an association between residual liver volume and clinical infection.*

[6] Clavien PA, Yadav S, Sindram D, et al. Protective effects of ischemic preconditioning for liver resection performed under inflow occlusion in humans. Ann Surg 2000;232:155–62. PMID: 10903590.
  *The first randomised clinical trial demonstrating benefit in clinical markers from ischaemic preconditioning of the liver in patients undergoing liver resection.*

[21] van de Poll MC, Wigmore SJ, Redhead DN, et al. Effect of major liver resection on hepatic ureagenesis in humans. Am J Physiol Gastrointest Liver Physiol 2007;293:G956–62. PMID: 17717046.
  *Clinical experimental study demonstrating the relationship between liver volume and urea synthesis in patients undergoing varying degrees of liver resection.*

# Perioperative care for hepato-pancreato-biliary surgery

**3**

Helen M.E. Usher | Elizabeth M.E. Cole

## INTRODUCTION

Hepato-pancreato-biliary (HPB) surgery can present many challenges during the perioperative period. With an ageing population, there are increasing numbers of patients with significant comorbid conditions presenting for surgery. Although patient outcomes have improved with a number of advances in perioperative technique, there remains significant morbidity and mortality associated with major HPB surgical procedures.[1] As a result, it is essential to ensure thorough preoperative assessment of patients, optimisation of medical conditions and consideration of multimodal prehabilitation interventions. These measures may not be possible for all, particularly in the emergency setting; however, the involvement of a multidisciplinary team (MDT) from the point of diagnosis can optimise the patient's perioperative journey.[2] In addition, adherence to Enhanced Recovery After Surgery (ERAS) programmes has been shown to reduce morbidity, length of hospital stay and cost in a number of surgical settings.[3–5]

### INTRODUCTION TO PERIOPERATIVE MEDICINE

Perioperative medicine is a cross-specialty collaboration focussed on the patient experience from the preoperative period until their discharge home and full recovery. In addition to improving the overall patient experience, good perioperative care can reduce complication rates, average length of hospital stay, mortality, readmission rates and per capita cost.[6]

Evidence-based protocols as part of ERAS pathways are now widely used across a variety of surgical specialties, including liver and pancreatic surgery.[3,4] They aim to achieve earlier recovery by optimising preoperative physiological function, reducing the surgical stress response and facilitating postoperative recovery. Evidence for ERAS in patients with cirrhosis or obstructive jaundice is still fairly limited.

Focus on the preoperative period has become increasingly important for the surgeon and anaesthetist, with an aim to identify those at particular increased risk for significant perioperative morbidity or even mortality.

### PREOPERATIVE PERIOD

Patient engagement is a vital part of the perioperative journey and starts with the first encounter. 'Making Every Contact Count' is a national approach to use the multitude of interactions patients have with the healthcare team to encourage positive change in their physical and mental health and wellbeing.[7] It is important to put patients at the centre of their care and by gaining their confidence, it is hoped they will improve engagement with prehabilitation and preparation for both their operation and the recovery period.

## RISK STRATIFICATION

Preoperative risk scoring systems and risk prediction models can be used in both the elective and emergency settings to estimate adverse postoperative outcomes. These figures can then be used to guide discussions both within the MDT and with the patient to make more meaningful and informed decisions about the proposed procedure.

Child–Pugh scoring was developed in the 1960s to predict mortality in patients with cirrhosis undergoing portosystemic shunts and is still used today as a broad measure of perioperative risk in patients with liver failure.[8] The Child–Pugh score was further developed for use in liver transplantation but has since been replaced with the Model for End-stage Liver Disease (MELD) or United Kingdom Model for End-Stage Liver Disease (UKELD) score, which includes a wider range of variables.[9,10]

The National Surgical Quality Improvement Program (NSQIP) collects data on morbidity and mortality based on 135 clinical variables for patients undergoing major surgical procedures from the preoperative period to 30 days postoperatively.[11] The data from this large-scale audit has led to the development of the surgical risk calculator, which predicts outcomes based on the proposed surgery and individual patient risk factors. Other perioperative scoring systems used are the ASA (American Society of Anaesthesiology) score, P-POSSUM (Portsmouth Physiological and Operative Severity Score for the enumeration of Morbidity and Mortality) and SORT (Surgical Outcome Risk Tool). These vary in complexity, although the rise in app-based technology makes the majority of these scores quick and easy to calculate.

Risk is also evaluated in the preoperative assessment clinic using a range of techniques designed to determine cardiopulmonary reserve. The 6-minute walk test (6MWT) is a simple test which measures the distance patients can walk on a flat surface at normal pace in 6 minutes. In thoracic and major general surgery, the distance was found to be predictive of postoperative complications and length of stay.[12] Cardiopulmonary exercise testing (CPET) provides an objective assessment of exercise capacity and determines where the limitation lies (Fig. 3.1). During graded exercise on a static cycle, CPET records data on oxygen consumption, anaerobic threshold and extrapolates stroke volume. This can be used to differentiate causes of dyspnoea, prognosticate for cardiopulmonary disease and detail the patient's functional status.[13]

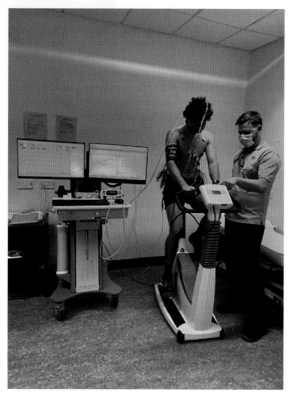

**Figure 3.1**  Cardiopulmonary exercise testing.

Information from all of the above can be used to inform MDT decision-making, direct prehabilitation efforts, guide intraoperative anaesthetic and surgical management and assist in the triage of postoperative care.

## PREOPERATIVE COUNSELLING

Whilst there are no studies specifically evaluating the effect of preoperative counselling before hepato-biliary surgery, there is evidence that managing patient expectations and providing written information increases the patient's engagement with the decision-making process.[14]

The Academy of Medical Royal Colleges host the 'Choosing Wisely' campaign—a global initiative aimed at improving conversations between patients and healthcare staff.[15] The framework encouraged for use by patients in consultations is BRAN:

- What are the **B**enefits?
- What are the **R**isks?
- What are the **A**lternatives?
- What if I do **N**othing?

Following the Montgomery ruling, it is now not only unacceptable but also unlawful to fail to provide patients with adequate information to allow them to make an informed decision and to provide consent for a procedure.[16]

## MULTIDISCIPLINARY TEAM

Shared decision-making is now the cornerstone of patient-centred care. MDT input comprising surgeons, physicians, anaesthetists, oncologists, specialist nurses, physiotherapists and dieticians provides a coordinated approach to the management of the patient and a sharing of expertise. Whilst there is little high-grade evidence to suggest that MDT meetings improve clinical outcomes, they allow discussion of the available options, which may include a non-operative approach such as interventional radiological procedures or chemotherapy. It is imperative that patient's wishes and expectations are known and that these are considered when planning treatment. Health-related quality of life is of greater importance to the individual patient than many of the traditionally used outcome measures, and there is increasing focus on developing validated tools to assess this.

## OPTIMISATION OF COMORBIDITIES AND PREHABILITATION

Major surgery evokes a stress response, the impact of which varies upon the pre-morbid physiological and psychological reserves of the patient. More vulnerable patients will experience greater morbidity, mortality and longer stays in hospital. Increasing efforts are being made to optimise patients before surgery to improve outcomes with a multimodal prehabilitation approach.

### PULMONARY PREHABILITATION

Chronic obstructive pulmonary disease (COPD) is the second most common lung disease in the UK, after asthma, and the prevalence increases with age.[17] Expiratory airflow limitation is the principal pathophysiology, characterised by reduced forced expiratory volume in 1 second (FEV1) and forced vital capacity (FVC). This group of patients are at particular risk for anaesthetic-related complications and postoperative respiratory infections. The British Thoracic Society have long promoted pulmonary rehabilitation as a key management strategy in chronic respiratory disease. Early referral should be made for anyone with COPD for pulmonary rehabilitation to improve symptoms, exercise tolerance, muscle strength and overall health status.[18] Medication should also be reviewed and optimised by the patient's respiratory physician prior to surgery.

### CARDIAC PREHABILITATION

Cardiac prehabilitation programmes have developed due to the increasing prevalence of ischaemic heart disease (IHD). There remains a high mortality associated with IHD despite advances in medical, radiological and surgical techniques. Patients with known IHD are at increased risk of a perioperative myocardial infarction (MI), which can be mitigated with appropriate investigation and intervention. Patients with angina, heart failure or structural heart disease should have surgery delayed where possible to optimise medical therapy and/or undergo interventions such as percutaneous coronary intervention (PCI), coronary artery bypass grafting (CABG) or valve repair/replacement. Cardiac prehabilitation programmes also focus on education, counselling, graduated exercise training and lifestyle modifications such as smoking cessation.[19]

### HYPERTENSION

Hypertension is increasingly common in elective surgical patients and if uncontrolled, it increases the risk of perioperative MI, stroke, bleeding and death. Blood pressure should be optimised prior to elective surgery, with sufficient time to allow autoregulatory mechanisms to reset and promote adequate organ perfusion. ACE inhibitors should be withheld on the day of surgery to prevent exaggerated hypotension during induction of anaesthesia. Beta-blockers, if established, should be continued to prevent rebound tachyarrhythmias and an increase in myocardial oxygen demand.

## ANAEMIA

Anaemia is multifactorial and is common in patients presenting for surgery. Even mild anaemia increases postoperative morbidity and mortality, and is associated with longer hospital stay and increased risk of allogenic blood transfusion. The introduction of Patient Blood Management (PBM) has shifted the focus from the use of blood products to optimisation of the patient.[20] The three pillars of PBM strategies are: 1) improving red cell mass with iron or erythropoietin-stimulating agents; 2) minimising blood loss by optimising surgical and anaesthetic techniques; and 3) optimising patient tolerance of anaemia by improving preoperative cardiopulmonary function. Surgery should be delayed where possible to allow for oral iron supplementation. Increasing numbers of centres have the facility to provide intravenous (IV) iron infusions preoperatively. However, in 2020, a randomised controlled trial (RCT) did not show a clinically significant reduction in blood transfusion following preoperative IV iron therapy.[21]

✓✓ Results of the recent PREVENTT trial did not demonstrate a clinical benefit for preoperative IV iron therapy in patients undergoing major abdominal surgery.[21]

## DIABETES

Diabetes affects nearly 10% of the global population, although it is estimated that a far greater number of people are undiagnosed.[22] Diabetes is a multisystem disease, associated with poor surgical outcomes. Improving glycaemic control and optimising associated complications will protect against further insults.

## FRAILTY

Frailty is gaining increasing recognition in perioperative medicine, although remains difficult to quantify. A number of objective assessment techniques, such as the Clinical Frailty Scale (CFS) or Edmonton Frail Scale (EFS) are widely used, but there is no set of agreed criteria for diagnosing frailty.[23] Increasing awareness of the challenges of frailty have led to the introduction of specific perioperative services such as the Proactive care of Older People undergoing Surgery (POPS) clinics which support individuals who would most benefit from prehabilitation services.

## LIFESTYLE INTERVENTIONS

### SMOKING

Smoking increases the risk of pulmonary and cardiovascular complications, primarily by reducing the availability of oxygen to tissues. Nicotine also stimulates the surgical stress response, increasing blood pressure, heart rate and systemic vascular resistance. Surgically, smoking impairs wound healing and increases the risk of anastomotic leaks.[24] There is evidence that abstinence for approximately 4 weeks reduces both respiratory and wound-healing complications.[25] The use of smoking cessation services and nicotine replacement therapy (NRT) has a twofold benefit by providing the patient a central role in their overall risk management.

✓✓ Smoking cessation for a minimum of 4 weeks prior to surgery has been shown to result in a reduction in respiratory complications and fewer wound-healing complications.[25]

### ALCOHOL

Alcohol consumption is rising globally, and in addition to being a contributing factor in a number of hepatobiliary and pancreatic diseases, it is also associated with a multitude of perioperative complications. It can increase the risk of infection, cardiopulmonary complications and bleeding. Immunosuppression is common amongst those drinking more than three units daily, and there is an increase in the neuroendocrine stress response to surgery.[26,27] Patients should be screened preoperatively for alcohol dependence using tools such as the well-validated FAST tool or the more detailed AUDIT tool.[28] Abstinence from alcohol for 4-8 weeks prior to elective surgery may reduce postoperative complications.[29,30] In the acute setting, patients need to be managed with pabrinex and thiamine supplementation to prevent Wernicke's encephalopathy, and benzodiazepines for withdrawal symptoms following the Clinical Institute Withdrawal Assessment for Alcohol (CIWA) protocol.[31]

### NUTRITION

Nutritional medicine has evolved dramatically over the past two decades, and it is now recognised that preoperative malnutrition, particularly low muscle mass, is an independent predictor of increasing morbidity and mortality.[32] The European Society for Clinical Nutrition and Metabolism (ESPEN) recommend that all surgical patients should have a nutritional risk score (NRS) performed at least 10 days preoperatively.[33] Patients with weight loss in excess of 10% over a 6-month period (or > 5% over 3 months), low body mass index (BMI; < 18.5 kg/m$^2$) or serum albumin less than 30 g/L should be given 7 days of oral supplements.[34] If weight loss is greater than 10%, surgery should be postponed for a minimum of 2 weeks where possible to allow adequate nutritional input, either enterally or parentally if indicated.

Conversely, obesity has now become a global epidemic, with over 4 million deaths annually as a result of being overweight or obese.[35] Defined as a BMI ≥ 30, obesity is a multisystem disease causing a wide range of perioperative complications. Weight loss should be encouraged and supported preoperatively to improve both operating conditions for the surgical team and to prevent or treat comorbidities that make anaesthesia increasingly challenging. Preoperative continuous positive airway pressure (CPAP) can help to reduce complications related to obstructive sleep apnoea, including by lowering blood pressure.[36] Weight loss either by calorie restriction or intragastric balloon has been reported to reduce liver bulk by 14% and 32%, respectively, thereby improving surgical access.[37] The Obesity Surgery

Mortality Risk Score (OS-MRS) predicts death in obese patients and can be used to determine both intraoperative risk and postoperative destination.[38]

## MEDICATION MANAGEMENT

### ANTICOAGULANTS

Long-term oral anticoagulation is increasingly prevalent for both primary and secondary prophylaxis. The British Committee of Standards for Haematology have published detailed guidelines for the perioperative management of anticoagulation and antiplatelet therapy, which should be used in conjunction with local haematology and cardiology advice.[39] The main factors to consider are if and when drugs should be discontinued, how to manage a patient who is fully anticoagulated, and when to restart agents postoperatively.

### WARFARIN

Warfarin is a vitamin K antagonist and should be withheld 5 days prior to elective surgery. The international normalised ratio (INR) should be less than 1.5 prior to surgery. If haemostasis is satisfactory, warfarin can be restarted at the normal maintenance dose the evening of surgery, or the next day. If the risk of thrombosis is high, bridging therapy with low molecular weight (LMWH) or unfractionated heparin (UFH) may be required. LMWH should be stopped at least 24 hours prior to surgery. In the emergency setting, warfarin should be reversed with IV vitamin K, prothrombin concentrate and fresh frozen plasma (FFP).

### DIRECT ORAL ANTICOAGULANTS

The management of direct oral anticoagulants (DOACs) depends on the half-life of the agent, taking into account renal dysfunction which may prolong this considerably. There are no widely available monitoring tests for measuring their anticoagulant activity and importantly, no direct antidotes routinely available at present. Renal function (creatinine and estimated glomerular filtration rate [eGFR]) should be measured and the time from the last dose determined. Apixaban and rivaroxaban (factor Xa inhibitors) should be withheld for 24 hours prior to low bleeding risk procedures or 48 hours prior to high bleeding risk surgery or neuraxial anaesthesia, and for 72 hours if the eGFR is < 30 ml/min/1.73m$^2$. Dabigatran (a direct thrombin inhibitor) should be withheld for 48 hours, or for 96 hours if eGFR is < 50 ml/min/1.73m$^2$. Surgery should be delayed where possible to allow one half-life from the most recent dose to pass. Prothrombin concentrate may be used if more urgent reversal is required and tranexamic acid can be considered. DOACs have good oral absorption and reach peak activity within a few hours; therefore, restarting should be within 24 hours if there is a low bleeding risk and no epidural catheter, or 48–72 hours if there is a high bleeding risk and an epidural catheter has been removed.

### ANTIPLATELET AGENTS

Aspirin should be continued for most invasive procedures and neuroaxial anaesthesia unless there is a perceived high bleeding risk. Clopidogrel is given in combination with aspirin following PCI or in acute coronary syndrome. Dual antiplatelet therapy is recommended for 6 weeks for bare metal stents and 6–12 months for drug-eluting stents. During this time, the risk of thrombosis is high. if the surgery is a low-bleeding risk it can continue without stopping the antiplatelets. If it is high-risk, it should be postponed where possible and if not, clopidogrel should be stopped 7 days prior to surgery. This should always be discussed with the patient's cardiologist. In emergency situations, tranexamic acid should be used and in the case of excessive bleeding, platelets should be administered.

### ORAL HYPOGLYCAEMIC AGENTS AND INSULIN

Diabetes is associated with an increase in perioperative complications, higher mortality and increased length of stay. All patients should have a recent HbA1c and if greater than 69 mmol/mol, patients should be referred to their diabetologist for review. Major surgery, prolonged fasting, poor control and emergency surgery is likely to lead to the use of a variable rate insulin infusion (VRII) for adequate glycaemic control. Short fasting times and minor surgery can be managed by making adjustments to their normal medications. Diabetic agents work either by lowering glucose concentrations (sulphonylureas, meglitinides, insulin) or by preventing it from rising (metformin, GLP-1 analogues, DPP-IV inhibitors). The latter can therefore be continued without risking hypoglycaemia.

## DAY OF SURGERY

Increasingly patients are admitted on the day of surgery having been seen in a preassessment clinic. This has a number of benefits but leaves only a narrow window for identification and management of any unanticipated problems.

## FASTING AND CARBOHYDRATE LOADING

Fasting reduces the risk of aspiration during induction of general anaesthesia.[40] However, modern practice recognises the complications associated with prolonged fasting, including increased nausea and vomiting, symptoms of malaise and anxiety, dehydration and hypovolaemia.[41] Current guidelines recommend fasting for 6 hours for solid food and 2 hours for clear fluid, including black tea or coffee.[42]

Carbohydrate loading is well-established within ERAS protocols, albeit with no demonstrable impact on surgical complications. Patients are prescribed a carbohydrate-rich drink the evening before surgery and 2 hours prior to anaesthesia. This reduces insulin resistance, promoting an anabolic rather than catabolic state. There is some interest that reducing insulin resistance may be beneficial in liver regeneration.[43]

## PREMEDICATION

The routine use of preoperative anxiolytic medication has been declining with increasing numbers of patients being admitted on the day of surgery. Administering preoperative medications with the aim of reducing patient anxiety in the anaesthetic room can have unwanted effects postoperatively, particularly in elderly patients in whom it may contribute to postoperative cognitive dysfunction. In addition, benzodiazepines rely on hepatic metabolism and can therefore have a prolonged duration of action in patients who develop hepatic insufficiency following liver resection. An alternative approach has been to provide consistent preoperative information with a clear explanation of the planned procedure.[3]

A small dose of an IV short-acting agent can then be used in the anaesthetic room to facilitate regional anaesthesia if required.

## VENOUS THROMBOEMBOLISM PROPHYLAXIS

Patients undergoing major hepatobiliary or pancreatic surgical procedures are at increased risk of venous thromboembolism (VTE), which is responsible for significant perioperative morbidity as well as mortality from fatal pulmonary embolism (PE). In addition to the risk factors of malignancy, immobility, prolonged general anaesthetic and transient dehydration, pancreaticoduodenectomy and liver resection procedures are independent risk factors for VTE.[3,4,44–46] In particular, following major liver resection, the thrombotic risk may not be accurately indicated by laboratory measures of coagulation.[46] This has led to a recommendation for antithrombotic prophylaxis to be commenced preoperatively and to continue until hospital discharge at the earliest.[3,4] Risk of bleeding should also be considered, as well as whether neuraxial blockade is to be undertaken as this will affect the timing of administration.

Mechanical prophylaxis in the form of antiembolism stockings and intermittent pneumatic compression devices should be used unless there is a contraindication such as peripheral arterial disease.[3,4]

Pharmacological prophylaxis using LMWH or UFH should be commenced 2–12 hours preoperatively. If neuraxial block is to be undertaken for surgery, administration of prophylactic LMWH should be 12 hours prior to this to reduce the risk of vertebral canal haematoma, which is a rare but a potentially devastating complication.[47]

Thromboprophylaxis should be continued until discharge from hospital, and extended prophylaxis for 28 days may be considered in this setting due to the increased risk factors of malignancy and major abdominal surgery.[48] There is moderate quality evidence from a Cochrane review (updated 2019) which supports prolonged thromboprophylaxis following hospital discharge, with no increase in bleeding complications, which has led to this recommendation in the 2018 NICE guidelines on thromboprophylaxis.[48,49]

✔✔ Continuing LMWH prophylaxis for 28 days following major abdominal or pelvic surgery has been shown to significantly reduce the risk of VTE compared with standard protocols for administration during hospital admission only.[48]

## ANTIBIOTICS AND ANTISEPTIC SKIN PREPARATION

Surgical site infection (SSI) is a significant cause of postoperative morbidity affecting up to 5% patients.[50] In many cases, this will be limited to a localised infection of the surgical wound; however, occasionally it can become much more serious, leading to deeper infection, abscess formation, and in some cases death.[50,51] It is associated with increased length of hospital stay and consequently increased costs.

A number of risk factors for the development of SSI are non-modifiable, such as increasing age of patient and recent radiotherapy. Others may be modifiable with significant lifestyle interventions as discussed above, such as obesity, smoking and the presence of diabetes. However, significant alterations in these factors are often limited by the constraints of timing of surgery in the majority of hepatobiliary and pancreatic procedures.

A number of recommendations have been made to prevent SSI, which include antibiotic prophylaxis and antiseptic skin preparation.[3,4,50,51]

For major HPB surgery, including liver resection and pancreaticoduodenectomy, a single dose of IV antibiotics is recommended to be given less than 1 hour prior to skin incision. The choice of antibiotic will vary depending on local hospital protocols, and may require repeat dosing perioperatively depending on the duration of surgery.[3,4,50,51]

There is no indication to continue antibiotics postoperatively following most major abdominal surgical procedures, including liver resection.[50–52] However, patients undergoing pancreaticoduodenectomy are at increased risk of postoperative SSI, particularly following preoperative biliary drainage. There is evidence to suggest that these patients should have targeted antibiotics based on organisms from bile instrumentation or patient cultures, and that prophylactic postoperative antibiotics should be considered.[4,53] Prior to incision, skin should be prepared with 2% chlorhexidine.[3,4,50]

## INTRAOPERATIVE CARE

### GENERAL ANAESTHESIA

The majority of patients undergoing major HPB surgery will have a general anaesthetic. The aims of general anaesthesia are to produce a safe, reversible loss of consciousness, optimise the physiological response to surgery and provide good operating conditions. Maintenance of general anaesthesia may be with an inhaled volatile anaesthetic or with total intravenous anaesthesia (TIVA) using propofol.

Undertaking surgical resection of a tumour may be associated with metastasis of tumour cells. There has been growing interest in whether the choice of anaesthetic technique can influence cancer recurrence and the development of metastases due to differing effects on immunity and cancer-signalling pathways. Some studies have shown the beneficial effects of a TIVA technique; however, there have been mixed results and few large randomised studies. A 2019 meta-analysis of studies in breast, oesophageal and non–small cell lung cancers found that TIVA was associated with improved recurrence-free as well as overall survival compared with volatile anaesthesia.[54] A retrospective cohort study of patients with hepatocellular carcinoma (HCC) who underwent hepatectomy found overall improved survival in those administered TIVA compared with volatile anaesthetic.[55] However, overall results have been variable and there remains a need to undertake large, randomised trials to examine if choice of anaesthetic agent has a significant effect on patient outcome.

### POSTOPERATIVE ANALGESIA

Good postoperative analgesia is an essential component of the surgical pathway as it can facilitate early mobilisation, optimise respiratory function and assist in postoperative recovery and return to normal activity. When planning the postoperative analgesic regimen, a number of factors need to be considered, such as the nature of the proposed surgery, patient factors and preferences, as well as their comorbidity.

Thoracic epidural analgesia (TEA) is achieved by a continuous infusion of local anaesthetic, such as (levo-) bupivacaine or ropivacaine, often in combination with an opioid, into the epidural space. This can provide excellent analgesia and lower rates of gastrointestinal dysfunction after abdominal surgery.[4,56] In addition, by avoiding large doses of IV opioid analgesics which can cause sedation and respiratory depression, TEA can help optimise respiratory function and reduce the risk of postoperative pulmonary complications.[57]

There are a number of significant side effects associated with TEA, such as urinary retention, hypotension and motor block which can delay mobilisation. This has led to interest in alternative analgesic strategies for HPB surgery.

Intrathecal opioid injection is an alternative technique which can be used in liver resection, particularly those that are performed laparoscopically.[58] This technique also avoids the potential challenge of removing an epidural catheter if a patient develops deranged coagulation following liver resection.

Local anaesthetic wound infusion catheters in conjunction with opioid patient-controlled analgesia (PCA) was shown to reduce the time until discharge criteria were met in the RCT of patients undergoing open liver resection.[59]

✔✔ Local anaesthetic wound infiltration combined with opiate PCA can reduce the time taken for patients to reach discharge criteria compared with epidural analgesia.[59]

The ERAS recommendations for liver surgery state that there is no evidence for the use of TEA over other analgesic strategies such as wound catheter, PCA or intrathecal opioid, and the choice will therefore depend on specific surgical and patient factors.[3]

TEA is recommended in pancreaticoduodenectomy due to improved postoperative pain control combined with a reduction in stress response which continues for the duration of infusion.[4,60] When TEA is used for postoperative analgesia, motor block can be reduced by careful titration of local anaesthetic and opioid doses. Epidural-associated hypotension due to peripheral vasodilatation should be managed with a protocol for vasopressors and cautious IV fluid administration to prevent fluid overload. In addition to the strategies above, a multimodal analgesia approach should be undertaken for all major HPB surgeries.

Paracetamol (acetaminophen) is inexpensive and effective, and can be administered by the oral, IV and rectal routes. The bioavailability following oral dosing is very good, and IV dosing should therefore be reserved for situations where the oral route is not available. Caution should be taken when prescribing to patients undergoing significant liver resection.

Clonidine and dexmedetomidine are $\alpha_2$-adrenoceptor agonists that are increasingly being used as adjuncts in the management of perioperative pain as they can reduce opioid requirements. However, their use is limited by the side effects of sedation, hypotension and bradycardia.

Ketamine has a role in multimodal analgesia for postoperative pain through its action on central pain pathways and opioid receptors, when given in low doses by IV or subcutaneous infusion. It stimulates the cardiovascular system through activation of the sympathetic nervous system, and causes increases in heart rate, blood pressure and cardiac output.

## POSTOPERATIVE NAUSEA AND VOMITING

Postoperative nausea and vomiting (PONV) is common, affecting 20–30% surgical patients, and can result in delayed recovery. It is essential to assess each individual undergoing surgery, as the physiology is complex. Risk factors are multifactorial and include female sex, non-smokers and a history of anxiety or prior motion sickness. Laparoscopic surgery can also increase the incidence of PONV. ERAS protocols for liver surgery and pancreaticoduodenectomy recommend the use of two antiemetics which act in different ways.[3,4] Ondansetron, a serotonin antagonist, can be particularly effective when used in conjunction with a corticosteroid such as dexamethasone. If a patient is at very high risk for PONV, IV anaesthesia with propofol should be considered as this is associated with a lower incidence of PONV than maintenance with inhalational anaesthetic agents.[61]

✔✔ Maintenance of anaesthesia with propofol reduces the incidence of PONV compared with volatile anaesthesia and is recommended for patients who are at higher risk of this complication.[61]

## HYPOTHERMIA

Patients undergoing major surgery are susceptible to perioperative hypothermia (core temperature less than 36°C) through a number of mechanisms. General anaesthesia results in a redistribution of body heat to peripheral tissues, and reduces the body's thermoregulatory control mechanisms of shivering and vasoconstriction. The addition of a neuraxial technique compounds these effects. Elderly patients and those with a low BMI are particularly susceptible, as are those having major surgery that lasts longer than 30 minutes. Large surgical incisions also contribute to heat loss.

Adverse effects of hypothermia include an increase in wound infection through mechanisms of reduced tissue perfusion and impaired immune responses, reduced scar formation and potential for wound dehiscence.[62] Cardiac arrhythmias are more common and drug effects may be prolonged. In major HPB surgery particularly, there are concerns of increased bleeding through impairment in platelet aggregation and the enzymes involved in coagulation, with subsequent increased transfusion requirements.[63]

Core temperature should be monitored throughout surgery, for example with a nasopharyngeal temperature probe.[64] Active warming using forced air or circulating water heating systems should be used, and where possible, these should be commenced either preoperatively or in the anaesthetic room, particularly when there are additional procedures to be undertaken such as invasive line insertion.[65] In addition, IV fluids should be warmed, particularly if transfusing red cell concentrate from fridge storage.

## INTRAOPERATIVE MONITORING

Inadequate oxygen delivery to the tissues during and after surgery can contribute to postoperative morbidity and mortality. Patients with poor cardiovascular and respiratory reserve or anaemia are less able to increase oxygen delivery and are therefore at increased risk of associated complications. Oxygen delivery depends on both the cardiac output and oxygen content of arterial blood, and it is therefore important to monitor and optimise these throughout surgery.

An arterial catheter provides continuous measurement of blood pressure as well as allowing blood sampling to ensure adequate oxygenation and haemoglobin, correction of biochemistry and monitoring of lactate which is of particular relevance during liver surgery. A central venous catheter (CVC) gives a continuous measurement of central venous pressure (CVP) and allows infusion of vasopressors and inotropes if required. In addition, for some major procedures, intraoperative cardiac output monitoring can be beneficial. This can be undertaken with pulse contour analysis systems using an arterial catheter (LiDCO, FloTrac), with oesophageal Doppler or increasingly, with the use of transoesophageal echocardiography (TOE) (Fig. 3.2). Pulmonary artery catheters (PACs) are also still used in some centres for cardiac output monitoring during major surgery.

## INTRAOPERATIVE FLUIDS

Goal-directed fluid therapy (GDFT) uses haemodynamic targets to guide perioperative IV fluid administration, inotropic and vasopressor therapy, blood transfusion and supplemental oxygen. There has been extensive research undertaken to determine if this strategy is associated with improved postoperative outcomes, and a systematic review and meta-analysis in 2021 found that GDFT reduces postoperative complications but not perioperative mortality.[66]

It remains unclear what the optimal types of fluid, inotropic and vasopressor agents are, and which patients are most likely to benefit. However, it is important to avoid fluid overload as this can cause bowel wall oedema and postoperative pulmonary complications. Therefore, monitoring of intravascular volume status and fluid responsiveness is recommended in major hepatobiliary surgery.[3,4,64] In addition, fluid restriction techniques may be used intraoperatively during liver resection surgery, and this needs to be taken into account within a GDFT protocol.

✅✅ GDFT reduces the incidence of postoperative complications but not mortality.[66]

## CENTRAL VENOUS PRESSURE CONTROL

Intraoperative control of CVP to less than 5 $cmH_2O$ during liver resection has been shown to reduce blood loss by decreasing hepatic congestion during parenchymal transection.[67,68] Although a Cochrane review in 2009 found that there was a reduction in blood loss with this technique, there was no difference in red cell concentrate transfusion or mortality.[69] However, a meta-analysis in 2014 showed that intraoperative control of CVP during liver resection was associated with lower blood loss as well as reduction in transfusion requirements.[70] Hughes et al.[71] conducted a systematic review and meta-analysis of the evidence and found that although there was a reduction in blood loss and transfusion requirements, there was no difference in morbidity or

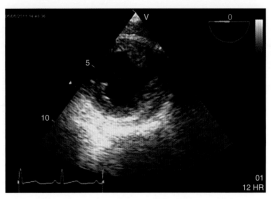

**Figure 3.2**  Transoesophageal echocardiography transgastric view.

hospital length of stay. Methods used to control CVP during liver resection include fluid restriction, venodilatation, diuretics and the use of epidural anaesthesia, as well as careful attention to airway pressures and avoidance of high positive end-expiratory pressure (PEEP). Importantly, the technique has not been shown to have a significant effect on hepatic or renal function.

✅✅ Low CVP surgery is associated with reduced blood loss and blood transfusion but not a reduction in morbidity.[71]

## BLEEDING, COAGULATION AND BLOOD TRANSFUSION

Although there have been many improvements in the surgical and anaesthetic techniques for major HPB surgery, there remains a significant risk of haemorrhage in some procedures. In patients undergoing pancreaticoduodenectomy, preoperative investigations including CT and endoscopic ultrasonography are often able to identify if a pancreatic mass involves vascular structures such as the portal, splenic or mesenteric veins which will increase the risk of intraoperative bleeding. In patients undergoing liver resection, there is a risk of sudden rapid bleeding during parenchymal transection. This will depend on the extent of the resection and patient factors such as underlying steatosis or preoperative chemotherapy. Intraoperative factors that affect bleeding include the use of the Pringle technique to temporarily occlude hepatic blood inflow.

For this reason, patients undergoing major HPB surgery should have large-bore IV access placed, with a wide-bore central catheter if necessary. A rapid infuser with the ability to warm infusion fluids and a cell salvage system are important to have available in case of significant blood loss.

The use of point-of-care viscoelastic coagulation testing has become more widely available and can be very helpful in HPB surgery, particularly in liver resection when laboratory coagulation measures may not reflect the ongoing situation.[72,73] Fig. 3.3 shows a ROTEM® Analysis, demonstrating the measured parameters of a blood clot. This analysis can inform clinicians which component of haemostasis is contributing to bleeding, which is of particular use in an acute setting such as intraoperative haemorrhage.

To undertake viscoelastic testing, different reagents are added to a blood sample to run different channels contemporaneously, to indicate whether bleeding is due to

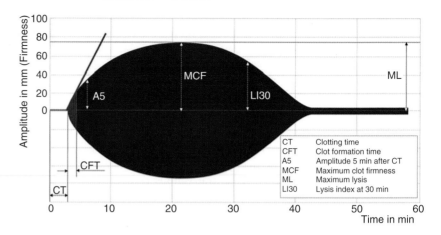

**Figure 3.3**  Parameters of ROTEM analysis.

thrombocytopaenia, a reduction in fibrinogen or coagulation factors, a heparin effect or fibrinolysis. This allows appropriate targeted use of blood products, factor concentrates, tranexamic acid or other medications to manage haemorrhage, and therefore reduce unnecessary transfusion.[72–75] Blood transfusion can have a number of unwanted effects, such as transfusion-related acute lung injury (TRALI) and fluid overload. In addition, there are concerns about the immunomodulatory effects of blood transfusion, and a systematic review of red blood cell transfusion in patients undergoing liver resection found that transfusion may have an effect on long-term cancer outcomes.[76] Further work has also shown an association between blood transfusion and cancer recurrence in patients having liver resection for HCC,[77] and therefore a targeted approach to transfusion using point-of-care testing should be undertaken where possible.

## GLYCAEMIC CONTROL

Both diabetic and non-diabetic patients undergoing major surgery may develop hyperglycaemia due to the surgical stress response. The resulting insulin resistance may be minimised in part by reduced fasting times and the provision of carbohydrate drinks which are part of ERAS pathways. Perioperative hyperglycaemia has been shown to be related to adverse outcomes in major surgery, in particular SSI, delayed wound healing and increased length of hospital stay.[3,4,78,79] During liver resection, there may be rapid changes in glucose concentration during Pringle occlusion of hepatic blood inflow whilst some patients may develop new-onset diabetes after pancreatic resection.[80] It is recommended that patients undergoing major HPB surgery should have insulin management to maintain normoglycaemia.

## MINIMALLY INVASIVE SURGERY

Minimally invasive surgery is one of the key features of established ERAS pathways, and evidence for its use in HPB surgery is increasing. The advantages of a laparoscopic technique are a reduction in the stress response to surgery, improved postoperative recovery and shorter length of stay. A literature review of laparoscopic liver resection in 2009 analysed 127 studies and found the technique to be safe with similar survival outcomes for patients with HCC or metastases from colorectal malignancy.[81] Further studies

have shown significantly fewer postoperative complications and reduced length of hospital stay in patients undergoing laparoscopic liver resection compared with open surgery, with no effect on tumour resection margins or long-term survival.[82,83] However, there remain a number of factors which may contribute to difficulties in laparoscopic liver surgery, such as the site and size of lesion, neoadjuvant chemotherapy and whether a patient has undergone previous resection.[84] Laparoscopic pancreatic surgery was originally undertaken to manage pseudocysts in pancreatitis and staging in pancreatic malignancy.[85] Open techniques are continued to be favoured for major pancreatic surgery, such as pancreaticoduodenectomy, due to the number and complexity of anastomoses involved. However, in large, high-volume centres, both laparoscopic and robotic techniques have been found to be safe and may be associated with reduced length of stay.[4,86]

## POSTOPERATIVE CARE

### HEPATIC INSUFFICIENCY FOLLOWING LIVER RESECTION

Although the liver is capable of significant regeneration after liver resection surgery, patients may be at risk of developing hepatic insufficiency or post hepatectomy liver failure (PHLF). Risk factors include the presence of steatosis, fibrosis or cirrhosis, preoperative chemotherapy, patient age and renal insufficiency. In addition, the extent of resection, dissection technique and intraoperative blood loss are associated with increased risk of hepatic insufficiency.[87] There are a number of techniques which aim to increase the volume of the liver remnant preoperatively, such as portal vein embolization; however, there is no direct correlation between liver volume and function, and patients may still develop this complication.

Therefore, patients undergoing liver resection, particularly those with the above risk factors, should be carefully monitored postoperatively to identify any clinical or biochemical indications of hepatic insufficiency. High lactate measurements can be an early indication of liver dysfunction as a result of reduced clearance.[88,89] However, lactate concentrations may be raised postoperatively for several reasons, including tissue hypoxia, anaerobic metabolism and the use of vasopressor medications.[89] Hyperbilirubinaemia and raised INR are used in the consensus definition of PHLF and therefore liver function tests and coagulation should be monitored postoperatively, with viscoelastic testing considered as discussed above.[73,87]

Management of PHLF will involve critical care support of multiorgan failure. Although a number of artificial liver support systems such as the Molecular Adsorbent Recirculating System (MARS) have been developed, there is currently no conclusive evidence to support their routine clinical use.[87] Some patients may be discussed for consideration of rescue orthotopic liver transplantation. However, attention to preoperative risk factors and intraoperative conditions remain the leading principles in mitigating the risk of PHLF developing.

## DRAINS

There has been a move away from the routine insertion of abdominal drains as part of many ERAS pathways. As well as contributing to postoperative pain and impaired pulmonary function, they may be a potential site for infection. Following liver resection, there is currently no consensus on prophylactic abdominal drainage.[3] In patients undergoing pancreaticoduodenectomy, there is a risk of postoperative pancreatic leaks and fistulae, which can be detected early by examination of drain fluids.[90] The ERAS guidelines suggest a conservative approach in selected patients with plan for early drain removal within 72 hours if drain amylase is < 5000 U/L on postoperative day 1.[4,90]

## NASOGASTRIC DRAINAGE, NUTRITION AND STIMULATION OF BOWEL MOVEMENT

Routine nasogastric (NG) tube insertion is no longer recommended in HPB surgery, and it is suggested that these should be removed before leaving theatre.[3,4] They can cause patient discomfort, and there is some evidence that they may cause an increase in pulmonary complications postoperatively.[91] Although patients undergoing pancreaticoduodenectomy may have gastric emptying problems due to the nature of the surgery, a randomised clinical trial in 2020 showed no difference in postoperative complications in patients with NG drainage, supporting current ERAS guidelines that they should be removed before the end of anaesthesia.[4,92]

 Routine postoperative NG drainage does not reduce complications in patients undergoing pancreaticoduodenectomy.[92]

Early oral intake is now recommended as part of HPB ERAS protocols, with an aim to establish a normal diet as soon as possible where tolerated.[3,4] Although it is recognised that there may be a delay in gastric function following pancreaticoduodenectomy, early postoperative oral intake should still be attempted. In some patients who are particularly malnourished at the time of surgery, nutritional support should be considered, with a preference for the enteral route wherever possible.[4,93]

A number of components of the HPB ERAS pathways are thought to contribute to earlier recovery of normal bowel function and the avoidance of ileus. These include minimally invasive surgical techniques with reduced bowel handling, the optimisation of fluid balance to avoid bowel oedema and early

postoperative oral intake.[3,4] Chewing gum has been suggested as a means to accelerate the return of normal bowel function by stimulating vagal reflexes, and although not recommended after hepatic surgery, it is felt to be a safe intervention which may be considered following pancreaticoduodenectomy.[94,95]

Alvimopan is a mu-receptor antagonist that reportedly helps with recovery of bowel function following abdominal surgery and should be considered following pancreaticoduodenectomy.[96]

## MOBILISATION

Early mobilisation should be encouraged as soon as possible following major HPB surgery, ideally from the first postoperative day. Prolonged immobility contributes to muscle atrophy and is a risk factor in development of VTE. Where possible, physiotherapy assistance should be offered to patients, particularly those who have been deconditioned prior to surgery.[3,4,64]

### Key points

- There are increasing numbers of patients with significant comorbidities presenting for major HPB surgery.
- Involvement of the MDT from the point of diagnosis can optimise the patient's perioperative journey.
- Risk stratification, multimodal prehabilitation and optimisation of medical conditions should be undertaken preoperatively wherever possible.
- ERAS pathways specific to HPB surgery have been developed with evidence-based recommendations for the perioperative care of patients.

🌐 References available at http://ebooks.health.elsevier.com/

### KEY REFERENCES

[21] Richards T, Baikady RR, Clevenger B, et al. Preoperative intravenous iron to treat anaemia before major abdominal surgery (PREVENTT): a randomised, double-blind, controlled trial. Lancet 2020;396(10259):1353–61.
  *A double-blind, parallel-group randomised trial did not demonstrate any difference in mortality or the rate of blood transfusion in the perioperative period in patients given preoperative intravenous iron therapy compared with placebo group.*
[25] Wong J, Lam DP, Abrishami A, et al. Short-term preoperative smoking cessation and postoperative complications: a systematic review and meta-analysis. Can J Anaesth 2012;59(3):268–79
  *A systematic review and meta-analysis of 25 studies demonstrated that smoking cessation for 4 weeks prior to surgery results in fewer respiratory and wound-healing complications.*
[48] Felder S, Rasmussen MS, King R, et al. Prolonged thromboprophylaxis with low molecular heparin for abdominal or pelvic surgery. Cochrane Database Syst Rev 2019:CD004318
  *A Cochrane Review of RCTs found that prolonged thromboprophylaxis with LMWH is associated with a significantly reduced risk of VTE compared with thromboprophylaxis during hospital admission only. This review of patients undergoing major abdominal surgery did not find any increase in bleeding complications or mortality.*
[59] Revie EJ, McKeown DW, Wilson JA, et al. Randomized clinical trial of local infiltration plus patient-controlled opiate analgesia vs. epidural analgesia following liver resection surgery. HPB 2012;14(9):611–8
  *An RCT of patients undergoing open liver resection found that local anaesthetic wound infiltration combined with opiate PCA reduced the time taken for patients to reach hospital discharge criteria. Analgesia from TEA was found to be superior; however, this benefit did not result in faster recovery.*

[61] Schraag S, Pradelli L, Alsaleh AJO, et al. Propofol vs inhalational agents to maintain general anesthesia in ambulatory and inpatient surgery: a systematic review and meta-analysis. BMC Anaesthesiol 2018;18(162):1–9

*A systematic review and meta-analysis found a reduction in PONV with the use of propofol for maintenance of anaesthesia in comparison with volatile anaesthetic.*

[66] Messina A, Robba C, Calabro L, et al. Association between perioperative fluid administration and postoperative outcomes: a 20-year systematic review and a meta-analysis of randomized goal-directed trials in major visceral/noncardiac surgery. Crit Care 2021;25(1):43

*A systematic review and meta-analysis of 21 RCTs found that GDFT reduces postoperative complications but is not associated with a reduction in mortality.*

[71] Hughes MJ, Ventham NT, Harrison EM, et al. Central venous pressure and liver resection: a systematic review and meta-analysis. HPB 2015;17(10):863–71

*A systematic review and meta-analysis of 8 RCTs found that surgery undertaken with low CVP control resulted in a reduction in blood loss and blood transfusion but not a reduced morbidity.*

[92] Bergeat D, Merdrignac A, Robin F, et al. Nasogastric decompression vs no decompression after pancreaticoduodenectomy: the randomized clinical IPOD trial. JAMA Surg 2020;155(9):e202291

*The IPOD (Impact of the Absence of Nasogastric Decompression After Pancreaticoduodenectomy) was an open-label, prospective, single-centre randomised clinical trial which found that routine nasogastric decompression did not result in a difference in postoperative complications.*

# The molecular biology of hepatopancreatobiliary cancer

**4**

Rachel V. Guest | T.R. Jeff Evans

## INTRODUCTION

As our understanding of the molecular mechanisms of cancer development and progression has advanced, we have seen significant improvements in therapeutic responses in patients. This arguably has been best illustrated in the field of breast cancer, where tamoxifen and trastuzumab (Herceptin) have transformed outcomes for millions of patients with disease once thought refractory to treatment. Furthermore, molecular profiling has enabled the stratification of tumours previously considered similar based on organ of origin or pathology into groups exhibiting variable prognostic risk or predicted response to therapy, allowing delivery of targeted treatments.[1]

Personalised or 'precision' cancer therapy aims to tailor therapies to specific targets to deliver 'the right drug(s) to the right person'.[2] Actionable targets include genes carrying somatic mutations leading to hyperactivation of oncogenic signalling, such as the V600E mutation in the *BRAF* gene, observed in more than half of malignant melanomas, which drives MAPK signalling to promote tumour growth. The pre-clinical development of BRAF inhibitors and their translation to the clinic for patients with advanced melanoma has been one of the greatest successes in surgical oncology of recent times.[3] It is also increasingly appreciated that such targets for therapy frequently reside within the stromal microenvironment of solid tumours as well as the cancerous epithelium, such as on cancer-associated fibroblasts (CAFs; e.g. TGFβ) or the neovasculature (e.g. VEGF receptors).[4]

Many barriers persist between currently available anticancer therapies and comprehensive individualised cancer care. Next-generation sequencing (NGS) technologies have revealed the true genomic complexity of tumours and have proven that cancer cells are not identical 'daughter' clones of a single genetically altered 'mother' cell, but rather a diverse community subject to Darwinian selective pressures where subpopulations carrying growth and survival advantages are selected ('driver mutations') and lineages carrying neutral or deleterious aberrations ('passenger mutations') persist due to genetic linkage with driver variants. Such spatial and temporal diversity within a single tumour ('intratumoral heterogeneity') means that targetable mutations frequently are only observed at low prevalence. As such, treatment selection biomarkers need to have sufficient sensitivity to detect low-frequency events, potentially spatially separated within different regions of the tumour. Serial biopsy from multiple tumour sites during the course of therapy is rarely clinically feasible. Consequently, it follows that exposure to targeted inhibitors can lead to emerging resistance over time and ultimately treatment failure.[5] Finally, to date many targets have simply proven undruggable, and the vast redundancy in cellular signalling networks means that surgery continues to play a pivotal role in the management of hepatopancreatobiliary cancers (Box 4.1).

## PANCREATIC DUCTAL ADENOCARCINOMA

### THE PDAC GENOME

Clinically relevant subtypes of pancreatic cancer have been identified; international collaborative studies have now sequenced a large number of sizeable patient cohorts and a signature of recurrent mutated genes in pancreatic ductal adenocarcinoma (PDAC) has emerged.[6–9] Alterations in the proto-oncogene *KRAS* are seen in > 95% patients, whilst 50% will exhibit mutations in the tumour suppressor *TP53*, *SMAD4* (a transcription factor mediating TGFβ signalling) and the cell cycle regulator *CDKN2A*.[10,11] A larger subset of mutations is expressed at 5–10% prevalence, including genes involved in chromatin remodelling (*ARID1A*, *MLL3*), DNA damage repair (*KDM6A*) and Wnt signalling (*RNF43*). By far, the majority of alterations occur at < 1% prevalence, however, often described as the 'long tail' of infrequent mutations.[8]

Metastatic pancreatic cancer is particularly refractory to systemic anticancer chemotherapy. A small proportion of patients have germline *BRCA1* or *BRCA2* mutations. Inhibitors of PARP (poly [adenosine diphosphate-ribose] polymerase), such as olaparib, have demonstrated activity in patients with breast and ovarian cancers with these germline mutations. In the POLO trial, maintenance olaparib provided a significant progression-free benefit to patients with a germline *BRCA* mutation and metastatic pancreatic cancer who had not progressed during platinum-based chemotherapy,[12] raising the tantalising possibility that molecular targeted therapy can enhance outcome in this hitherto refractory disease.

Recurrently observed mutations have been aggregated into 10–12 core pathways including Ras, TGFβ, Wnt, Notch, ROBO/SLIT signalling, SW1-SNF, chromatin modification, DNA repair and RNA processing. This has led to a suggested 'molecular taxonomy,' a proposed model with which we can better understand the mechanisms underpinning carcinogenesis in PDAC.[7,9,10] However, mutations between these mechanistic groups are not mutually exclusive and therefore at the time of writing such classifications have not yet led to clinical utility or a basis for trial design (Fig. 4.1).

The use of whole genome sequencing (WGS) to analyse somatic structural chromosomal rearrangements such as

## Box 4.1   Glossary of terms in molecular biology

**Glossary of terms in molecular biology**

| | |
|---|---|
| Genome | The totality of all genetic information in a cell. It includes the genes (coding regions), the non-coding regions and mitochondrial DNA. |
| Exome | The sequence of DNA (exons), which will be represented in mRNA after transcription. It includes the coding sequence and untranslated regions of mRNA. |
| Transcriptome | The set of all RNA transcripts in a cell (including coding and non-coding). |
| Epigenome | The record of chemical changes to the DNA and histone proteins in a cell unrelated to the nucleotide sequence of DNA that can be heritably passed to the daughter cell during mitosis or meiosis. |
| Next-generation sequencing (NGS) | A catch-all term used to describe large-scale technologies that can sequence the whole genome (whole genome sequencing, WGS), all exons within known genes (whole exome sequencing, WES) or only exons in selected genes (targeted panel). |
| Somatic mutation (variant) | A change in the DNA sequence of a cell (other than a gamete). |
| Germline mutation (variant) | A change in the DNA sequence of a gamete/germ cell which can be passed to offspring. |
| Precision medicine | A medical model that customises healthcare to a subgroup of patients or individual patient, often using genetic/molecular testing to select optimal therapies. |
| Polyploidy | A condition in which the cells of an organism have more than two paired sets of homologous chromosomes. |
| Aneuploidy | The presence of an abnormal number of chromosomes within a cell e.g. a human cell having 47 chromosomes rather than 46. |
| Single nucleotide polymorphism (SNP) | Variation between individuals in a population (>1%) at a specific nucleotide in their DNA sequence. |
| Genome-wide association study (GWAS) | An observational study of genome-wide genetic variations to see if a variant is associated with a trait/disease. |
| Histone | A group of abundant (and highly basic) proteins rich in arginine and lysine which form the nucleosome cores around which DNA is wrapped in eukaryotic chromosomes. |
| Nucleosome | The 'bead-like' structures in eukaryotic chromatin; composed of a short length of DNA wrapped around an octameric core of histone proteins. |
| Microsatellite instability (MSI) | A condition of increased susceptibility to mutation usually resulting from defective DNA mismatch repair. |
| DNA methylation | The addition of methyl groups to the DNA molecule, which can result in a change in gene expression (usually repression of transcription) without altering the DNA sequence. |
| CpG island | Regions of DNA with a high frequency of CpG sites (cytosine nucleotide followed by a guanine nucleotide in the linear sequence). Cytosines in CpG dinucleotides can be methylated to form 5-methylcytosines. Frequently found in gene promoters. |
| Immunotherapy | The treatment of a disease by exploiting the immune system. |
| Tyrosine kinase | An enzyme with the ability to transfer phosphate groups from ATP to the tyrosine residues of a protein within a cell. |
| Tumour neoantigen | Antigens presented by MHC class I or II molecules on the surface of tumour cells. Antigens only found on tumour cells are called tumour-specific antigens (TSAs). |
| Long non-coding RNA (lncRNA) | A species of RNA with transcripts > 200 nucleotides that are not translated into protein. |
| Micro RNA (miRNA) | Small single-stranded RNA species that act to regulate gene expression at the post-transcriptional level. |
| Liquid biopsy (circulating tumour DNA ctDNA) | The sampling of non-solid biological tissue (frequently blood), often to detect tumour-derived fragmented DNA that is freely circulating in the bloodstream. |
| CRISPR gene editing | A genetic engineering technique that allows modification of the genome. It is based on the bacterial CRISPR/Cas9 antiviral defence system, whereby the Cas9 nuclease is delivered using a synthetic guide RNA (gRNA) to cut the genome at a certain location and remove or add desired genes. |
| Basket trial | A type of clinical trial in which a drug is tested in patients who have different types of cancer based on the organ of origin, but who share the same molecular target or selection biomarker. |

insertions, deletions, translocations and amplifications in a cohort of 100 samples has similarly led to a suggested classification of PDAC into four subtypes.[8]

- 'Stable' tumours (20%) exhibit < 50 structural variation events and aneuploidy suggesting defective mitosis.
- 'Scattered' tumours (36%) show a moderate range of non-random chromosomal damage and < 200 'structural events'.
- 'Unstable' tumours (14%) display a large number (200–558) of structural events suggesting a defect in DNA maintenance (and perhaps therefore sensitivity to DNA damaging therapeutics).
- 'Locally rearranged' tumours (30%) are characterised by a significant focal event on one or two chromosomes (8).

Such a classification might be exploited clinically as a surrogate marker for therapeutic sensitivity. For example,

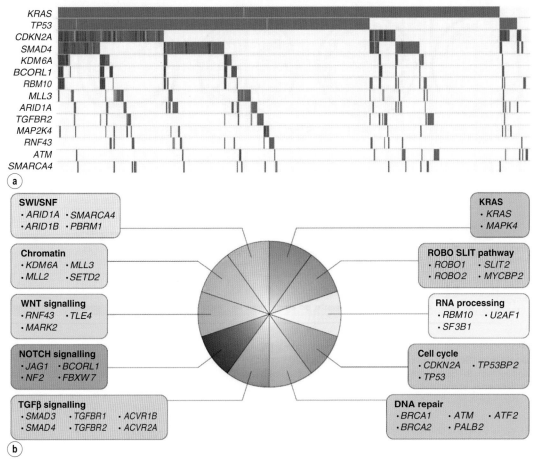

**Figure 4.1** **(a)** Mutations in the proto-oncogene *KRAS* are almost ubiquitous in pancreatic ductal adenocarcinoma. Approximately 50% of specimens exhibit mutations in *TP53*, *SMAD4* and *CDKN2A*. A smaller group of genes are mutated at 5–10% prevalence, but by far the majority of variants occur at < 1% frequency, making precision targeting with therapeutics highly challenging. **(b)** Recurrent observed mutations can be grouped into core molecular pathways according to mechanism. (Reproduced with permission from [1].)

cancers with an 'unstable' phenotype frequently exhibit mutations in *BRCA1*, *BRCA2* or a described mutational signature associated with the BRCA phenotype[13] and therefore a defective DNA damage response (DDR) which might imply susceptibility to agents targeting DDR deficiency (Fig. 4.2).[14]

Mutations in *KRAS* have been demonstrated to be associated with poor clinical outcomes and specifically the *KRAS G12D* mutation with the worst survival (a single point mutation in codon 12 resulting in substitution of the amino acid glycine for aspartate and constitutive activation of downstream signalling).[15,16] In a cohort of 356 patients, median overall survival (OS) was 20.3 months (IQR 11.3–38.3) in the presence of *KRAS* mutation compared with 38.6 months (IQR 16.6–63.1) in patients with wild-type tumours.[17] The accumulation of alterations in the other four principal driver genes (*KRAS*, *TP53*, *SMAD4*, *CDKN2A*) negatively affects clinical outcomes further. The use of multivariable Cox proportional hazard regression to analyse the effects of combinatorial gene alterations with survival concluded that inferior disease-free survival and OS is observed in patients with three or four mutations versus those with one or two alterations (after adjustment for age, sex, nodal status, tumour grade, lymphovascular invasion, receipt of perioperative treatment, resection margin status and institution).[17]

For many years RAS was considered 'undruggable', but there has been a co-ordinated effort in recent times to develop novel approaches to RAS blockade including mutant-specific covalent inhibitors,[18,19] the first of which (AMG-510) has now entered clinical trials in non-small cell lung cancer (https://clinicaltrials.gov/ct2/show/NCT04625647). Pre-clinical studies however have demonstrated immense redundancy in RAS signalling systems and experiments using pancreatic cancer cells with *KRAS* inhibition using gene editing with CRISPR/Cas9 retain active downstream signalling driving cell proliferation via the PI3K/MAPK pathway.[20] To effectively treat RAS-driven cancers, the MAPK pathway must be completely supressed and combination of RAS inhibitors with additional kinase inhibitors may be required as in other cancer types, e.g. melanoma.[21] Finally, RAS may also prove useful clinically as a biomarker, such as in the detection of early metastatic disease or recurrence. Studies assessing the utility of 'liquid biopsy' (the detection of circulating tumour DNA [ctDNA] in the blood) have demonstrated that detectable *KRAS G12D* in plasma was associated with inferior survival.[16]

The large number of low prevalence drivers in PDAC has led to concerns that previous trials testing targeted inhibitors in unselected patient populations might have failed to

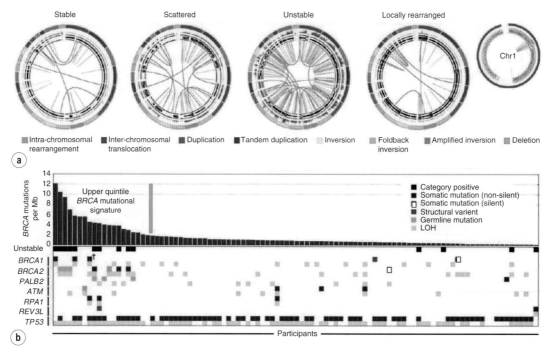

**Figure 4.2** **(a)** Four subtypes of pancreatic ductal adenocarcinoma (PDAC) have been described according to patterns in structural chromosomal rearrangements: 'Stable' (<50 events), 'Scattered' (50–200 events), 'Unstable' (>200 events) or 'Locally rearranged' (focal events on one or two chromosomes). **(b)** Significant overlap has been observed between Unstable phenotype PDAC and the BRCA mutational signature, suggesting that a deficiency in the DNA damage response occurs in a significant minority of PDACs, offering potential for therapeutic targeting. (Reproduced with permission from [8].)

detect an existing underlying benefit 'signal'. This has led to the development of novel research platforms whereby NGS can be used to characterise tumour genomes and detect actionable targets prior to study enrolment. PRECISION-Panc in the UK and PRECISION-Promise in the USA aim to perform personalised molecular analysis and drug response studies on individual samples to inform trial recruitment i.e. 'the right trial for the right patient'.[22] This 'precision oncology' model of patient selection to enter trials according to personalised tumour sequencing has also now been adopted in other cancers including hepatocellular cancer (HCC) and biliary tract cancer (BTC).[23,24]

## THE PDAC TRANSCRIPTOME

In addition to characterisation of the PDAC genome, transcriptomic analyses have been conducted to assess how genetic alterations are transcribed to the RNA level and define the networks of gene expression associated with tumorigenesis.[9,25,26] Studies have examined both whole tumour and microdissected samples and observed enrichment of gene programmes that cluster into subtypes which may correlate with clinical features including histopathology and survival. These have been named in one study of 456 PDACs as 'Squamous', 'Progenitor', 'Immunogenic' and 'Aberrantly Differentiated Endocrine Exocrine' (ADEX).[9] Other studies have identified overlapping subtypes in independent cohorts, using both actual and virtual microdissection to minimise contamination from stromal or normal pancreas tissue.[25,26] Further work is ongoing to corroborate the applicability of such classifications to wider cohorts and identify the potential clinical utility of gene expression analyses (Fig. 4.3).

## THE PDAC EPIGENOME

We now know that alterations in DNA molecules themselves (mutations) account for only a proportion of the tumour heterogeneity observed in solid cancers. Epigenetics has been defined as the study of inherited phenotypes through mechanisms that do *not* involve the coding capacity of the DNA sequence.[27] Such events involve the covalent addition of methyl groups to DNA or modification to histones (highly alkaline proteins that associate with DNA to form the nucleosome and regulate gene expression), including phosphorylation, acetylation, ubiquitylation, and sumoylation. These modifications are observed on genes involved in a wide range of cellular activities including cell growth and differentiation. Some histone modifications are observed at actively transcribed gene promoters (H3K4me3, H3K27Ac), whereas others are thought to be repressive for transcription (H3K27me3, H3K9me3). In healthy development and adult tissue homeostasis, epigenetic regulation ensures that the correct gene is expressed at the correct time and in the correct context to give rise to a particular phenotype. It is therefore easy to appreciate how dysregulation of such modifications plays a role in cancer via effects on proliferation, apoptosis, senescence and invasion. Indeed, the epigenetic landscape has been shown to be profoundly altered in neoplastic cells.

Our understanding of the complexities of how the epigenome is regulated is still evolving and the mechanisms by which epigenetic changes contribute to cancer are still to be elucidated. Mutations in oncogenes, e.g. *KRAS,* can alter histone and DNA modifications via direct regulation of histone proteins and modifying enzymes.[28] Somatic mutations in genes responsible for nucleosome remodelling, such as

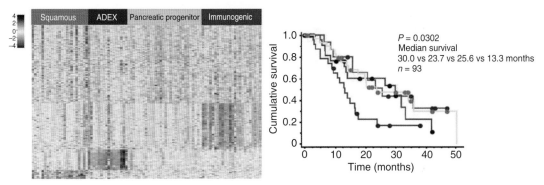

**Figure 4.3**  RNA sequencing has identified four classes of PDAC based on gene expression signatures: squamous *(blue)*; ADEX (abnormally differentiated endocrine exocrine) *(brown)*; pancreatic progenitor *(yellow)*; immunogenic *(red)*. Kaplan-Meier analysis shows that patient survival stratifies by transcriptional subclass. (Reproduced with permission from 9.)

*ARID1A, MLL2* and *KDM6A*, have been observed in PDAC.[8] Furthermore, dysregulation of non-coding RNAs (ncRNAs; RNA species directly able to regulate the epigenome) is similarly described and some specific species (e.g. *LINC00673*) may be associated with clinical outcomes.[29]

In PDAC, analysis of DNA methylation patterns can distinguish between transcriptional subtypes of the disease, including the 'classical' and 'basal' classification described by The Cancer Genome Atlas.[30] Specific 'super enhancers' (regions of the genome comprising multiple enhancers or lengths of DNA that bind transcription factors) have been demonstrated to be driven by distinct upstream regulators resulting in altered gene expression networks between subtypes.[31,32] For example, high levels of the transcription factor GATA6 is associated with the classical subtype, whereas super-enhancers in PDAC exhibiting the basal subtype appear to be regulated by the hepatocyte growth factor receptor (MET).[32,33] Indeed, some have argued that as these phenotypes cannot be distinguished based on their somatic variants (mutations), precision medicine platforms should also incorporate RNA-seq analyses.[34] Furthermore, epigenetic markers are able to distinguish tumours that appear identical at the genomic level, e.g., metastatic deposits and the primary tumour.[35] Others have similarly characterised the epigenetic remodelling that occurs at different phases of disease progression; the formation of metastases is associated with global enrichment of H3K27ac chromatin.[36] Large-scale mapping projects aim to further characterise the methylation, histone modifications and other epigenetic hallmarks of PDAC; these will require integration with genomic and phenotypic data before we fully understand how the epigenome contributes to the clinical behaviour of patients with pancreatic cancer and how best to use therapies, such as inhibitors of histone deacetylases or of DNA methylation.

## MICROSATELLITE INSTABILITY AND IMMUNOTHERAPY

Microsatellite instability (MSI) refers to a state of 'hypermutability' or heightened susceptibility to mutation, arising as a result of defective DNA mismatch repair (MMR). Loss of function of one or more genes encoding the MMR proteins (*MSH1, PMS2, MLH1, MSH6*) leads to an inability to correct mistakes that occur during DNA replication, resulting in accumulation of thousands of errors and generation of microsatellite fragments (short,1-6 base pair repetitive sequences of DNA, frequently GT or CA repeats) that recur throughout the genome. For example, 15% patients with colorectal cancer have a deficiency of DNA MMR, most commonly as a result of sporadic hypermethylation of the *MSH1* promoter, or due to germline mutation of the *MLH1* or *MSH2* genes as occurs in Lynch syndrome. Also, 1–2% of surgically resected PDACs exhibit MSI or defective DNA MMR.[37] Lynch syndrome is associated with an 8.6-fold (C95% CI 4.7–15.7) increased risk of PDAC compared with the general population, and these cancers frequently exhibit a medullary/colloid phenotype with lymphocytic infiltrate and unlike conventional PDAC, are typically wild type for *KRAS/TP53*.[37,38] The potential benefits of surveillance for PDAC in Lynch syndrome remain unknown and since the absolute risk is thought to be relatively low, it is not advocated by current guidelines.[39]

Much interest has been generated by the success of immune checkpoint inhibitors in colorectal cancers exhibiting MSI.[40] These agents include humanised monoclonal antibodies targeted to the immune checkpoint receptors programmed death-1 (PD-1; e.g. pembrolizumab) or cytotoxic T-lymphocyte-associated protein 4 (CTLA-4; e.g. ipilimumab). Blockade of these receptors promotes CD8+ cell-mediated killing of cancer cells and since tumours exhibiting MSI have a high mutational burden, they are considered to have increased 'neoantigen load'. They are therefore thought to be more susceptible to immune surveillance and hence are predicted to exhibit an enhanced response to immune checkpoint inhibition. Initial trials of these agents as monotherapy in PDAC have produced mixed results,[41,42] although the more recent multicentre KEYNOTE-158 study which included exclusively patients with MSI high tumours reported a RECIST overall response rate (ORR) of 18.2% (95% C.I. 5.2–40.3) in advanced PDAC.[43] Further studies investigating checkpoint inhibitors in combination with other immunomodulators are proving to offer more promise. The COMBAT trial was a phase IIa, dual cohort study evaluating the safety and efficacy of the checkpoint inhibitor pembrolizumab in combination with an antagonist of the chemokine receptor 4 (CXCR4), BL-8040. Patients were given the above combination either in isolation or with chemotherapy, observing an ORR of 32% when combined with cytotoxic chemotherapy.[44] It should be noted that subjects in this trial had microsatellite stable disease, and further randomised trials are needed to fully evaluate the role for immunotherapy in PDAC (Fig. 4.4).

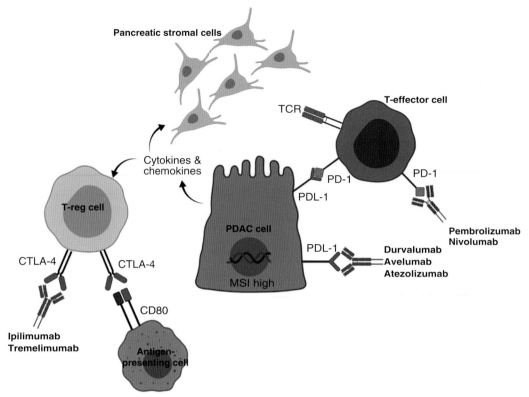

**Figure 4.4** Current molecular targets for immunotherapy in pancreatic ductal adenocarcinoma (PDAC). *CD80+,* Cluster of differentiation 80; *CLTA-4,* cytotoxic T-lymphocyte-associated protein 4; *PD-1,* programmed death-1; *PDAC,* pancreatic ductal adenocarcinoma; *PDL-1,* programmed death ligand-1; *MSI,* microsatellite instability; *TCR,* T cell receptor.

## PANCREATIC INTRAEPITHELIAL NEOPLASIAS

Many epithelial adenocarcinomas are known to arise from non-invasive precursor lesions which accumulate genetic and epigenetic changes.[45] PDAC most commonly arises from precursor epithelial proliferations known as pancreatic intraepithelial neoplasias (PanINs), which have been classified as 'low grade' (PanIN-1, PanIN-2) or 'high grade' (PanIN-3), exhibiting increasing features of cytological atypia, and dissection of pancreata harbouring PDAC will very commonly reveal multiple advanced PanINs.[46,47] The majority of PanINs harbour *KRAS* mutations and as lesions progress into invasive carcinoma, other driver alterations are accumulated later (*TP53, SMAD4, CDKN2A*).[48] Genetic studies sequencing PanINs and PDAC from the same pancreas have shown that there can be clonal expansion of a single ancestral cell that gives rise to more than one lesion which then accumulate additional driver mutations to form an invasive cancer.[49]

Less commonly PDAC arises from cystic lesions of the pancreas: intraductal papillary mucinous neoplasms (IPMNs) or mucinous cystic neoplasms (MCNs) (see Chapter 18). As is seen with PanINs, IPMNs can be multifocal and can involve the entire pancreatic duct. The majority follow an indolent course, with a 1-, 5- and 10-year survival rate of 100%, 100% and 94.2%, respectively.[50] The role of cancer susceptibility genes in IPMN and MCN remains poorly understood.

## BIOMARKERS

Genetic analyses of metastatic PDAC deposits compared with their primary tumour indicate that there is considerable latency between the appearance of the primary malignant clone and seeding of the index metastasis (6.8 years on average in one study).[51] This suggests significant opportunity for the early detection of pancreatic cancer; however, unfortunately a sensitive and specific serum assay for the diagnosis and prevention of early PDAC has not yet been developed.

Serum carbohydrate antigen (CA) 19-9 is a sialylated Lewis blood group antigen produced by PDAC cells and is the most commonly used biomarker worldwide.[52] Approximately 6% of the White population and 22% of the Black population in the USA do not generate the specific sialyl antigen and do not produce CA19-9.[52] Furthermore, CA19-9 can be raised in biliary obstruction, pancreatitis and extra-pancreatic malignancies and does not have sufficient specificity or sensitivity to act as a screening tool for early detection in asymptomatic populations.[53,54] A meta-analysis of 11 studies encompassing 2316 individuals estimated a pooled sensitivity of 0.80 (95% CI 0.77–0.82), specificity of 0.80 (95% CI 0.77–0.82) and area under the curve of 0.87 for the diagnostic accuracy of CA19-9 in patients with PDAC.[55] CA19-9 is therefore used rather for disease monitoring and levels have been shown to predict tumour stage, resectability, OS and response to therapy.[56–58]

Carcinoembryonic antigen (CEA), a glycoprotein widely used for disease monitoring in colorectal cancer, is also used as a biomarker for pancreatic cancer. CEA has an inferior sensitivity/specificity profile, cited by one meta-analysis to be 0.43 (95% CI 0.39–0.47) and 0.82 (95% CI 0.79–0.84), respectively, and consequently CA19-9 remains the only approved serum diagnostic biomarker.[59] CEA is however frequently measured as part of fluid analysis as part of endoscopic evaluation of pancreatic cysts. A threshold of 192 ng/dL is widely used as a cut-off for diagnosis of mucinous pancreatic cystic lesions; however, CEA levels cannot distinguish benign from malignant cystic lesions.[60,61]

Research into novel biomarkers has moved towards assessing the utility of ctDNA and panels of multiple blood-based markers as diagnostic 'signatures' to boost test sensitivity, as well as the role of microRNAs and genomic or transcriptomic data from biopsies to predict response to therapy.

## HEREDITARY PANCREATIC CANCER

Up to 10% of patients presenting with pancreatic cancer will have a family history with at least one relative with the disease.[62] The genetic basis for the majority of the familial clustering of pancreatic cancer remains unclear; however, several susceptibility genes have been identified which include the DNA repair pathway genes *ATM, BRCA1, BRCA2, PALB2*,[63] genes encoding DNA MMR machinery *MLH1, MSH2, MSH6, PMS2*,[38] germline variants which lead to hereditary pancreatitis *PRSS1, STK11*[64] as well as classic tumour suppressor genes such as *TP53* and *CDKN2A* (also known as p16).[65]

Furthermore, PDAC is observed in a number of hereditary tumour predisposition syndromes, most of which follow an autosomal dominant inheritance (Table 4.1).

Studies have now demonstrated the survival benefit from screening high-risk individuals with a positive family history or known germline mutation status,[66,67] and the International Cancer of the Pancreas Screening (CAPS) consortium have published consensus guidelines which recommend annual surveillance (in the absence of symptoms) commencing from the age of 50 or 10 years earlier than the youngest family member using MRI/MRCP and EUS.[68] Such recommendations are intended to improve the detection of early-stage PDAC and pre-malignant lesions harbouring high-grade dysplasia (PanIN/IPMN) (Table 4.2).

## HEPATOCELLULAR CANCER

### THE HCC GENOME

Molecular profiling is not yet recommended as standard of care in HCC; to date no recurrently observed mutations predict therapeutic clinical response. However, agents that target C-MET and the FGF19/FGFR4 signalling pathways are currently in clinical development in selected patient populations. The most frequently detected alterations in HCC are mutations in the promoter of *TERT* gene (telomerase reverse transcriptase) in 60% of cases, the cell cycle regulator *TP53*, key components of the Wnt signalling pathway (*CTNNB* [β-catenin], *AXIN1* and *AXIN2*), and the chromatin regulators *ARID1A* and *ARID2*.[69,70] As is observed in many solid tumours including PDAC, there are also a large number of low-frequency somatic mutations observed in genes controlling cell proliferation/cell cycle regulation, differentiation, epigenetic regulation, oxidative stress and signalling pathways including TGFβ.[71]

WGS studies have shown that mutations are progressively acquired in hepatocytes following the repeated cycles of injury and repair that ultimately lead to liver cirrhosis, and regenerative nodules arise as clonal expansions of hepatocytes surrounded by bands of 'bridging fibrosis'.[72] Mutations in the *TERT* promoter specifically trigger reactivation of telomerase and thus unrestrained proliferation of hepatocytes/tumour cells and is therefore intimately related to the stepwise development of hepatocarcinogenesis, with one study identifying *TERT* mutations in 6% of low-grade dysplastic nodules, 19% of high-grade dysplastic nodules, 61% of early HCCs and 42% of advanced HCCs (Fig. 4.5).[73]

It has been proposed that different aetiologies of background liver disease predispose to the acquisition of different genetic alterations; for example, there is evidence that alcohol consumption is associated with *CTNNB* mutations; aflatoxin B1 with *TP53* mutations and the *TERT* promoter is a frequent side of insertion for the HBV genome.[75–77] Specific enrichments of mutations have not been identified in HCV, haemochromatosis or NAFLD. These associations are by no means non-overlapping, and the complex interaction between mutational signatures and environmental risk factors remains incompletely understood.

As we have seen in pancreatic cancer, HCC has been similarly classified according to the structural chromosomal rearrangements observed within tumours. A large proportion

**Table 4.1   Inherited tumour predisposition syndromes associated with germline mutations conferring an increased risk of pancreatic ductal adenocarcinoma**

| Tumour predisposition syndrome | Mutation | Inheritance | Phenotype |
|---|---|---|---|
| Peutz-Jeghers syndrome | *STK11* (formerly *LKB1*) | Autosomal dominant | Gastrointestinal hamartomatous polyposis, mucocutaneous pigmentation, increased cancer risk of small bowel, colon, pancreas, lung, testis, ovary, breast, endometrium |
| Familial atypical multiple mole melanoma and pancreatic cancer syndrome (FAMMM) | *CDNK2A* (p16) | Autosomal dominant | Multiple atypical melanocytic naevi, melanoma, pancreas |
| Lynch syndrome (formerly hereditary non-polyposis colorectal cancer, HNPCC) | *MSH2, MLH1, MSH6, PMS, PMS2* | Autosomal dominant | Colon, endometrium, ovary, pancreas, stomach, small bowel, bile duct, gallbladder |
| Breast and ovarian cancer syndrome | *BRCA1, BRCA2, PALB1* | Autosomal dominant | Breast, ovary, colon, prostate, pancreas |
| Ataxic telangiectasia | *ATM* | Autosomal recessive | Progressive ataxia in children, conjunctival telangiectasia, leukaemia, lymphoma, ovary, stomach, brain, colon, pancreas |
| Li-Fraumeni syndrome | *TP53* | Autosomal dominant | Sarcoma, breast, osteosarcoma, leukaemia, glioma, adrenocortical, pancreas |

**Table 4.2** Summary of CAPS Consortium consensus guidelines for screening high-risk individuals for pancreatic cancer. Age, family history and mutation status are the main criteria for determining eligibility for pancreatic surveillance.[68] *Consensus as to when to start surveillance was not reached.

**Who?**

- All patients with Peutz-Jeghers syndrome (carriers of a germline *LKB1/STK11* gene mutation)
- All carriers of a germline *CDKN2A* mutation
- Carriers of a germline *BRCA1, BRCA2, PALB2, ATM, MLH1, MSH2* or *MSH6* gene mutation with at least one affected first-degree blood relative
- Individuals who have at least one first-degree blood relative with pancreatic cancer who in turn also has a first-degree relative with pancreatic cancer (familial pancreatic cancer kindred)

**When (at what age)?**

- Age to initiate surveillance depends on individual's gene mutation status and family history

Familial pancreatic cancer kindred (without a known germline mutation) — Start at age 50 or 55* or 10 years younger than the youngest affected blood relative

Mutation carriers: For *CDKN2A*, Peutz-Jeghers syndrome, start at 40; *BRCA2, ATM, PALB2, BRCA1, MLH1/MSH2* start at age 45 or 50 or 10 years younger than the youngest affected blood relative

- There is no consensus on the age to end surveillance

**How?**

| | |
|---|---|
| At baseline | • MRI/MRCP + EUS + fasting blood glucose and/or HbA1C |
| During follow-up | • Alternate MRI/MRCP + EUS (no consensus how to alternate)<br>• Routinely test fasting blood glucose and/or HbA1c |
| On indication | • Serum CA19-9 — • If concerning features on imaging<br>• EUS-FNA only for — • Solid lesions of ≥ 5 mm<br>• CT only for — • Cystic lesions with worrisome features<br>• Asymptomatic MPD structures (with or without mass)<br>• Solid lesions, regardless of size<br>• Asymptomatic MPD structures of unknown aetiology (without mass) |

**Intervals and surgery**

| | |
|---|---|
| 12 months | • If no abnormalities, or only non-concerning abnormalities (e.g. pancreatic cysts without worrisome features) |
| 3 or 6 months | • If concerning abnormalities for which immediate surgery is not indicated |
| Surgery | • If positive FNA and/or a high suspicion of malignancy on imaging |

- When surgery is indicated, perform an oncological radical resection at a specialty centre

**Goals**

| | |
|---|---|
| The goal of surveillance is to detect and treat the following pathological lesions | • Stage I pancreatic cancer, confined to the pancreas, resected with negative margins<br>• Pancreatic cancer precursor lesions with high-grade dysplasia (PanIN or IPMN) |

*CA19-9,* Carbohydrate antigen 19-9; *CT,* computed tomography; *EUS,* endoscopic ultrasound; *FNA,* fine needle aspirate; *IPMN,* intraductal papillary mucinous neoplasm; *MPD,* main pancreatic duct; *MRCP,* magnetic resonance cholangiopancreatogram; *MRI,* magnetic resonance imaging; *PanIN,* pancreatic intraepithelial neoplasia.

of hepatocytes in the healthy human liver exhibit polyploidy —a condition in which the normally diploid cell acquires one or more additional sets of chromosomes. This is suggested to have arisen as an evolutionary phenomenon that generates genetic diversity within the liver and has been termed the 'ploidy conveyer'.[78] This presence of multiple gene copies within individual hepatocytes appears to be protective against '*loss of function*' mutations, in particular loss of tumour suppressor genes, and '*gain of function*' mutations are therefore proportionally more prevalent in HCC than

in other solid tumours.[74] Aneuploidy (the presence of an abnormal number of chromosomes within a cell) arises due to an increased rate of whole chromosome mis-segregation during mitosis or structural aberrations (translocations or deletions)—a phenomenon known as chromosomal instability (CIN). Aneuploidy is detected in > 90% of HCC, and this karyotypic diversity is thought to confer cells with greater phenotypic variance in terms of response to cytotoxic agents and enhanced tolerance of the accumulation of a greater number of mutations.[79–81]

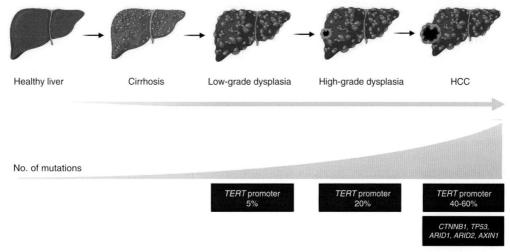

Healthy liver     Cirrhosis     Low-grade dysplasia     High-grade dysplasia     HCC

No. of mutations

TERT promoter
5%

TERT promoter
20%

TERT promoter
40-60%

CTNNB1, TP53,
ARID1, ARID2, AXIN1

**Figure 4.5** The stepwise development of hepatocellular cancer (HCC) in the cirrhotic liver: the development of low-grade through to high-grade dysplastic nodules is associated with the accumulation of somatic mutations. Some, in particular *TERT* mutations, can arise in pre-malignant lesions, whereas others (e.g. *TP53*) are more frequently observed in advanced invasive cancer. (Adapted from [74].)

## HERITABLE PREDISPOSITION TO HCC

HCC rarely arises within a truly healthy liver microenvironment and is generally not observed in cancer predisposition syndromes (case reports exist of HCC arising in patients with germline *APC* mutations and as part of the BAP-1 tumour predisposition syndrome). HCC can occur, however, as the end result of a heritable disorder that accelerates chronic liver disease. Such conditions include haemochromatosis (C282Y mutation of the *HFE* gene), Wilson disease (mutation of the copper transporting gene *ATP7B*), α-antitrypsin deficiency (*SERPINA1* mutation) and metabolic disorders, for example, tyrosinemia (*FAH* mutation).[82]

Biallelic germline mutations in the *HNF1A* gene (hepatocyte nuclear factor 1 alpha) (also known as *TCF1* [transcription factor 1]) are associated with the occurrence of benign hepatocellular adenoma (HCA), which can be numerous, and have potential to transform into HCC.[83] Three molecular subtypes of HCA have been identified based on genomic analyses[84]:

- HCAs inactivated for *HNF1α* (H-HCA) account for 30–40% of HCAs and the majority of patients carry somatic rather than germline mutations. *HNF1α* is a gene required for hepatocyte differentiation, regulating the downstream transcription of other hepatocyte identity genes. These can be differentiated from other types of HCA by the absence of liver fatty acid binding protein (*LFABP*) and morphological steatosis.
- Inflammatory HCAs (I-HCA) account for 40–50% and exhibit a spectrum of somatic mutations, all of which result in downstream activation of the JAK-STAT pathway. They occur in association with alcohol consumption, obesity and the metabolic syndrome.
- β-CATENIN–activated HCAs (β-HCA) account for 10–20% of HCAs and harbour somatic *CTNNB1* mutations in exon 3, 7 or 8. They are proportionately more common in males and have the highest rate of transformation to malignancy.

There is currently no guideline that advocates genomic subtyping of HCAs following pathological assessment;

however, all HCAs > 5 cm that increase in size (≥ 20% in accordance with RECIST criteria), exhibit exophytic protrusion or that arise in men should be considered for resection.[84]

Several single nucleotide polymorphisms (SNPs) have been identified to be associated with HCC development. SNPs are substitutions of single nucleotides at certain positions in the genome that are observed in the general population at a frequency of > 1%. Numerous studies including genome-wide association studies (GWAS) have identified SNPs in genes involved in pathways governing oxidative stress, detoxification, inflammation, DNA repair, cell cycle regulation and hormonal metabolism; however to date, this has not yet led to the implementation of genetic screening strategies.[85]

## FIBROLAMELLAR HEPATOCELLULAR CARCINOMA

Fibrolamellar carcinoma is a well-described but rare variant of HCC observed in adolescents and young adults, most frequently without co-existing liver disease. Its name describes its histological morphology of thick bands of fibrous stroma that surround and embed the epithelial tumour cells. These patients exhibit a higher rate of lymph node metastases and tumours are frequently large at presentation, although curative resection can still be offered in up to 70% of patients. The molecular event driving fibrolamellar HCC is now established as a large segmental (400 kb) deletion on chromosome 19 that results in an 'in-frame' fusion between part of the DnaJ heat shock protein family member B1 gene (*DNAJB1*) and the protein kinase cAMP-activated catalytic subunit alpha gene (*PRKACA*). This signature gene fusion (*DNAJB1-PRKACA*) acts as an oncogenic driver and is required for tumour initiation,[86,87] although this has not yet been exploited therapeutically.

## THE HCC TRANSCRIPTOME

HCC can be divided into two principal classes according to gene expression, each constituting approximately 50% of patients.[88] HCCs of the *low proliferation class* tend to exhibit a well-differentiated morphology and are generally small without satellite nodules or vascular invasion. They include a subclass characterised by high expression of the Wnt/β-catenin signalling (and a higher rate of *TERT* mutations) as well as a subclass with a gene expression profile very close to that of normal liver. These HCCs have been associated with alcohol and HCV aetiologies and tend to have better clinical outcomes.

HCCs of the *high proliferation class* tend to exhibit a more aggressive phenotype, with CIN and overexpression of genes involved in cell survival/proliferation with activation of the PI3K/Akt pathway and *TP53* mutations. Patients with proliferative HCCs tend to have higher serum alpha feto-protein (αFP) levels and tumours are poorly differentiated histologically.[82,89]

*Angiogenesis and anti-angiogenic therapies:* The majority of systemic therapies for advanced HCC target anti-angiogenic pathways. Tumour hypoxia stimulates hypoxia-inducible proteins which upregulate pro-angiogenic factors including vascular endothelial growth factor (VEGF)-A, B, C and D, fibroblast growth factors (FGF), platelet-derived growth factors (PDGF), angiopoietins and hepatocyte growth factor (HGF) which trigger signalling cascades via their respective tyrosine kinase receptors in the cancerous endothelium. This stimulates intracellular signalling via MAPK or PI3K/Akt/mTor to sustain endothelial cell survival signals and promote proliferation. The result is dysregulated vessel growth and maturation leading to disordered and fragile vascularity (Fig. 4.6).[90]

*First-line agents:* The oral multi-tyrosine kinase inhibitor (TKI) sorafenib which targets VEGFRs (1, 2 and 3), PDGFR-β, RAF-1 and B-RAF has been the cornerstone of systemic therapy in HCC for more than a decade.[92] The phase III SHARP trial comparing sorafenib with placebo demonstrated survival benefit in patients with advanced disease (median OS

10.7 vs 7.9 months; HR 0.69 95% CI 0.55–0.87; $P < 0.001$).[93] A modest survival benefit was also seen in a parallel phase III trial in Asian patients, principally with HBV-related HCC.[94] The greatest responses are observed in patients with disease confined to the liver and to those with HCV-aetiology. Toxicities of sorafenib include hand-foot syndrome, diarrhoea, weight loss and hypophosphataemia, and 10–15% of patients eventually become intolerant to the drug. European Association for the Study of the Liver (EASL) and European Society for Medical Oncology (ESMO) guidelines continue to recommend sorafenib as first-line therapy in patients who have well-preserved liver function (Child-Pugh A) with Barcelona Clinic Liver Cancer (BCLC) stage C disease or stage B disease who have progressed on locoregional therapy.[95]

Lenvatinib is a multi-kinase inhibitor with activity against VEGFR1, 2 and 3, FGFR1, 2, 3 and 4, PDGFRα, RET and c-Kit, and has been tested against sorafenib in a phase III non-inferiority randomised controlled trial of patients with treatment-naïve, unresectable HCC.[96] A total of 954 patients were randomised across 20 countries, with a median OS of 13.6 months (95% CI 12.1–14.9) seen in the lenvatinib arm, which was statistically non-inferior to 12.3 months (95% CI 10.4–13.9) in the sorafenib arm, and with superior secondary endpoints including objective response, time to disease progression and progression-free survival (PFS). Common adverse events in the lenvatinib group were diarrhoea, hypertension, weight loss, reduced weight and fatigue. This trial excluded patients with > 50% liver occupancy or main portal vein invasion and therefore some have argued this cohort had less advanced disease than in some other trials. Lenvatinib is recommended as an alternative first-line option for systemic therapy in advanced HCC.[97]

*Second-line agents:* Regorafenib is a multi-kinase inhibitor that targets VEGFR, C-KIT, RET, B-RAF, PDGFR and FGFR1.

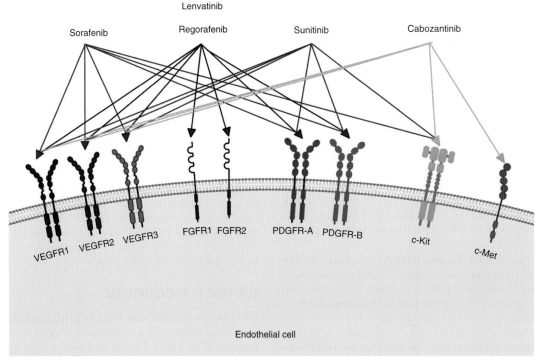

**Figure 4.6**    Receptor targets of anti-angiogenic tyrosine kinase inhibitors in hepatocellular cancer. (Adapted from [91].)

It was the first agent to demonstrate survival benefit in patients who have progressed on sorafenib, shown in 573 patients with well-preserved liver function in the phase III RESORCE trial.[98] Patients in the regorafenib arm demonstrated median OS of 10.6 months (95% CI 9.1–12.1) compared with 7.7 months for patients receiving placebo (95% CI 6.3–8.8). Regorafenib is now the standard of care in patients who have tolerated sorafenib but whose disease has progressed.

Cabozantinib targets c-Met in addition to VEGFR, C-KIT, RET, FLT-3, Tie2 and Axl receptors. Following the results of the phase III CELESTIAL trial, it can be considered for use in patients who have progressed on one or two systemic therapies but continue to exhibit well-preserved liver function and good performance status.[99]

Unlike the TKIs discussed above which are small molecules, ramucirumab (RAM) is a monoclonal antibody targeted to VEGFR2. The REACH trial (ramucirumab versus placebo as second-line treatment) failed to show an improvement in OS except in a subgroup of patients with an αFP > 400 ng/mL.[100] The REACH-2 trial has demonstrated a survival benefit in patients who have progressed on or are intolerant of sorafenib with an αFP > 400 ng/mL.[101]

## IMMUNOBIOLOGY AND IMMUNOTHERAPY

HCC is a prototypical cancer arising from an inflammatory microenvironment: HCC in the absence of cirrhosis or chronic liver disease is rare. The liver is a key anatomical site of immune recognition and its low-pressure sinusoids are the largest reticuloendothelial system in the human body. Liver sinusoidal endothelial cells (LSECs) are able to present antigen and activate the adaptive immune response as well as dampen immunogenicity and induce tolerance by downregulation of MHC class II and production of anti-inflammatory cytokines.[102] It has been established that infiltration of CD8+ and CD4+ T cells is associated with OS and PFS in HCC, but these cells become 'exhausted' and regulatory T cells begin to accumulate with disease progression and/or metastasis.[103] Co-expression of multiple tumour-associated antigens (TAAs) including αFP, EpCAM, GPC3 in HCC is associated with favourable differentiation status, smaller tumour size, greater NK cell and B cell infiltration (which drive anti-tumour immunity) and enhanced survival.[104]

Conventional systemic chemotherapy has proven ineffective against HCC, with no survival benefit observed after treatment with FOLFOX (fluorouracil/leucovorin/oxaliplatin), doxorubicin or gemcitabine.[105] Given the success of immune checkpoint inhibitors in other cancer types, trials have rapidly extended to HCC and immunotherapy is now recommended for consideration in patients who are intolerant to or have progressed on TKIs.[97]

*Monotherapy:* The fully human anti-CTLA-4 monoclonal antibody tremelimumab was the first immune checkpoint inhibitor to be tested in HCC, but effects on survival were modest and large phase III studies of this and other anti-CTLA4 agents as monotherapy have not yet been undertaken, leaving their efficacy undetermined.[106]

The human anti-PD1 monoclonal antibody nivolumab was assessed as monotherapy by the non-comparative CheckMate-040 phase I/II trial which demonstrated acceptable

safety profiles and objective response rates (ORR) of 20% in sorafenib-naïve/intolerant patients or sorafenib progressors.[107] The follow-up CheckMate-459 trial comparing nivolumab with sorafenib as first-line therapy in unresectable HCC failed to demonstrate superiority.[108] Keynote-224 and Keynote-240 were phase II and III trials, respectively, comparing the humanised anti-PD-1 monoclonal antibody pembrolizumab against placebo in sorafenib-intolerant patients or patients who had progressed on sorafenib.[109,110] In Keynote-240, 413 patients with Child's A cirrhosis received treatment for up to 35 cycles or until interruption due to progression or unacceptable toxicity. Improvements were seen in the co-primary endpoints of OS (HR = 0.78, 95% CI 0.61–0.99, P = 0.0238) and PFS (HR = 0.78, 95% CI 0.61–0.99, P = 0.0209); however, these did not meet the pre-specified statistical threshold for significance of an OS of 0.65 due to longer than predicted survival in the placebo group. This was thought to be due to use of several drugs approved during the study period including nivolumab and regorafenib in the placebo group following disease progression. Pembrolizumab is advocated by ESMO for second-line treatment for patients who progress on or are intolerant of sorafenib.[97]

Studies looking at anti-programmed death ligand 1 (PD-L1) agents as monotherapy in HCC have included a phase I/II studies of the monoclonal antibodies durvalumab and avelumab as second-line therapies following progression or intolerance of sorafenib. These have demonstrated an acceptable safety profile and promising survival data.[111,112]

*Combination therapy:* There is much interest in using combination therapy to enable the targeting of multiple co-inhibitory receptors to enhance the clinical response. Dual immune checkpoint blockade aims to combine PD-1 and CTLA-4 inhibition as has been successfully seen in melanoma and non-small cell lung cancer. A subgroup analysis of data from the Checkpoint-040 study was undertaken to assess the safety and efficacy of nivolumab (anti-PD1) and ipilimumab (anti-CTLA) in combination. The rate of adverse events was 37%, however the discontinuation rate for toxicity was just 5%. The ORR of 31% compared favourably to ORR for nivolumab monotherapy from the same study (14%).[113] Similarly, encouraging phase I/II results from combination durvalumab (anti-PDL1) and tremelimumab (anti-CTLA4) have led to the opening of the phase III HIMALAYA trial which aims to enrol 1054 participants and will complete in 2022.

The IMbrave150 phase III trial randomised 501 patients with treatment-naïve advanced HCC to receive either atezolizumab (humanised monoclonal antibody to PD-L1) in combination with bevacizumab (monoclonal antibody targeting VEGF-A) or sorafenib until unacceptable toxicity was encountered or loss of clinical benefit.[114] Intention to treat analysis demonstrated a hazard ratio for death of 0.58 (95% CI 0.42–0.79, P = <0.001) in the atezolizumab/bevacizumab arm, with OS at 12 months of 67.2% (95% CI 61.3–73.1) compared with 54.6% (95% CI 45.2–64.0) in the sorafenib arm. The rate of adverse events was similar in both groups. The combination of atezolizumab and bevacizumab significantly improved both of the co-primary endpoints of OS and PFS and is now licensed as a first-line therapy option in patients with untreated advanced HCC. It should be noted that approximately 70% of patients in both arms of this study had a

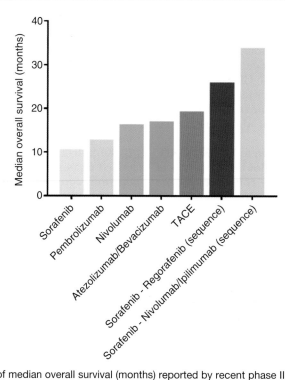

**Figure 4.7**   Schematic representation of median overall survival (months) reported by recent phase III trials of systemic therapies in advanced hepatocellular cancer (note that trial populations are heterogenous and should not be directly compared).

background of viral hepatitis. Non-viral HCC, and especially non-alcoholic steatohepatitis (NASH) HCC, might be less responsive to immunotherapy, probably owing to NASH-related aberrant T-cell activation causing tissue damage that leads to impaired immune surveillance.[115] The LEAP-002 study seeks to test combination lenvatinib with pembrolizumab in BCLC stage B or C patients not amenable to locoregional therapy, which has also shown promising results in phase I.[116]

Excitingly, it has been predicted that combining immunotherapy with existing locoregional treatments might offer potential for synergistic effects on tumour cell death through enhancing tumour-specific antigen release and presentation via dendritic cells (DCs).[117,118] A proof-of-concept study in 30 patients combined the anti-CTLA-4 agent tremelimumab with radiofrequency ablation and demonstrated a partial response with reduction in HCV viral load, a clear increase in CD8+ T cells and improvement in PFS.[119] Clinical trials are now underway to evaluate the use of TACE with nivolumab (TACE-3 study) or TACE with atezolizumab/bevacizumab combination therapy (DEMAND study).[120] It is predicted that systemic therapy is likely to soon exceed the survival benefits of TACE and some have advocated the use of immunotherapy first line in order to identify patients with treatment-resistant disease early on who would gain the most benefit from TACE.[121] Indeed, studies are now examining the role of immunotherapy in early disease; for example the currently recruiting KEYNOTE-937 trial aims to evaluate the efficacy of adjuvant pembrolizumab following surgical resection or ablation (Fig. 4.7).[122]

## CELL THERAPY

As an even more sophisticated strategy to therapeutically target tumour neoantigens, 'immune primers' such as ilixadencel have been developed consisting of monocyte-derived allogeneic DCs which have been stimulated with a combination of pro-inflammatory cytokines and can be injected intra-tumorally to stimulate recruitment of immune cells. Such agents either as monotherapy or in combination with sorafenib or other agents are in early-phase trials.[123]

Furthermore, genetically engineered T-cell-based immunotherapies including CAR-T cells (chimeric antigen receptor) and SPEAR-T cells (specific peptide enhanced affinity receptor, TCR) targeting HCC tumour antigens including αFP, EpCAM and GPC3, are in early development with initially promising results.[124,125]

## BILIARY TRACT CANCER

BTC is a term that encompasses the spectrum of cancers arising from the intrahepatic biliary tree (intrahepatic cholangiocarcinoma, ICC), the gallbladder (gallbladder cancer, GBC) and the extrahepatic bile ducts (extrahepatic cholangiocarcinoma, ECC) which includes both perihilar or 'Klatskin' tumours (pCCA) and the distal bile ducts (dCCA). There is increasing clinical and molecular evidence that these cancers behave and respond to treatment very differently, and the design of clinical trials for new therapies is beginning to take account of such differences. Although previously considered rare, the incidence of BTC is increasing, principally due to a rise in ICC, and the majority (>65%) are unresectable at presentation. In patients who are treated with curative surgery, there is a high rate of relapse and therefore OS rates remain very poor (5–15%).

## THE BTC GENOME

It is only in the last decade that the NGS technology has been applied to BTC. Arguably, the most significant discoveries have been the identification of mutations in the isocitrate dehydrogenase genes (*IDH1* and *IDH2*) and the fibroblast growth factor receptor 2 gene, (*FGFR2*), both of which represent clinically 'druggable' targets. These mutations arise at similar frequencies, are seen most commonly in intrahepatic tumours (15–20% ICC), but appear to be for the most part non-overlapping. IDH1 and IDH2 are cytoplasmic enzymes involved in cellular metabolism and NADPH generation, which when mutated, result in the production of an 'oncometabolite', 2-hydroxyglutarate (2-HG).[126] In the FGFR2 locus on chromosome 10, translocation events occur at a consistent breakpoint, resulting in the fusion of the disrupted FGFR2 gene with several gene partners (*BICC1*, *PPHLN1*, *TACC3*, *MGEA5*) and gain of function with activation of oncogenic signalling; the precise mechanisms of which are the subject of ongoing research.[127,128] ICC also appears to exhibit a propensity for mutations in the epigenetic regulator *BAP1* and the ephrin receptor *EPHA2*. Integrative analyses have demonstrated a degree of mutation clustering in BTC; for example, an association has been observed between *FGFR2* fusions and *BAP1* mutations.[129] Patients with this mutational profile appear to exhibit more indolent disease and a more favourable prognosis.[130]

Mutations in the classical oncogene *KRAS* and tumour suppressor *TP53* are observed in all subtypes of BTC.[131] ECC and GBC appear to exhibit a propensity for developing aberrations in the HER gene family, especially the ERBB receptors, fusion events in the protein kinases *PRKACA* and *PRKACB* and, as is observed in ampullary cancer, mutations in the epithelial tumour suppressor *ELF3*.[132] Finally, a wide range of mutations are observed with low frequency in genes associated with kinase signalling (*BRAF*, *PTEN*, *PIK3CA*, *STK11*), DNA damage (*CDKN2A*, *CCND1*, *ROBO2*, *BRCA1*, *BRCA2*), epigenetic regulation (*ARID1A*, *ARID1B*, *ARID2*, *MLL2*, *MML3*), Wnt signalling (*RNF43*, *CTNNB1*, *APC*) and Hippo signalling *NF2*) (Fig. 4.8).[133]

Genomic studies have revealed not only the molecular differences between tumours arising at different anatomical sites but also differences according to aetiology. As discussed in Chapter 14, a significant proportion of the worldwide burden of BTC arises secondary to chronic inflammatory states associated with biliary parasites (*Clonorchis sinensis*, *Opisthorchis viverrini*) or hepatolithiasis. These tumours exhibit a higher mutational rate than the sporadic disease seen in the West (median 4700 mutations per tumour vs 3143) and show a higher frequency of mutations in the tumour suppressors and cell cycle regulators *BAP1* and *TP53*, the regulator of TGFβ signalling *SMAD4*, and amplifications in *ERBB2* (also known as *HER2*).[131,134,135]

## THE BTC EPIGENOME

The discovery in BTC of somatic mutations in genes whose functions include regulation at the epigenetic level including, *IDH1/2*, *KMT2C*, *ARID1A* and *BAP1*, has been striking. Such events influence multiple cellular processes affecting heritable information including DNA and RNA modification, miRNA biogenesis, histone modification and chromatin remodelling.[129,136] Methylation is the most common DNA modification and we now know this is one of the earliest events in tumorigenesis. Methyl groups are enzymatically transferred to CpG dinucleotides, so-called 'CpG islands' and these domains co-localise with various regulatory elements to modulate transcription. An association has been observed between liver fluke–associated BTC and CpG island hypermethylation, with fluke-negative BTCs associated with hypermethylation of CpG shores (regions of the genome immediately flanking CpG islands).[131] Fluke-associated

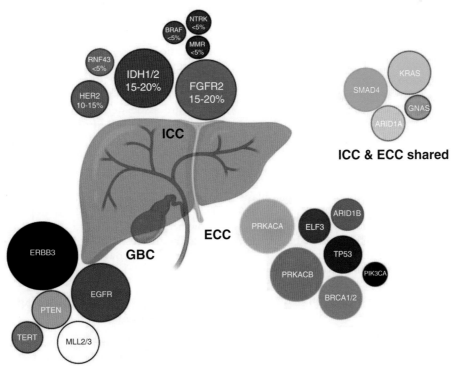

**Figure 4.8** Frequency of targetable mutations in biliary tract cancer vary by anatomical location. (Adapted from [24].) *ECC*, Extrahepatic cholangiocarcinoma; *GBC*, gallbladder cancer; *ICC*, intrahepatic cholangiocarcinoma.

BTCs also have higher mutation rates, downregulation of the DNA demethylation enzyme TET1 and upregulation of the histone modification enzyme EZH2, suggesting that early inflammatory events cause epigenetic dysregulation. This is important as epigenetic signatures might offer potential for exploitation as future diagnostic markers in early disease or in patients at high risk. In sporadic disease, genome-wide methylation analyses have so far identified differentially methylated regions in promoters of genes associated with the Wnt, TGFβ and PI3K signalling pathways.[137]

ncRNAs are key regulators of the transcriptome, which are themselves not transcribed into protein, but which nonetheless affect a huge variety of cellular systems. They include both long non-coding RNAs (lncRNAs), which are generally involved in repression of transcription and small ncRNAs, which include microRNAs (miRNAs) and small interfering RNAs (siRNAs). Of these, miRNAs are the best studied in BTC and in particular high levels of miR-21 have been identified in patient tissue and serum.[138] Conflicting data exist on the role played by the miR-200 family, with both oncogenic and tumour suppressive roles suggested in different patient cohorts and systems, which may reflect the ability for miRNAs to assume differing roles depending on cellular context.[139,140] Comprehensive large-scale 'RNome' studies are awaited and the complex role of these species on BTC pathogenesis is yet to be fully elucidated.

## THE BTC TRANSCRIPTOME

Whole transcriptome analyses have classified BTC into two phenotypes: 'inflammatory' (38%) or 'proliferative' (62%), depending on whether enrichment of inflammatory or oncogenic pathways are observed.[141] Patients who exhibit a proliferative transcriptional subtype appear to have a reduced OS (24.3 months vs 47.2 months, $P = 0.048$) compared to those with the inflammation expression pattern. A number of molecular signalling pathways are upregulated in BTC and have established pre-clinical and translational evidence to support them as key drivers of the disease. The best described of these are Notch, Wnt, PI3K/AKT, IL-6, EGFR/HER, Hedgehog and Hippo-Yap.

The Notch signalling pathway is a highly conserved cell-to-cell regulator that controls cell proliferation, differentiation and the maintenance of stem cell populations. Named after the 'notched' appearance seen on the wings of *Drosophila* following genetic deletion, this pathway is a critical regulator of the embryonic development of the bile ducts in mammals. Notch plays two key roles in this context: first, it induces ductal differentiation of bipotential hepatoblasts in the embryonic liver, inducing cells to a biliary/cholangiocyte (rather than hepatocyte) phenotype[142]; second, later in development it stimulates branching of the biliary tree, enabling the arborisation of the developing ductular network.[143] During liver injury in the adult liver, Notch signalling can be reactivated in bipotential liver progenitor cells to induce cholangiocyte differentiation for repair in biliary disease.[144] It is therefore unsurprising that Notch is also upregulated in BTC and it has been shown that it is wild-type signalling that is driving disease: Notch receptors and their ligands are not mutated. Notch pathway expression correlates with cancer progression and poor survival, and genetic overexpression and deletion studies have shown that the Notch 1 and Notch 3 receptors are the key mediators of this effect.[145,146] This pathway has proven challenging to target pharmacologically, but inhibitors of gamma-secretase (an enzyme complex required for effecting Notch signalling) show some promise and clinical trials are underway.[147]

Wnt signalling, a further tightly controlled molecular pathway key to the regulation of embryonic development and adult tissue homeostasis, is frequently aberrant in solid tumours. This is archetypally described in colorectal cancer whereby mutational inactivation of the adenomatous polyposis coli (APC) tumour suppressor leads to disruption of the β-catenin destruction complex, β-catenin accumulation and unopposed pathway activation. In BTC, the β-catenin gene CTNNB1, and other pathway mutations e.g. in APC are infrequent; more commonly, wild-type Wnt signalling is activated through release of Wnt ligands by tumour-associated macrophages in the cancer stroma or DNA methylation of Wnt pathway components e.g. SOX17.[148,149] Pharmacological Wnt inhibitors targeting Wnt ligands (including inhibitors of the enzyme Porcupine that drives Wnt ligand secretion), frizzled receptors and β-catenin have shown efficacy in preclinical models and are being explored in clinical trials.

The Hippo-Yap pathway is a regulator of mammalian organ size and genetic overexpression of YAP results in dramatic overgrowth of the liver.[150] As with Notch and Wnt, mutations of this pathway are uncommon (5% exhibit mutations in Salvador and 3% in NF2),[129] but increased wild-type YAP signalling is seen in BTC, thought to be triggered by proliferative signals from the tumour stroma including IL-6, PDGF and FGF. Furthermore, YAP expression appears to correlate with worse clinical outcomes. As we have seen in other evolutionarily conserved pathways, safe pharmacological targeting without excess toxicity can be problematic due to the ubiquity of these signals in tissue homeostasis and in this case the therapeutic approach has been to target other pathways known to interact with YAP such as FGFR inhibition.[151]

Upregulation of numerous pathways involved in inflammation and fibrosis have been described in BTC, promoting cholangiocarcinogenesis through tumour-stromal interactions. A plethora of inflammatory cytokine and chemokines are found in the desmoplastic stroma and many are associated with poor clinical outcomes.[152] IL-6, the best characterised of these, is found at high levels in the blood and bile of patients with BTC and is directly mitogenic to biliary epithelia through its downstream effector STAT3 as well as supporting tumour growth through methylation of several genes including EGFR.[153] CAFs secrete paracrine factors including IL-1ß, stromal cell-derived factor 1 (SDF-1), PDGF and heparin-binding epidermal growth factor (HB-EGF).[154] Finally, accumulation of bile acids themselves, although not directly carcinogenic, promotes tumour growth through bile duct proliferation and inflammation.[155]

## MICROSATELLITE INSTABILITY AND IMMUNOTHERAPY

Patients with the worst prognosis in BTC exhibit high mutational load and an abundance of tumour-specific neoantigens; the so-called 'MSI phenotype'.[128] Expression of immune checkpoint molecules including PD-L1, which repress the host immune response against tumour cells, has been shown to be highest in this group. One study examining 1502 BTCs concluded that ICCs and GBCs have stronger expression of immune checkpoint molecules and greater mutational burden than ECCs.[157] This suggests that at least a subgroup of patients with BTC might be susceptible to immunotherapy with a potential opportunity for targeting.

Phase II clinical trials have evaluated immune checkpoint blockade with pembrolizumab monotherapy in patients exhibiting MMR deficiency (arising either genetically, in patients with Lynch syndrome, or sporadically, in patients who have acquired somatic mutations in, or epigenetic silencing of one of the four MMR genes). Studies including patients with non-colorectal MMR-deficient tumours including biliary tract have demonstrated an encouraging responsiveness to anti-PD1 blockade as measured by biochemical (Ca19-9) and radiological response.[158] The PD-L1 inhibitor nivolumab has been trialled in 54 patients with BTC and has shown modest response rates (independent ORR 11%); however, all responders were found to express PD-L1 and demonstrated prolonged PFS.[159] A host of trials are therefore now underway evaluating immunotherapy in combination with existing chemotherapy regimens or other immunotherapy agents.[160]

## PRECISION ONCOLOGY IN BTC

The above evidence indicates that 40% of patients with BTC harbour a genetic alteration that is clinically targetable with a currently available therapeutic.[128] This is of particular importance in a cancer in which the survival benefits of both adjuvant and palliative chemotherapy continue to remain modest.[161,162] Ivosidenib is an oral selective reversible inhibitor of mutant IDH1 and has been evaluated in patients with advanced IDH1 mutant BTC in phase I studies and the phase III 'ClarIDHy' trial.[164,165] These have demonstrated significantly improved PFS (median 2.7 months for ivosidenib vs 1.4 months placebo), with 32% of ivosidenib-treated patients progression free at 6 months and low rates of toxicity. Regulatory approval is awaited for use of ivosidenib after ineffective standard therapy in patients with advanced IDH-mutant BTC.

FGFR translocation events (fusions or rearrangements, which occur in 20% of ICCs) can be targeted using inhibitors of FGFR1-3 which can be either ATP-competitive, reversible inhibitors (erdafitinib, infigratinib, pemigatinib, derazantinib) or non-ATP covalent inhibitors (futibatinib). The phase II 'FIGHT-202' study of pemigatinib in treatment refractory advanced BTC demonstrated disease stabilisation or regression in patients with FGFR rearrangements/fusions; with a response rate of 35.5% and median PFS of 6.9 months.[166] Trials of infigratinib have shown similar response rates (31%) and median PFS (6.8 months).[167] Such agents are associated with some toxicities, including hyperphosphataemia (which may require pre-emptive phosphate binders), fatigue and ophthalmological adverse events. Pemigatinib has now been approved by the Food and Drug Administration and the European Commission for advanced or metastatic BTC with confirmed FGFR rearrangement which has progressed on first-line therapy. Trials are underway to evaluate the role of these drugs as first line agents in treatment-naïve disease, comparing for example pemigatinib with gemcitabine/cisplatin in the 'FIGHT-302' phase III study.[168] In addition to translocations and fusions, it is worth remembering that FGFR2 point mutations can arise as resistance mutations following therapy with ATP-competitive inhibitors and here non-ATP covalent inhibitors such as futibatinib may play a role for acquired resistance.

A total of 5% of patients with ICC harbour BRAF-V600 mutations. BRAF inhibitors are well-studied using 'basket trials'—clinical trials testing new drug(s)/agent(s) in patients who have different types of cancer all with the same mutation or biomarker and include patients with BTC. Exclusive to BTC, the 'ROAR study' has evaluated the safety and efficacy of combination BRAF inhibitor dabrafenib and MEK inhibitor trametinib. An ORR of 51% was seen with a manageable safety profile.[169]

Finally, the neurotrophic receptor kinase (NRK)1-3 is known to undergo fusion events in BTC (3.5%) leading to constitutively acting, ligand-independent signalling.[170] These can be targeted with the TRK inhibitors, entrectinib and larotrectinib, as has been done in basket studies which have included patients with BTC, including the STARTRK-2 study which is yet to report.[171]

## FUTURE DIRECTIONS

The above molecular characterisations illustrate the achievements that have been attained in advancing our understanding of the biology of hepatopancreatobiliary cancers and the rapidly evolving nature of this field. In particular, the use of immunotherapy in HCC and 'precision' or target-directed, individualised treatments in PDAC and BTC are beginning to change the landscape of therapies available to the HPB MDT and as more phase III trials report, we can have real optimism in seeing significant improvements in the outcomes of these patients.

> ## Key points
>
> - 'Precision oncology' aims to identify somatic mutations present in an individual's tumour that can be specifically targeted with pharmacological agents to deliver 'personalised' anti-cancer treatment.
> - Pancreatic ductal adenocarcinoma (PDAC) can be classified according to the functional pathways of somatic mutations identified and/or structural rearrangements of chromosomal abnormalities present.
> - Surgical resection should be offered to patients with hepatic adenomas (HCAs) considered 'high risk' (HCAs > 5 cm, increase in size ≥ 20%, exhibit exophytic protrusion or arising in men).
> - Immunotherapies are currently being trialled and show promising initial results in the treatment of patients with advanced HCC.
> - Biliary tract cancer (BTC) exhibits different mutational profiles according to the site of disease and shows much promise for developing targeted precision therapy.

*Images created in* BioRender.com.

 References available at http://ebooks.health.elsevier.com/

# 5 Benign liver lesions

Marcel den Dulk | Cornelius H.C. Dejong

## INTRODUCTION

Benign liver tumours are common and frequently found coincidentally. Most benign liver lesions are asymptomatic, although larger lesions can cause non-specific complaints such as vague abdominal pain. Although rare, some of the benign lesions, e.g. large hepatic adenomas, can cause complications such as rupture or bleeding.

Ultrasound, computed tomography (CT), magnetic resonance imaging (MRI), and positron emission tomography (PET)-CT of the liver are the routine imaging modalities for the liver. Ultrasound is often a good screening investigation and can differentiate a cystic from a solid lesion. CT (with contrast enhancement) and MRI can be used to study the number and size of lesions, and often provide further characterisation of lesions. However, even with these imaging modalities, it may be challenging to differentiate between a benign liver lesion, such as a hepatic adenoma, and a malignancy, such as a well-differentiated hepatocellular carcinoma. Liver biopsies are in general only undertaken if there is doubt about the diagnosis and if results of the biopsy could influence the management strategy.

Asymptomatic lesions are often managed conservatively by observation. Surgical resection can be performed for symptomatic lesions or when there is a risk of malignant transformation. The type of resection is variable, from small, simple, peripheral resections or enucleations, to large resections or even liver transplantation for severe polycystic liver disease (PLD). Historically liver resections were performed as open operations, whereas nowadays many interventions are performed as laparoscopic or sometimes as robotic procedures.

This chapter will focus on the description of benign liver lesions in the normal liver. These lesions can be classified by their origin, as is shown in Table 5.1.

## HEPATOCELLULAR LIVER LESIONS

### FOCAL NODULAR HYPERPLASIA

#### GENERAL
Focal nodular hyperplasia (FNH) is the second commonest benign solid liver tumour, with a prevalence of approximately 0.2%.[1] It has a higher incidence in females, mainly between 20 and 40 years of age, but also occurs in men and even in children. It is a rare finding in children but is more commonly observed after treatment for childhood cancer, with haematopoietic stem cell transplantation as the most important risk factor. Because of the predominant occurrence in females and the young age at onset, a role for female hormones has been suggested, but a relationship with oral contraceptives has not been clearly demonstrated.[2] In men, the lesions are often smaller and less typical.[3]

#### CLINICAL PRESENTATION
FNH lesions are often asymptomatic and found during imaging for unrelated reasons.[4] However, a small proportion of patients experience symptoms such as abdominal pain or a palpable mass.[3] In up to 20%, other liver lesions are found, such as hepatic haemangiomata or adenomas.[3] Although FNH is commonly observed, complications are very rare; there are only a few published cases of spontaneous rupture resulting in intraperitoneal haemorrhage.

#### DIAGNOSIS
Ultrasound is often the initial imaging investigation when a hepatic lesion is found. There is only a subtle difference in echogenicity between FNH and the surrounding normal liver.[5] Although the accuracy of the diagnosis increases with the use of contrast-enhanced ultrasound and colour Doppler, ultrasound is currently not the modality of choice for characterisation of an FNH.

On CT, FNH is usually homogeneous and isoattenuating to the normal liver before contrast injection. FNH lesions are hypervascular in the arterial phase and typically have a central scar (hypodense).[5] In the portal phase, a typical FNH returns to isoattenuating compared to the normal liver.[5] In the delayed phase, hyperattenuation of the central scar and septae are often seen.

MRI has a higher sensitivity (70%) and specificity (98%) for FNH than ultrasonography or CT.[6] Typically, FNH is iso- or hypointense on T1-weighted images, is slightly hyper- or isointense on T2-weighted images, and has a hyperintense central scar on T2-weighted images (Fig. 5.1). A typical FNH demonstrates intense homogeneous enhancement during the arterial phase of gadolinium-enhanced imaging and enhancement of the central scar during later phases.[6]

#### PATHOLOGY
FNH is typically a lobulated lesion composed of nodules surrounded by fibrous septa originating from a central scar in an otherwise normal liver (Fig. 5.1).[6] On histological analysis, a classic FNH shows nodular hyperplastic parenchyma. The hepatic plates may be moderately thickened (two or three cells in thickness) with normal-appearing hepatocytes. The central scar contains fibrous connective tissue,

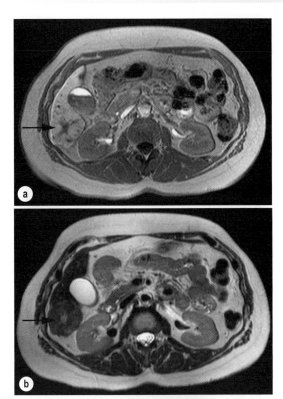

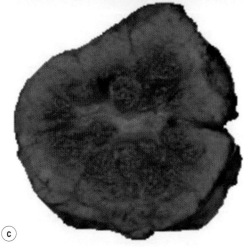

**Table 5.1   Classification of benign liver lesions by their origin**

| Hepatocellular | Focal nodular hyperplasia |
| | Hepatocellular adenoma |
| | Nodular regenerative hyperplasia |
| | Dysplastic nodules |
| Cholangiocellular | Bile duct cysts (simple or polycystic) |
| | Mucinous biliary cystadenoma |
| | Bile duct adenoma (biliary hamartoma/ Von Meyenburg complexes) |
| | Intraductal papillary neoplasm of the bile duct |
| Mesenchymal | Cavernous haemangioma |
| | Lipoma |
| | Angiolipoma |
| Inflammatory | Hepatic abscess (pyogenic, amoebic) |
| | Hydatid cysts |
| Others | Mesenchymal hamartoma |
| | Focal fatty infiltration |
| | Hepatic pseudotumours |

**Figure 5.1**  Focal nodular hyperplasia (FNH) caudal in the right liver lobe (segment 6). On MRI T1-weighted images **(a)** late phase after Primovist administration, FNH may be iso- to hypointense on T1, with a hypointense central scar, indicated by an *arrow*. On the T2-weighted images **(b)**, the FNH is mainly slightly hyper- to isointense, with a hyperintense scar, indicated by an *arrow*. A cross-sectional image of the resection specimen of the same patient is seen in **(c)**, showing the central scar.

that triggers a response from hepatic stellate cells to produce the typical central scar.[7]

## MANAGEMENT

In general, the diagnosis can be made on MRI or CT, and routine biopsy is not indicated.[7] However, when imaging is not typical or if there is doubt about the diagnosis, e.g. with a differential diagnosis of hepatic adenoma or hepatocellular adenocarcinoma, a biopsy can be considered. FNH is currently not considered premalignant.[5]

In asymptomatic patients with typical features of FNH on imaging, no further treatment or follow-up is required. However, further evaluation is recommended for symptomatic lesions when the diagnosis cannot be firmly established. The current American College of Gastroenterology guidelines recommend follow-up with an annual ultrasound for 2–3 years in women diagnosed with FNH who wish to continue using oral contraceptives. In individuals with a firm diagnosis of FNH who are not using oral contraceptives, follow-up imaging is not required.[7]

✓ The diagnosis of FNH can be made on MRI or CT, and routine biopsy is not indicated. However, when imaging is not typical or if there is doubt about the diagnosis, e.g. with a differential diagnosis of hepatic adenoma or hepatocellular adenocarcinoma, biopsy can be an option. FNH is not a precursor of malignancy. In asymptomatic patients with typical features of FNH on imaging, no further treatment or follow-up is required. However, further evaluation is recommended for symptomatic lesions in which the diagnosis cannot be firmly established.

## HEPATOCELLULAR ADENOMA

### GENERAL

Hepatocellular adenomas (HCAs) are rare benign hepatic neoplasms in otherwise normal livers, with a prevalence of around 0.04% on abdominal imaging.[1] HCAs are predominantly found in women of child-bearing age (second to fourth decade) with a history of oral contraceptive use; they

cholangiolar proliferation with surrounding inflammatory infiltrates and malformed vessels of varying calibre, including tortuous arteries with thickened walls and capillaries, but no portal veins. Approximately 50% of lesions show some degree of fatty infiltration compared with the surrounding liver. In less than 20% of FNH lesions, the liver shows signs of steatosis.[6]

The development of FNH is thought to be caused by an injury to the portal tract resulting in the formation and enlargement of arterial to venous shunts.[7] This in turn causes hyperperfusion in local arteries resulting in oxidative stress occur less frequently in men.[8,9] The association between oral contraceptive usage and HCA is strong, and the risk for HCA increases if an oral contraceptive with high hormonal potency is used, and if it is used for over 20 months. Long-term users of oral contraceptives have an estimated annual incidence of HCA of 3–4 per 100,000.[8] More recently, an increase in incidence in men has been reported, probably related to the increase in obesity, which is reported as another risk factor for developing HCA. In addition, anabolic steroid usage by body builders and metabolic disorders such as diabetes mellitus or glycogen storage disease type I are associated with HCAs. HCAs in men are generally smaller but have a higher risk of malignant transformation.

In the majority of patients, HCAs are solitary, but in a minority of patients more than 10 lesions have been described (also referred to as liver adenomatosis).

## CLINICAL PRESENTATION

Small HCAs are often asymptomatic and found on abdominal imaging being undertaken for other purposes, during abdominal surgery or at autopsy. Some patients present with abdominal discomfort, fullness or (right upper quadrant) pain due to an abdominal mass. It is not uncommon that the initial symptoms of an HCA are acute onset of abdominal pain and hypovolaemic shock due to intraperitoneal rupture. In a series of patients who underwent resection, bleeding was reported in up to 25%.[10,11] The risk of rupture is related to the size of the adenoma.[11] Exophytic lesions (protruding from the liver) have a higher chance of bleeding than intrahepatic or subcapsular lesions (67% vs 11% and 19%, respectively, $P < 0.001$).[12] Lesions in segments II and III are also at higher risk of bleeding than lesions in the right liver (35% vs 19%, respectively, $P = 0.049$).

## DIAGNOSIS

HCAs are often detected first by ultrasound during investigation of right upper quadrant discomfort. The high lipid content of adenomas may contribute to the hyperechoic appearance of these lesions.[13] The ultrasound appearance is often heterogeneic due to haemorrhage, necrosis and fat content. Colour Doppler ultrasound can be used to differentiate HCA from FNH. However, the diagnosis of adenoma is not usually made definitely at ultrasonography, and subsequent CT or other imaging modalities are often required to confirm the diagnosis.[13]

Multiphasic helical CT allows more accurate detection and characterisation of focal hepatic lesions. The degree of attenuation of the adenoma relative to the background liver depends on the composition of the tumour and liver.[13] CT may demonstrate a hypoattenuating mass due to the presence of intratumoural fat, or the lesion may be nearly isoattenuating relative to normal liver on unenhanced, portal venous-phase and delayed-phase images (most of the adenomas; Fig. 5.2). Alternatively, the lesion may be hyperattenuating in all phases of both contrast enhanced and unenhanced images in fatty livers.[13] Due to the presence of large subcapsular feeding vessels, peripheral enhancement may be seen on contrast-enhanced CT, with a centripetal pattern of enhancement. Small HCAs may enhance rapidly and are often hyperattenuating relative to the liver. The enhancement usually does not persist in adenomas due to arteriovenous shunting. Larger HCAs may be more

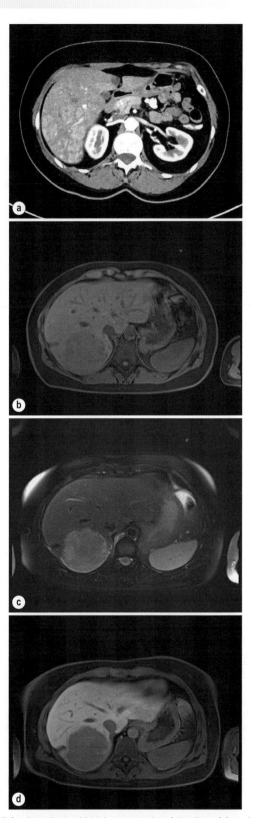

**Figure 5.2** A patient with adenomatosis of the liver **(a)** and another patient with a hepatocellular adenoma posteriorly in the right liver lobe (segment 7; **b**, **c** and **d**). **(a)** shows CT appearance of multiple heterogenous hyperdense lesions during the arterial phase. On MRI, the signal of the adenoma depends both on the fat composition of the liver and the adenoma. This adenoma is isointense on the T1-weighted images **(b)**, is heterogeneous hyperintense on T2-weighted images **(c)**, and there is no substantial uptake or retention after administration of Primovist (hepatocellular-specific contrast agent; **d**).

heterogeneous than smaller lesions, and their CT appearance is less specific.[13]

On MRI, HCAs are usually heterogeneous in appearance. They are typically bright on T1-weighted MRI, and predominantly hyperintense relative to liver on T2-weighted images (Fig. 5.2).[13] Almost one-third of adenomas have a peripheral rim corresponding to a fibrous capsule (Fig. 5.2). Some groups use PET-CT scan with [18]F-fluoromethylcholine to differentiate between HCA and FNH (sensitivity 100%, specificity 97%).[14] Alternatively, a biopsy can be considered in very selected cases when there is persistent doubt about the diagnosis.[15]

## PATHOLOGY

HCAs are typically nodular lesions with a size ranging from microscopic to lesions as large as 20 cm.[9] They are relatively uniform, although areas of congestion, necrosis, haemorrhage or fibrosis can be observed. Often large subcapsular vessels are seen as well as intratumoural fat. On microscopic examination, HCA is defined as a tumoural monoclonal proliferation of well-differentiated, usually bland-looking hepatocytes arranged in sheets and cords that are usually one, or at most two, cells in width.[9]

More recently, molecular classification has revealed four major subtypes of HCA (the Bordeaux classification): HNF1A (coding for hepatocyte nuclear factor 1a) inactivating mutations (30–40%), inflammatory adenomas (40–50%), β-catenin-mutated HCAs (β-HCA; 10–15%) and unclassified HCAs (10%).[16] Inflammatory HCAs can also be β-catenin activated (10%). It is important to differentiate between these subclasses, as β-catenin mutations appear to be associated with a higher risk of malignant transformation.[16]

## MANAGEMENT

HCAs have a risk of spontaneous rupture and malignant transformation. The risk of rupture is related to the size of the adenoma.[11] In a group of 124 patients, 25% of HCAs ruptured, but no rupture was observed in lesions < 5 cm.[11] Recent hormonal treatment is also a risk factor for haemorrhage.[11] Mortality after spontaneous rupture is approximately 5–10%.

Stoot et al.[17] performed a systematic review and studied 1635 HCAs. They concluded that only 4.2% of patients with HCA had malignant transformation, and malignant transformation in lesions < 5 cm was a very rare finding. The risk of malignant transformation is much higher in men, and in some studies, it is reported to be as high as 47%.[18]

There is no guideline for the treatment of HCAs, although there are general agreements. In men, all lesions should be considered for surgical resection independent of size, given the high risk of malignant transformation, while taking into account comorbidity and location of the lesion. Resection should also be considered in patients with HCAs due to a metabolic disorder.[15] In women, lesions < 5 cm can be observed with sequential imaging after cessation of oral contraceptive treatment.[19] In larger tumours, treatment strategies vary. Some clinicians have proposed non-surgical management if hormone therapy is stopped and patients are followed up with serial radiological examinations. The time period of waiting is still under debate; however, recent studies indicate that a waiting period of longer than 6 months could be justified.[20–22] Others have advocated resection of adenomas because of the risk of haemorrhage and malignancy.[7] Alternatively, elective transarterial embolisation could be a valid approach in women.[23]

Hepatic arterial embolisation can be effective for controlling bleeding in patients who present with acute haemorrhage.[24] If the lesion is atypical, resection could be considered; however, if there is no suspicion of a malignancy, it is best to wait for resorption of the haematoma before further therapy.[24] HCAs tend to grow during pregnancy.[15] In a prospective study of 48 women with 51 pregnancies with HCA < 5 cm, progression was seen in a quarter of pregnancies with a median increase of 14 mm. One woman with HCA that grew to > 7 cm was treated successfully with a transarterial embolisation at week 26 of pregnancy to prevent further growth.[25] Therefore, pregnancy should not be discouraged in the presence of a small HCA; however, close sonographic surveillance is recommended.[15,25]

Orthotopic liver transplantation has been performed for HCAs. However, liver transplantation should be reserved for exceptional cases, such as for hepatic adenomatosis in patients with a metabolic liver disease (e.g. glycogen storage disease) or in patients with hepatic adenomatosis and (a suspicion of) malignant transformation.

More recently, the subtypes of the Bordeaux classification of HCA have been studied related to their risk of complications. Some groups report that percutaneous core needle biopsy is of limited value because the therapeutic strategy is based primarily on patient sex and tumour size.[26] Others report a different therapeutic approach based on subtype. Thomeer et al.[15] concluded that there was no evidence to support the use of subtype classification in the stratification and management of individual patients related to risk of bleeding. Size still remains the most important feature to predict those at risk of bleeding during follow-up. However, malignant transformation does seem to be related to differences in subtypes. β-catenin-mutated HCAs trigger a potent mitogenic signalling pathway that is prominent in HCC.[15] Cases of inflammatory HCAs can also show activation of the β-catenin pathway with a risk of developing malignancy.[9] Therefore, β-catenin-mutated and inflammatory HCAs are prone to malignant degeneration, and particularly if > 5 cm.[15] In these circumstances, invasive treatment should be considered.

✔ There is currently no guideline for the treatment of HCAs, although there are some general agreements. In men, all lesions should be considered for surgical resection independent of size, given the high risk of malignant transformation, while taking into account comorbidity and location of the lesion. Resection should also be considered in patients with HCAs due to a metabolic disorder. In women, lesions < 5 cm can be observed with sequential imaging after cessation of oral contraceptive treatment. In larger tumours, treatment strategies vary. Some advocate non-surgical management in which hormone therapy is stopped and patients are followed up with serial radiological examinations, whereas others combine this strategy with transarterial embolisation. The waiting period should be at least 6 months, although recent publications have shown that a longer period is necessary. Others resect larger adenomas because of the risk of haemorrhage and malignancy. More recently, it was found that the HCA subtype with a β-catenin mutation is more prone to malignant transformation, and invasive treatment should be considered in these patients. For patients with acute haemorrhage from a HCA, hepatic arterial embolisation can be effective for controlling bleeding, after which either resection or observation (with or without biopsy) could be considered.

## NODULAR REGENERATIVE HYPERPLASIA

Nodular regenerative hyperplasia (NRH) is the transformation of normal hepatic parenchyma into small regenerative nodules, also known as micronodular transformation.[7] This condition should not be confused with regeneration nodules found in cirrhotic patients, which are different entities. NRH nodules are thought to be related to altered blood flow; obstructive portal venopathy causes ischaemia, which in turn leads to hyperplasia of hepatic acini with adequate blood flow in order to compensate for atrophied hepatocytes.[27] In a retrospective study, NRH was found in 2.1–2.6% of autopsies; all middle-aged to elderly adults with a female-to-male ratio of 2:1.[28] NRH has been associated with immunological and haematological disorders, cardiac and pulmonary disorders, several drugs and toxins, neoplasia and organ transplantation.[27] It has been suggested by some that NRH is a premalignant condition, although others think that NRH is a condition secondary to HCC or its treatment.

NRH is often discovered incidentally. The majority of patients are asymptomatic, although some patients have signs of portal hypertension.[7] The nodules have variable echogenicity on ultrasonography and are often hypodense on CT without significant enhancement. Unfortunately, even MRI may not be helpful to distinguish the lesions as they are often small and difficult to characterise.[7] Therefore, histological examination is necessary to make the diagnosis of NRH. A correct diagnosis is often difficult using percutaneous needle biopsy, and in these cases laparoscopically guided liver biopsy or wedge biopsy for diagnosis may be considered.[7]

The management depends on the presenting symptoms, but should at least focus on treating the underlying condition.[7,27] If there is portal hypertension, treatment options include medication or sometimes portosystemic shunt procedures, but it may also be necessary to treat complications such as ascites or oesophageal varices. Liver failure is a rare complication for which liver transplantation may be the only solution.[27]

## CHOLANGIOCELLULAR LIVER LESIONS

## SIMPLE CYSTS OF THE LIVER

### GENERAL
Hepatic cysts are relatively common and seen in approximately 6% of ultrasound procedures.[1] The incidence increases with age, with more than half of patients over 60 years of age having one or more simple cysts.[29] These non-parasitic cysts can occur as single, multiple or diffuse cysts (PLD will be discussed separately). Cysts can range from 1 mm to > 20 cm (containing several litres of fluid). Some groups report that cysts are more frequent in women with a female-to-male ratio of approximately 2:1, but others indicate a more even distribution. Symptomatic cysts are reported up to 10 times more commonly in women than in men.[30]

Simple cysts contain clear, bile-like fluid, but have no communication with bile ducts. As bile duct epithelium covers the cyst inner lining, it is hypothesised that simple cysts arise during embryogenesis when intrahepatic ductules fail to connect with intra- or extrahepatic ducts.[29]

### CLINICAL PRESENTATION
In the majority of patients, the cysts are discovered incidentally.[29] A small fraction of patients, mainly with large cysts, experience symptoms such as abdominal pain, early satiety, nausea and vomiting due to a mass effect.[29] Physical examination may reveal a palpable abdominal mass or hepatomegaly. Complications such as haemorrhage, rupture and biliary obstruction are rare and are more likely in larger cysts.[29]

### DIAGNOSIS
The diagnosis of a simple cyst can be made by ultrasound. Ultrasound has a sensitivity and specificity of approximately 90% for diagnosing cysts.[29] CT shows a well-demarcated, water-attenuated, smooth lesion without an internal structure, and no enhancement with contrast (Fig. 5.3).[7] MRI T1-weighted sequences show low signal intensity, whereas T2-weighted sequences show extremely high signal intensity, which does not enhance after contrast injection. MRI has a diagnostic accuracy of 97% for cysts. Aspiration of the cyst for diagnosis is not needed or recommended.[7]

If intracystic haemorrhage occurs, ultrasound typically shows a hyperechogenic pattern with suggestion of septations or solid portions.[29] In general, when irregularities and nodules in the cystic wall are identified, these should be considered neoplastic.[29] Simple cysts rarely have calcifications and this is more characteristic of hydatid cysts.

### MANAGEMENT
Asymptomatic cysts do not require treatment, but symptomatic cysts may require intervention. Percutaneous aspiration does not provide definitive treatment as the cyst typically recurs; however, it may help to clarify if abdominal pain is related to a cyst.

Percutaneous aspiration sclerotherapy is recommended by many as the preferred first treatment.[29,31] Wijnands et al.[31] performed a systematic literature review and reported excellent results with respect to long-term efficacy and safety after aspiration sclerotherapy of hepatic cysts. Recurrence rates of aspiration sclerotherapy range between 20% and 30%. A primary surgical approach should be considered if it is difficult to rule out cystadenoma or malignancy. Surgery may also be indicated if there is biliary communication and infection, when sclerotherapy has been ineffective, and in patients with recurrence.[32]

Surgical deroofing or fenestration of the cystic wall results in excellent reduction of symptoms.[33] Historically, this was done as an open procedure, but nowadays a laparoscopic approach can be performed safely with minimal morbidity (Fig. 5.3). Recurrence rates of 10–25% are reported.[33] Excision of a simple cyst is usually not necessary and can result in additional morbidity and mortality as there is often no dissection plane between the cyst and crucial structures in the liver. However, in selected cases a more radical resection with emphasis on preserving functional hepatic parenchyma may be necessary. If histology of the partially removed cyst wall is abnormal or suggestive of a cystadenoma, hepatic resection is indicated.

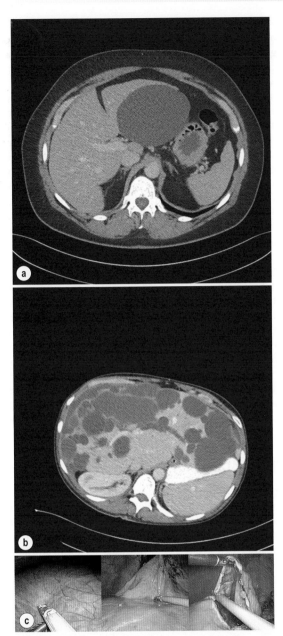

**Figure 5.3** **(a)** CT of a solitary liver cyst in segment 2/3. **(b)** CT of a patient with polycystic liver disease. **(c)** Laparoscopic cyst fenestration.

## POLYCYSTIC LIVER DISEASE

### GENERAL

PLD is a condition which is characterised by the development of multiple hepatic cysts.[34] Similar to simple liver cysts, it is a congenital malformation of biliary ducts. Three PLD entities are recognised in adults: (1) Von Meyenburg complexes (biliary hamartoma; hepatic cystic hamartoma) with characteristic small, non-hereditary nodular cystic lesions; (2) isolated PLD with innumerable hepatic cysts (autosomal dominant; PCLD); and (3) autosomal dominant polycystic kidney disease (ADPKD) with cysts in both kidneys and in many cases hepatic cysts. The incidence of Von Meyenburg complexes is estimated at 0.7–5.6%, the prevalence of ADPKD 1/400 to 1/1000, and the prevalence of PCLD is 1/100,000 to 1/1,000,000.[34] Von Meyenburg complexes will

be addressed later in this chapter. This section will focus on the other two entities.

Variants of three genes have been associated with PCLD and are present in approximately 25% of cases: protein kinase C substrate 80 K-H (PRKCSH), SEC63 homologue (SEC63), and low-density lipoprotein receptor-related protein 5 (LRP5).[35,36] Variants in two genes are responsible for ADPKD in virtually all cases: polycystic kidney disease 1 (PKD1; 85%) and polycystic kidney disease 2 (PKD2; 15%).[35–37] Studies have shown that between families with PLD, the clinical course can be heterogeneous, and that in families there is a considerable phenotypic variability of hepatic cysts.[34]

### CLINICAL PRESENTATION

The majority (> 80%) of patients with PLD are clinically asymptomatic.[36] When symptoms arise, they are associated with the extent of hepatomegaly or due to compression of neighbouring organs. Symptoms include pain, abdominal discomfort, pyrosis, early satiety, weight loss and anorexia. In general, women present with larger-sized liver cysts and are more frequently symptomatic, suggesting that a hormonal component may play a role.[36]

Complications can occur, such as cyst haemorrhage, rupture and infection. These complications appear to occur more frequently in ADPKD than in PCLD.[34] Rupture and jaundice have only occasionally been described. In advanced stages, portal hypertension, ascites and liver failure can be found.

The main difference between ADPKD and PCLD is the presence of polycystic kidneys. The prognosis of these diseases is different, as the majority of ADPKD patients develop enlarged kidneys and end-stage renal disease. In patients with PCLD, a few renal cysts may be present, but this does not result in renal failure.[34]

Imaging is similar to that for simple cysts and typically includes assessment by MRI or CT (Fig. 5.3). However, it should be remembered that in patients who present with multiple liver cysts, imaging of the kidneys should also be performed. Several clinical classifications have been proposed to grade the severity of PLD, e.g. Gigot's classification, Qian's classification and Schnelldorfer's classification. These classifications use factors such as symptoms, number and size of cysts to grade the severity of PLD.[38]

### MANAGEMENT

The primary aim of treatment of PCLD and ADPKD is to reduce symptoms.[34] Treatment varies depending on the phenotype of PLD; patients with a few large cysts require a different approach to those with many small cysts.

In asymptomatic patients, no therapy is warranted. Women should be advised to stop oral contraceptives. More recently, treatment with somatostatin analogues has shown a reduction in liver volume after 6 months of therapy, but only a modest improvement in quality of life.[36,39] Analgesics can be administered for symptomatic relief of pain.

In patients with large symptomatic dominant cysts, invasive treatments may be considered. Several studies have shown beneficial effects of invasive treatments, including aspiration sclerotherapy or laparoscopic cyst deroofing.[34,36] However, recurrence and reintervention rates are high, showing that indications for an intervention in PLD should be considered carefully.[36] In selected cases, hepatic resection combined with fenestration may be an option.[38] Liver transplantation for PLD is uncommon. Indications for liver transplantation are progressive sarcopenia from inability to eat combined with pain and immobility due to a massive liver, and Budd–Chiari-like syndrome with the development of ascites. In patients with both complicated PLD and kidney failure, a combined liver and kidney transplant is often performed.

## CYSTADENOMA

### GENERAL

Cystadenomas of the liver are rare tumours, accounting for < 5% of biliary tumours.[7] They are solitary, usually multilocular, almost always found in women, with a preference for presentation in the fourth decade of life. No association between cystadenomas and oral contraceptive use has been found.[40] Cystadenomas > 20 cm in diameter have been reported. In the majority of cases (95%), the content of the cyst is mucin.[7]

Histologically, cystadenomas are multilocular with benign cuboidal to columnar epithelium. In the past it was thought that all lesions had an ovarian-like stroma, but cystadenomas without ovarian-like stroma have been reported in 15% of patients.[40]

Various hypotheses about the origin of the ovarian-like stroma in hepatic cystadenomas exist. One explanation is that during embryological development, when the gonads are located directly under the diaphragm, on the left side distally from liver, pancreas and spleen ectopic ovarian cells migrate to the liver and eventually form the lesion. This would explain the predominance of cystadenomas in segment 4. Furthermore, a diagnosis of cystadenoma should be considered in females if cystic lesions are present in both the liver and the pancreas.[41,42] Another hypothesis is that cystadenomas may be remnants of ectopic tissue destined to form the gallbladder due to the resemblance between ovarian stroma and embryonic mesenchyma of the embryonic gallbladder and large bile ducts.

Cystadenoma is thought to be a precursor of cystadenocarcinoma.[7] Malignancy has been identified in approximately 10% of resections for presumed cystadenoma.[43] In contrast to cystadenomas, hepatic cystadenocarcinomas are found more equally distributed in men and women. Furthermore, cystadenocarcinoma follows a more aggressive course in men (more often in a cystadenoma without ovarian-like stroma). Therefore, a lesion that is considered to be a cystadenoma in a man should always raise the suspicion of a malignancy.

### CLINICAL PRESENTATION

Cystadenomas are often found incidentally. Larger cysts can be symptomatic and present with abdominal pain, abdominal fullness, early satiety and weight loss. Laboratory values are usually normal.[43]

### IMAGING

On ultrasonography, cystadenomas typically have irregular walls and internal septations forming loculi (small spaces or cavities within the main cystic lesion).[7] If a complex cyst is found on ultrasound investigation, cross-sectional imaging with CT and MRI should always be obtained. CT and MRI can help identify heterogeneous septations, irregular papillary growths and thickened cyst walls (Fig. 5.4). The cysts are typically hyperintense on T2 weighting, although they may appear heterogeneous because of mucinous content.[7]

It is difficult to differentiate cystadenomas from cystadenocarcinomas preoperatively on imaging. However, the presence of calcifications along with mixed solid and cystic components on imaging is associated with cystadenocarcinoma.[7] Also, a mural or septal nodule and a nodule diameter > 10 mm on conventional ultrasound are suggestive of cystadenocarcinoma. Aspiration or biopsy is not recommended as it has limited sensitivity and there is a risk of disseminating malignancy if there is an underlying cystadenocarcinoma.[7] Besides, it does not alter the management strategy as the recommended treatment for both is resection.

### MANAGEMENT

If a cystadenoma is diagnosed, complete tumour excision is the standard treatment, both to obtain a definitive histological diagnosis and to prevent malignant transformation. Recurrence rates are low with either standard hepatic resection or enucleation, but are approximately 60% following aspiration or partial resection.[43] Therefore, if cyst fenestration has been performed for what was thought to be a simple cyst, but the definitive histology confirms a cystadenoma, resection is indicated. After excision of a cystadenoma, long-term outcome is good; however, the prognosis for patients with a cystadenocarcinoma is worse.[43]

## BILE DUCT ADENOMA

Bile duct adenomas, also referred to as bile duct hamartomas or Von Meyenburg complexes, are benign bile duct malformations. They are composed of dilated intrahepatic bile ductules embedded in fibrous stroma and usually appear as subcapsular or parenchymal nodules < 10 mm in diameter. In general, these lesions do not cause clinical symptoms, but they can cause a diagnostic dilemma when liver metastases

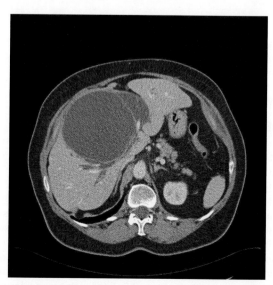

**Figure 5.4** CT showing central cystic liver lesion with a thickened wall and separations with secondary biliary duct dilatation. Histology confirmed a cystadenoma.

are suspected. When found during surgery, a biopsy may be necessary to differentiate between a bile duct adenoma and hepatic malignancies, such as cholangiocarcinoma or metastasis. Treatment is usually not required.

## INTRADUCTAL PAPILLARY NEOPLASM OF THE BILE DUCT

Intraductal papillary neoplasm of the bile duct (IPNB) is a rare bile duct tumour and is, along with biliary intraepithelial neoplasia, thought to be a precursor lesion of cholangiocarcinoma. It is characterised by papillary growth within the bile duct lumen and is regarded as a biliary counterpart of intraductal papillary mucinous neoplasm (IPMN) of the pancreas.

Patients present with repeated episodes of abdominal pain, jaundice and acute cholangitis, although some patients experience no complaints (mainly in the group of patients with non-mucinous-producing biliary papillomatosis).[44] The most common radiological findings for IPNB are bile duct dilatation and intraductal masses. The patterns of bile duct dilatation are diffuse duct ectasia, localised duct dilatation and cystic dilatation.[44] Some groups recommend cholangioscopy to confirm the histology and view the extent of the tumour.[45]

All patients with IPNB should be considered for treatment. IPNB (and associated mucin) often cause recurrent cholangitis and obstructive jaundice, even if these tumours are not malignant.[45] Patients without distant metastasis should be considered for surgical resection. Intraoperative frozen section of the resection margin of the bile duct and regional lymph node excision are recommended.[45] Patients treated by curative resection have a good prognosis.[44]

## MESENCHYMAL LIVER LESIONS

### HAEMANGIOMATA

#### GENERAL

Haemangiomata are the commonest benign non-cystic liver lesions, with an incidence of approximately 3%.[1,46] Liver haemangiomata are more frequently observed in women than in men (ratio 5:1).[2] The mean age at diagnosis is around 50 years.[1] The size of the lesions varies from some millimetres to > 20 cm. In a study of more than 45,000 hospital patients undergoing liver ultrasonography, the mean diameter of haemangiomata was 2 cm.[1] Classically, giant haemangiomata were defined as haemangiomata greater than 4–5 cm in diameter.[47] However, in more recent years, several groups are defining giant haemangiomata as lesions > 10 cm.[4] These giant haemangiomata are mainly found in women, and a role for female hormones in progression has been considered, although a strong association with the oral contraceptive pill has not been demonstrated.

In the majority of cases (77%), haemangiomata are solitary lesions, but a minority (1.6%) of patients have > 5 haemangiomata.[1] A few cases of familial cavernous liver haemangiomata have been described, with similar lesions in other organs such as cerebral cavernous malformations.

## CLINICAL PRESENTATION

Haemangiomata are most frequently found incidentally during abdominal ultrasonography for unrelated reasons.[5] Most haemangiomata are small. Sometimes patients with larger haemangiomata present with non-specific abdominal complaints such as vague abdominal pain, fullness, early satiety, nausea or vomiting. This might be explained by compression of adjacent organs or stretch of Glisson's capsule.

Presentation with spontaneous rupture or bleeding from a haemangioma is rare; in a large retrospective cross-sectional study, it was observed mainly in large, peripherally located exophytic growing haemangiomata.[46] Even if symptoms are present, the majority of patients have other explanations for these complaints. In a study by Farges et al.[48] 54% of patients with symptoms had another cause for their symptoms. Furthermore, half of the patients with no other explanation for their complaints were still symptomatic after treatment (resection [n = 8], embolisation [n = 5] and hepatic artery ligation [n = 1]), which questions whether the haemangioma itself was the real cause of the initial complaints.[48] However, some patients do present with pain from haemangiomata; these lesions are often located on the surface of the liver and resection of the haemangioma may result in resolution of symptoms.

A rare presentation in patients with a giant haemangioma is thrombocytopenia and hypofibrinogenaemia caused by consumption of coagulation factors, also known as Kasabach–Merritt syndrome. This is a serious complication and mortality ranges between 10% and 37%.

## DIAGNOSIS

As the majority of patients are asymptomatic, haemangiomata are often found by coincidence during imaging studies. The majority of haemangiomata can be diagnosed accurately by imaging alone. On ultrasonography, haemangiomata typically appear as well-defined, lobulated, homogeneous hyperechoic masses, but may also have hypoechoic portions due to haemorrhage, fibrosis or calcification. The diagnostic accuracy of ultrasound is reported to be 70–80%.[5] However, unenhanced ultrasound alone cannot differentiate a small haemangioma from a hepatocellular carcinoma, liver cell adenoma, FNH or solitary metastasis. Contrast-enhanced ultrasound has been found to increase accuracy to > 90%.

The 2014 American College of Gastroenterology guidelines strongly recommended that an MRI or CT is undertaken to confirm the diagnosis of haemangioma.[7] On CT prior to administration of intravenous contrast, haemangiomata appear as a well-demarcated hypodense mass. After intravenous contrast, haemangiomata classically have peripheral nodular enhancement and progressive centripetal fill-in (Fig. 5.5).[7] The best imaging modality for haemangiomata is MRI, with a reported sensitivity and specificity of > 90% (Fig. 5.5). It has been suggested that MRI is used when lesions are < 3 cm, close to the heart, or close to intrahepatic vessels.[27] Haemangiomata are bright on T2-weighted imaging and on enhanced T1-weighted imaging show a similar pattern as found on enhanced CT with peripheral nodular enhancement.

Single-photon emission CT (SPECT) using technetium-99 m-labelled red blood cells was previously found

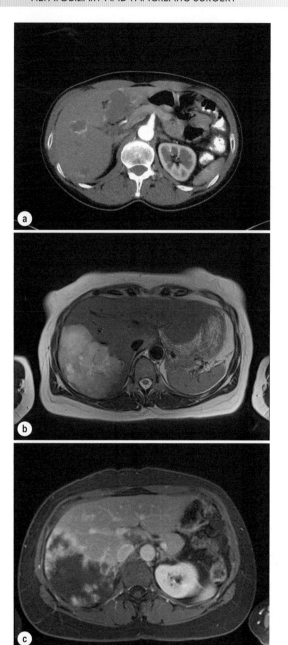

**Figure 5.5** **(a)** CT after intravenous contrast administration in the arterial phase shows several haemangiomata as nodular, discontinuous enhancements. In portal and late venous phase, there is progressive centripetal filling (not shown on this image). **(b)** T2-weighted MRI of a patient with a giant haemangioma. The haemangioma is seen as a hyperintense lesion. **(c)** Enhanced T1-weighted image (gadolinium enhancement) in the same patient. The lesion does not show uptake of the contrast and a peripheral nodular enhancement pattern is seen.

to be a helpful tool in the diagnosis of larger haemangiomata and those not located near large vessels. However, with improved technology, increased availability and decreased costs of MRI, there is now only a limited role for SPECT.

## PATHOLOGY

Macroscopically, haemangiomata are well-circumscribed compressible tumours with a dark colour.[5] Microscopically,

they are composed of multiple blood vessels lined by a single layer of endothelial cells within a thin, fibrous stroma.[4] Their blood supply is from the hepatic artery.

Needle biopsy is not necessary and should only be considered in exceptional cases if the findings are atypical. It is debatable whether a needle biopsy of a hypervascular tumour, like a haemangioma, can be safely performed. In a retrospective study of 38 patients with haemangiomata ranging from 1 cm to 13.5 cm in size, no haemorrhage was reported after percutaneous needle biopsy.[49] However, others have reported bleeding after needle biopsy.

## MANAGEMENT

Trastek et al.[50] retrospectively studied 36 patients with hepatic haemangiomata > 4 cm that were managed conservatively. They found no need for surgery after an observation period of up to 15 years (mean 5.5 years). Furthermore, the majority of haemangiomata remained stable over time.[48] Complications are very rare, and therefore conservative management is in general appropriate.[7]

For larger or symptomatic lesions, the risk of intervention should be weighed against the benefit of resection. Surgical intervention can be considered in patients with a growing lesion that becomes very large (> 10 cm) or if the patient begins to report symptoms such as recurrent pain. Follow-up imaging is not required for classical haemangiomata.

If intervention for a haemangioma is performed, complete surgical resection or enucleation of the lesion is the best treatment option.[47] If possible, enucleation of the lesion is preferred rather than hepatic resection, to avoid loss of functional liver tissue, to reduce blood loss and reduce the risk of postoperative complications.[47,51] Surgical intervention for hepatic haemangiomata should not be underestimated as it carries a high risk of major perioperative bleeding.

Nowadays, transarterial embolisation is rarely used as the only treatment. In a small prospective series, selective transarterial embolisation of haemangioma as the only treatment appeared to improve symptoms, although the size of the lesions did not change.[52] In a recent meta-analysis of 1450 patients, transarterial embolization was found to be safe and associated with reduction in the size of haemangiomas and alleviation of symptoms.[53] However, in the uncommon case of rupture of a (giant) haemangioma (1–4% of cases), initial embolisation of the haemangioma to temporarily control the bleeding before resection should be performed. Others use this strategy for elective resections of giant haemangiomata. Other treatment options such as radiofrequency ablation (RFA) with or without preoperative arterial embolisation have been used successfully.[51] Although very rare, liver transplantation has been performed for technically unresectable, complicated, giant haemangiomata.

✔ Conservative management is appropriate for asymptomatic haemangiomata < 4 cm in diameter. For larger or symptomatic lesions, the risk of intervention should be weighed against the benefit of resection. Surgical intervention can be considered in patients with a growing lesion that becomes very large (> 10 cm) or if the patient has symptoms such as recurrent pain. Follow-up imaging is not required for classic haemangiomata.

## HEPATIC LIPOMA AND ANGIOLIPOMA

Lipomatous tumours, such as hepatic angiomyolipoma or hepatic lipoma, are very rare benign tumours.[5] They are often asymptomatic, although abdominal discomfort could be a presenting symptom. Hepatic angiolipomas may be part of the clinical manifestations of tuberous sclerosis (also called Bourneville-Pringle disease, a rare genetic disease that causes benign tumours to grow in different organs including brain, skin, kidney and liver). For atypical cases, it may be necessary to perform a biopsy to differentiate them from other hypervascular tumours, including HCC, FNH and haemangiomata.[5] The prognosis of these tumours is favourable, although resection may be necessary due to symptoms.

## INFLAMMATORY LIVER LESIONS

## PYOGENIC LIVER ABSCESS

### GENERAL

Liver abscess is a rare but potentially lethal condition, which in the USA at the end of the last century accounted for approximately 20 per 100,000 hospital admissions.[54] The aetiology has changed over time. Historically, the commonest cause of a liver abscess was acute appendicitis, but in the era of modern surgery and antibiotics, this cause has declined drastically in importance. Other causes for hepatic abscesses include diverticular disease and inflammatory bowel disease (e.g. Crohn's disease). However, biliary causes are now the most frequent known cause of pyogenic liver abscesses. In earlier reports, benign obstruction of the bile duct, commonly due to choledocholithiasis, was the predominant cause of liver abscesses, whereas in later publications there is an increase in malignant biliary obstruction as the main aetiological factor.[54] Other rarer, non-gastrointestinal sources of hepatic abscesses include bacterial endocarditis, urinary sepsis, pneumonia, osteomyelitis and intravenous drug abuse. Direct extension into the liver from perforation of an adjacent organ, such as from the gallbladder, colon, stomach or duodenum are other sources of a hepatic abscess.

### CLINICAL PRESENTATION

The commonest presenting features are vague non-specific symptoms. Patients present with fever, chills, right upper quadrant pain, jaundice, anorexia and malaise.[54] Almost all patients will have an elevated C-reactive protein (CRP), most will have an elevated white blood cell count, and more than half of patients will have abnormal liver enzymes with cholestatic parameters.

### DIAGNOSIS

Ultrasonography generally demonstrates a fluid-filled cavity. It can provide information on the number of lesions, the diameter and anatomical location, as well as information on the presence of bile duct dilatation. CT can be helpful to further evaluate the liver for the number of abscesses and to provide anatomical information required to make treatment decisions (Fig. 5.6). Gas in the abscess is only observed in approximately 20% of cases. An MRI or MRCP should be considered if a biliary cause of a hepatic abscess is suspected,

such as in patients with distended bile ducts or obstructive liver function tests.

### MANAGEMENT

Hope et al.[55] studied 107 patients with hepatic pyogenic abscesses managed in a single centre and found that abscesses < 3 cm could be treated successfully with antibiotics only. For abscesses > 3 cm that were unilocular, a combination of antibiotics and percutaneous drainage was successful in 83%, whereas for complex multiloculated abscesses > 3 cm this regimen was only successful in 33% of patients. Given the non-significant difference in mortality in this last group between patients drained percutaneously and those undergoing surgery, the authors suggested that this last group of abscesses should be treated by surgery. In our opinion, all hepatic abscesses that are not caused by a malignancy should be first treated with antibiotics and (multiple) percutaneous (catheter) drainage (Fig. 5.6). If this fails, an operation can

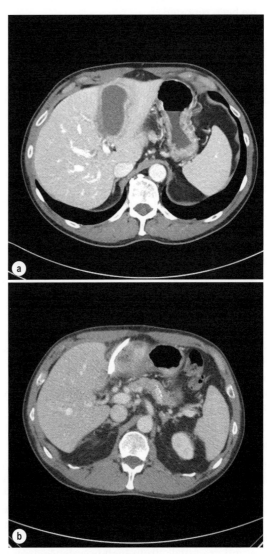

**Figure 5.6** CT in the portal-venous phase after intravenous contrast enhancement (**a** and **b**). (**a**) A hypodense lesion measuring 10 × 8.2 × 4.6 cm in the left lobe of the liver with a thick wall with contrast enhancement suggestive of a liver abscess, probably originating from diverticular disease. (**b**) CT after percutaneous drainage of the abscess with the drain located in the abscess.

be considered, e.g. video-assisted abscess debridement, laparoscopic drainage, or resection in exceptional cases.

A meta-analysis comparing percutaneous needle aspiration with catheter drainage concluded that both techniques are safe methods to manage liver abscesses.[56] However, percutaneous catheter drainage was more effective as it facilitated a higher success rate and reduced the time required to achieve clinical relief. It is recommended that drained pus is sent for analysis to determine the responsible microorganisms and to ensure appropriate antibiotics are administered. Virtually all micro-organisms have been cultured, although enteric organisms are most commonly identified (*Escherichia coli* and *Klebsiella pneumoniae*).

In addition to treating the hepatic abscess, the underlying cause should also be treated. Although mortality has dropped drastically with current treatment regimens, mortality for patients with liver abscesses is still relatively high, with mortality rates of approximately 7–10%. For those admitted to the intensive care unit, mortality rates of up to 28% have been reported.[57]

## AMOEBIC LIVER ABSCESS

### GENERAL

Amoebic liver abscesses caused by *Entamoeba histolytica* account for 10% of liver abscesses and are predominantly found in areas were *E. histolytica* is endemic, such as in tropical areas.[58] In Mexico 8.4% of the population have serum antibodies against *E. histolytica*. Only 10% of patients experience symptoms, mainly of amoebic colitis. Liver abscesses are the commonest extraintestinal manifestation of this infection. They are found in 1% of clinically infected patients, and primarily affect men between the ages of 18 and 50 years.[59]

*E. histolytica* trophozoites normally remain confined to the bowel lumen. However, some virulent trophozoites can migrate through the mucosa of the bowel and reach the liver through the portal system. There they can provoke enzymatic focal necrosis of hepatocytes and multiple micro-abscesses that eventually coalesce to form a single lesion. The central cavity contains a homogeneous thick liquid, with typically reddish-brown and yellow colour similar to 'anchovy paste'.[60] This material is almost always sterile, except when a secondary infection has occurred, and this allows differential diagnosis from a pyogenic abscess. The amoebae can be found at the edge of the lesion, but are rarely detected in the pus or within the abscess cavity itself.[60]

### CLINICAL PRESENTATION

Right upper quadrant pain, fever and hepatomegaly are the predominant symptoms of hepatic amoebiasis, which can occur without any symptom of intestinal amoebiasis.[59,60] Patients with an amoebic abscess are usually more acutely ill than patients with a pyogenic abscess, have high fever and abdominal pain in the right upper quadrant. They are also younger and are usually from high-prevalence areas or recent travellers to such areas. Amoebic abscesses are more often found in individuals with suppressed cell-mediated immunity. Jaundice is an unusual symptom and is found in patients with multiple lesions or very large abscesses, and is associated with an adverse prognosis.[60]

Both ultrasound and CT are sensitive in the detection of amoebic liver abscesses. In many patients, it is difficult to differentiate amoebic abscesses from pyogenic abscesses, but epidemiologic and clinical information in conjunction with positive amoebic titres may suggest the diagnosis. The lesion is typically oval or round and located near the liver capsule. On contrast-enhanced CT, amoebic abscesses usually appear as rounded well-defined lesions, with an enhancing wall 3–15 mm in thickness, and a peripheral zone of oedema around the abscess that is somewhat characteristic. The central abscess cavity may contain multiple septa or fluid-debris levels.

The diagnosis can be confirmed by demonstrating *E. histolytica* trophozoites in aspirated pus, or more frequently from the necrotic material obtained by needle biopsy of the edge of the lesion. However, the amoeba will be found in only a small percentage of cases.[60] In contrast, serum antibodies to *Entamoeba* species are present in > 90% of cases.[59] False-negative serology tests may be obtained early in the infection (first 7–10 days), but repeated tests usually will come back positive.[58]

### MANAGEMENT

Most amoebic liver abscesses can be treated with metronidazole treatment alone.[58,59] The role of therapeutic aspiration remains controversial. It is reasonable to reserve aspiration for individuals in whom the diagnosis is uncertain, when there is no response to metronidazole, in individuals with large left lobe abscesses (because of the risk of rupture into the pericardium), and in severely ill patients.[59] Individuals with an amoebic liver abscess should also be treated to eliminate intestinal colonisation by *E. histolytica*.[58,59]

## HYDATID CYSTS

### GENERAL

Echinococcosis or hydatid disease is a parasitic illness caused by the tapeworm *Echinococcus*. The liver is the most commonly infected organ.[61] Hepatic echinococcosis is (if not treated on time) a life-threatening disease caused by *Echinococcus granulosus* or *Echinococcus multilocularis* causing a cystic and alveolar form, respectively.[62] Infection with *E. granulosus* is more common, whereas *E. multilocularis* infection is more serious.[61]

*E. granulosus* has a worldwide distribution, with the highest prevalence found in Mediterranean countries, Russia, China, North and East Africa, South America and Australia.[62] The parasite life cycle involves dogs (or coyotes, dingoes and red foxes) as definitive hosts and ungulates (sheep, pigs, goats and horses) as intermediate hosts. Humans can accidently become 'aberrant' intermediate hosts, after ingestion of *Echinococcus* eggs excreted by infected carnivores. The eggs grow inside the host organs (mainly the liver) and form a cyst (hydatid cyst). Hydatid cysts are round in shape and are usually filled with a clear fluid. The inner part of the cyst features a germinating membrane, whereas the outer part features a laminated layer.[61] In time, the parasite cysts expand and cause a granulomatous inflammatory reaction which leads to the cyst becoming walled off by fibrous tissue.[61,62] Maturing cysts may develop daughter cysts (cyst in a cyst) and septations.[5,62] Peripheral calcifications are common in both viable and non-viable cysts.[5]

*E. multilocularis* is endemic in the northern hemisphere, including North America, Asia and some European countries (mainly France, Switzerland, Austria and Germany).[62] However, due to migration of refugees, the disease is increasingly found in non-endemic areas. The definitive hosts are wild carnivores (such as the red fox) and domestic cats and dogs, intermediate hosts are small rodents, whereas humans are aberrant hosts who ingest embryonated eggs.[62] Echinococcal larvae form alveolar structures with multiple vesicles of different sizes within the liver.[61] Alveolar echinococcosis may spread locally or metastasise to the brain, bones or lungs via the blood.[61]

### CLINICAL PRESENTATION

The majority of patients are asymptomatic since the cyst grows only slowly in the liver (1–5 mm per year).[61,62] Liver lesions are therefore often found incidentally. The most common presenting symptoms are right upper quadrant discomfort and loss of appetite.[61] Complications from hydatid cysts include cyst leakage or rupture resulting in anaphylaxis, cholangitis due to obstruction of bile ducts by daughter cysts or rupture of a cyst into a biliary duct, or secondary infection of the cysts.[61,62] *E. multilocularis* is initially found in the liver (usually the right lobe), but metastasis to lung, brain, bones and local extension of the lesion (in the abdomen, retroperitoneum, or diaphragm) may be found later in the infection.[62] In late-stage disease, patients with alveolar echinococcosis may present with liver failure.

### DIAGNOSIS

Ultrasound is a good tool for screening and follow-up. With ultrasound imaging, hydatid sand (scolices in the cyst fluid from ruptured vesiculae which form a white sediment), floating membranes, daughter cysts and vesicles inside the cyst can be identified. CT can identify cyst wall or septal calcifications, and internal cystic structures and can be used to assess for complications (Fig. 5.7). MRI is superior for demonstrating cyst wall defects, biliary communication and neural involvement. Serological diagnosis is useful to confirm a radiological diagnosis and may also be an important tool for follow-up after surgical or pharmacological treatment. However, not all patients with cystic echinococcosis have a detectable immune response as this is dependent on the degree of echinococcal antigen secretion.[62]

### MANAGEMENT

The treatment options for cystic echinococcosis include surgery, percutaneous treatments and medical treatment with a benzimidazole (such as albendazole or mebendazole), and should be undertaken in a centre with expertise in this disease.[61,62] The most appropriate treatment option depends on multiple variables such as disease-specific characteristics (cyst number, size, site and presence of cystobiliary communication) and clinical condition of the patient.

Surgery is currently reserved for complicated cysts (biliary fistula), multiseptated cysts, cysts with daughter cysts and large superficial cysts with a high risk of perforation.[61] If feasible, surgical removal of hydatid cysts offers the best chance to completely cure the disease.[62] A benzimidazole is often given to reduce the risk of anaphylaxis and secondary cystic echinococcosis.

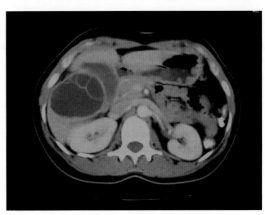

**Figure 5.7** CT of a patient with *Echinococcus granulosus* showing a non-calcified hydatid cyst with daughter cysts.

Another treatment option is the PAIR method; an acronym which stands for Puncture, Aspiration, Injection, Reaspiration. With this strategy, the cyst is punctured under ultrasound guidance, the cyst fluid is aspirated, a protoscolicidal agent (e.g. hypertonic saline or ethanol) is injected and the fluid re-aspirated. In selected patients, a success rate of up to 97% has been reported, but this method is less suitable for cysts that have daughter cysts.[61] Furthermore, PAIR should not be used if a cystobiliary communication is present, due to the risk of developing sclerosing cholangitis. To minimise the risk of secondary echinococcosis, concurrent treatment with a benzimidazole is recommended. This is usually given 4 hours before the puncture and continued for a month.[62] An alternative percutaneous method is placement of a broad tube to remove the solid components of the cysts as well as the daughter cysts.[61]

Medical treatment without surgery or PAIR may be used for patients with small cysts (< 5 cm) without daughter cysts or septations. Otherwise, this treatment should be restricted to patients who cannot undergo surgical or percutaneous treatment.[61,62] It is reported that complete cure (i.e. cyst disappearance) only occurs in approximately one-third of patients treated with a benzimidazole alone.[62]

*E. multilocularis cysts* are treated with surgery or pharmacotherapy. Surgery is the first-choice option in all operable patients.[61,62] Liver transplantation may be an option in patients with advanced liver failure. Albendazole treatment should be given for a prolonged period after surgery (at least 2 years) and patients should be monitored for recurrent disease. For patients not suitable for surgery, the optimal duration of therapy is not clear and a benzimidazole could even be necessary for life.[62]

## OTHER LIVER LESIONS

Mesenchymal hamartoma is an uncommon benign liver lesion that mainly occurs in young children (< 2 years of age), although cases in adults have been reported. These lesions consist of a mixture of epithelial and mesenchymal structures. If the lesions enlarge, surgical resection is recommended. Transformation to undifferentiated (embryological) sarcoma has rarely been described.

Focal steatosis and fatty sparing (also referred to as focal fatty change of the liver) are frequent findings on liver imaging and can mimic solid lesions. Regional variations in the degree of fat accumulation in the liver can be related to vascular anomalies, metabolic disorders, use of certain drugs or coexistence of hepatic masses. If the diagnosis is made (with or without biopsy), no further treatment is necessary.

Inflammatory hepatic pseudotumours are rare hepatic lesions that can mimic malignant lesions. They can occur at all ages. The aetiology is unclear, but an underlying infectious cause has been suggested. Patients can present without any symptoms or with fever, weight loss or upper abdominal pain. A biopsy can be necessary to differentiate the lesion from other tumours. On histological examination myofibroblasts, polyclonal plasma cells and fibrous tissue can be found. The course of the disease is unpredictable. Spontaneous regression has been reported, although recurrence after regression has also been described.[63] Treatment with antibiotics or steroids should be considered.

## Key points

- Benign liver lesions are common and often asymptomatic.
- Asymptomatic lesions can usually be managed conservatively.
- Haemangiomata are the commonest benign non-cystic liver lesion and can be > 10 cm in diameter (giant haemangioma). They are more common in females.
- Haemangiomata are managed conservatively, although in patients with recurrent pain and very large lesions, resection might be considered.
- Focal nodular hyperplasia (FNH) is the second commonest benign non-cystic liver tumour. If the diagnosis is certain, neither a resection nor follow-up of asymptomatic patients is necessary.
- Hepatocellular adenomas are rare hepatic tumours, mainly found in women of child-bearing age and are associated with the use of oral contraceptives.
- The risk of bleeding and malignant transformation increases with hepatocellular adenomas > 5 cm in diameter; the risk of malignancy is higher in men.
- Hepatic cysts are common, and if asymptomatic, need no further treatment.
- Cystadenomas are rare benign cystic tumours of the liver that should be considered for resection.
- Cystadenomas are more frequently found in women, and if found in men carry a higher risk of a malignancy.
- Hepatic liver abscesses should be treated with antibiotics and/or percutaneous drainage.
- Amoebic liver abscesses should be treated initially with metronidazole.
- Hepatic echinococcosis is a parasitic illness, in which humans are an accidental intermediate host. Although the disease is mainly found in endemic areas, it is increasingly found in non-endemic areas due to migration of refugees and should be managed in centres with expertise in the disease.

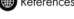 References available at http://ebooks.health.elsevier.com/

## KEY REFERENCES

[7] Marrero JA, Ahn J, Rajender Reddy K, et al. ACG clinical guideline: the diagnosis and management of focal liver lesions. Am J Gastroenterol 2014;109:1328–47; quiz 48. PMID: 25135008.
  *In this guideline of the American College of Gastroenterology, the authors provide an evidence-based approach to the diagnosis and management of a focal liver lesion, discussing not only malignant liver lesions but also benign solid and cystic liver lesions such as haemangioma, focal nodular hyperplasia, hepatocellular adenoma and hepatic cysts.*

[15] Thomeer MG, Broker M, Verheij J, et al. Hepatocellular adenoma: when and how to treat? update of current evidence. Therap Adv Gastroenterol 2016;9:898–912. PMID: 27803743.
  *Review that discusses the decision-making processes and associated risk analyses for hepatocellular adenoma based on lesion size and subtype. Hepatocellular adenomas > 5 cm present for 6 months after stopping oral contraceptives, lesions with a β-catenin mutation or lesions in male patients, associated with steroid use, glycogen storage disease or underlying viral hepatitis should be considered for an intervention.*

[16] Blanc JF, Frulio N, Chiche L, et al. Hepatocellular adenoma management: call for shared guidelines and multidisciplinary approach. Clin Res Hepatol Gastroenterol 2015;39:180–7. PMID: 25434466.
  *Describes the molecular subtypes of hepatocellular adenomas and their potential relevance for management. β-catenin-mutated hepatocellular adenomas are associated with a higher risk of malignancy, but also other mutations in the heterogenic group of hepatocellular adenomas are discussed.*

[17] Stoot JH, Coelen RJ, De Jong MC, et al. Malignant transformation of hepatocellular adenomas into hepatocellular carcinomas: a systematic review including more than 1600 adenoma cases. HPB 2010;12:509–22. PMID: 20887318.
  *A systematic review of hepatocellular adenomas focusing on malignant transformation. The authors conclude that malignant transformation of hepatocellular adenomas is rare (4.2%) and is mainly observed in lesions > 5 cm.*

[29] Lantinga MA, Gevers TJ, Drenth JP. Evaluation of hepatic cystic lesions. World J Gastroenterol 2013;19:3543–54. PMID: 23801855.
  *This review article describes the literature and an algorithm to guide clinicians in characterising hepatic cystic lesions. The diagnosis of simple liver cysts is based on typical ultrasound characteristics, whereas serodiagnostic tests and microbubble contrast-enhanced ultrasound are invaluable in differentiating complicated cysts, echinococcosis and cystadenoma/cystadenocarcinoma when ultrasound, CT and MRI show ambiguous findings.*

[36] Zhang ZY, Wang ZM, Huang Y. Polycystic liver disease: classification, diagnosis, treatment process, and clinical management. World J Hepatol 2020;12:72–83. PMID: 32231761.
  *This review mainly focuses on polycystic liver disease (PLD) classification, clinical manifestation, diagnosis and treatment. Only a small number of patients have symptoms that require treatment. At present, the treatment of PLD is mainly drugs intervention, cyst puncture and sclerotherapy, fenestration, transcatheter arterial embolization, liver resection and liver transplantation.*

[47] Hoekstra LT, Bieze M, Erdogan D, et al. Management of giant liver hemangiomas: an update. Expert Rev Gastroenterol Hepatol 2013;7:263–8. PMID: 23445235.
  *A literature review on giant haemangiomata, defined as > 5 cm. In patients with a giant liver haemangioma, observation is justified in the absence of symptoms, whereas surgical resection could be considered in selected patients with abdominal (mechanical) complaints or complications, or when diagnosis remains inconclusive.*

[56] Cai YL, Xiong XZ, Lu J, et al. Percutaneous needle aspiration versus catheter drainage in the management of liver abscess: a systematic review and meta-analysis. HPB 2015;17:195–201. PMID: 25209740.
  *A systematic review and meta-analysis on the treatment of liver abscesses. Percutaneous catheter drainage is more effective than percutaneous needle aspiration because it facilitates a higher success rate and reduces the time required to achieve clinical relief.*

[59] Stanley Jr SL. Amoebiasis. Lancet 2003;361:1025–34. PMID: 12660071.
  *Describes epidemiology, diagnosis and treatment of amoebiasis. Amoebic liver abscesses grow inexorably and, at one time, were almost always fatal, but now even large abscesses can be cured by one dose of antibiotic.*

[61] Mihmanli M, Idiz UO, Kaya C, et al. Current status of diagnosis and treatment of hepatic echinococcosis. World J Hepatol 2016;8:1169–81. PMID: 27729953.
  *Reviews the diagnosis and treatment of E. granulosus and E. multilocularis infections. The available treatment options for E. granulosus infection include open surgery, percutaneous interventions and pharmacotherapy, whereas E. multilocularis is treated with aggressive surgery as the first-choice treatment, while pharmacotherapy is used as an adjunct to surgery.*

# Primary malignant tumours of the liver

## 6

Cecilia G. Ethun | Michael I. D'Angelica

## INTRODUCTION

Primary liver malignancies comprise a group of tumours, some very rare, that have traditionally been divided into three main categories based on the cell type of origin—hepatocellular (hepatocellular carcinoma [HCC]), biliary (intrahepatic cholangiocarcinoma [ICC]), and mesenchymal (angiosarcoma, epithelioid haemangioendothelioma).[1] Yet, as our understanding of the molecular genetics and tumorigenesis of primary liver malignancy evolves, the once clear distinction between and uniformity within categories continue to blur. Subtypes, such as fibrolamellar HCC, demonstrate morphomolecular and clinical features distinct from typical HCC, and mixed hepatocellular-cholangiocellular carcinoma represents the merging of two traditionally different tumour types from different cell lineages.[2,3] As such, primary malignant tumours of the liver often exist as part of a continuum, with some falling somewhere within a spectrum of cellular and genomic differentiation.[4]

✓✓ Understanding the underlying pathogenesis of primary malignant liver tumours is imperative for appropriate diagnosis, and has implications for management, treatment response and prognosis.

## HEPATOCELLULAR CARCINOMA

HCC is the most common primary liver tumour, accounting for 75–85% of primary liver malignancies. It is the sixth most commonly diagnosed cancer overall and in 2020, was third leading cause of cancer mortality, with an estimated 830,000 deaths reported worldwide.[5] The rates of HCC incidence and mortality are two to three times higher among men than women, and vary widely between geographical regions. In many countries in Eastern Asia, South-Eastern Asia, and Northern and Western Africa, HCC is the most commonly diagnosed malignancy and leading cause of cancer-related deaths.[5,6]

Less common risk factors include $\alpha_1$-antitrypsin deficiency, hereditary hemochromatosis, primary biliary cirrhosis and autoimmune hepatitis. Due in large part to widespread public health efforts to improve vaccination against HBV, limit hepatitis B and C viral transmission and reduce aflatoxin exposure, the incidence and mortality rates of HCC have mostly decreased over the last several decades, particularly in high-risk countries of Eastern and South-Eastern Asia, and Eastern Sub-Saharan Africa.[7,8] In patients with chronic viral hepatitis who have already developed cirrhosis, successful antiviral therapy for both HBV and HCV has been demonstrated to significantly reduce, although not entirely eliminate, the risk of developing HCC across both low- and high-risk regions.[9–12] As such, antiviral treatment for patients with chronic infections from HBV and HCV should follow the recommendations of existing European Association for the Study of the Liver (EASL) guidelines.[13,14] In other areas, the major risk factors for HCC appear to be in transition. For example, in low-risk regions, such as Europe, North America and South America, there has been an increase in the incidence of HCC in recent years, which may reflect increases in non-alcoholic fatty liver disease (NAFLD) related to the increased prevalence of obesity, diabetes and metabolic syndrome in these populations.[8,15] The effect of risk modification on the development of HCC in patients with NAFLD is unclear.

✓ The main risk factors for the development of HCC include chronic infection from HBV and HCV, exposure to foods contaminated with aflatoxins, heavy alcohol consumption, obesity, type 2 diabetes and smoking.

✓ Shifting patterns in the incidence of HCC worldwide reflect geographic differences in risk factors, vaccination and screening protocols. While the incidence of HCC is decreasing in many high-risk countries, it is increasing in previously low-risk regions, such as Europe, North America and South America.

✓✓ Treatment with antiviral therapies have demonstrated efficacy in preventing progression to cirrhosis and decreasing the incidence of HCC and are recommended in all patients with chronic hepatitis due to HBV and HCV.

### PATHOGENESIS OF HCC

The association between HCC and cirrhosis is well established—while only an estimated 1–3% of patients with cirrhosis develop HCC annually, approximately 90% of patients with HCC have underlying cirrhosis. Repeated rounds of cellular injury followed by regeneration in the setting of chronic inflammation contributes to the development of liver fibrosis, cirrhosis and eventually HCC in a multi-step process estimated to take approximately 20 to 40 years. These sustained cycles of hepatocyte injury and repair, compounded by the host inflammatory response to viral infection, increase the risk of genomic alterations and contribute to oxidative stress, DNA damage and chromosome instability.[16] The role of the host immune system in the development of cirrhosis and eventual HCC in patients with NAFLD is less well understood, but is thought to be mediated by metabolic pathways, insulin resistance and lipotoxicity.[17]

✓ The accumulation of genetic aberrations within cirrhotic nodules from repeated injury and repair promotes progressive atypia and eventual malignant transformation to HCC.

71

## SCREENING FOR HCC

Because HCC develops over decades, often silently, screening and surveillance in high-risk individuals is one of the most important components in a comprehensive HCC program. The primary goal of screening is to detect HCC in early stages when effective treatment and long-term cure are still possible. There is currently only a single, randomised controlled trial (RCT) examining the impact of screening compared with no screening on survival. Performed in China, 18,816 patients with HBV were randomly assigned to either a screening program, which consisted of serum α-fetoprotein levels (AFP) and liver ultrasound (US) every 6 months, or no screening. Despite only a 68% adherence, their results still demonstrated a 37% reduction in HCC-related mortality with biannual screening protocol.[18] Additional population cohort studies and cost-effectiveness analyses have largely reinforced the benefits of biannual screening in high-risk patients, leading to this practice being universally accepted.[19–22] How high-risk is defined and what the true cost-effectiveness of screening is in certain patient populations, such as those with advanced liver disease who are not candidates for transplantation, high-risk non-cirrhotics or those with NAFLD, is less clear.

Several tests may be used for surveillance, including both imaging and serological studies. The most widely used exam for HCC surveillance is liver US, as it is non-invasive, poses little risk to the patient, has a relatively moderate cost and can detect additional related conditions, such as ascites or portal vein thrombosis, which may need prompt treatment. A meta-analysis of 19 studies demonstrated that US surveillance detected the majority of HCC tumours before clinical presentation, with a pooled sensitivity of 94%. However, the sensitivity of US to detect early-stage HCC was only 63%.[20] The use of contrast-enhanced US has been proposed in an effort to improve the detection of small, early-stage HCC tumours; however, this has not been proven and its use has not been widely adopted.[23] While multidetector computed tomography (CT) and dynamic magnetic resonance imaging (MRI) can be valuable studies in circumstances where US is less effective, such as in fatty liver disease, their associated high-cost, radiation exposure, need for contrast agents and considerably high false-positive rates have limited their role in long-term surveillance schemes.[24] Several serological tests have been investigated to aid early diagnosis of HCC, including AFP, prothrombin induced by vitamin K absence II (PIVKA II), the ratio of glycosylated AFP (L3 fraction) to total AFP, α-fucosidase, and glypican. Although AFP is the most widely used biomarker for HCC, it has largely been a tool of diagnosis rather than surveillance. Indeed, studies examining the utility of AFP for surveillance have been disappointing, and current guidelines recommend against its routine use in HCC screening.[25] Other serum markers have primarily been studied as diagnostic or prognostic aids, and insufficient evidence exists to recommend their use for screening purposes.

✔✔ Screening for HCC should be performed by experienced personnel in all high-risk individuals using abdominal US every 6 months.

## DIAGNOSIS OF HCC

Non-invasive imaging forms the cornerstone of diagnosis for HCC in the cirrhotic liver. Image-based diagnosis relies on a high pre-test probability in the setting of cirrhosis, combined with the presence of hallmark radiographic findings that are typical of HCC—arterial phase hyperenhancement and non-peripheral wash-out on portal venous and/or delayed phases (Fig. 6.1a–d).[26] Adopted in 2011 by the American College of Radiology, the Liver Imaging Reporting and Data System (LI-RADS) provides a set of standardised terminology and establishes a framework for the classification of liver lesions in the setting of cirrhosis, ranging from LR-1 (definitely benign) to LR-5 (definitely HCC) (Table 6.1).[27] The accuracy of the radiographic diagnosis of HCC relies on two major factors—tumour size and imaging modality. Because small tumours are more challenging to diagnose, the EASL and European Organisation for Research and Treatment of Cancer (EORTC) developed a sequential algorithm for the work-up of tumours < 10 mm and 10–20 mm in size (Fig. 6.2).[25,28]

While several imaging modalities may be used to diagnose HCC, multiphasic contrast-enhanced CT and MRI are the most widely used and studied. In general, MRI appears to have a higher sensitivity than CT, although this depends on tumour size.[29,30] A recent prospective, multicentre study of 544 nodules in 381 patients demonstrated an increased sensitivity and specificity with contrast-enhanced MRI (72.3% and 89.4%, respectively) compared with CT (67.9% and 76.8%, respectively) for lesions 10–20 mm in size; for lesions 20–30mm in size, the sensitivity and specificity of contrast-enhanced MRI and CT were comparable (70.6% and 83.2% vs 71.6% and 93.6%, respectively). Importantly, this study also found that the combination of CT and MRI resulted in a specificity of 100%, but a sensitivity of only 55%, supporting the recommendation against routine dual imaging for small lesions.[30]

The use of contrast-enhanced ultrasound (CEUS) for the diagnosis of HCC is controversial. Although refinements in the definition of the typical hallmark features of HCC on CEUS have led to improved diagnostic capacity, its sensitivity remains significantly lower than CT or MRI, missing roughly 13% of HCCs seen on cross-sectional imaging.[31] Furthermore, because CEUS does not provide a panoramic view of the liver, does not carry the added benefit of staging and is not easily reviewed across imaging software platforms, it is not recommended as a first-line imaging technique for the diagnosis of HCC.[25] Still, it may be beneficial when used to characterise one or a few nodules seen on conventional US, or when both CT and MRI are either contraindicated or inconclusive.

✔✔ The diagnosis of HCC in cirrhotic patients with tumours larger than 1 cm is largely based on non-invasive criteria using four-phase multidetector CT or dynamic contrast-enhanced MRI. The typical hallmark features of HCC include a hypervascular tumour in the arterial phase with washout in the portal venous or delayed phases.

✔ In situations where CT or MRI are inconclusive, imaging suggests a malignancy other than HCC, or in non-cirrhotic patients, pathologic confirmation should be obtained.

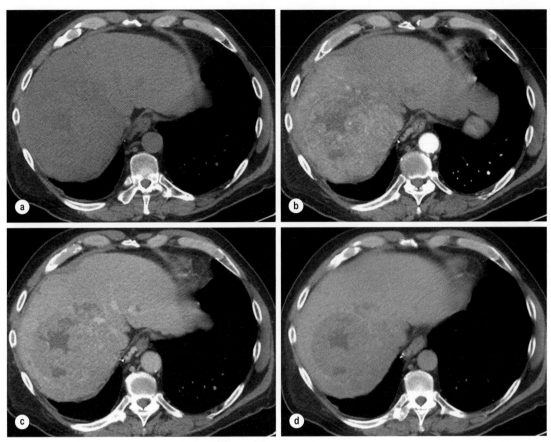

**Figure 6.1**  Characteristic imaging findings of hepatocellular carcinoma on four-phase contrast-enhanced computed tomography. (a) Pre-contrast phase, showing an iso-intense lesion in the right liver. (b) Arterial phase, showing arterial hyperenhancement. (c) Portal venous phase, showing non-peripheral wash-out. (d) Delayed venous phase, showing continue washout and a partial capsule.

**Table 6.1  American College of Radiology Liver Reporting & Data System (LI-RADS) for CT and MRI imaging for hepatocellular carcinoma (HCC)**

| LI-RADS | Description | Management |
|---|---|---|
| Negative | No observations detected | Return to surveillance in 6 months |
| LR-NC | Not categorizable due to image degradation or omission | Repeat or alternative imaging in < 3 months |
| LR-1 | Definitely benign observation | Return to surveillance in 6 months |
| LR-2 | Probably benign | Consider repeat diagnostic imaging in 6 months |
| LR-3 | Intermediate probability of malignancy | Repeat or alternative imaging in 3–6 months |
| LR-4 | Probably HCC | Multidisciplinary discussion for further work-up |
| LR-5 | Definitely HCC | Multidisciplinary discussion for management consensus |
| LR-M | Probably/definite malignancy not HCC specific | Multidisciplinary discussion. Consider biopsy |
| LR-TIV | Definite tumour in vein | Multidisciplinary discussion. May include biopsy |

## HCC STAGING SYSTEMS

Many staging systems for HCC exist, each utilising different combinations of clinicopathologic factors and displaying varying degrees of applicability, tumour-specific focus and prognostic value. The American Joint Committee on Cancer (AJCC) TNM classification is the standard staging system for cancer worldwide. In HCC, the TNM classification focuses on four major clinicopathologic factors—tumour size, multifocality, vascular invasion and extrahepatic spread.[32] Although

it is widely referenced for HCC, TNM system relies on pathologic characteristics of resected specimens only, and fails to incorporate underlying liver function and patient-specific factors. The Barcelona Clinic Liver Cancer (BCLC) staging system is clinically-based, applicable to all stages of disease and has been externally validated in different clinical settings.[25,33] Based on tumour stage, liver function and performance status, it stratifies patients with HCC into four categories—early, intermediate, advanced and terminal—and makes treatment recommendations for each (Fig. 6.3).[33,34]

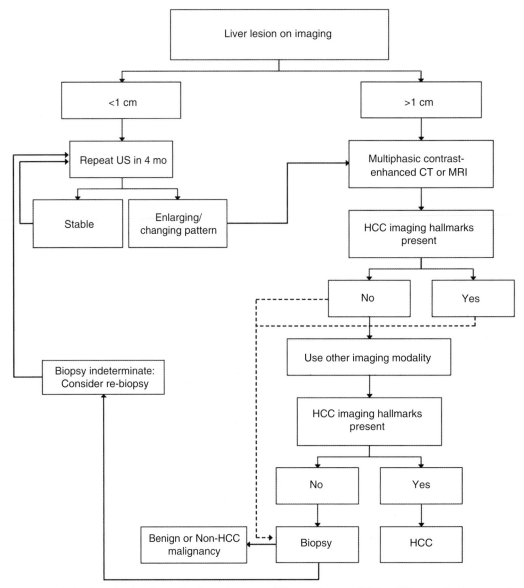

**Figure 6.2** Recommended algorithm for the diagnosis of small hepatocellular carcinomas (HCCs). *CT,* computed tomography; *MRI,* magnetic resonance imaging; *US,* ultrasound. (Adapted from [25].)

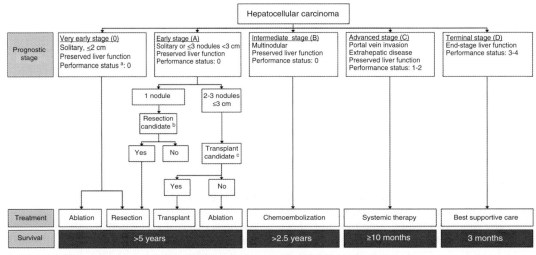

**Figure 6.3** The modified Barcelona Clinic Liver Cancer (BCLC) staging system.
[a]Performance status based on the Eastern Cooperative Oncology Group performance status evaluation.
[b]Determination of resectability should be based on whether or not the future liver remnant will be of sufficient quantity and quality, with adequate inflow, outflow and biliary drainage, in order to sustain function postoperatively.
[c]Determination of transplant candidacy should be based on validated criteria, such as the Milan criteria, and specific institutional protocols for liver transplantation. (Reprinted with permission from Elsevier. A. Forner, M. Reig, J. Bruix. Hepatocellular carcinoma. Lancet [2018]; Volume 391, Issue 10127: 1301–1314.)

✅ Due to the unique nature of the disease, any clinical staging system for HCC should include tumour-specific factors, underlying liver function, and patient performance status.

✅✅ The BCLC staging system is the most widely used staging system for HCC and is the recommended system for prognosis and treatment allocation in Europe.

## SURGERY

Surgery is considered first-line therapy for HCC and is the only potentially curative treatment option, with 5-year survival ranging from 60–80% in well-selected patients. The choice of resection or transplantation is generally dictated by the degree of underlying liver dysfunction and the burden of disease.

### LIVER RESECTION

Liver resection for HCC is unique, in that it requires consideration of not just technical and biologic resectability, but also underlying liver dysfunction. In liver surgery, the technical resectability of a tumour is defined not only by what can be removed, but more importantly, by what will be left behind. Hepatic artery and portal vein inflow, hepatic vein outflow, biliary drainage, and the quantity and quality of the future liver remnant (FLR) must be adequate in order to maintain hepatic function and allow for regeneration following resection.[35] Inflow, outflow and biliary drainage can be determined using high-quality cross-sectional imaging.

The Child-Pugh score is the most commonly used measurement of liver quality and function. Liver resection is still considered safe and appropriate in patients with a Child-Pugh A score without evidence of portal hypertension. Other measurements that may be helpful in improving patient selection for resection include the model for end-stage liver disease (MELD), MELD-Na, indocyanine green kinetics, liver stiffness measurement and cholinesterase/bilirubin ratio.[36–38] The assessment of liver quantity can be performed by evaluating the expected postoperative FLR as a ratio of the total liver volume (minus the tumour volume). Ratios of at least 25% are considered safe in healthy, non-cirrhotic livers. An FLR of at least 30–40% is recommended in patients with chronic liver disease and a Child-Pugh A score.[39] In patients whose FLR may be inadequate, but who are otherwise candidates for liver resection, pre-operative portal vein embolisation (PVE) should be considered.

The biologic principles of resection for HCC largely focus on four factors—tumour size, multifocality, vascular invasion and extrahepatic spread. As previously mentioned, these factors form the basis of the AJCC TNM staging system, and are incorporated into various other clinical staging systems, such as the BCLC.[26,32,33] However, unlike transplantation for HCC, specific oncologic criteria are not as well defined for resection and in practice, the determination of resectability from a tumour biology standpoint can vary widely. For example, resection may still be considered feasible in select patients with large tumours (size > 5 cm) or limited multifocal disease. The benefit of resection in patients with major vascular invasion, however, is questionable and should be pursued only in highly selected patients. With few exceptions, the presence of extrahepatic disease, including regional lymph node metastasis, is a contraindication to resection in patients with HCC.

With regards to underlying liver dysfunction, liver resection is the treatment of choice in non-cirrhotic patients with HCC. Challenges arise in patients with HCC in the setting NAFLD and metabolic syndrome, but without significant fibrosis or cirrhosis, as postoperative morbidity following resection is increased compared to those with normal livers. Still, postoperative mortality remains less than 2% and patients demonstrate prolonged long-term survival compared to patients with cirrhosis undergoing resection.[40,41] In patients with cirrhosis, the decision to proceed with liver resection should rely on a combination of tumour-related factors, the degree of underlying liver dysfunction, and the extent of resection required to achieve complete tumour extirpation. In 2012, the EASL and EORTC developed a set of guidelines for resection of HCC in patients with cirrhosis—solitary tumours and well-preserved liver function, platelet count > 100,000/mL or the absence of portal hypertension.[28]

✅ Technical resectability, tumour biology, underlying hepatic dysfunction and patient comorbidities must all be considered prior to resection in patients with HCC.

✅ Resection is the treatment of choice for HCC in the non-cirrhotic liver.

### LIVER TRANSPLANTATION

HCC is the only malignancy for which solid organ transplantation is widely accepted. The Milan criteria (solitary tumour ≤ 5 cm or ≤ 3 tumours each ≤3 cm in size, without vascular invasion) is the most widely accepted and reliable tool for determining transplantability.[42,43] Patients within Milan criteria have an expected 5-year survival rate that ranges from 65% to 80%, and have a longer survival than patients who fall outside the criteria.[44] In centres where the conventional Milan criteria is used, patients beyond Milan may still be offered transplantation if they can be successfully down-staged into the accepted criteria.[45] In order to limit dropout and improve the success rate of downstaging strategies, restricted eligibility for downstaging protocols using tumour number, size and AFP is recommended.[25,46]

Several expanded criteria have been developed and externally validated, and demonstrate similar post-transplant survival to the Milan criteria (Table 6.2).[47–51] While there is no consensus on the applicability of any single expanded criteria, surrogate markers of tumour biology, such as AFP, and response to neoadjuvant therapy are likely to replace conventional, morphology-based criteria to determine transplant eligibility. Regardless of the criteria used, major vascular invasion and extrahepatic disease are absolute contraindications to liver transplantation for patients with HCC.[25,46]

Due to challenges with organ availability and allocation, wait times can be significant, and patients with HCC who are candidates for liver transplantation are at risk of tumour progression while waiting. Neoadjuvant 'bridging' therapy using various combinations of ablation and transarterial techniques has been shown to reduce dropout due to progression of disease and has become nearly universally accepted.[52–54] This is particularly true in regions where the expected wait time is greater than 6 months.[55]

**Table 6.2   Summary of validated selection criteria for liver transplantation in patients with hepatocellular carcinoma**

| System | Criteria | Survival[a] |
|---|---|---|
| Milan[42,43] | • Solitary tumour < 5 cm, OR<br>• 2–3 tumours, all < 3 cm<br>• No vascular invasion or extrahepatic disease | 4-yr OS: 85% |
| UCSF[47,98] | • Solitary tumour < 6.5cm, OR<br>• 2–3 lesions, all < 4.5 cm, with total tumour diameter < 8 cm<br>• No vascular invasion or extrahepatic disease | 5-yr OS: 75% |
| Up-to-7[48] | • Up to 7 tumours, with largest tumour < 7 cm<br>• No vascular invasion or extrahepatic disease | 5-yr OS: 71% |
| TTV + AFP[49] | • Total tumour volume 115 cm$^3$<br>• AFP < 400 ng/mL<br>• No vascular invasion or extrahepatic disease | 4-yr OS: 75% |
| AFP-French model[50] | • Points based on largest tumour diameter, number of nodules and AFP level<br>• No vascular invasion or extrahepatic disease | 5-yr OS: 68% (low-risk score)<br>5-yr OS: 48% (high-risk score) |
| Toronto[51] | • Any size, any number of tumours<br>• No poorly differentiated tumours<br>• No cancer-related systemic systems<br>• No vascular invasion or extrahepatic disease | 5-yr OS: 68% |

[a]All studies reported no statistically significant difference between patients within Milan and those outside Milan, but within the proposed criteria, among the respective study cohorts.
*AFP,* alpha-fetoprotein; *OS,* overall survival; *TTV,* total tumour volume; *UCSF,* University of California, San Francisco.

✓✓ Liver transplantation is the recommended first-line treatment for patients who fall within Milan criteria and are not eligible for resection.

✓ There is no consensus on the use of expanded criteria for transplantation in HCC.

✓ Patients beyond Milan criteria may be considered candidates for liver transplantation after successful downstaging.

✓✓ Major vascular invasion and the presence of extrahepatic disease are absolute contraindications to liver transplantation in HCC.

✓ In patients with HCC who are transplant candidates, the use of locoregional and liver-directed therapies to bridge the patient while on the wait list is recommended.

## LOCOREGIONAL THERAPIES

✓✓ Locoregional therapy is the recommended treatment approach for patients with HCC who are not candidates for resection or transplantation.

### ABLATION

Tumour necrosis using ablative techniques can be achieved using either chemical ablation (percutaneous ethanol injection [PEI]), thermal ablation (radiofrequency [RFA] or microwave ablation [MWA]) or cryoablation. All ablative procedures may be done using a percutaneous, laparoscopic or open approach. In order to improve the efficacy of ablation, image guidance using US, CT, or cone-beam CT should be used. Caution should be used, however, when lesions are close to important structures as thermal spread can lead to injury to major bile ducts and surrounding organs.

PEI is one of the most common techniques for treating small, well-circumscribed HCC, and can achieve complete necrosis in 90% of tumours < 2 cm in size. However, PEI is less successful in tumours larger than 2 cm, may demonstrate inconsistent distribution within the tumour, and is associated with a high recurrence rate.[56] Studies comparing PEI with RFA have consistently demonstrated improved overall survival (OS), disease-free survival and recurrence-free survival with RFA.[57]

RFA uses high-frequency alternating currents to generate frictional heat, inducing cell death. The heat produced by RFA creates a coagulative necrosis, which can be applied beyond the boundaries of the tumour, treating a margin potentially containing microscopic tumour cells. Outcomes with RFA vary widely but are generally favourable for early HCC, with an estimated 3-year OS of 76% and RFS of 46% for tumours < 3 cm in size.[58] Larger tumours may still be successfully treated with RFA by using multipolar approaches or by combining RFA with transarterial chemoembolisation (TACE).[59,60] Multiple studies have been performed comparing RFA with surgery for HCC. A 2017 Cochran review comparing RFA with surgery for small, solitary HCC found no difference in survival between the two. Surgery was associated with fewer HCC recurrences, while RFA was associated with fewer adverse events and shorter hospital length of stay.[61] For tumours > 5 cm or multifocal tumours > 3 cm, surgery is associated with improved survival compared with RFA, and should be the treatment of choice in resectable patients.

MWA uses electromagnetic energy to heat tissue. One of the benefits of this technique is that it is less affected by nearby vessels, and thus, less prone to heat sink than RFA. Although data are still emerging, MWA has been shown in several studies to be at least equivalent to RFA in terms of survival, recurrence and adverse events, and may be considered an alternative to RFA in patients with small or unresectable HCC.[62]

Irreversible electroporation (IRE) is an emerging ablative technique that delivers non-thermal, high-voltage electric pulses to tumour cells, resulting in increased cell membrane permeability and subsequent apoptosis. Similar to MWA, IRE is less likely to demonstrate heat sink and is safe to use near blood vessels, bile ducts and other critical structures.[63] Still, high-quality data examining the long-term effectiveness of IRE for HCC are lacking.

✓✓ RFA is the standard of care for patients with early-stage HCC tumours that are not otherwise suitable for surgical resection.

✓ In patients with small (<3 cm), solitary tumours in favourable locations, RFA may be considered an alternative to surgery.

✓✓ Ethanol injection is an option in tumours < 2 cm when thermal ablation is not technically feasible.

✓ MWA is associated with acceptable local control and survival, comparable to RFA, but long-term data are still needed.

## TRANSARTERIAL THERAPIES

Arterial-directed therapy involves the selective catheter-based infusion of particles targeting the feeding arteries of the tumour-containing portion of liver. By taking advantage of HCC's primarily arterial-dependent inflow, transarterial therapies are able to selectively target HCC while sparing much of the surrounding liver, which is primarily fed by the portal venous system. Transarterial therapies currently being used include transarterial embolisation (TAE), TACE, TACE with drug-eluding beads (TACE-DEB) and selective internal radiation therapy (SIRT).

TACE is the most common primary treatment for unresectable HCC. In addition to the ischaemic effects from arterial embolisation, as seen in TAE, TACE also demonstrates cytotoxic effects through the intra-arterial infusion of chemotherapy. While TACE has shown superior efficacy to supportive care, two RCTs directly comparing TACE with TAE have failed to demonstrate any differences in response, recurrence or survival between the two.[64,65]

The most common drugs used during conventional TACE, either alone in combination, are doxorubicin or epirubicin, and/or cisplatin or miriplatin. In order to improve the efficacy of cytotoxic agents, iodised oil (Lipiodol) is combined with the chemotherapy agents, increasing their concentration in the tumour cells. Other techniques include TACE-DEB, which uses calibrated doxorubicin microspheres to both deliver tumour-specific drugs and achieve permanent embolisation. While initial results for TACE-DEB were promising, subsequent data comparing conventional TACE with TACE-DEB have been mixed, without any clear indication for one over the other.[66,67]

TACE should not be performed in patients with liver decompensation, hyperbilirubinaemia (bilirubin > 2 mg/dL), bilioenteric anastomosis, impaired kidney function, or when the tumour burden is > 50% of the total liver volume. Portal vein thrombosis is a relative contraindication to TACE, although it may still be safely performed if the thrombosis does not involve the main portal and the treatment is selective.

SIRT, also known as radioembolisation, involves catheter-based arterial infusion of radioisotopes, such as 131-Iodine-labelled Lipiodol or yttrium-90 (Y90) microspheres (either resin or glass), and may be performed in a lobar, sectoral or segmental approach, depending on tumour size and location. Given the hypervascularity of HCC, particles are preferentially delivered to areas containing tumour, emitting high-energy,

low-penetration radiation. There are no large RCTs comparing SIRT with TACE or TACE-DEB, but two recent meta-analyses demonstrated that SIRT was associated with longer time to progression, less toxicity and less post-treatment pain. Response rates and long-term survival between techniques, however, was similar.[68,69] In addition, SIRT is safe for tumours close to critical structures and in the setting of portal vein thrombosis, and may be done as an outpatient procedure.

✓✓ TACE is considered first-line for patients with BCLC stage B HCC.

✓✓ Conventional TACE and TACE-DEB show similar benefit and safety profile.

✓✓ TACE should not be used in the setting of decompensated or advanced liver disease, major venous invasion, or extrahepatic metastases.

✓ SIRT using yttrium-90 microspheres has an acceptable safety profile and may be used alone or in combination with TACE or TACE-DEB. High-quality data defining specific subsets of patient who may benefit most from SIRT over other locoregional therapies are lacking.

## SYSTEMIC THERAPY

Due to success of locoregional therapies available to treat patients with unresectable HCC, systemic therapy has traditionally been reserved as a last resort of patients with particularly advanced or metastatic disease.

### SORAFENIB

Sorafenib is an oral multikinase inhibitor that suppresses angiogenesis and tumour cell proliferation and is the most widely studied systemic therapy for HCC. The SHARP trial was a randomised, placebo-controlled, phase III study that randomised 602 patients with advanced HCC to either receive sorafenib or best supportive care. Median and 1-year OS was longer in the sorafenib arm than the placebo arm (10.7 months and 44% vs 7.9 months and 33%, respectively). Disease control rate was also improved in the sorafenib arm.[70] The Asia-Pacific study was a trial that randomised 226 patients with advanced HCC to sorafenib or placebo arms, and similarly found improved OS and disease control with sorafenib compared with placebo.[71]

### LENVATINIB

Lenvatinib is an inhibitor of multiple growth signalling targets, including vascular epithelial growth factor (VEGF), fibroblast growth factor and platelet-derived growth factor. In a randomised, phase III, non-inferiority trial (REFLECT), 954 patients with unresectable HCC were randomized to receive either lenvatinib or sorafenib as first-line therapy. Lenvatinib was found to be non-inferior to sorafenib (13.6 months vs 12.3 months, respectively) and is considered an alternative to sorafenib as first-line therapy in patients with unresectable HCC.[72]

### ATEZOLIZUMAB AND BEVACIZUMAB

Bevacizumab is a VEGF inhibitor that has previously demonstrated a modest effect in patients with HCC. In a phase III trial with 501 patients with unresectable HCC, the combination of atezolizumab and bevacizumab demonstrated improved 1-year OS compared with sorafenib as first-line (67.2% vs 54.6%, respectively).[73]

First-line systemic therapy for patients with advanced HCC includes sorafenib, lenvatinib and atezolizumab plus bevacizumab.

## FIBROLAMELLAR CARCINOMA

Fibrolamellar carcinoma (FLC) is a rare variant of HCC, defined by the presence of well-differentiated, polygonal hepatic tumour cells with an eosinophilic granular cytoplasm surrounded by a fibrous lamellar stroma. It is most frequently observed in the Western hemisphere, where it accounts for approximately 1% of all HCCs. These tumours occur at a younger age than HCC (20–35 years), preferentially in women, and do not arise in a background of chronic liver disease.

Typically large at the time of diagnosis (8–10 cm), the common symptoms related to FLC are a palpable mass, abdominal pain, weight loss, malaise and anorexia. AFP is elevated in patients with FLC less than 10% of the time. On imaging, FLC presents as a large, solitary, hypervascular, heterogeneous liver mass with a central hypodense region due to central necrosis or fibrosis (Fig. 6.4). On MRI, the central scar has low attenuation on T2 images, whereas the central scar of focal nodular hyperplasia has high attenuation. They have well-defined margins and calcification is present in 68%. Histology demonstrates deeply eosinophilic, polygonal neoplastic cells surrounded by a dense, layered fibrous stroma.

Complete resection is the primary treatment for FLC. Because portal lymph node involvement is common (60%), a portal lymphadenectomy is recommended at the time of resection. Prognosis is better than that of HCC overall, with a 5-year survival of 50–75% following resection.[74] Locoregional and distant disease recurrence is common, occurring in approximately 80% of patients at 5 years. Thus, close long-term follow-up is recommended. In young, otherwise healthy individuals, repeat resection for disease recurrence may be offered.

True FLC should be differentiated from mixed FLC–HCC, defined as conventional HCC displaying some distinct area with FLC features.[75] Liver transplantation may be an alternative option in selected cases and survival rates of 48% can be obtained in patients transplanted for FLC–HCC.[76] No effective systemic therapy has been demonstrated.

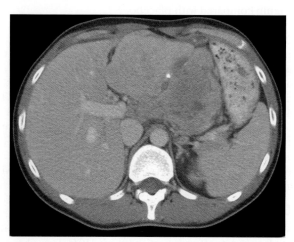

**Figure 6.4** Characteristic imaging findings of fibrolamellar hepatocellular carcinoma on contrast-enhanced computed tomography. Large left hepatic mass with central hypoenhancement and calcification.

FLC is a variant of HCC that typically occurs in younger women without underlying liver dysfunction.

Resection is the mainstay of treatment for FLC. Although recurrence is common, the disease presents with an indolent course and survival rates are favourable compared with HCC.

## INTRAHEPATIC CHOLANGIOCARCINOMA

ICC arises from the peripheral intrahepatic biliary radicles and is the second most common primary tumour of the liver. In the Western world, the incidence of ICC is 0.3–3 per 100 000 per million, and occurs with equal frequency in men or women between the age of 55 and 75 years. Recent reports suggest that the incidence is increasing, particularly in the USA, UK, France, Italy, Japan and Australia. Although this increase may be real, it is likely explained, in part, by improvements in the diagnosis of this tumour and changes in the rules for how they should be coded according to the International Classification of Diseases for Oncology (ICD).[77]

### RISK FACTORS

The traditional risk factors for ICC include chronic biliary inflammation such as primary sclerosing cholangitis, chronic choledocholithiasis, hepatolithiasis, parasitic biliary infestation and choledochal cysts. However, in most patients with ICC (more than 95%), none of these risk factors can be identified. The exception occurs in some areas of Asia, and in particular, north-eastern Thailand, where the parasite *Opisthorchis viverrini* is prevalent.

New risk factors are emerging, including NAFLD, HBV infection, HCV infection, diabetes and metabolic syndrome.[78] However, in contrast to HCC, most ICCs develop without a background of liver disease. In a surgical series, 75% of patients had normal livers, 16% had chronic hepatitis/liver fibrosis and 9% had cirrhosis.

### DIAGNOSIS OF ICC

ICC tends to be diagnosed at an advanced stage because the tumour remains clinically silent in its early stages. Symptoms, when present, include abdominal pain, malaise, night sweats, asthenia, nausea and weight loss. Unfortunately, by the time symptoms are apparent, the tumour is often unresectable.

Patients may present with an elevation in liver enzymes, in particular alkaline phosphatase or γ-glutamyltransferase, although these are fairly non-specific. Jaundice may be present if the tumour compresses or invades the biliary confluence and is typically a sign of unresectable disease.

While routinely drawn, the benefit of serum markers for ICC is unclear. Carcinoembryonic antigen (CEA) exceeds 20 ng/mL in 15% and carbohydrate antigen (CA) 19–9 is > 300 U/mL in 40% of cases. AFP exceeds 200 ng/mL in only 6% of patients.

Multiphasic contrast-enhanced CT and MRI with MR cholangiopancreatography (MRCP) are the imaging modalities of choice for evaluating ICC. On CT, ICC presents as a hypodense lesion with irregular, infiltrative margins, no arterial enhancement and variable delayed enhancement in the portal venous phase (Fig. 6.5a and b). On MRI, ICC appears as a hypointense lesion on T1-weighted images and a hyperintense lesion on

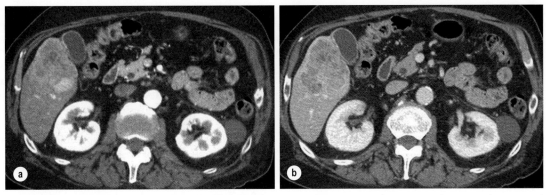

**Figure 6.5**    Characteristic imaging findings of hepatocellular carcinoma on multi-phase contrast-enhanced computed tomography. (a) Arterial phase, showing arterial hyper-enhancement. (b) Portal venous phase, showing incomplete peripheral enhancement with central washout.

T2-weighted images, with pooling of contrast on delayed images. There is often peripheral biliary dilatation seen on cross-sectional imaging. MRCP can be valuable to determine the extent of biliary involvement. In cases where the diagnosis is still unclear after high-quality cross-sectional imaging, biopsy may be considered. CT chest must be obtained to rule out pulmonary metastases. Positron emission tomography may also be used to assess for distant metastatic disease. Additional work-up to rule out other malignancies, including esophagogastroduodenoscopy and colonoscopy, should also be considered.

✔ Multiphasic contrast-enhanced CT and MRI with MRCP are the primary imaging modalities for evaluation and surveillance of ICC.

✔ Percutaneous biopsy should only be performed if the diagnosis is unclear on high-quality cross-sectional imaging or if the result will change clinical management.

## CLASSIFICATION AND STAGING

There are three primary subtypes of ICC based on tumour growth patterns: mass-forming, the most common type found in approximately 60% of cases; periductal-infiltrating, which spreads along the bile ducts; and intraductal-growth type with intraluminal spread. Tumours may also have mixed components, in particular a combination of mass-forming and periductal-infiltrating. The clinical significance of these growth patterns is unclear.

The eighth edition of AJCC TNM staging for ICC is based on the number of tumours (solitary vs multiple), tumour size (<5 cm or >5 cm), vascular invasion (major vascular and/or microscopic invasion) and extension into the visceral peritoneum.[79]

## SURGERY

Complete resection is the only potentially curative treatment option in patients with ICC. The goal of resection should be to achieve a negative margin while leaving behind an FLR that is of adequate quality and quantity. In situations where the size of the FLR is in question, PVE may be performed preoperatively. Bilateral inflow or outflow involvement, multifocal disease and distant metastases should be considered unresectable. A diagnostic laparoscopy may be considered at the time of or prior to resection to assess for unresectable or disseminated disease. The presence of lymph node metastases is one of the most important prognostic indicators. As such, a portal lymph node dissection should be routinely performed for adequate staging.[80] There are no data to support any therapeutic benefit to lymphadenectomy in patients with ICC.

Five-year survival following an R0 resection for ICC ranges from 23% to 42%. Recurrence is high and is found in roughly 50% of patients. For patients in whom complete resection is not possible, 5-year survival approaches 0%.[81]

✔ Resection with negative margins is the only potentially curative treatment option in patients with limited and resectable ICC.

✔ Because lymph nodes involvement provides important prognostic information, a portal lymphadenectomy should routinely be performed for all patients undergoing resection.

## ADJUVANT THERAPY

The role of adjuvant therapy following resection in patients with ICC is unclear, as studies examining its benefit have had mixed results and include a heterogenous population of patients with all biliary cancers. The PRODIGE 12–ACCORD 18 trial was a French multicentre RCT that examined the benefit of adjuvant gemcitabine-oxaliplatin (GEMOX) versus surveillance in patients with resected biliary tract cancers. Of the 194 patients randomized, 43% had ICC. There was no difference in OS or recurrence-free survival between the two arms, and the use of adjuvant GEMOX was not recommended.[82] The BILCAP trial was a UK multicentre RCT that investigated adjuvant capecitabine for resected biliary tract cancers. Of the 447 patients randomised, only 19% had ICC. In the intention-to-treat analysis, there was no difference in OS between the two arms; however, in the per-protocol analysis, capecitabine was associated with improved OS compared with observation (53 vs 36 months, respectively).[83] Based on the results of BILCAP, many surgeons and medical oncologists have adopted the use of capecitabine in the adjuvant setting for ICC. The ACTICCA-1 trial is a Dutch multicentre RCT that compares adjuvant gemcitabine plus cisplatin to adjuvant capecitabine in patients with resected biliary tract cancers. Accrual began in 2014 and is estimated to be completed in 2023, with an anticipated sample size of 781 patients.[84]

Based on data from two large USA-based cancer registries, adjuvant chemoradiation may be used in patients with positive microscopic margins or metastatic lymph nodes; however, further research is needed to better define the role of chemoradiation for resected ICC.[85,86] There are no data to support the use of other locoregional therapy for ICC in the adjuvant or neoadjuvant settings in otherwise resectable patients.[87]

✅✅ Adjuvant capecitabine should be considered in all patients who undergo resection of ICC.

✅ Adjuvant chemoradiation may be used in patients with positive microscopic margins or lymph node metastases.

## ADVANCED DISEASE

### CHEMOTHERAPY

The combination of gemcitabine and cisplatin is considered the standard-of-care treatment for patients with advanced or metastatic ICC. This recommendation is based on the results from the phase III ABC-02 trial, which demonstrated improved OS and progression-free survival with gemcitabine plus cisplatin over gemcitabine alone in patients with advanced biliary tract cancers.[88] There are currently insufficient data to support a recommendation of any specific second-line regimen in ICC.

### LOCOREGIONAL THERAPY

Locoregional therapies, including TACE, TACE-DEB, SIRT with yttrium-90 microspheres, and radiation therapy have all been demonstrated to be safe and effective in patients with unresectable ICC in retrospective series and small cohort studies. The use of locoregional therapy in ICC to successfully downsize tumours and convert initially unresectable disease to being resectable has also been described; however, data are extremely limited and are insufficient to recommend conversion strategies in patients with ICC.

The use of hepatic arterial infusion (HAI) chemotherapy with floxuridine for unresectable liver-confined ICC has demonstrated promising results. In a meta-analysis that included 20 studies comparing HAI with TACE, TACE-DEB and SIRT, HAI was associated with improved OS and tumour response, with a response rate of 57%.[89] HAI chemotherapy may also be combined with systemic chemotherapy. In a large retrospective series of patients with unresectable ICC, the combination of HAI and systemic chemotherapies was associated with improved OS compared with systemic chemotherapy alone (30.8 vs. 18.4 months).[90] Despite the encouraging results, HAI chemotherapy should be limited to use in experienced centres or in a trial setting.

### TARGETED THERAPY

The most common genetic alterations in ICC are isocitrate dehydrogenase (*IDH*) mutations and fibroblast growth factor-2 (*FGFR2*) fusions. Thus, the most promising targets currently under investigation for use in the advanced and adjuvant setting for ICC are *IDH* inhibitors for *IDH*-mutant tumours and drugs targeting *FGFR2* gene fusions. While preliminary data are encouraging, further studies are still needed and use of these targeted therapies should be limited to experienced centres in the setting of a clinical trial.

✅✅ Gemcitabine plus cisplatin is currently the standard-of-care, first-line treatment regimen for patients with advanced and metastatic ICC.

✅ The use of any specific second-line regimen, locoregional therapy and/or chemoradiation should be decided on in a case-by-case basis after discussion in a multidisciplinary conference.

## EPITHELIOID HAEMANGIOENDOTHELIOMA

Epithelioid haemangioendotheliomas (EHEs) are neoplasms of vascular origin that arise predominantly from soft tissues, bones and visceral organs, in particular from the lung and the liver. Hepatic EHE develops from the endothelial cells lining the sinusoids and progresses along the sinusoids and vascular pedicles. It is extremely rare (no more than 200 cases have been reported), with an incidence of less than 1 per million population. It does not arise on a background of liver disease and there is no identified causative factor. Mean age at presentation is 42 years with a female-to-male ratio of 3:2.[91] Half of patients present with right upper quadrant pain, while a quarter of patients are diagnosed incidentally. The remainder of patients present with severe symptoms, such as ascites, jaundice, weakness and weight loss. Liver failure as a result of massive infiltration has also been described but is rare. Unfortunately, these tumours are usually discovered at an advanced stage; almost 90% are multifocal and often involve both lobes. Approximately one-third of patients have extrahepatic spread to regional lymph nodes, peritoneum, lung and spleen.

### DIAGNOSIS

Work-up for EHE can be challenging and patients are frequently misdiagnosed until specific immunohistochemistry is performed on biopsy specimens. Laboratory parameters are non-specific and tumour markers are normal. On imaging studies, the lesions are frequently confused with cholangiocarcinoma, metastatic carcinoma, sclerosing haemangioma or inflammatory pseudotumours. They are usually hypoechoic or heterogeneous on US, hypodense on CT with peripheral and/or central marginal enhancement on the arterial phase becoming isodense during the later phase and may display a halo or target pattern of enhancement. On MRI, they are hypointense on T1-weighted images, and heterogeneously hyperintense on T2-weighted images with similar contrast enhancement as that seen on CT. Multiplicity of lesions (especially if coalescent), their subcapsular location with liver capsule retraction and the presence of calcification (10–30%) or central necrotic and haemorrhagic areas should raise the suspicion of the diagnosis, especially in young patients. Histologic examination shows a tumour composed of epithelioid and dendritic cells in variable proportions with a propensity for invasion of hepatic and portal veins, an overall ill-defined growth pattern and infiltrative margins. Immunostaining for factor VIII-related antigens is highly specific for EHE, and most tumours also stain positive for CD34 and CD31 endothelial markers. Epithelial markers, including cytokeratins, are negative.

### TREATMENT

Although exceptional, prolonged survival of more than 10 years has been reported without treatment, and both partial and complete spontaneous tumour regression has even been described. On the other hand, some patients die within 2 weeks of diagnosis and 20% are dead within 1 year. Overall, only 20–40% survive more than 5 years. Reports of favourable outcome with an estimated 5-year survival of 75% probably represent a highly selected subgroup.

Because of the rarity of this tumour and its highly variable course, there is no widely accepted therapeutic strategy. Partial hepatectomy is rarely feasible due to the invariable multifocal involvement of the liver. Palliative resection is not advocated.

The place of liver transplantation has recently been addressed by a multi-institutional analysis.[92] In 59 patients reported to the European Liver Transplant Registry, impressive 5- and 10-year survival rates of 83% and 74%, respectively, were reported. Invasion of lymph nodes and presence of restricted extrahepatic involvement had limited impact on survival and should therefore not be considered as contraindications to transplantation.[93] The current shortage of liver grafts and the prolonged waiting time may dictate that liver transplantation is indicated only in highly selected patients. Experience with locoregional or systemic chemotherapy is small and of limited value, especially as first-line therapy.

## ANGIOSARCOMA

Representing less than 1% of primary liver tumours, angiosarcomas of the liver are rare tumours with a dismal prognosis. Despite its rarity, it has received attention because of its frequent association with environmental carcinogens. There is clear association with prior exposure to thorium dioxide (Thorotrast), arsenicals and vinyl chloride. Association with androgenic anabolic steroids, oestrogens, oral contraceptives, phenelzine and cupric acid has also been reported. Overall, up to 50% of angiosarcomas are associated with previous exposure to a chemical carcinogenic agent.

These environmental risk factors may account for the male predominance (gender ratio of 3:1) and age at the time of diagnosis (50–70 years). Patients usually experience non-specific symptoms such as abdominal pain, weakness, fatigue, anorexia and weight loss, but an acute abdomen related to tumour rupture is a classical presentation. Biological abnormalities may include haemolytic anaemia and thrombocytopenia, which are related to microangiopathic haemolysis and intravascular coagulation, respectively.

Morphologically, angiosarcoma may present as a large solitary mass or as multinodular lesions. On CT, they are usually hypodense and remain so after contrast injection except for occasional focal areas of central or peripheral ring-shaped enhancement. On delayed imaging, the lesion continues to enhance compared with that of the early-phase images. On MRI, the lesions tend to be hyperintense on T2-weighted images and heterogeneous on T1-weighted images, with focal hyperintensity on a background of hypointensity. Enhancement on the arterial and portal phases is heterogeneous. Although the progressive enhancement could mimic that of haemangioma, angiosarcomas clearly differ in that they are usually multiple and more heterogeneous, and enhancement is of lower intensity than the aorta, whereas it is the same for angioma.

Angiosarcomas are rapidly growing and carry a poor prognosis, with an estimated median survival of 6 months among all patients. When localized, surgery is the mainstay of treatment for primary liver angiosarcomas and carries a 5-year OS of approximately 30%. Unfortunately, disease recurrence is common and most patients have multifocal or metastatic disease at presentation, most notably in the lung and spleen.[94,95] There are very few effective systemic therapy options; however, chemotherapy in the adjuvant setting may be associated with improved survival compared with surgery alone.[96,97] Due to frequent recurrence and poor survival, transplantation is not recommended.

## CONCLUSION

Primary liver malignancies are rare cancers that originate from various cell lines within the liver, most commonly, hepatocytes (HCC) and cholangiocytes (cholangiocarcinoma). Surgery, whether with transplantation or resection, is the only potentially curative treatment when indicated. While locoregional liver-directed therapies and systemic therapy are largely reserved for advanced disease and in patients who are not otherwise suitable for surgical intervention, they may also play a complimentary role in the neoadjuvant and adjuvant settings, underscoring the importance of multidisciplinary management for these unique diseases.

### Key points

- Hepatocellular carcinoma (HCC) and intrahepatic cholangiocarcinoma (ICC) are the most common primary liver malignancies.
- The diagnosis of primary liver malignancies largely relies on high-quality cross-sectional imaging, using either four-phase CT or contrast-enhanced MRI. Biopsy is indicated for unresectable tumours or when the diagnosis is in question.
- Resection and transplantation, in well-selected patients, are the only potentially curative treatment option for patients with primary liver malignancies, regardless of aetiology.
- For HCC, the choice between liver transplantation and resection primarily relies on tumour size, tumour number and the degree of underlying liver dysfunction. The BCLC is the most commonly used staging system for HCC and provides a framework for management strategies. The Milan criteria is considered the gold standard for selecting patients with HCC for liver transplantation, although expanded criteria may be used at select institutions.
- Beyond tumour biology and patient performance status, the technical considerations for liver resection include ensuring adequate quantity and quality of the future liver remnant and preservation of vascular inflow, outflow and biliary drainage.
- Liver-directed therapies such as ablation and chemoembolisation play an important role in the management of HCC, particularly in patients who have liver-only disease and are not candidates for either resection or transplantation. In select cases, liver-directed therapies may be used to bridge patients while awaiting transplantation or to convert them from outside to being within transplant criteria.
- Systemic therapy is typically reserved for patients with advanced disease who are not otherwise candidates for surgery. For ICC, capecitabine may be considered in the adjuvant setting, while gemcitabine plus cisplatin is the standard-of-care treatment for unresectable and metastatic disease. Sorafenib, lenvatinib and atezolizumab plus bevacizumab are all considered first-line systemic therapy for advanced HCC.

 References available at http://ebooks.health.elsevier.com/

### KEY REFERENCES

[10] Singal AK, Fontana RJ. Meta-analysis: oral anti-viral agents in adults with decompensated hepatitis B virus cirrhosis. Aliment Pharmacol Ther 2012;35(6):674–89.

*A meta-analysis of the oral nucleos(t)ide analogues in patients with decompensated HBV cirrhosis. Pooled 1-year data demonstrated improvement in Child-Turcotte-Pugh scores and superior transplant-free survival in patients with decompensated HBV cirrhosis treated with lamivudine compared to patients who were untreated. Undetectable viral loads were seen in up to 83% of patients treated. One-year transplant-free survival was as high as 95% with HBV treatment.*

[11] Morgan RL, Baack B, Smith BD, et al. Eradication of hepatitis C virus infection and the development of hepatocellular carcinoma a meta-analysis of observational studies. Ann Intern Med 2013;158(5):329–+.

*A systematic review of 18 studies assessing the association between response to HCV treatment and the development of HCC. Sustained viral response was associated with reduced risk for HCC.*

[18] Zhang BH, Yang BH, Tang ZY. Randomized controlled trial of screening for hepatocellular carcinoma. J Cancer Res Clin Oncol 2004;130(7):417–22.

*A randomized controlled trial of 18,816 patients with HBV infection or chronic hepatitis to assess the effect of screening on HCC mortality. Among the screened group, 58.2% completed the screening protocol. Compared to the control group, patients in the screened group had more frequently identified subclinical HCC (60.5% vs 0) and small HCC (45.3% vs 0), and were more likely to underwent surgical resection (46.5% vs 7.5%). Five-year overall survival was 46.4% in the screened group versus 0 in the unscreened group.*

[20] Singal A, Volk ML, Waljee A, et al. Meta-analysis: surveillance with ultrasound for early-stage hepatocellular carcinoma in patients with cirrhosis. Aliment Pharmacol Ther 2009;30(1):37–47.

*A meta-analysis of the performance of ultrasound surveillance for HCC, specifically for small HCC. Surveillance US demonstrated a pooled sensitivity of 94% for detecting the majority of subclinical tumours; however, only a 63% sensitivity for detecting early HCC. Meta-regression analysis demonstrated a significantly higher sensitivity for early HCC with ultrasound every 6 months than with annual surveillance.*

[21] Trinchet JC, Chaffaut C, Bourcier V, et al. Ultrasonographic surveillance of hepatocellular carcinoma in cirrhosis: a randomized trial comparing 3- and 6-month periodicities. Hepatology 2011;54(6):1987–97.

*A multicentre, randomized trial comparing screening US at 3-month vs 6-month intervals in 1,278 patients with histologically confirmed compensated cirrhosis. The incidence of small focal lesions (<10 mm) was higher in patients screened at 3-month vs 6-month intervals (41% vs 28%); however, there was no difference in the incidence of HCC between groups.*

[29] Lee YJ, Lee JM, Lee JS, et al. Hepatocellular carcinoma: diagnostic performance of multidetector CT and MR imaging-a systematic review and meta-analysis. Radiology 2015;275(1):97–109.

*A systematic review and meta-analysis of 40 studies of the diagnostic performance of CT and MRI for evaluating HCC in patients with chronic liver disease. MR imaging showed higher per-lesion sensitivity than multidetector CT.*

[30] Aube C, Oberti F, Lonjon J, et al. EASL and AASLD recommendations for the diagnosis of HCC to the test of daily practice. Liver Int 2017;37(10):1515–25.

*A multicentre prospective trial to evaluate the performance of CT, MRI, and contrast-enhanced US alone or in combination for the diagnosis of HCC between 10 and 30 mm in 381 cirrhotic patients. Among tumors 10-20 mm, sensitivity was highest in MRI (70.6%) and CT (67.9%), while specificity was highest in contrast-enhanced US (92.9%). The best sequential approach was with MRI followed by contrast-enhanced US.*

[33] Llovet JM, Bru C, Bruix J. Prognosis of hepatocellular carcinoma: the BCLC staging classification. Semin Liver Dis 1999;19(3):329–38.

*A staging classification for HCC, which comprises four stages that select the best candidates for the best therapies currently available: Early stage (A) includes patients with asymptomatic early tumors suitable for radical therapies--resection, transplantation or percutaneous treatments; Intermediate stage (B) comprises patients with asymptomatic multinodular HCC; Advanced stage (C) includes patients with symptomatic tumors and/or an invasive tumoral pattern (vascular invasion/extrahepatic spread). Stage B and C patients may receive palliative treatments/new agents in the setting of phase II investigations or randomized controlled trials; End-stage disease (D) contain patients with extremely grim prognosis that should merely receive symptomatic treatment.*

[42] Mazzaferro V, Regalia E, Doci R, et al. Liver transplantation for the treatment of small hepatocellular carcinomas in patients with cirrhosis. N Engl J Med 1996;334(11):693–9.

*A retrospective study of 48 patients with cirrhosis and small, unresectable HCC who underwent liver transplantation. Demonstrated that patients with either a single tumour <5 cm or no more than three tumours each < 3 cm was associated with improved overall and recurrence-free survival compared to patients with tumours that fell outside of those criteria.*

[44] Mazzaferro V, Bhoori S, Sposito C, et al. Milan criteria in liver transplantation for hepatocellular carcinoma: an evidence-based analysis of 15 years of experience. Liver Transpl 2011;17(Suppl. 2):S44–57.

*A systematic review and meta-analysis assessing the value of the Milan Criteria as an independent prognostic factor for liver transplant in patients with HCC based on 90 studies.*

[60] Wang X, Hu Y, Ren M, et al. Efficacy and safety of radiofrequency ablation combined with transcatheter arterial chemoembolization for hepatocellular carcinomas compared with radiofrequency ablation alone: a time-to-event meta-analysis. Korean J Radiol 2016;17(1):93–102.

*A meta-analysis comparing the efficacy and safety of combined RFA and TACE with RFA alone in patients with HCC based on six randomised controlled trials. The results demonstrated that the combination of TACE and RFA was associated with significantly higher overall survival and recurrence-free survival compared to RFA alone, without increase in major complications.*

[61] Majumdar A, Roccarina D, Thorburn D, et al. Management of people with early- or very early-stage hepatocellular carcinoma: an attempted network meta-analysis. Cochrane Database Syst Rev 2017;3:CD011650.

*A meta-analysis of 18 trials to compare the benefits of various interventions used in the management of early and very early HCC. Results demonstrated no difference in all-cause mortality between surgery and RFA in patients with early HCC, although evidence was of low or very low quality.*

[71] Cheng AL, Kang YK, Chen Z, et al. Efficacy and safety of sorafenib in patients in the Asia-Pacific region with advanced hepatocellular carcinoma: a phase III randomised, double-blind, placebo-controlled trial. Lancet Oncol 2009;10(1):25–34.

*A phase III, randomized, placebo-controlled trial assessing the efficacy and safety of sorafenib in 226 patients from the Asia-Pacific region with advanced HCC. Patients were randomized 2:1 to either sorafenib (n=150) or placebo (n=76). Compared to placebo, sorafenib demonstrated improved median OS (6.5 months vs 4.2 months, p=0.014) and median time to progression (2.8 months vs 1.4 months, p=0.0005).*

[72] Kudo M, Finn RS, Qin S, et al. Lenvatinib versus sorafenib in first-line treatment of patients with unresectable hepatocellular carcinoma: a randomised phase 3 non-inferiority trial. Lancet 2018;391(10126):1163–73.

*A phase III, multicentre, non-inferiority trial comparing the efficacy of Lenvatinib to sorafenib as first-line treatment for patients with unresectable HCC. Lenvatinib was found to be non-inferior to sorafenib for overall survival (13.6 months vs 12.3 months, respectively).*

[73] Finn RS, Qin S, Ikeda M, et al. Atezolizumab plus bevacizumab in unresectable hepatocellular carcinoma. N Engl J Med 2020;382(20):1894–905.

*A phase III, randomized controlled trial comparing the efficacy of atezolizumab plus bevacizumab to sorafenib in patients with unresectable HCC. Patients were randomized 2:1 to receive either atezolizumab-bevacizumab (n=336) to sorafenib (n=165). Patients receiving atezolizumab-bevacizumab demonstrated improved 12-month survival (67.2%) and median progression-free survival (6.8 months) compared to those who received sorafenib (54.6% and 4.3 months, respectively).*

[83] Primrose JN, Fox RP, Palmer DH, et al. Capecitabine compared with observation in resected biliary tract cancer (BILCAP): a randomised, controlled, multicentre, phase 3 study. Lancet Oncol 2019;20(5):663–73.

*A phase III, randomized, controlled trial assessing the efficacy of adjuvant capecitabine compared to observation in 447 patients in the UK with resected biliary tract cancers. Following curative-intent resection, patients were randomized 1:1 to receive either capecitabine (n=223) or undergo observation (n=224). The study failed to meet its primary endpoint, demonstrating no difference between groups in the intention-to-treat of overall survival; however, adjuvant capecitabine was associated with improved median overall survival compared to observation (53 months vs 36 months, p=0.028) in the pre-specified sensitivity and pre-protocol analyses.*

[88] Valle J, Wasan H, Palmer DH, et al. Cisplatin plus gemcitabine versus gemcitabine for biliary tract cancer. N Engl J Med 2010;362(14):1273–81.

*A phase III, randomized, controlled trial assessing the efficacy of gemcitabine plus cisplatin compared to gemcitabine alone in 410 patients with advanced biliary tract cancers. Patients were randomly assigned 1:1 to receive either gemcitabine-cisplatin (n=204) or gemcitabine alone (n=206). Gemcitabine-cisplatin was associated with improved median overall survival and median progression-free survival compared to gemcitabine alone (11.7 months vs 8.1 months, p<0.001; and 8.0 months vs 5.0 months, p<0.001, respectively). Patients treated with combination therapy also demonstrated improved tumor control compared to those treated with monotherapy (81.4% vs 71.8%, p=0.049).*

# Colorectal liver metastases

**7**

Jordan M. Cloyd | Timothy M. Pawlik

## INTRODUCTION

Despite recent advances in screening, diagnosis and management, colorectal cancer (CRC) remains the second leading cause of cancer death in Western countries. In 2018, 1.8 million new CRC cases were estimated to have occurred worldwide.[1] Almost two-thirds of patients with CRC develop distant metastases and the liver is the most frequent site of metastatic disease. Although as many as 25% of patients will present with synchronous metastases at the time of diagnosis, another 20% will develop metachronous metastases during the next 3 years of follow-up.[2,3] The extent of liver disease is a key determinant of survival in patients with isolated colorectal liver metastases (CRLMs).[4] Surgical resection of CRLMs, especially when combined with modern systemic chemotherapy, is associated with the best long-term survival outcomes. In turn, efforts to improve the surgical management of CRLMs are critical. Given major advances in CRC over the past several decades, this chapter will provide a concise but comprehensive review of the diagnosis, evaluation, management and outcomes of patients with CRLM.

✔✔ While the median survival of patients with advanced CRLM has improved over the last several decades with the introduction of more efficacious chemotherapy, surgical resection remains the cornerstone of potentially curative therapy.[5–8]

## DIAGNOSIS

The diagnosis of CRLM is usually based on imaging during the staging of patients with CRC. Guidelines recommend cross-sectional imaging of the chest, abdomen and pelvis at the time of diagnosis, as well as every 6–12 months in follow-up of patients with treated CRC. Although the diagnosis may be confirmed via percutaneous image-guided biopsy, most often a thorough history and physical examination, as well as laboratory tests (e.g. carcinoembryonic antigen [CEA] level) and characteristic imaging of the lesion are adequate to substantiate a diagnosis of CRLM. Occasionally, the diagnosis of CRLM will be made inadvertently at the time of surgery for presumed localised CRC, either because incomplete imaging was performed in the setting of an emergency presentation, or occult liver metastases were not visualised on preoperative imaging. Nevertheless, the diagnosis, staging and operative planning of CRLM is dependent on high-quality imaging. Multiple different imaging modalities can be used to assess patients with CRLM (Table 7.1).[9,10]

Transabdominal ultrasonography (US) is a relatively inexpensive test that can provide general information about the number, location and extent of liver metastases. The addition of duplex can increase US sensitivity to define the proximity of lesions to adjacent vital structures, such as the portal vein and inferior vena cava.

✔✔ US is **not** a sensitive diagnostic test for CRLM and can fail to identify over 50% of metastatic lesions.

A major limitation of US is reliance on the skill and knowledge of the operator. In addition, other factors such as the patient's body habitus, presence of steatosis and the inability to detect extrahepatic disease hamper the diagnostic yield and utility of US. In contrast to transabdominal US, intraoperative US (IOUS) has a much higher sensitivity to detect CRLM through high-resolution imaging of the liver. However, with the increasing use of magnetic resonance imaging (MRI) and positron emission tomography–computed tomography (PET-CT), detection of new unsuspected lesions by IOUS has decreased. Nevertheless, IOUS does help identify new lesions in a subset of patients and is also essential to provide real-time guidance of the resection plane at the time of surgery. Some surgeons have proposed using contrast-enhanced IOUS to improve the sensitivity of detecting CRLM, but this is not routinely performed.[11,12]

At most centres, triple-phase contrast multidetector CT is the modality of choice for CRC staging and surveillance. CRLM typically appear as hypoattenuating lesions and are best identified in the portal venous phase (Fig. 7.1). Arterial phase images are typically used to distinguish metastatic disease from benign vascular lesions and also to identify the liver vascular anatomy for pre-surgical planning, or if placement of a hepatic arterial infusion pump is being considered (Fig. 7.2). Additionally, extrahepatic metastases may be detected by obtaining chest, abdomen and pelvic images. The major disadvantage of CT is its lower sensitivity to recognise small (<1 cm) liver lesions, especially among patients with background liver parenchymal disease, such as steatosis.

In contrast, MRI provides high-resolution assessment of the liver and can be superior to CT in detecting and characterising indeterminate small lesions (Figs. 7.1 and 7.3) with sensitivity rates of 91–97%, compared with 71–73% for CT. MRI is also more accurate to differentiate benign versus malignant subcentimetre liver lesions, with a specificity of 97.5% versus 77.3% for CT. Importantly, MRI tends to be more accurate in detecting and characterising CRLM if there is underlying liver parenchymal disease. Recent advances in MRI techniques, including the introduction of tissue-specific contrast agents such as gadobenate

**Table 7.1** Advantages and limitations of various imaging modalities in evaluating liver metastases

| Modality | Advantages | Pitfalls |
|---|---|---|
| US | Low cost<br>Availability | High operator dependence<br>Body habitus dependence<br>Low sensitivity in<br>    Liver steatosis<br>    Small lesions<br>    Extrahepatic spread |
| IOUS | Localisation of deep-seated lesion<br>Mapping vasculature<br>Real-time guidance for surgical plane<br>Guiding RFA | Increases duration of surgery |
| CT | Availability<br>Relatively low cost<br>High sensitivity and specificity<br>Extrahepatic spread evaluation<br>Vascular mapping<br>Liver volume estimation<br>Planning targeted therapies<br>Therapy monitoring | Poor confidence in<br>    Detecting < 1 cm lesions<br>    Lesion detection in chemotherapy-<br>      induced liver steatosis<br>    Distinction of malignant from benign<br>Not suitable for<br>    Contrast allergies<br>    Compromised renal function |
| MRI | Increased sensitivity and specificity for<br>    Detection of small lesions (<1 cm)<br>    Detection of lesions after chemotherapy-induced fatty changes<br>    Lesion characterisation<br>Treatment planning<br>Therapy response monitoring | Not suitable for patients with<br>    Claustrophobia<br>    Implants (pacemaker, stents, etc.)<br>    Impaired renal function (CE-MRI)<br>    Non-compliance |
| PET | Accurate extrahepatic site detection<br>Superior sensitivity and specificity when combined with CT/CE-CT<br>Therapy response monitoring<br>Detection of residual or recurrent disease | Limited accessibility<br>High cost<br>Poor detection of lesions<br>    <1 cm<br>    After chemotherapy |

*CE*, Contrast-enhanced; *CT*, computed tomography; *IOUS*, intraoperative ultrasonography; *MRI*, magnetic resonance imaging; *PET*, positron emission tomography; *RFA*, radiofrequency ablation; *US*, ultrasonography.
Reproduced from Sahani DV, Bajwa MA, Andrabi Y, et al. Current status of imaging and emerging techniques to evaluate liver metastases from colorectal carcinoma. Ann Surg 2014;259(5):861–72.

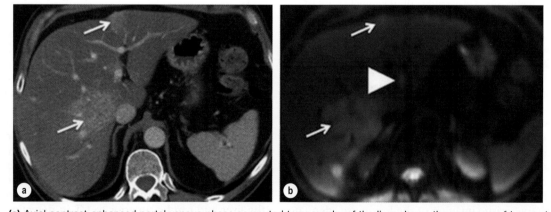

**Figure 7.1** **(a)** Axial contrast-enhanced portal venous phase computed tomography of the liver shows the presence of two metastases *(thin arrows)*; **(b)** diffusion MRI (b = 100 s/mm²): identification of an additional metastasis in segment 2 *(arrowhead)*. (From Legou F, et al. Diagn Interv Imaging 2014;95(5):505–12. Copyright © 2014 Elsevier Masson SAS. All rights reserved.)

dimeglumine and gadoxetate (Gd-EOB-DTPA; Primovist in Europe and Eovist in the USA), as well as diffusion-weighted imaging (DWI), have further enhanced the diagnostic yield of CRLM (Figs. 7.4 and 7.5). An important consideration is the evaluation of CRLM among patients who have received systemic chemotherapy. Preoperative chemotherapy can affect the liver parenchyma and limit the sensitivity of cross-sectional imaging for detecting CRLM. Meta-analyses have suggested that MRI is the best modality for detecting CRLM following systemic chemotherapy.[13]

PET is another commonly used imaging modality which can supplement CT or MRI. PET utilises intravenously

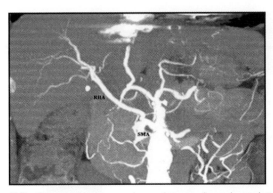

**Figure 7.2** Computed tomography angiogram. A maximum intensity projection rendered coronal three-dimensional image demonstrating a replaced right hepatic artery (RHA) from superior mesenteric artery (SMA) in a patient scheduled for right hepatectomy for colorectal liver metastases. (From Sahani DV, Bajwa MA, Andrabi Y, et al. Current status of imaging and emerging techniques to evaluate liver metastases from colorectal carcinoma. Ann Surg 2014;259(5):861–72. PMID: 24509207.)

administered radioactive fluorodeoxyglucose (FDG) to identify metabolically active metastatic lesions. The metabolic activity of a lesion can be quantified by measuring the standardised uptake value (SUV). While the routine use of PET in CRC staging is limited due to insufficient anatomic detail, poor sensitivity of lesions smaller than 1 cm, and false-positive results in the setting of inflammation (Fig. 7.6), the primary advantage of PET-CT or PET-MRI is the superior detection of extrahepatic disease (Fig. 7.7) and evaluation of indeterminate lesions. PET-CT is also effective at diagnosing CRLM, with one meta-analysis highlighting a sensitivity and specificity of 74.1% and 93.9%, respectively.[14] Whether PET should be routinely considered in the preoperative evaluation of potentially resectable CRLM is more controversial. A randomised controlled trial of 150 patients with CRLM noted that the number of futile laparotomies was reduced with the addition of preoperative FDG-PET.[15] Thus, PET remains an important imaging modality in the evaluation of patients with possible CRLM and selection of patients for surgery.

## PATIENT SELECTION FOR HEPATIC RESECTION

The definition of resectability has evolved considerably since Ekberg et al.[16] in 1986 proposed that surgery for CRLM was only indicated if all of the following criteria were met: <4 metastases, no extrahepatic disease, and ability to obtain resection margins ≥ 10 mm. Though these criteria have evolved over the past four decades, there remains considerable variability in the definition of resectability among liver surgeons. Since the ability to undergo hepatic resection is one of the most important prognostic factors for patients with CRLM, the determination of resectability and candidacy for metastasectomy has significant implications. Therefore, defining which patients are candidates for surgery, as well as employing efforts to safely expand the indications for resection, are critical to extend the benefits of surgery to more patients.

☑☑ According to the Americas Hepato-Pancreato-Biliary Association (AHPBA) most recent expert consensus statement and also the National Comprehensive Cancer Network (NCCN) guidelines, CRLM is considered resectable as long as the tumour can be removed completely (R0 resection), the predicted future liver remnant (FLR) function is adequate to prevent postoperative liver failure, extrahepatic sites of the disease are controllable, and the primary tumour can be resected for cure.[17]

Practically, determinations of resectability are best made by a multidisciplinary team of CRC specialists. As outlined by the AHPBA consensus statement, resectability should be determined along two domains: oncologic and technical. Oncologic resectability refers to the selection of patients most likely to benefit from major liver resection based on underlying tumour biology. Relevant factors may include the burden of liver metastases, the presence of extrahepatic disease, the disease-free interval and/or the response to neoadjuvant therapy. Increasingly, given its prognostic importance, tumour mutation status may influence the determination of oncologic resectability. Technical resectability refers to the ability to perform a margin-negative resection while preserving an appropriate FLR with adequate vascular inflow and outflow and biliary drainage. Patients with normal hepatic function can safely tolerate resection with a planned FLR size of > 20%. However, in order to minimise the risk of posthepatectomy liver failure (PHLF), patients with compromised liver function (obesity, receipt of chemotherapy for greater than 12 weeks, diabetes mellitus), an FLR > 30% is advised. An FLR > 40–50% of total liver volume is necessary to minimise the risk of PHLF in patients with cirrhosis.[18] For patients with insufficient FLR volume, several augmentation strategies can be utilised to optimise patients for liver resection.[19]

☑☑ Patients who do not meet FLR requirements may benefit from additional preoperative procedures to induce hypertrophy of the FLR, such as portal vein embolisation (PVE) or associating liver partition and portal vein ligation for staged hepatectomy (ALPPS).[20–22]

## CURRENT ISSUES IN THE SURGICAL MANAGEMENT OF CRLM

### MARGIN STATUS

While a margin width < 1 mm is typically defined as R1 margin status, the optimal R0 margin width at the time of liver resection remains controversial. Pawlik et al.[22] found that R1 margin status was associated with worse overall survival (OS) following liver resection, but that greater margin widths (1–4 mm, 5–9 mm, or ≥1 cm) were not associated with improved OS, recurrence risk or site of recurrence. Similarly, Sadot et al.[23] found no benefit of margins > 1 mm but that even submillimetre margin widths were associated with improved OS compared with microscopically involved margins. On the other hand, a systematic review and meta-analysis suggested that wider surgical margins were associated with improved outcomes and margins > 1 cm should

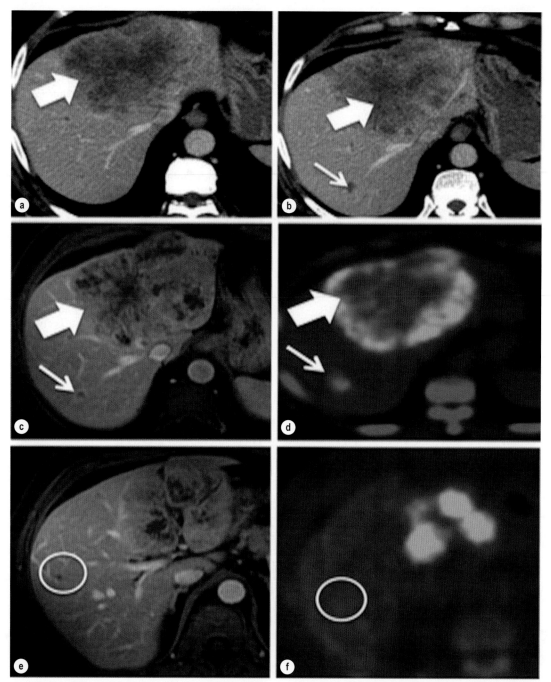

**Figure 7.3** **(a)** Portal venous phase contrast-enhanced liver CT: necrotic mass, with fibrous enhancement centred on segments 2–4 *(thick arrow)*; **(b)** a second hypodense lesion on CT scan is visible in segment 7 *(thin arrow)*; **(c)** MRI shows peripheral enhancement of both lesions *(arrows)*; **(d)** both lesions are hypermetabolic on PET-CT *(arrows)*; **(e)** discovery of an additional lesion on portal venous phase contrast-enhanced MRI *(circle)*; **(f)** this third lesion was not seen on CT or PET-CT *(circle)*. *CT,* computed tomography; *MRI,* magnetic resonance imaging; *PET,* positron emission tomography. (From Legou F, et al. Diagn Interv Imaging. 2014 May;95(5):505-12. Copyright © 2014 Elsevier Masson SAS. All rights reserved.)

be considered if possible.[24] Several observations suggest that the influence of margin status on outcomes more likely represents a biological effect. First, patients with RAS mutations are more likely to have positive margins.[25] Second, the prognostic significance of R1 margin status is mitigated among patients with a significant radiographic or pathologic response to neoadjuvant therapy.[26] Finally, conversion of an R1 margin to R0 by intraoperative re-resection has not been associated with improved outcomes.[27] Thus, while microscopically negative margins ≥ 1 mm remain the objective of any resection for CRLM, the direct impact of margin status on patient outcomes may be less impactful than other biological factors (Fig. 7.8).

## PARENCHYMAL-SPARING APPROACHES

The objective of parenchymal-sparing hepatectomy (PSH) is to maintain oncologic principles of margin-negative resection while maximising the remaining liver remnant. In

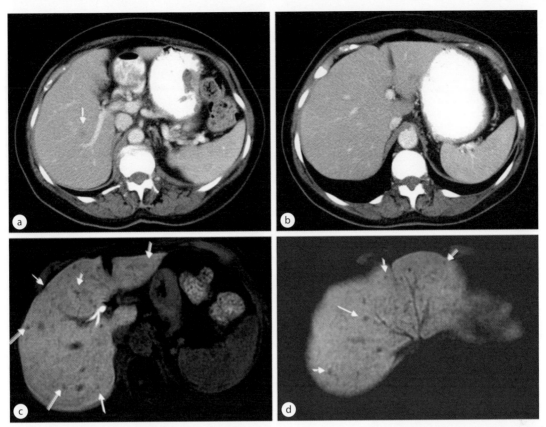

**Figure 7.4** A 44-year-old man, with stage III colon cancer who underwent resection 1 year previously followed by adjuvant chemotherapy. Follow-up restaging CT **(a, b)** showed reduced liver attenuation in comparison with spleen due to steatosis and a possible lesion in the right lobe *(arrow)*. Liver MRI was performed with hepatobiliary contrast agent Eovist. On 10-minute delayed hepatobiliary phase, T1-weighted fat saturation MR images **(c, d)** demonstrate enhancing liver parenchyma and numerous non-enhancing, small metastases scattered within the right and left lobe of liver *(arrows)*. *CT,* computed tomography; *MRI,* magnetic resonance imaging. (From Sahani DV, Bajwa MA, Andrabi Y, et al. Current status of imaging and emerging techniques to evaluate liver metastases from colorectal carcinoma. Ann Surg 2014;259(5):861–72. PMID: 24509207.)

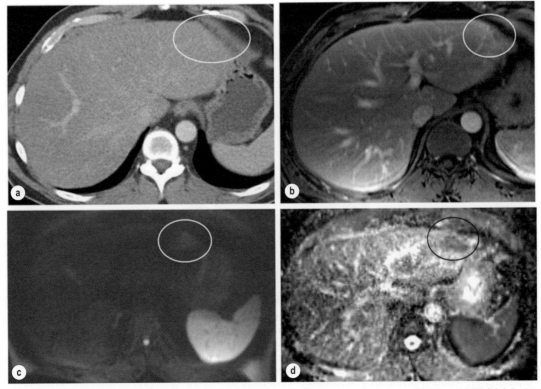

**Figure 7.5** A 51-year-old man with colorectal liver metastases receiving chemotherapy. Follow-up CT **(a)** and MRI **(b)** failed to demonstrate left lateral section metastasis that is more obvious on diffusion-weighted MRI **(c)** as a focal bright area with associated restricted diffusion on apparent diffusion coefficient image **(d)**. *CT,* computed tomography; *MRI,* magnetic resonance imaging. (From Sahani DV, Bajwa MA, Andrabi Y, et al. Current status of imaging and emerging techniques to evaluate liver metastases from colorectal carcinoma. Ann Surg 2014;259(5):861–72. PMID: 24509207.)

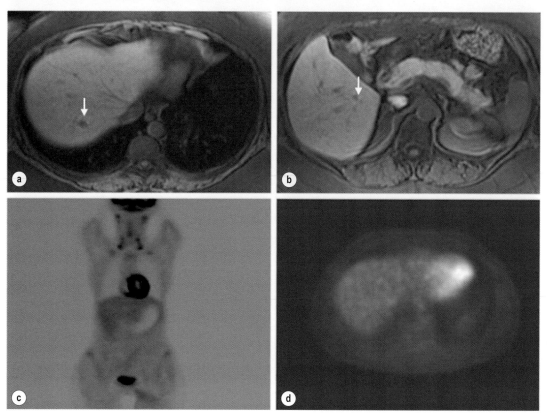

**Figure 7.6** Small colorectal liver metastasis without increased FDG uptake in a 47-year-old woman. MRI of the liver shows two small metastatic deposits *(arrow)* in the right liver **(a, b)**. Representative coronal and axial images from a whole-body FDG-PET examination **(c, d)** show no corresponding focal increased FDG uptake in the liver. *FDG,* fluorodeoxyglucose; *MRI,* magnetic resonance imaging; *PET,* positron emission tomography. (From Sahani DV, Bajwa MA, Andrabi Y, et al. Current status of imaging and emerging techniques to evaluate liver metastases from colorectal carcinoma. Ann Surg 2014;259(5):861–72. PMID: 24509207.)

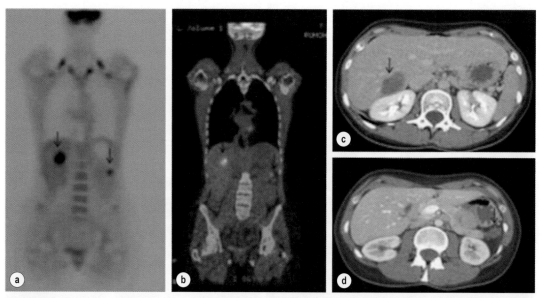

**Figure 7.7** Whole-body PET-CT was performed on a 49-year-old woman with rectal cancer. Coronal FDG-PET **(a)** and fused PET-CT **(b)** images from whole-body PET-CT show a focus of intense FDG uptake in the liver *(arrows)*. Corresponding axial image **(c)** acquired during CT shows the metastatic deposit in the right liver *(arrow)*. Another discrete extrahepatic peritoneal metastatic deposit is evident in the left side of upper abdomen on the FDG-PET and fused PET-CT image *(arrow)* that on corresponding axial CT image **(d)** is located adjacent to the tail of pancreas *(arrow)*. *CT,* computed tomography; *FDG,* fluorodeoxyglucose; *PET,* positron emission tomography. (From Sahani DV, Bajwa MA, Andrabi Y, et al. Current status of imaging and emerging techniques to evaluate liver metastases from colorectal carcinoma. Ann Surg 2014;259(5):861–72. PMID: 24509207.)

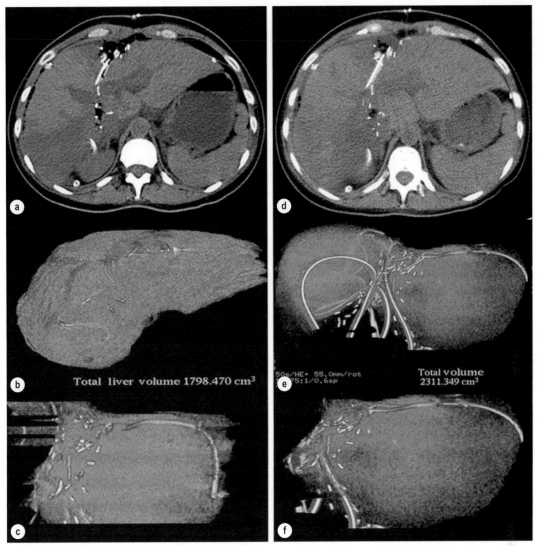

**Figure 7.8** A 48-year-old female, with a history of rectal cancer and liver metastases underwent right portal vein ligation and *in situ* liver-splitting surgery. The postoperative axial **(a)** and volumetric computed tomography (CT) images of the liver (b, c) show total liver volume (TLV) = 1798 cm³ **(b)**, and left liver volume **(c)** = 612 cm³. Axial **(d)** and volumetric CT images obtained after 1 week **(e, f)** show an increase in TLV to 2311 cm³ **(e)** and left liver volume to 908 cm³ **(f)**, corresponding to 35% increase in volume. (From Sahani DV, Bajwa MA, Andrabi Y, et al. Current status of imaging and emerging techniques to evaluate liver metastases from colorectal carcinoma. Ann Surg 2014;259(5):861–72. PMID: 24509207.)

practice, PSH usually emphasises resection of one or more liver segments rather than an entire hemiliver. While anatomic resections, such as segmentectomy or sectionectomy, are often used in parenchymal-sparing approaches, these procedures can also often be achieved by more limited non-anatomic resections, occasionally termed wedge resections. PSH is associated with not only reduced incidence of PHLF but also salvageability in the case of liver recurrence.[28,29] Systematic reviews of PSH are suggestive of perioperative benefits with no difference in long-term outcomes.[30] On the other hand, recent literature has called into question the role of PSH for patients with **KRAS**-mutant CRLM, although this remains controversial.[31]

✓✓ Surgeons should aim for microscopic negative margins > 1 mm. Parenchymal-sparing approaches are acceptable when feasible and may be associated with improved short-term outcomes and salvageability in the case of hepatic recurrence.

## EXTRAHEPATIC DISEASE AND ROLE OF SURGERY

The lungs, intra-abdominal lymph nodes and peritoneum are the most common sites of CRC metastases following the liver. The presence of extrahepatic metastases has been associated with poor outcomes and traditionally considered a contraindication for hepatic resection.[32] However, with recent advances in surgical techniques and systemic medical treatment, hepatic resection can be considered in patients with extrahepatic disease, particularly those individuals amenable to local treatment (e.g. resection, ablation or radiation). For example, Shah et al.[33] demonstrated that an aggressive multidisciplinary approach to treat combined lung and liver metastases resulted in prolonged OS. Nevertheless, consideration can be given to surgical resection of CRLM even for selected patients with limited unresectable extrahepatic metastases that can be controlled with maintenance systemic therapy. For example, Mise et al.[34] reported worse OS among patients who underwent resection of CRLM alone than patients who underwent resection of liver and lung metastases, but better than a similar cohort of patients who received chemotherapy alone. Patients with extrahepatic disease who are being considered for liver resection should be managed in a multidisciplinary setting and generally should be treated with preoperative therapy to help define tumour biology.

## MINIMALLY INVASIVE SURGERY

Technical advances in minimally invasive surgery have expanded the indications for laparoscopic and robotic liver resections. Indeed, over the past several decades, the indications for minimally invasive surgery and proposed management guidelines have been generated at several international consensus conferences. Regarding resection of CRLM, the OSLO-COMET trial randomised patients with resectable CRLM to either open or laparoscopic PSH. Laparoscopic liver resection resulted in improved short-term outcomes with no differences in margin status or OS.[35,36] Subset analysis of tumours in more technically challenging posterosuperior segments demonstrated similar results.[37,38] Systematic reviews and consensus guidelines support the use of laparoscopic approaches to resection of CRLM.[39,40] Robotic approaches to surgery for CRLM appear to result in similar short- and long-term outcomes compared with laparoscopic liver resection.[41]

## MANAGEMENT OF BILOBAR CRLM

The management of bilobar CRLM has undergone significant advances in recent years. Extending the benefits of surgery to patients with advanced bilobar CRLM represents a prime opportunity to improve outcomes of patients with metastatic CRC.[42] The choice of surgical strategy for patients with bilateral CRLM depends on the burden and location of the tumour. A one-stage approach with multiple PSHs is a safe and effective technique in management of small and favourably positioned bilateral CRLM.[43] When CRLMs in the right hemiliver are peripheral but the central in the left hemiliver, then a formal left hepatectomy may be combined with PSHs of the right-sided peripheral lesions. Alternatively, ablation of a central left tumour along with PSHs of the right tumours could be performed. Either approach can be performed in a single-stage fashion. In general, combination resection-ablation is safe and may be associated with decreased blood loss, shorter hospital stay and less morbidity compared with aggressive resectional approaches.[44]

For bilobar CRLM where extended right hepatectomy is required, careful attention to the FLR is necessary. In general, ablation/resection of metastases in the left liver remnant should be avoided.[45]

Patients with inadequate FLR may be considered for two-stage hepatectomy (TSH). In the first stage, the FLR is cleared of metastatic disease followed by PVE. A second curative-intent stage of the operation is performed after hypertrophy of the contralateral liver when there has been adequate increase of the FLR volume. The long-term survival of patients who complete both stages is comparable to patients with more limited disease treated by a conventional single–stage strategy.[46] An alternative to TSH is ALPPS. In this two stage approach, a right portal vein ligation is first combined with parenchymal transection and clearance of the FLR of metastases. The second stage is performed during the same hospital admission 1–2 weeks later and involves completion hemihepatectomy. ALPPS is associated with high morbidity and mortality, but accumulating evidence suggests it is a reasonable option for well-selected healthy patients with bilobar CRLM.[47]

## TUMOUR MUTATIONS

Due to advances in next-generation sequencing and an improved understanding of the molecular underpinnings of CRC pathogenesis, molecular biomarkers are increasingly being used to determine prognosis and management of patients with CRLM. *KRAS* is the most commonly mutated gene in patients with CRLM and carries an adverse prognostic impact on OS.[48] Similarly, BRAF, SMAD4 and TP53 mutations are associated with worse survival compared to patients with wild-type genes.[49] Emerging evidence suggests that double mutations interact in a negative synergistic fashion. For example, concomitant RAS and TP53 mutations are independently associated with worse outcomes following resection of CRLM, while simultaneous APC and PIK3CA mutations are also associated with worse outcomes among patients with CRLM.[50,51] Although growing evidence demonstrates the prognostic ability of tumour mutations, further research is needed to clarify their role in treatment decisions.

# PREOPERATIVE CHEMOTHERAPY

The role of preoperative chemotherapy in the management of CRLM can be discussed in three categories of patients: resectable metachronous, unresectable metachronous, and synchronous disease.

## RESECTABLE METACHRONOUS CRLM

Current data regarding neoadjuvant chemotherapy in patients with resectable metachronous CRLM are conflicting. Several theoretical advantages exist relative to the use of neoadjuvant chemotherapy: potential downstaging to facilitate margin-negative resection of large tumours or resection via a parenchymal-sparing or minimally invasive approach; assessment of tumour response to chemotherapy; and patient selection based on tumour biology prior to major surgery. In contrast, progression of disease and chemotherapy-associated liver toxicity are potential drawbacks. The EORTC 40983 phase III trial investigated the efficacy of perioperative chemotherapy.[52] In this prospective randomised controlled trial, 364 patients with up to four CRLMs were randomly assigned to either immediate liver resection or six cycles of preoperative FOLFOX4, surgery, then six cycles of postoperative chemotherapy. After 3 years, the absolute increase in progression-free survival (PFS) with chemotherapy was 8.1% in eligible patients (from 28.1% in the surgery alone group to 36.2% in the chemotherapy group; HR 0.77; $P = 0.041$). In the latest update of the trial, 5-year PFS still remained higher in eligible patients who received perioperative chemotherapy, while 5-year OS was not significantly different between the two groups.[53] Of note, the incidence of postoperative complications (25%) and PHLF (8%) was higher among patients treated with perioperative chemotherapy compared with surgery alone (16% and 4%, respectively) though postoperative mortality was not significantly different between the two groups. On the other hand, the rate of non-therapeutic laparotomy was lower among patients who received perioperative chemotherapy (5% vs 11%). While additional trials are necessary to investigate the role of preoperative chemotherapy among patients with resectable CRLM, selection of neoadjuvant therapy needs to be based on factors that include tumour biology, risk of underlying liver insufficiency, and difficulty of the resection.

✓✓ When utilised, the recommended duration of neo-adjuvant therapy is typically four to six cycles and liver resection is typically delayed for at least 4 weeks after completion of chemotherapy. Although FOLFOX, FOLFIRI or XELOX chemotherapy regimens are all acceptable, the optimal regimen has not been established.[54,55]

✓✓ The addition of bevacizumab (VEGFR inhibitor) to a front-line oxaliplatin-containing regimen leads to improved pathologic response, but EGFR inhibitors such as cetuximab and panitumumab should not be used in the perioperative setting for resectable patients given trials demonstrating OS detriment.[56–59]

## UNRESECTABLE METACHRONOUS CRLM

Preoperative systemic chemotherapy has the potential to downsize unresectable CRLM and convert initially inoperable lesions to resectable tumours. Such conversion has been reported in as high as 40% of patients with unresectable disease and may vary due in part due to the subjective definition of unresectability and chemotherapy used.[60] FOLFOX and FOLFIRI are two suggested regimens for induction therapy, with a high objective response rate (RR). Higher resectability rates have been reported for regimens that contain both oxaliplatin and irinotecan, such as FOLFOXIRI. The addition of biologic agents such as cetuximab, panitumumab or bevacizumab may increase response in some patients.[61]

When employing preoperative 'conversion' chemotherapy, liver resection should be performed when the metastases become clearly resectable, but typically delayed at least 4 weeks after completion of chemotherapy. According to NCCN guidelines, response to conversion therapy should be evaluated every 2 months.[55] Traditionally, the RECIST criteria are used to assess changes in tumour size.[62,63] Although novel CT-based morphologic criteria and PET functional imaging have been proposed as indicators of a response for targeted therapies, their application as standard measures requires further validation and confirmation.[64–66] It is also important to note that complete radiological response is not always equivalent to complete pathological response. The incidence of viable cancer cells after a complete radiological response occurs in 40–50% of patients and thus resection is still recommended if the area of metastasis can be identified.[67]

## SYNCHRONOUS CRLM

Compared with metachronous disease, synchronous CRLM is associated with worse prognosis. Among patients with resectable synchronous CRLM, preoperative systemic chemotherapy has the potential to select patients without aggressive tumour biology for aggressive surgical strategies. Widespread tumour progression on chemotherapy may be a contraindication to subsequent liver resection. In patients with unresectable synchronous CRLM, preoperative chemotherapy should be given in an attempt to convert the lesions to being resectable. Thus, the use of preoperative systemic chemotherapy should be strongly considered for patients with synchronous CRLM and asymptomatic (i.e. no obstruction or bleeding) primary tumours.

For patients with synchronous CRLM, the timing of hepatic resection is another controversial topic. Options include liver-first staged approach, colorectal-first staged approach and simultaneous approach. In general, systematic reviews demonstrate that simultaneous resection of the primary with the liver metastases, when feasible, tends to be associated with a shorter total length of hospital stay and less morbidity but with comparable 5-year survival.[68,69]

## ADJUVANT CHEMOTHERAPY

The main goal of adjuvant chemotherapy is to reduce the risk of disease recurrence that can occur in up to 60–70% of patients following resection of CRLM.

### SYSTEMIC CHEMOTHERAPY

Two phase III trials with similar design, FFCD and EORTC/NCIC, investigated the benefit of 5-fluorouracil (5FU)-based chemotherapy following resection of CRLM.[70,71] Although preliminary results demonstrated a trend toward better disease-free survival (DFS) and OS in the group of patients who received adjuvant chemotherapy, both trials were closed prematurely due to slow accrual. In a pooled analysis of both trials ($n = 278$), Mitry et al.[72] reported that adjuvant chemotherapy was associated with better median PFS (27.9 months vs 18.8 months, $P = 0.058$) and OS (62 months vs 47 months, $P = 0.095$) than surgery alone. In another randomised clinical trial of 180 patients who underwent curative CRLM resection, the 3-year DFS was improved with uracil-tegafur/leucovorin adjuvant therapy; however, OS was similar.[73] More recently, the JCOG0603 trial randomised 300 patients to either surgery alone or surgery with adjuvant mFOLFOX. While DFS was improved among patients who received adjuvant chemotherapy, OS was worse potentially due to more deaths in the adjuvant chemotherapy arm after recurrence.[74]

### HEPATIC ARTERY INFUSION CHEMOTHERAPY

The main rationale for hepatic artery infusion (HAI) chemotherapy is that liver metastases derive their blood supply predominantly from the hepatic artery. A few small randomised trials have demonstrated a benefit with HAI chemotherapy alone in patients with CRLM in terms of OS and intrahepatic recurrence-free survival (RFS).[75,76] In contrast, several studies have demonstrated the therapeutic advantage of adjuvant HAI combined with systemic chemotherapy. Kemeny et al.,[77] in a randomised trial of 109 patients with potentially resectable CRLM, reported that combined systemic and regional HAI therapy was associated with a better 4-year intrahepatic RFS (67%) and overall RFS (46%) than surgery alone (43% and 25%, respectively). In another study, 2-year intrahepatic RFS and 2-year OS of patients treated with combined therapy after hepatic resection were superior to patients who received systemic therapy alone.[78] The benefit persisted long term at 10-year follow-up.[79] Recent studies have also demonstrated the survival benefit of adjuvant HAI-floxuridine in addition to modern systemic chemotherapy using oxaliplatin or irinotecan.[80,81]

Due to evidence predominantly accumulated at only a few institutions, the potential toxicity associated with HAI chemotherapy, possible surgical complications of pump placement, challenges with maintaining the pumps and administering HAI chemotherapy, and the improved effectiveness of modern systemic chemotherapy regimens, HAI has not gained universal acceptance. However, HAI chemotherapy with or without systemic 5FU is a reasonable approach in the management of CRLM following liver resection at institutions with experience.

## SURVIVAL AND PROGNOSIS

✓ Prior to the availability of current chemotherapeutic agents, the 5-year OS of patients with CRLM ranged from 30% to 40%.[6] With improvements in the multidisciplinary management of CRLM and the advent of new systemic chemotherapies, the 5-year OS of many patients with CRLM can now exceed 60%.[82]

Several studies have identified perioperative clinicopathological factors, including primary tumour stage, CEA level, number of CRLM, size of the largest lesion, presence of extrahepatic disease and margin status as predictors of postoperative prognosis.[6,83–85] In one of the earliest efforts, Nordlinger et al.[84] developed a scoring system composed of age, size of largest metastasis, CEA level, stage of the primary tumour, disease-free interval, number of liver nodules and resection margin status. By giving one point to each of these factors, the authors classified patients into three risk groups with different 2-year survival. Subsequently, in an analysis of 1001 patients with CRLM who underwent liver resection, Fong et al.[6] identified seven criteria as independent predictors of poor outcome: positive margin ($P$ = 0.004), extrahepatic disease ($P$ = 0.003), node-positive primary ($P$ = 0.02), disease-free interval from primary to metastases < 12 months ($P$ = 0.03), number of hepatic tumours > 1 ($P$ = 0.0004), largest hepatic tumour > 5 cm ($P$ = 0.01) and CEA > 200 ng/ml ($P$ = 0.01). The authors used the last five factors to create a clinical risk score (CRS) that was predictive of outcome. Although several other predictive systems have been developed, the clinical value of most scoring systems is undetermined. In a study by Nathan et al.,[86] only poor-to-moderate prognostic discriminatory ability of the Fong, Nordlinger and MSKCC predictive scoring systems was reported with C-statistics of just 0.57, 0.56 and 0.57, respectively. Scoring systems might provide useful clues toward disease prognosis and guide patient selection and surveillance, but should not be relied upon to exclude patients from being considered for curative-intent resection.

✓✓ A study by Roberts et al.[87] assessed the prognostic value of eight different scores and noted that only the Rees postoperative index was a significant predictor of DFS and disease-specific survival. Nodal status of the primary tumour, differentiation degree of the primary tumour, presence of extrahepatic disease, tumour diameter, CEA level and resection margin status are the six main components of the Rees postoperative index.[83]

✓✓ Sasaki et al.[88] introduced in 2018 an externally validated 'Metro-ticket' tumour burden score model as an accurate tool to predict long-term survival of patients with CRLM undergoing resection with excellent prognostic discriminatory power.

## SURVEILLANCE

Although surgery improves survival of patients with CRLM, recurrence is common. The liver and lung are the most common sites of tumour recurrence, with the liver being the only site in 35–40% of cases.[89,90] Repeat resection can be considered in selected patients. The 5-year survival of patients who undergo repeat hepatic resection for recurrent liver metastases is reported to be 40–50% with acceptable perioperative morbidity and mortality.[91] The duration of relapse-free interval and the number of lesions are the main predictors of prognosis. In the future, surveillance strategies may be tailored to distinct clinicopathologic and molecular characteristics. For example, *KRAS* status might predict the pattern of recurrence and hence guide surveillance strategies.[92,93]

✓ Post-hepatectomy monitoring is recommended to identify early and potentially resectable recurrences. Repeat physical examination, serum CEA measurement and CT of chest, abdomen and pelvis every 3–6 months for the first 2 years, and then every 6 months for up to 5 years is recommended.

## MANAGEMENT OF UNRESECTABLE CRLM

### SYSTEMIC CHEMOTHERAPY

Palliative chemotherapy in patients with unresectable CRLM can relieve symptoms, improve quality of life and prolong survival. The advent of targeted molecular therapies has further improved the efficacy of current regimens (Table 7.2). Either irinotecan- or oxaliplatin-based regimens (e.g.

**Table 7.2  Most commonly used chemotherapy regimens in patients with colorectal liver metastasis and their components**

| Regimen | Irinotecan | Oxaliplatin | Leucovorin | Fluorouracil/capecitabine |
|---------|------------|-------------|------------|---------------------------|
| FOLFIRI | ✓ | | ✓ | ✓ |
| FOLFOX | | ✓ | ✓ | ✓ |
| XELOX | | ✓ | | ✓ |
| FOLFOXIRI | ✓ | ✓ | ✓ | ✓ |

FOLFOX, FOLFIRI or XELOX) can be administered as a first-line therapy with relatively similar efficacy. Several studies have failed to show the superiority of FOLFOX over FOLFIRI, and selection is usually made based on the regimen toxicity profile as well as patient fitness.[94,95] However, if the patient has already received adjuvant oxaliplatin-containing therapy in the previous 12 months, FOLFIRI is the preferred treatment. Capecitabine can be substituted for 5FU plus leucovorin; the combination XELOX increases patient convenience with comparable RR, PFS and OS.[96,97]

Triple regimen therapy, FOLFOXIRI, is recommended in young patients with severe symptoms, high tumour burden, or contraindications to biologic agents such as *RAS/BRAF* mutations. In a phase III trial of 244 patients with unresectable CRLM, FOLFOXIRI was associated with improved RR, PFS and OS compared with FOLFIRI.[98] Similarly, Cremolini et al.[99] demonstrated that median OS in patients treated with FOLFOXIRI plus bevacizumab was longer than that with FOLFIRI plus bevacizumab (29.8 months vs 25.8 months, respectively; HR 0.8; $P = 0.03$).

The addition of molecular-targeted therapies to a first-line chemotherapy regimen can also be a reasonable approach. In a pooled analysis of seven randomised controlled trials, Hurwitz et al.[100] demonstrated that the addition of bevacizumab to chemotherapy was associated with an increase in OS (HR 0.80; 95% CI 0.71–0.90) and PFS (HR 0.57; 95% CI 0.46–0.71). In a phase III study of 1401 patients with metastatic CRC, Saltz et al.[101] concluded that bevacizumab in combination with oxaliplatin-based chemotherapy improved PFS. There was no difference in RR and OS with combination therapy. In contrast, other studies have challenged the therapeutic benefit of bevacizumab.[102] Furthermore, several trials have confirmed the efficacy of adding anti-EGFR medications like cetuximab or panitumumab to first-line chemotherapy regimens in the palliation of patients with inoperable wild-type *KRAS* metastatic CRC.[103] The choice of bevacizumab or anti-EGFR agents depends upon several factors. In patients with *RAS/BRAF* mutated tumours or patients who have markers of anti-EGFR resistance, bevacizumab is the preferred medication. Likewise, patients with right-sided primary tumours are less likely to benefit from cetuximab. The administration of bevacizumab should be carefully considered in elderly patients with a history of intra-arterial thromboembolic events or patients with recent major surgical intervention.

## HEPATIC ARTERY INFUSION THERAPY

The role of HAI chemotherapy in the management of advanced inoperable CRLM is typically limited to patients with isolated liver lesions that are not amenable to surgical resection or ablation. In general, the primary tumour should have been removed and there should be no or minimal extrahepatic disease. The infusion catheter is usually inserted into the gastroduodenal artery; as such, hepatic artery thrombosis, biliary toxicity, incomplete perfusion of the liver, and misperfusion to the stomach or duodenum with ulcers are all possible complications.[104] Floxuridine is the most thoroughly studied agent used in HAI therapy, but recently some investigators demonstrated the safety of delivering modern chemotherapy agents such as oxaliplatin and irinotecan via this route.[105] Although several studies have demonstrated the superiority of HAI therapy over 5FU-based systemic therapies, a demonstrable survival advantage has been inconsistent.[106,107] Considering that irinotecan- or oxaliplatin-based systemic therapy was not used in most of these trials, the true superiority of HAI chemotherapy over standard systemic therapy for patients with unresectable CRLM remains uncertain.

Other hepatic artery–based therapeutic strategies, including yttrium-90 transarterial radioembolisation (Y-90 TARE) and transarterial chemoembolisation (TACE), have been investigated (Fig. 7.9). These therapies are most commonly used following induction systemic chemotherapy in liver-dominant metastatic CRC. The SIRFLOX trial randomised 549 patients with unresectable CRLM to either first-line chemotherapy or chemotherapy with Y-90 TARE. There was no difference in OS, yet the TARE group experienced greater adverse events.[108]

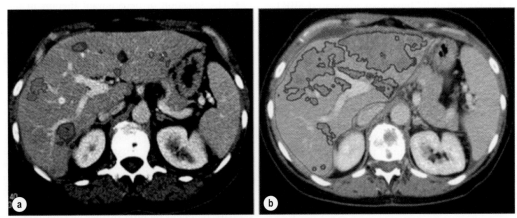

**Figure 7.9** Multifocal colorectal liver metastases in a 50-year-old female treated with radioembolisation. **(a)** Processed CT image before radioembolisation shows segmentation of metastatic lesion and liver for estimation of tumour burden and liver volume, respectively. **(b)** Processed CT image from the same patient approximately 2 months afterwards shows substantial interval increase in tumour. (From Sahani D, Bajwa MA, Andrabi Y, et al. Current status of imaging and emerging techniques to evaluate liver metastases from colorectal carcinoma. Ann ... 2014;259(5):861–72. PMID: 24509207.)

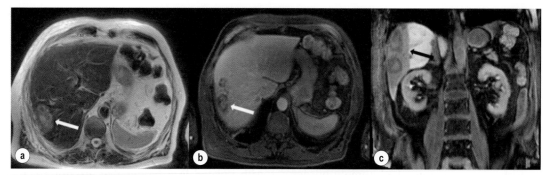

**Figure 7.10** A 56-year-old man with colorectal liver metastases **(a)** *(white arrow)* who underwent proton radiation therapy. Images from follow-up magnetic resonance imaging **(b, c)** show reduced enhancement on the dynamic contrast-enhanced images indicating response to therapy on 10-minute delayed hepatobiliary phase *(white arrow)*. A sharp demarcation between treated liver from uninvolved liver *(black arrow)* is evident **(c)**. (From Sahani DV, Bajwa MA, Andrabi Y, et al. Current status of imaging and emerging techniques to evaluate liver metastases from colorectal carcinoma. Ann Surg 2014;259(5):861–72. PMID: 24509207.)

## ABLATION THERAPY

Tumour ablation is an alternative locoregional therapy for patients with unresectable isolated liver metastasis. Radiofrequency ablation (RFA) was previously the most common method of local ablation therapy but has been recently surpassed by microwave ablation (MWA). Both can be performed by open, laparoscopic or percutaneous approaches. While most often utilised in combination with resection, ablation can be used to treat oligometastatic unresectable CRLM. Several limitations to ablative therapy exist, including proximity to major blood vessels and other vital structures, as well as the decreased efficacy at tumour size > 3 cm.

## RADIATION THERAPY

The effective antitumour dosage of traditional external beam radiation therapy (EBRT) is very toxic to the normal liver parenchyma. Development of radiation techniques utilising targeted radiation such as stereotactic body radiotherapy (SBRT) or proton beam therapy (PBT) has provided a new opportunity for local control of CRLM (Fig. 7.10). In a phase II trial of 42 patients with inoperable CRLM, SBRT was associated with a promising median OS of 29.2 ± 3.7 months.[109] Van der Pool et al.[110] have also advocated SBRT as a treatment option for lesions not amenable for resection or RFA. Radiation is most often indicated for patients with oligometastatic unresectable disease > 3 cm who have stable disease following induction systemic chemotherapy.

## CONCLUSION

The treatment of CRLM has evolved significantly over the last several decades. The cornerstone of potentially curative therapy remains surgical resection, and advances in perioperative and surgical techniques have expanded the number of patients eligible for curative-intent operations. Multidisciplinary care that involves thoughtful utilisation of perioperative chemotherapy is also critical to optimise the potential for long-term survival. Options for patients with advanced unresectable disease have expanded and now include more effective combined systemic chemotherapy with targeted biologic agents, as well as locoregional liver-directed therapies.

Toronto HPB video atlas – http://pie.med.utoronto.ca/TVASurg/all-cases/.

## Key points

- The liver is the most frequent site of metastases in patients with colorectal cancer, and the extent of liver disease is a key determinant of patient survival.
- The diagnosis of CRLM is usually based on imaging findings and percutaneous biopsy may be used to confirm the diagnosis.
- Surgical resection with negative microscopic margins (R0 resection) offers patients with CRLM the best chance for long-term survival. With recent advancements in multidisciplinary management of patients, CRLM may be considered resectable as long as the tumour can be removed completely, the predicted future liver remnant function is adequate to prevent postoperative liver failure, extrahepatic sites of the disease are controllable, and the primary tumour has been resected for cure.
- The advent of portal vein embolisation (PVE), staged hepatectomy with portal vein ligation, parenchymal-sparing hepatectomy with serial liver resections, and combining surgery with ablation has increased the number of patients with CRLM who might benefit from surgical resection. Advances in minimally invasive surgery as well as perioperative management have improved the short-term outcomes of liver surgery.
- The selection of neoadjuvant therapy in management of patients with resectable CRLM needs to be considered individually, based on tumour biology, risk of liver insufficiency and difficulty of any potential resection.
- In patients with unresectable CRLM, preoperative systemic chemotherapy has the potential to downsize lesions and convert initially unresectable disease to resectable disease.
- The main goal of adjuvant chemotherapy is to reduce the risk of disease recurrence that can occur in up to 60–70% of patients following resection of CRLM.
- Either irinotecan- or oxaliplatin-based regimens (e.g. FOLFOX, FOLFIRI, or XELOX) can be administered as a first-line systemic chemotherapy in patients with unresectable CRLM with relatively similar efficacy. The benefit of additional molecular-targeted therapies to first-line chemotherapy regimens requires further investigation.
- A multidisciplinary approach involving a medical oncologist, surgeon, radiation oncologist, radiologist, interventional radiologist, and pathologist is critical for optimising outcomes of CRLM.

 References available at http://ebooks.health.elsevier.com/

## KEY REFERENCES

[5] Stangl R, Altendorf-Hofmann A, Charnley RM, et al. Factors influencing the natural history of colorectal liver metastases. Lancet 1994;343(8910):1405–10.

*Provided natural outcome of patients with CRLM who did not receive any treatment and introduced six factors (percentage liver volume replaced by tumour [LVRT], grade of malignancy of the primary tumour, presence of extrahepatic disease, mesenteric lymph node involvement, serum carcinoembryonic antigen [CEA] and age) as independent determinants of survival.*

[6] Fong Y, Fortner J, Sun RL, et al. Clinical score for predicting recurrence after hepatic resection for metastatic colorectal cancer: analysis of 1001 consecutive cases. Ann Surg 1999;230(3):309–18;discussion 18–21. PMID: 10493478.

*Provided a clinical score to predict outcome of patients with CRLM following surgical resection.*

[9] Sahani DV, Bajwa MA, Andrabi Y, et al. Current status of imaging and emerging techniques to evaluate liver metastases from colorectal carcinoma. Ann Surg 2014;259(5):861–72. PMID: 24509207.

*A review of the role of current imaging modalities in diagnosis and management of CRLM.*

[17] Adams RB, Aloia TA, Loyer E, et al. Selection for hepatic resection of colorectal liver metastases: expert consensus statement. HPB (Oxford) 2013;15(2):91–103. PMID: 23297719.

*Expert consensus about the criteria of resectability and selection of patients with CRLM for hepatic resection.*

[20] Abdalla EK. Portal vein embolization (prior to major hepatectomy) effects on regeneration, resectability, and outcome. J Surg Oncol 2010;102(8):960–7. PMID: 21165999.

*Described the role of PVE in liver regeneration and prevention of hepatic insufficiency after hepatectomy.*

[21] de Santibañes E, Clavien PA. Playing Play-Doh to prevent postoperative liver failure: the 'ALPPS' approach. Ann Surg 2012;255(3):415–7. PMID: 22330039.

*The ALPPS procedure and its role in prevention of post-hepatectomy liver failure.*

[35] Fretland Å A, Dagenborg VJ, Bjørnelv GMW, et al. Laparoscopic versus open resection for colorectal liver metastases: the OSLO-COMET randomized controlled trial. Ann Surg 2018;267:199–207.

*Randomised controlled trial demonstrating improved perioperative outcomes with laparoscopic liver resection for colorectal liver metastases compared with open liver resection.*

[36] Aghayan DL, Kazaryan AM, Dagenborg VJ, et al. Long-term oncologic outcomes after laparoscopic versus open resection for colorectal liver metastases : a randomized trial. Ann Intern Med 2021;174(2):175–82.

*Above randomised controlled trial showing no difference in long-term outcomes with laparoscopic liver resection.*

[52] Nordlinger B, Sorbye H, Glimelius B, et al. Perioperative chemotherapy with FOLFOX4 and surgery versus surgery alone for resectable liver metastases from colorectal cancer (EORTC Intergroup trial 40983): a randomised controlled trial. Lancet 2008;371(9617):1007–16. PMID: 18358928.

*The randomised trial demonstrated the role of perioperative chemotherapy in management of patients with CRLM who underwent liver resection.*

[53] Nordlinger B, Sorbye H, Glimelius B, et al. Perioperative FOLFOX4 chemotherapy and surgery versus surgery alone for resectable liver metastases from colorectal cancer (EORTC 40983): long-term results of a randomised, controlled, phase 3 trial. Lancet Oncol 2013;14(12):1208–15. PMID: 24120480.

*Long-term follow-up results of previous study.*

[54] Van Cutsem E, Cervantes A, Adam R, et al. ESMO consensus guidelines for the management of patients with metastatic colorectal cancer. Ann Oncol 2016;27(8):1386–422. PMID: 27380959.

*Guidelines of European society for medical oncology in comprehensive management of patients with metastatic colorectal cancer.*

[56] Primrose J, Falk S, Finch-Jones M, et al. Systemic chemotherapy with or without cetuximab in patients with resectable colorectal liver metastasis: the New EPOC randomised controlled trial. Lancet Oncol 2014;15(6):601–11. PMID: 24717919.

*Addition of cetuximab to chemotherapy and surgery for resectable CRLM in KRAS exon 2 wild-type patients results in shorter progression-free survival.*

[68] Kelly ME, Spolverato G, Le GN, et al. Synchronous colorectal liver metastasis: a network meta-analysis review comparing classical, combined, and liver-first surgical strategies. J Surg Oncol 2015;111(3):341–51. PMID: 25363294.

*This meta-analysis demonstrated that there is no clear statistical surgical outcome or survival advantage towards any of three available approaches in management of patients with synchronous CRLM.*

[87] Roberts KJ, White A, Cockbain A, et al. Performance of prognostic scores in predicting long-term outcome following resection of colorectal liver metastases. Br J Surg 2014;101(7):856–66. PMID: 24817653.

*Compared the value of different prognostic scores in predicting long-term outcome of patients with CRLM following hepatic resection.*

[88] Sasaki K, Morioka D, Conci S, et al. The tumor burden score: a new 'Metro-ticket' prognostic tool for colorectal liver metastases based on tumor size and number of tumors. Ann Surg 2018;267(1):132–41. PMID: 27763897.

*Introduced a prognostic tool based on maximum tumour size and number of lesions for patients undergoing hepatic resection of CRLM.*

[108] Wasan HS, Gibbs P, Sharma NK, et al. First-line selective internal radiotherapy plus chemotherapy versus chemotherapy alone in patients with liver metastases from colorectal cancer (FOXFIRE, SIRFLOX, and FOXFIRE-Global): a combined analysis of three multicentre, randomised, phase 3 trials. Lancet Oncol 2017;18:1159–71.

*Randomised controlled trial of first-line y-90 radioembolisation did not improve survival outcomes compared with chemotherapy alone.*

# 8 Non-colorectal hepatic metastases

Chaya Shwaartz | Steven Gallinger | Carol-Anne Moulton

## INTRODUCTION

Colorectal cancer (CRC) is the second most common cancer diagnosed in women and the third most common cancer diagnosed in men worldwide.[1] The majority of CRC-related mortality is due to metastatic disease with the liver being the most common site (80%).[2] Fifty percent of patients with CRC have liver metastases at presentation; however, the majority of these liver metastases are unresectable.[2] Although CRC is the most common source of secondary hepatic tumours, almost any solid malignancy can metastasise to the liver. Tumour cells from gastrointestinal (GI) tract malignancies may reach the liver directly via the portal circulation and liver metastases may occur in apparent isolation, as is sometimes seen with CRC. In contrast, metastases from non-GI tumours may seed the liver via the systemic circulation and are generally indicative of disseminated disease.[3]

The success of hepatectomy in improving outcomes in metastatic CRC has generated renewed enthusiasm in considering resection of liver metastases for non-colorectal primary cancers. Liver resection has become the standard of care for colorectal liver metastases (CRLM) and many centres have adopted an increasingly aggressive approach, with reported 5-year survival rates exceeding 50% in selected series.[4,5] Furthermore, approximately 20% of patients are cured of their disease following hepatic resection.[6] The complementary use of staged resection such as portal vein embolisation (PVE) and associating liver partition and portal vein ligation for staged hepatectomy (ALPPS), and the use of radiofrequency ablation (RFA) has increased the proportion of patients eligible for resection.[7] At the same time, advances in surgical technique, postoperative care and knowledge of liver anatomy have significantly reduced the morbidity and mortality associated with major liver resection to less than 20% and 5%, respectively.[8,9]

Liver metastases of non-colorectal origin constitute a diverse group of tumours, most commonly arising from GI sites. These tumours can be broadly divided into neuroendocrine and non-neuroendocrine malignancies, encompassing unique and markedly varied natural histories. Neuroendocrine tumours (NETs) have historically been described as indolent malignancies with resection of NET liver metastases associated with 5-year overall survival (OS) rates of 61–74%.[8,10–12] While hepatectomy is an accepted management strategy for NETs, it is performed less frequently for non-NETs.

Evidence regarding hepatectomy for non-colorectal metastases originates largely from retrospective reviews spanning several decades of experience.[13–16] Many studies fail to distinguish between NET and non-NET metastases, and when that distinction is made, the non-NET metastases are usually considered a single entity despite comprising a heterogeneous set of pathologies. Reports focusing on a single tumour type are usually based on small case series. With advances in surgical techniques, and promising results observed for CRC and NET hepatic metastases, the role of surgical treatment for non-NETs has once again become an area of active interest.

✓ Due to the paucity of prospective, controlled data, the appropriate indications for liver resection for non-CRC metastases are unclear. Factors routinely associated with improved long-term outcomes include a long disease-free interval between treatment of the primary tumour and development of liver metastases, little or no extrahepatic disease, the projected future liver remnant and well- to moderately-differentiated cancer. Unfortunately, no single measure of tumour biology yet exists, although intensive research on molecular classification will lead to improved selection over the next decade.

## PATHOPHYSIOLOGY AND MOLECULAR BASIS OF LIVER METASTASES

Achieving cancer cure requires the complete eradication of all tumour cells. Thus, for most solid tumours, complete surgical excision is the cornerstone of treatment, often with adjuvant systemic treatment to treat microscopic disease. In the presence of metastases, there is an apparent contradiction in using a local therapy, i.e. surgery, to treat what is considered disseminated disease.

The rationale behind a surgical approach to metastatic disease is based on the concept of site-specific metastases. First proposed by Paget in 1889, this 'seed and soil' hypothesis argues that solid tumours have a distinct pattern of distant organ involvement created by the target organ microenvironment. Ewing proposed a 'mechanical' theory in which the metastatic pattern is determined by the venous drainage of the primary tumour.[17] Neither theory takes into account the complexity of the metastatic process, which requires that a cancer cell gains specific invasion and metastatic potential before it can disseminate. The clonal selection model of the metastatic process suggests that heterogeneity develops within a population of cancer cells through mutational events, allowing a subpopulation to randomly acquire the necessary traits to disseminate successfully.[18] Alternatively, it has been argued that within cancers of the same pathological type, i.e. breast cancer, some tumours are a priori more likely to develop metastases than others. This is supported by gene expression data where specific molecular signatures have been found to accurately predict prognosis in breast cancer,[19] ovarian cancer[20] and melanoma.[21] Similarly, in CRC the genotype of microsatellite instability correlates with a decreased likelihood of metastatic spread.[22]

A recent refinement to Paget's hypothesis, based on molecular genetic research, suggests that the primary tumour is itself capable of preparing the 'soil' by creating a 'premetastatic niche'.[23] Every cancer has a type-specific pattern of cytokine expression that appears to direct both malignant and non-malignant cells to specific distant organs. The influx and clustering of bone marrow-derived haematopoietic cells is one of the earliest events in the development of a metastatic deposit. This is closely followed by local inflammation and the release of matrix metalloproteinases. These local events appear to mediate remodelling of the extracellular matrix, creating a more permissive microenvironment for the eventual deposition and growth of malignant cells.[24] Thus, the primary tumour both chooses and alters the sites to which it metastasises. For reasons not yet understood, many solid tumours preferentially metastasise to the liver.

If the site-specific hypothesis of metastatic spread is correct, complete surgical excision of liver metastases can remove the only site of disease and offer a chance for cure. Nonetheless, residual micrometastatic disease may exist within the liver, and hepatic recurrences are a common cause of treatment failure following hepatectomy. Even in the presence of micrometastases, the removal of all macroscopic disease may have immunological benefits. The immune-suppressing effects of cancers are well accepted: malignant cells can induce both adaptive and innate immune suppression, facilitating tumour growth. The degree of immune suppression correlates with the tumour burden and if all gross metastatic disease can be removed, host defences may attack micrometastatic deposits more effectively. The use of neoadjuvant or adjuvant chemotherapy may improve cure rates by controlling micrometastases.[25–27]

The advent of next-generation sequencing technologies and high-density oligonucleotide arrays has further deepened our understanding of the metastatic process. Whereas the ability of a cancerous cell to metastasise was once believed to occur following the accumulation of multiple somatic mutations in many cancer-causing genes, new findings, specifically in pancreatic cancer, have challenged this belief. Studies by Yachida et al.[28] and Campbell et al.[29] describe the existence of multiple subclones within a primary pancreatic cancer, each containing a unique genetic signature corresponding to an eventual site of metastatic spread. These subclones are present many years before an eventual metastasis is clinically detected, when disease is at an early stage. Furthermore, metastases seen in different organs share many common genetic mutations as well as site-specific changes that confer a selective growth advantage in the respective tissue. Alternatively, Notta et al.[30] in 2016 have challenged the timing of tumour evolution of pancreatic cancer whereby a 'single cataclysmic' event, such as chromothripsis, spawns a highly metastatic clone capable of seeding multiple organs very rapidly.

Studies investigating single-nucleotide polymorphisms in genes associated with tumour dormancy and immune response checkpoints have associated certain mutations with survival outcomes in patients undergoing resection of CRLM.[31,32] These findings could assist oncology teams in better risk-stratifying patients for surgical resection and theoretically similar studies could be performed on patients with non-CRLM, though at present there are few validated data available. Future studies on the biology of metastases are likely to improve our understanding of this complex process, translating into more effective therapy.

## CLINICAL APPROACH TO NON-COLORECTAL LIVER METASTASES

Routine clinical, radiological and serological assessments for liver metastases should be guided by the propensity for liver metastases of each specific tumour type and the ability of potential treatments to alter the outcome of the metastatic disease. In imaging the liver, the choice of transabdominal ultrasound (US), contrast-enhanced ultrasound (CEUS), contrast-enhanced triphasic computed tomography (CT), magnetic resonance imaging (MRI) and positron emission tomography (PET) will be dictated by tumour type as well as local availability and expertise.

Functional imaging uses radiolabelled somatostatin analogues, such as indium pentetreotide scintigraphy (Octreoscan), and can detect NETs expressing somatostatin receptors with 80–90% sensitivity. Additionally, whole-body PET using a somatostatin analogue, Gallium (DOTA-TOC, DOTATATE or DOTANOC), has been found to be accurate for the detection of new metastases in NETs.[33–36] Occasionally, the initial presentation of a NET will be a liver metastasis from an unidentified primary. Biopsy will demonstrate NET and the investigative focus will be aimed at localisation of the primary tumour. When the primary site remains unknown despite imaging and endoscopy, extended immunohistochemistry staining for neuroendocrine markers or gene expression classifiers can distinguish small bowel from pancreatic NETs. Positive CDX2 staining suggests a midgut primary, whereas positive PAX6 or ISL1 staining suggests a pancreatic primaryA.[37–40] Some patients can be assessed for recurrence of non-CRLM using more targeted techniques and biochemical markers (e.g. CA-125 for epithelial ovarian cancer, chromogranin A, pancreastatin, neurokinin A, polypeptide, substance P, and neuron-specific enolase for NETs).

When a patient is considered for hepatic metastasectomy, the most critical component of the clinical assessment is an accurate determination of the extent of metastatic spread, including a thorough assessment for extrahepatic disease. The anatomical areas targeted for investigation (brain, lung, bone) will be determined by the known metastatic pattern of the primary tumour. Multidisciplinary input from specialists with expertise in hepatic surgery and management of the primary cancer is essential.

Certain tumours, such as gastric, breast and ovarian cancer, have a predilection for intraperitoneal spread. Although CT is the preferred modality for diagnosing peritoneal carcinomatosis, its accuracy is still limited. For many of these equivocal cases, diagnostic laparoscopy has been recommended and found to result in a change in management in 20% of cases and may be used selectively in preoperative staging.[41]

While the discussion that follows will review management and outcomes of liver resection for hepatic metastases based on primary tumour type, general considerations as proposed by Adam et al. in 2006 remain relevant. In their review of 1452 patients from 41 centres undergoing liver resection for non-colorectal and non-neuroendocrine primary tumours, age > 60 years, presence of extrahepatic disease, R2 resection and major hepatectomy were associated with decreased OS. These factors should be considered when contemplating liver resection for these patients.

## TREATMENT STRATEGIES

Several treatment modalities exist for metastatic disease, and the therapeutic approach must be tailored to the tumour type, the performance status of the patient and the extent of disease. Treatment decisions in this context can only be determined properly by a multidisciplinary oncology team. Non-surgical ablative strategies and systemic or locally delivered chemotherapy can be used as adjuncts to resection.

RFA has been reported to be safe and successful at achieving local control in patients with liver metastases from breast cancer,[42] ovarian cancer[43] and NETs.[44] The major limitation of RFA is the difficulty in achieving complete necrosis for tumours > 3 cm, as well as limited utility when tumours are close to major vascular or biliary structures. Novel techniques such as microwave ablation (MWA), stereotactic radiotherapy and irreversible electroporation (IRE) need to be assessed in prospective randomised trials as they may supplant surgical resection in some cases.[45–47]

Transarterial embolisation (TAE) takes advantage of the differential blood supply of liver metastases, which depends mainly on the hepatic arteries, and the normal parenchyma, which relies more heavily on the portal vein. Transarterial chemoembolisation (TACE) involves the local delivery of a drug prior to occluding the artery and allows prolonged exposure of the tumour to the agent without increasing systemic toxicity. Both TAE and TACE have been well described for the treatment of unresectable hepatocellular carcinoma[48] and the symptomatic relief of NETs.[49]

Finally, it behooves the surgical oncologist to keep abreast of the explosion of recent advances in systemic therapy, such as immunotherapy, to ensure proper selection of patients who will benefit from resection.

## MANAGEMENT OF LIVER METASTASES BY PRIMARY TUMOUR

### NEUROENDOCRINE TUMOURS

NETs represent a diverse group of tumours originating throughout the GI tract from cells of the neuroendocrine system. They are classified by site of origin and include GI and pancreatic histological subtypes.[10] NETs arise most commonly in the midgut and produce neurosecretory granules, express characteristic neuroendocrine differentiation markers, and may secrete vasoactive substances responsible for carcinoid syndrome.

About 30% of the patients with NETs present with metastatic disease, preferentially to the liver, and in many patients the liver remains the only site of metastatic disease for a prolonged period of time.[50,51] The majority of patients have multifocal, bilobar disease, of which less than 20% are candidates for surgery. Additionally, these patients have worse prognosis than patients with isolated locoregional disease.[10,51,52] (Fig. 8.1) Depending on the primary site, extent of the disease, and tumour characteristics, different treatment modalities such as liver resection, non-surgical liver-directed therapies, and systemic therapies are available. Liver resection may be performed with curative intent, symptom control or prolongation of survival in the palliative setting.

The choice of treatment for NET hepatic metastases is largely dependent on underlying tumour biology and pattern of metastatic spread.[53] In general, resection or cytoreduction is associated with improved survival, offers relief from hormonal symptoms and prevents sequelae of carcinoid syndrome. Resection has a clear advantage over medical treatment in regards to symptom relief and OS in patients that can be optimally cytoreduced.[54–58] In 2009, Frilling et al. classified the metastatic pattern of spread in the liver for NETs into three morphological subtypes[59–61]: (I) 'restricted metastases' involving one lobe or two adjacent segments; (II)

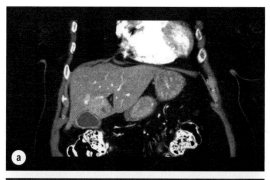

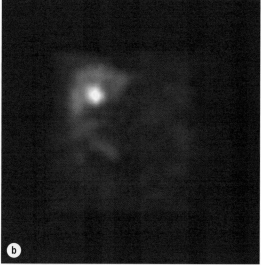

**Figure 8.1** **(a)** A 67-year-old female with a node-positive distal jejunal carcinoid tumour and synchronous solitary liver metastasis in segment 4B. **(b)** Octreotide scan of the same patient. Transaxial single-photon emission computed tomography (SPECT) demonstrates abnormal activity in segment 4B corresponding to known metastasis on CT.

'dominant lesion with bilobar metastases' whereby a single major focus is accompanied by multiple contralateral satellite lesions; (III) diffuse, multifocal liver metastases affecting multiple segments within and between lobes. These three groups differ significantly in terms of treatment strategies and clinical outcomes. Hence, patients with type I or II disease (25% and 15% of cases, respectively), in the absence of extrahepatic metastases, can be considered for curative surgical resection.[12] The aim of liver resection with curative intent in NETs is to leave no residual disease (R0 resection) in both primary and secondary sites, and this may be associated with 5-year survival rates of up to 85%.[52]

Hepatic resection for metastatic NETs results in improved OS compared with those receiving supportive care. There is still a debate regarding the resection margin. Some series show that there is improved progression-free survival (PFS) in patients who underwent complete resection. Sarmiento et al.[56] showed that R0 resection was associated with longer PFS than R1/R2 resections (median PFS 30 months vs 16 months, $P < 0.001$). However, few other studies have shown that margin status is not associated with risk of progression.[8,57,62] Furthermore, R1 and R2 resections result in 5-year survival rates of 70% and 60%, respectively, challenging the dogma that surgery should be reserved only for patients most likely to have an R0 resection.[54,63] The recommendation currently is to pursue surgical cytoreduction for both functional and non-functional tumours even when complete cytoreduction cannot be obtained.[64]

Historically, cytoreduction aimed to reduce tumour volume by at least 90% in situations where R0 resection was not feasible. Although there are no data from randomised trials, large series using historical controls or contemporary cases matched for stage have demonstrated that liver resection with optimal cytoreduction results in improved survival.[65–68] Recent data suggest that cytoreduction of 70% or greater of tumour burden effectively palliated symptoms and was associated with improved PFS.[62,69,70] Therefore, resection should be considered when a 70% debulking threshold is possible including in patients with multiple NET liver metastases, Ki-67 less than 20% and even in patients with extrahepatic disease as long as this threshold is achieved.[64,71] Importantly, patients with extensive liver replacement tumour burden > 50–70% or high-grade NET liver metastases may not benefit from surgery.[71] Additionally, patients with poor performance status and significant comorbidities, severe hepatic insufficiency or carcinoid heart disease may also not benefit from surgical intervention.[64]

✅ Cytoreduction can also offer effective and durable palliation from symptoms for patients with functional tumour syndromes. As a result, surgical debulking has been advocated for both functional and non-functional tumours. An aggressive approach, sometimes combining liver resection with other ablative strategies, is warranted (Fig. 8.2). Liver transplantation is an emerging option for NET liver metastases that are otherwise unresectable but is controversial.

In regard to the question of whether or not to resect the primary tumour in patients with unresectable metastatic disease, guidelines recommend evaluating the patients' symptoms, medical condition, grade and location of the tumour, and potential to improve response to peptide receptor radionuclide therapy (PRRT).[71]

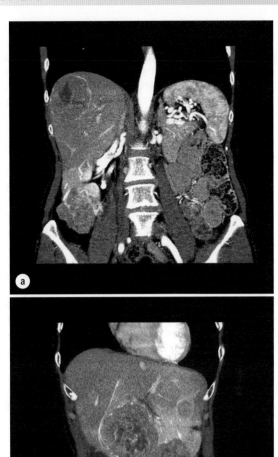

**Figure 8.2** **(a)** A 59-year-old female with an incidental finding of multiple neuroendocrine tumour metastases. There was no evidence of primary tumour on octreotide scan and endoscopy. Note multiple hypervascular, large metastases with central necrosis. **(b)** Same patient as in **(a)**. A debulking operation to remove 90% of tumour burden would be possible by performing an extended right hepatectomy with wedge resections from segment 2.

Despite resection, hepatic recurrence occurs in up to 84% of patients at 5 years post-surgery.[56,72] Sarmiento et al.[56] showed a 5-year recurrence rate of 76% even in patients who had R0 resection. This is partially due to underestimation of the tumour burden on preoperative imaging.[73] Recurrence is suspected by the elevation of tumour markers such as 5-hydroxyindoleacetic acid (5-HIAA) and chromogranin A. Chromogranin A is more sensitive than 5-HIAA in identifying disease progression, and high levels have been shown to predict poorer outcomes. A reduction in chromogranin A levels of > 80% predicts a good outcome following cytoreductive hepatectomy, even when complete resection has not been achieved.[74]

Non-surgical treatment modalities used for NET metastases include RFA, TAE and TACE. Ablation can be performed as an adjunct to resection and can minimize the loss of normal liver tissue and allows improved cytoreduction. RFA in isolation can achieve symptomatic relief and local control of variable duration in up to 80% of patients with NET hepatic metastases. Although studies comparing RFA with other modalities are limited, RFA has been advocated in patients with bilobar disease with up to 14 hepatic lesions of < 7 cm in diameter, involving up to 20% of liver volume.[72,75] Ablation seems to be effective for palliation of symptoms and may provide survival benefit with relatively low rate of complications.[76] TAE and TACE are more useful options for improving hormonal symptoms and slowing tumour growth in patients with NET liver metastases. Both appear to deliver comparable results and thus one modality is not favoured over the other. Embolisation is usually indicated for more extensive hepatic disease or for tumours in close proximity to biliary structures precluding RFA.[72,77] Duration of response is typically short as the tumour rapidly develops collaterals and thus repeat treatments are often required.[78] Embolisation is contraindicated in patients with 50–75% liver involvement due to the risk of precipitating acute hepatic failure. In general, aggressive multimodal therapy with embolic, ablative and systemic strategies is recommended to debulk or downstage metastatic NETs. Symptom control with non-surgical approaches, recognising that repeat treatments may be required, can limit the need for cytoreductive surgery in many patients.

Liver transplantation has been advocated for patients with extensive, unresectable liver metastases with no extrahepatic disease. The two largest reports from US and European registries reported only 150 cases in 20 years and 213 cases in 27 years, respectively.[79,80] The 5-year survival rates were relatively poor at 52% with a 5-year disease-free survival (DFS) of approximately 30% in both studies. Additionally, a systematic review found that recurrence after liver transplantation for NET liver metastases ranged from 31% to 57%.[81] In 2016, Mazzaferro et al.[82] conducted a retrospective, non-randomized study of patients with NET considered for liver transplantation from 1995 to 2010. Transplant eligibility included a primary tumour with curative resection of all extrahepatic disease along with criteria for the best transplant outcomes: low-grade (G1-2) histology, <50% tumour involvement of the liver, stable disease for more than 6 months and age up to 60 years. They reported significantly improved long-term outcomes in the transplantation group compared with controls, with 5-year survival rates of 97% versus 88% and 10-year survival rates of 51% versus 22%, respectively. Concerns remain regarding tumour recurrence in the context of immunosuppression, so while liver transplantation does appear to confer long-term survival in carefully selected patients, optimal patient selection criteria remain in evolution.[53,83]

NETs are graded based on mitotic rate and Ki-67 proliferative index on a scale from 1 to 3. Grade 1 and 2 tumours are considered to have indolent growth patterns. Despite this benign description, 46–93% of patients with NETs will have liver involvement at the time of diagnosis, with a 5-year untreated survival of 0–20%.[52] Systemic chemotherapy with platinum-based regimens has shown a response rate of up to 67% in grade 3 NETs and is generally indicated for patients with high-grade NETs. However, overall the survival benefit of chemotherapy is limited and associated with significant toxicity and response rates of approximately 30%.[53,75]

Somatostatin analogues such as octreotide and lanreotide can achieve symptomatic relief in 70–80% of patients with functional tumours.[84–86] Both have also been shown to confer improvement in PFS compared with placebo as well as stabilized tumour size.[84] There is emerging evidence that pasireotide, a somatostatin analogue that binds more somatostatin receptors than octreotide or lanreotide, may have an even greater antiproliferative effect.[87] Furthermore, molecularly targeted therapies, such as the vascular endothelial growth factor inhibitor sunitinib and the mammalian target of rapamycin (mTOR) inhibitor everolimus, have shown promise in patients with metastatic NETs.[88] Furthermore, PRRT is a treatment option for patients who progress on somatostatin analogues.[89]

## GASTROINTESTINAL STROMAL TUMOURS

Liver metastases may be observed in approximately 16% of patients with retroperitoneal sarcomas and about 60% of patients with visceral sarcomas.[90] Gastrointestinal stromal tumours (GISTs) are the most common GI mesenchymal malignancies and the most common source of hepatic metastases. GISTs originate from the interstitial cells of Cajal and approximately 70–80% of GISTs harbour a mutated c-Kit proto-oncogene, which results in the constitutive activation of the receptor tyrosine kinase leading to unregulated cell growth. Two-thirds of c-Kit mutations are located on exon 11. c-Kit exon 9 and platelet-derived growth factor receptor α (PDGFRA) mutations, encompassing a wild-type kinase domain that modulates receptor inhibitor sensitivity, account for another 5–10% of GISTs.[91]

Primary GISTs represent 1% of all GI malignancies, and arise in the stomach (55–60%), small intestine (30–35%), colon/rectum (5–10%) and oesophagus (5%).[92,93] The primary tumour can be classified into four prognostic categories ranging from very low risk to high risk, according to site of the primary lesion, size of the primary lesion, and the number of mitotic figures identified on histology. Resection remains the standard treatment of primary GIST. For GIST metastatic to the liver, the therapeutic modalities include systemic therapies such as chemotherapy and targeted therapy, including tumour ablation, TAE and resection.

GIST metastatic to the liver is usually unresponsive to cytotoxic agents with response rates as low as 5%.[94] However, targeted therapy directed against the oncogenic KIT and PDGFR tyrosine kinases has been shown to be very effective. Imatinib mesylate is a selective tyrosine kinase inhibitor (TKI) that has revolutionised the treatment of GIST. Despite complete surgical resection with microscopic negative margins, recurrence (local or distant) occurs in 50% of patients.[95] The use of imatinib in the adjuvant setting was investigated in the phase III ACOSOG placebo-controlled trial (Z9001) for patients with resected GIST > 3 cm in size. A statistically significant 1-year recurrence-free survival (RFS) of 98% in the treatment group versus 83% in the placebo group was observed, prompting the inclusion of imatinib as an adjuvant treatment modality in patients with moderate- to high-risk primary tumours.[95] Response to imatinib is greatest in tumours that harbour the c-Kit exon 11 mutation, with resistance rates higher in patients harbouring exon 9 or PDGFRA mutations.[95] Demetri et al.

showed that the median OS was 57 months with imatinib in a study population of which 95% had liver metastasis. Importantly, approximately 18% had primary resistance to imatinib as well as secondary resistance that developed at a median of 2 years due to development of secondary mutations.[96,97] Second- (e.g. sunitinib) and third-line agents (e.g. nilotinib and masitinib) have shown promise in patients resistant to imatinib.[98]

Percutaneous ablation and intra-arterial therapies are used for palliative purposes or combined with resection. There are very scarce data regarding these modalities for the treatment of liver metastasis from GIST.[99–106]

In the era of imatinib as an effective systemic therapy for GIST, the primary goal is to remove macroscopic disease. The efficacy and low side-effect profile of imatinib prompted initial enthusiasm for the combined use of surgery and imatinib in the management of metastatic GIST. Additionally, resection is sometimes performed in order to remove disease that is progressing while leaving macroscopic disease that is responding to therapy with imatinib. Overall, surgery is recommended after 6–9 months from the initiation of imatinib for maximal treatment response and is usually appropriate for patients with response to preoperative imatinib treatment.

Although evidence guiding surgical management in metastatic GIST is limited, a single-institution randomized controlled trial combining neoadjuvant imatinib with surgery and adjuvant imatinib in patients with previous R0 resection of the primary tumour has shown favourable 3-year OS (90% vs 60%).[107] A recent Dutch study evaluated 48 patients who underwent liver resection for GIST metastases, 36 of whom received TKI therapy either pre- or postoperatively. Median survival was 7.5 years and 5-year OS was 76%. Multivariate analysis demonstrated that R0 resection of the liver metastasis was the only significant predictor of survival.[108] A multicentre European study retrospectively evaluated 239 patients undergoing hepatic metastasectomy, all of whom received adjuvant imatinib. R0/R1 resection was found to be a significant predictor of survival and median survival in this group was 8.7 years. Other significant predictors of survival were female sex and metastases confined to the liver (compared to patients with liver and peritoneal disease).[109] Metastatic disease to the liver, peritoneum and/or other sites had a median time to progression of 3 months following surgery.[110]

✔ GIST liver metastases are usually unresectable and therefore imatinib is generally accepted as the first-line treatment for metastatic disease. The efficacy and low side-effect profile of imatinib has promoted enthusiasm for the combined use of surgery and imatinib in the management of metastatic GIST. High-quality evidence is lacking, but retrospective series studying the combination of surgery with imatinib in patients with resectable metastases have demonstrated good results with 5-year survival rates of > 70%.

Disease progression is managed by imatinib dose escalation followed by second- and third-line agents. In the event of tumour rupture or haemorrhage, surgery or hepatic artery embolisation may be performed in an emergency setting. Imatinib therapy for 6–12 months is recommended for patients with unresectable hepatic metastases and if the tumour responds, resection can be considered if an R0 resection can be anticipated.[92]

# BREAST CANCER

The liver is the third most common site of breast cancer metastases after bone and the lungs.[111] The widely held concept that liver metastases in breast cancer reflects diffuse systemic disease has led to a nihilistic view of the role of liver resection in this setting. However, an aggressive surgical approach has been proposed for patients presenting with the liver as the sole site of involvement. The data are mostly retrospective and are based on heterogeneous indications, making it difficult to provide strong evidence-based guidelines. Of note, the National Comprehensive Cancer Network guidelines do not recommend liver resection for breast cancer liver metastasis; however, the ESOESMO International Consensus Guidelines for Advanced Breast Cancer (ABC 4) recommend resection in selected patients.

Although metastatic breast cancer is common, isolated liver lesions in metastatic breast cancer are seen in less than 10% of patients.[112,113] In a Japanese series of 11,000 breast cancer patients treated over an 18-year period, only 34 patients had resectable liver metastases.[114] Selection criteria for such metastases are inconsistent in surgical series, with some centres considering resection only for disease confined to the liver, while others advocate a more liberal approach. In short, there are no clear selection criteria for resection. Oestrogen receptor-positive primary tumours and a prolonged disease-free interval of > 48 months before development of metastases have been associated with improved survival.[111] Response to chemotherapy also appears to be an important predictor of survival. In one study, patients who progressed during pre-hepatectomy chemotherapy had a 5-year survival rate of 0% versus 11% in responders.[115] Therefore, surgery should only be considered in patients who have responded to preoperative chemotherapy and/or hormonal therapy.

✔ Isolated liver metastases from breast cancer are rare. Previous response to systemic therapy appears to be an important predictor of survival following liver resection for metastatic breast cancer.

In a series of 52 patients with breast cancer liver metastasis, the reported postoperative 3-year survival of patients who developed breast cancer liver metastasis within 48 months of the primary breast cancer was lower than the group who had a longer disease-free interval following liver resection (45% vs 82%). Additionally, in the same series the authors reported that patients who had N1b-N2 disease at the time of first diagnosis of breast cancer had 83% 3-year intrahepatic recurrence compared with 41% among patients with N0/N1 disease.[116]

A meta-analysis of 36 studies including 1025 patients undergoing liver resection for breast cancer metastases showed a median OS of 41 months (data from 25 studies) after curative intent surgery with a median time to recurrence of 11.5 months (from six studies).[111] Five-year OS rates range from 25% to 60%.[111,114,117,118] Five-year DFS rates are lower than OS rates, suggesting that liver resection may function as a cytoreductive rather than curative procedure in these highly selected patients.[111,119]

Most of these data come from retrospective surgical case series. A recent study of patients with isolated hepatic metastases from the Memorial Sloan Kettering Cancer Center compared the outcomes of 69 patients treated with resection or ablation with 98 patients treated with systemic therapy. The surgery group had a lower hepatic disease burden, a longer disease-free interval from primary diagnosis to the diagnosis of liver metastasis and were more likely to have oestrogen receptor-positive tumours. In this series, the median OS of the surgical cohort was 50 months, which was similar to the 45 months for the chemotherapy cohort. This finding persisted after propensity score matching of 49 patients in each group. However, 10 (15%) of the surgically treated patients had a DFS of > 5 years, indicating there are selected patients who benefit from an aggressive surgical approach.[113] This was reinforced by a French report of 19 patients who underwent repeat hepatectomy for breast cancer metastases with 5-year OS (following the second liver resection) of 46% and a median survival of 41 months.[120]

Feng et al.[121] used propensity-matching to compare the outcomes of patients who underwent liver resection with patients who received systemic chemotherapy alone. They reported that the mean survival and 3- and 5-year OS among patients who underwent hepatic resection were significantly better than the non-resection cohort with 61.8 versus 38.6 months, 54.7% versus 45.6%, and 54.7% versus 21.9%, respectively. Hepatic resection was also associated with improved intrahepatic PFS with a 5-year PFS of 41% versus 3.8% in the non-surgical group. Multivariate analysis identified hormonal receptor status and hepatic resection as independent prognostic factors. The authors concluded that hepatic resection might offer a survival benefit compared with systemic treatment alone, especially among patients with positive hormonal receptors.

Based on current limited data, liver resection of breast cancer liver metastasis should be recommended for women with limited disease in the liver, long disease-free interval between primary diagnosis of breast cancer and liver metastasis, and patients with HER2 positive and triple-negative disease that responded to systemic chemotherapy. All patients should be discussed in a multidisciplinary meeting.

## OVARIAN CANCER

Epithelial ovarian cancer represents the most common malignancy of the ovary, and cytoreductive surgery and platinum-based chemotherapy are the mainstays of treatment. In ovarian cancer, the liver is the most common site of metastasis followed by the lung, bone and brain.[122,123] A recent retrospective analysis using the SEER database showed that patients with liver metastasis from ovarian cancer had higher survival than patients with bone and brain metastasis.[123] Residual disease following cytoreduction surgery for ovarian cancer is a major negative prognostic factor for survival.[124] Unfortunately, most patients develop chemoresistance after 24–36 months and the median survival for advanced disease is 3.5 years.[125–127] Aggressive surgical debulking is advocated in advanced cases, with optimal cytoreduction targeted at < 1 cm of residual disease.[128] A meta-analysis by Chang et al.[124] showed that there was an inverse correlation between the amount of residual disease after cytoreductive surgery and survival. They showed that with every 10% increase in cytoreduction to no visible disease, there was a survival benefit of 2.3 months. Intraperitoneal chemotherapy has been demonstrated to further improve survival compared with intravenous therapy and requires optimal debulking in order to be effective.[129] Successful

cytoreduction is thus a crucial step in the management of advanced ovarian cancer.

Ovarian cancer can involve the liver through the development of peritoneal lesions on the surface of the liver (stage III – Fig. 8.3) or intraparenchymal metastases (stage IV – Fig. 8.4). Peritoneal metastases that invade the liver parenchyma may be difficult to distinguish from parenchymal metastases that spread haematogenously and can reflect different disease biology and response to therapy, including liver resection.[126,127] If this distinction can be made preoperatively, those with haematogenous liver metastases can be considered to have advanced disease (similar to those with pulmonary metastases) and are treated with palliative systemic therapy rather than surgery.[126,127] Although the liver is rarely the only site of metastatic disease in ovarian cancer, hepatectomy can be an important component of a primary cytoreduction strategy. Survival is improved for patients with stage IV disease who have undergone adequate debulking surgery including hepatectomy.[130] In a retrospective review, Bristow et al.[130] reported a median survival of 50.1 months in patients with stage IV ovarian cancer who underwent hepatic cytoreduction for liver metastasis (1 cm residual disease). Interestingly, optimal hepatic cytoreduction was only achieved in 16% of patients, resulting in a median survival of 27 months. Furthermore, the number of parenchymal liver lesions correlated with survival; median survival was 20.9

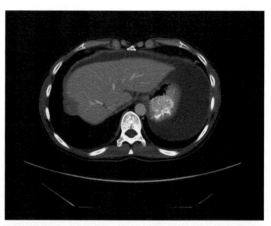

**Figure 8.3** Stage III ovarian cancer with hepatic involvement. Note direct invasion of liver capsule by peritoneal tumour plaque.

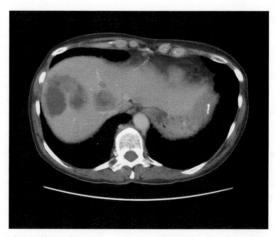

**Figure 8.4** Stage IV ovarian cancer with intraparenchymal liver metastases.

months for 1–2 lesions compared with 6.4 months when 31 lesions were present. Although the study has significant limitations given the small sample size, it demonstrates the difficulty in achieving optimal hepatic cytoreduction.

The use of neoadjuvant chemotherapy in the management of advanced ovarian cancer is an area of debate. There are four randomized clinical trials regarding the use of neoadjuvant chemotherapy in patients with advanced ovarian cancer. Overall results from these studies showed no difference in regard to OS or PFS. However, in regard to adverse events, neoadjuvant chemotherapy was favoured. Additionally, neoadjuvant chemotherapy also reduced the need for bowel resection and stoma formation, and was associated with lower perioperative mortality rates.[131–134]

Survival following primary surgical debulking is inversely correlated with volume of residual disease, disease stage and tumour differentiation. Similarly, survival following hepatectomy for recurrent disease is dependent on optimal cytoreduction, negative margin status, greater pelvic than abdominal disease and a longer recurrence-free interval. It has been demonstrated that when complete cytoreduction of recurrent disease is possible, hepatic resection should be considered as the median survival is improved.[126] TACE and RFA offer potential alternative therapeutic options in achieving local control in patients with contraindications to resection or as adjuncts to systemic therapy.[126,135,136]

## RENAL CELL CARCINOMA

Renal cell carcinoma (RCC) accounts for about 3% of malignancies. Surgery is the only curative treatment for this malignancy. Approximately 20–30% of patients with RCC present with synchronous metastatic disease and another 20–40% of patients with previous nephrectomy will develop metastatic disease.[137,138] The prognosis for metastatic RCC is poor with a 5-year OS of 5–10%.[139] Liver metastases are seen in about 20% of patients with RCC and fewer than 5% of patients have metastases restricted to the liver.[140,141] Additionally, liver metastases are associated with a poor prognosis of 7–12 months.[142,143] Systemic therapy options for RCC are limited. Interleukin-2 and interferon-α were previously used as first-line therapy for metastatic RCC and were not found to be active against liver metastases.[143,144] Current regimens employ TKIs like sunitinib, which is associated with an improved PFS in phase III trials, and emerging data suggest that immune checkpoint inhibitors are effective in metastatic RCC.[144,145]

The available data on hepatic resection for RCC metastases are limited to retrospective reports. A study from the Netherlands examined 33 patients who underwent resection or ablative therapy for RCC hepatic metastases. The study documented no operative mortality, with 5-year DFS and OS of 11% and 43%, respectively. The median OS was 33 months.[137] A second retrospective study compared 68 patients who underwent surgery to a cohort of 20 patients who were eligible but refused an operation. Disease in these patients was mostly confined to the liver. Overall 5-year survival in the treatment arm was 62% in comparison with 29% in the control group.[146] A review of six studies including 140 patients who underwent liver resections reported 5-year OS rates ranging between 34% and 43% and a median survival of 16–48 months.[138] Factors associated with better survival included metachronous metastases, R0 metastasectomy and non-sarcomatoid histology.[137,138,143,146]

More contemporary series have examined liver resection for RCC metastases in the context of TKI use. In one series of 39 patients undergoing liver resection (37 patients) or ablation (2 patients), the overall median survival was 42 months. During a median follow-up period of 2.2 years, 74% of patients who received no targeted therapy recurred compared with 40% of patients maintained on postoperative treatment. Multivariate analysis identified postoperative TKI therapy as a predictor of survival.[147] Preoperative TKI therapy has also been shown to downsize unresectable RCC liver metastases in order to facilitate safe liver resection.[148]

## MELANOMA

Malignant melanoma can be of cutaneous, uveal or mucosal origin with different disease characteristics for each kind. Cutaneous melanoma is the most common and can metastasise to the liver in about 14% of patients; however, it is rarely confined to the liver.[149] Uveal melanoma is very rare.[150,151] As opposed to cutaneous melanoma, uveal melanoma often metastasises to the liver (89% of patients will have liver metastasis) and in about 45% of patients the liver is the only site of metastases. Mucosal melanoma is extremely rare[152,153] and 36% of patients with mucosal melanoma will have liver metastases.

Favourable results in patients undergoing metastasectomy in the lung, soft tissues or abdomen have provided some enthusiasm for surgery in a selected patient population. The available evidence for hepatectomy for metastatic melanoma is limited and consists largely of subset analyses from larger series of patients with non-CRLM. One retrospective study evaluated all patients who presented with metastatic melanoma over the last decade at a single Australian institution.[154] In this series, 13 patients underwent resection for liver metastases. Median disease-free interval from resection of the primary was 49 months, median DFS was 14 months and median OS was 21 months. An American series of 24 patients undergoing liver resection had similar results with a reported median DFS of 12 months and median OS of 28 months.[155] In a 2021 review paper, Höppener et al.[156] described the results of 37 studies investigating surgical treatment for metastatic melanoma.

A total of 947 patients treated with resection were described; 302 (32%) from cutaneous primary, 489 (52%) from uveal primary, 3 (<1%) from mucosal primary and 16 (2%) from unknown primary origin. In the remaining patients treated with resection, the origin was not reported. The seven studies that reported on debulking described a total of 221 patients. Complete microscopic resection was achieved in 83% (range 40–100%) of patients treated with resection. Perioperative mortality and morbidity after surgical treatment (both resection with curative intent and debulking) were approximately 2% (range 0–8%) and 14% (range 0–36%), respectively. In patients that were defined as free of disease after resection, recurrent disease was observed in 75%. Median PFS for resection was 12 (range 5–20) months. Median survival was 26 months after resection versus 11 (range 5–18) months after debulking.

The only study that directly compared resection (with hepatic arterial infusion [HAI]), debulking with HAI and systemic therapy/best supportive care found OS for resection (with HAI) to be significantly improved compared with the other treatments, with no difference observed between debulking with HAI and systemic therapy/best supportive care.[157] Survival following hepatectomy appears to be more favourable in this highly selected but rare group of patients with melanoma of ocular origin. Pawlik et al.[158] reported a 5-year survival rate of 21% for liver resection for ocular melanoma, with a 0% 5-year survival rate for cutaneous melanoma. However, 75% of resected patients in this study developed recurrent disease, and the rate of recurrence was similar between the ocular and cutaneous groups.

The prognosis for patients with metastatic melanoma is poor, and the median survival for patients with stage IV disease has historically been 6–9 months. GI and liver metastases occur in 2–4% of individuals with stage IV disease,[154] and palliative radiotherapy and systemic chemotherapy have largely been ineffective in conferring a survival advantage. Biological agents such as interferon-α and interleukin-2 have yielded modest response rates that are rarely durable and are associated with significant toxicity.[159,160]

Liver resection with postoperative tumour-infiltrating lymphocyte (TIL) therapy has been explored. TIL involves resection of metastatic lesions followed by extraction and culture of infiltrating lymphocytes ex vivo with interleukin-2. A direct comparison was performed between patients with complete surgical resection versus those with residual hepatic disease receiving postoperative TIL. The observed 3-year OS was 53% in the TIL cohort, with prognosis largely favoured by lack of extrahepatic disease and a single hepatic metastasis.[161]

New molecular therapies have become standard of care in treatment of metastatic melanoma. BRAF and MEK inhibitors (e.g. vemurafenib and trametinib, respectively) are used for patients with tumour mutations in the *BRAF* gene. Similarly to checkpoint inhibitors, BRAF and MEK inhibitors demonstrated superior survival compared with dacarbazine and proved most effective when combined.[162–165] Immunomodulators targeting CTLA-4 (e.g. ipilimumab) and PD-1 (e.g. nivolumab, pembrolizumab) are used increasingly in all patients with advanced melanoma. These agents collectively have improved OS for patients with advanced melanoma compared to interleukin-2 and conventional cytotoxic chemotherapy.[166] In a randomized phase III study of 834 patients with advanced cutaneous melanoma, pembrolizumab proved superior to ipilimumab in terms of PFS and OS, with less toxicity.[167] Combining CTLA-4 and PD-1 checkpoint inhibitors has proved even more effective. In a randomized phase III trial, 945 patients with advanced cutaneous melanoma were randomized 1:1:1 to either first-line nivolumab, nivolumab plus ipilimumab, or ipilimumab.[168] The widespread use of these agents may lead to an increased number of patients referred for consideration for resection of isolated hepatic metastases. It is difficult to estimate the impact that liver resection will have on these patients, but it seems reasonable to adopt a resectional approach in highly selected patients, i.e. those with a long disease-free interval from treatment of the primary tumour to development of metastases, and patients who can be rendered disease-free following surgery.

## NON-COLORECTAL GASTROINTESTINAL ADENOCARCINOMA

Liver metastases from non-colorectal GI adenocarcinomas can arise from the oesophagus, stomach, pancreas, gallbladder, ampulla of Vater, small bowel and bile duct. The main route for liver metastases from the GI tract is haematogenous spread through the portal venous system. Hepatic resection has generally been considered to be contraindicated in these cases unless it is for palliative purposes. Chemotherapy is the primary treatment modality for metastatic disease originating from the GI system. Locoregional therapy should be considered in a multidisciplinary meeting for selected patients. In a large series of 1452 patients, Adam et al.[169] reported GI primary tumours as the second largest subset of patients requiring liver resection for non-colorectal non-neuroendocrine liver metastases. They reported an overall 5-year survival of 31% and median survival of 26 months.

## OESOPHAGUS

Patients with liver metastases from oesophageal cancer have a worse prognosis following liver resection when compared with other GI malignancies. Metastatic oesophageal cancer is usually widely disseminated and is associated with a 5-year survival rate of 3–5% when multiple sites of disease are present and 7–8% when disease is limited to the liver.[170] There are limited data regarding hepatectomy for metastatic oesophageal cancer.[171] Two case reports in the English-language literature describe hepatectomy for isolated, synchronous liver metastases.[172,173] In both cases, hepatectomy was performed simultaneously with oesophagectomy and was followed by hepatic arterial chemotherapy. Both patients developed multiple liver metastases at 6 and 7 months postoperatively. These recurrences responded partially to systemic chemotherapy, and the patients were alive with disease at 14 and 18 months following hepatectomy. A report of four cases of liver resection for metachronous oesophageal cancer metastases has also been published. All patients received chemotherapy before liver resection. Two patients died at 10 and 21 months following liver resection, one was alive at 22 months, and one patient had prolonged survival of 92 months after chemotherapy and liver resection.[174] Sano et al.[175] reported regarding 51 patients who underwent liver resection for oesophageal cancer liver metastases with a median survival of 15 months and a 5-year OS of 15%. Adam et al.[169] evaluated 20 patients with liver metastases from oesophageal cancer and 25 patients from gastroesophageal junction cancer who underwent liver resection, reporting a 3-year survival of 32% and 12%, and a median survival of 16 and 14 months, respectively. Thus, although rarely feasible, hepatectomy may provide a limited survival benefit in chemosensitive oesophageal cancer with isolated liver metastases. Given the small number of cases in the literature, liver resection in this context should be offered rarely and only in highly selected patients.

## STOMACH

Gastric adenocarcinoma is the second most common cause of cancer-related death worldwide, and the liver is a major site of spread in 9–40%, though in most cases the metastatic pattern is diffuse involving the peritoneum and distant lymph nodes.[176–179] Additionally, hepatic metastases are diagnosed synchronously in 3–14% of patients with gastric cancer, and metachronously in up to 37% of patients after curative gastrectomy.[180] Among patients with GI non-colorectal non-neuroendocrine liver metastasis, liver metastases from gastric cancer are the leading indication for liver resection.[169] The 5-year OS in patients with liver metastases ranges 0–10% and surgery has historically been contraindicated. There is some emerging literature that liver resection or ablation may provide a therapeutic benefit in the rare situation when of a solitary hepatic metastasis. A meta-analysis of 23 retrospective studies including 802 patients reported a 5-year OS rate of 23.8% and a median survival of 22 months.[178] Size and number of hepatic metastases correlated with OS. A subsequent meta-analysis of 39 studies (many the same as in the previous study) including 909 patients had similar findings reporting a 5-year OS rate of 27.8% and median survival of 29 months with better outcomes seen in Asian studies than in Western series.[180]

A Japanese group reported on their experience using an aggressive approach to gastric cancer liver metastases, adopting the same patient selection criteria as for CRLM. Median RFS was similar between both groups (15.2 months for CRLM versus 16.4 months for gastric cancer metastases), while the 5-year OS rate in patients with CRC (193 patients) was 55% versus 14% in patients with gastric cancer (26 patients). Metachronous metastases, solitary metastases and moderate or well-differentiated tumours were associated with longer survival in the gastric cancer group.[179] A second Japanese group restricted liver resection to those patients with three or fewer metastases. In their series of 28 patients, 5-year OS rate was 32% and median survival was 49 months.[181] A contemporary series of 94 patients from 28 Japanese hospitals used a mix of resection and ablation for liver-only gastric metastases. They reported a 5-year OS rate of 42.3% with no differences between resection, ablation or combined approaches for the liver metastases. Patients with solitary liver metastases and < 3 positive lymph nodes had an improved survival.[182]

The Italian Research Group for Gastric Cancer has recently advocated resection of synchronous hepatic metastases if an R0 resection can be performed of both the primary and the metastases.[177,183] A cohort of 53 patients who underwent curative intent synchronous R0 resection had a median survival of 13 months and a 5-year OS rate of 9.3%. This was significantly improved compared with a median survival of 6.6 months in 98 contemporary patients undergoing palliative gastrectomy and a 3-month median survival for 44 patients who underwent surgical bypass. Montagnani et al.[184] evaluated 33 observational studies involving 1304 patients who underwent hepatic resection for gastric cancer liver metastases and reported a 5-year and 10-year OS rate of 22% and 11%, respectively. Cui et al.[185] reported similar results analysing 10 studies with 1287 patients (241 in the surgical group and 1046 in a non-surgical group). Markar et al.[180] reported improved OS for liver resection and a median 1-year, 3-year, and 5-year survival of 68%, 31%, and 27%, respectively, in an analysis of nine studies with 679 patients, 235 in the resection group and 444 in the non-resected group. Importantly, it appears that studies from eastern countries have reported better survival than western countries.[186]

Montagnani et al.[184] documented that the following factors are associated with better OS: lower T stages, absence or limited nodal involvement, no serosa or lymphatic or vascular involvement in the primary tumour, single or fewer than three metastases, unilobar disease, diameter of the largest lesion less than 5 cm and negative resection margins.

These results suggest that a highly selected subset of patients with gastric cancer liver metastases can achieve long-term survival with an aggressive surgical approach. Whether Asian results can be extrapolated to Western populations remains unclear.

## SMALL BOWEL

Primary small bowel malignancies represent an exceedingly rare but histologically diverse subgroup accounting for 2% of all GI malignancies.[187] Small bowel adenocarcinoma represents the majority of these tumours and is seen in up to 5% of patients with familial adenomatous polyposis (FAP). By virtue of its non-specific clinical presentation and the limitations of radiological and endoscopic diagnostic modalities to examine the small bowel, approximately 80% of patients present with advanced disease. In addition, the low prevalence of small bowel adenocarcinoma limits our understanding of the natural history of tumour spread, restricting the development of clear treatment guidelines. The ability of surgery to prolong PFS in hepatic small bowel adenocarcinoma metastases has been described in a single case report of an FAP patient with a PFS of 3 years following neoadjuvant chemotherapy and surgery.[187] Adam et al.[169] reported a series of 28 patients with small bowel primary tumours and 12 patients with non-ampullary duodenal tumours. Interestingly, patients with liver metastases from the small bowel had the best prognosis after resection among all GI tumours, with a 5-year OS of 49% and a median survival of 58 months, whereas patients who underwent resection of duodenal tumour metastases had a 5-year OS and median survival of 21% and 34 months, respectively. Rompteaux et al.[188] evaluated 34 patients who underwent curative intent resection of metastases from small bowel adenocarcinoma, 9 of whom (29.4%) had isolated liver metastases resected. Median survival was 28.6 months and 41.2% of the patients were alive after 3-year follow-up. The factors associated with worse prognosis after resection were poor differentiation, R1 margins and lymphatic invasion. The National Comprehensive Cancer Network Practice Guidelines for treatment of small bowel adenocarcinoma recommends that certain patients with small bowel adenocarcinoma and limited metastases to visceral organs may be candidates for metastasectomy.[189] Future studies examining liver resection in patients with metastatic small bowel adenocarcinoma will provide further guidance to its role in this disease.

## PANCREAS

Pancreatic ductal adenocarcinoma (PDAC) accounts for 90% of all histological subtypes of pancreatic cancer and confers a poor overall prognosis.[190] Over the last 50 years, PDAC has continued to rank as the 10th most common cancer in the Western world and the 4th leading cause of cancer death. PDAC presents in a non-specific manner, often when disease is already at an advanced stage. Improvements in chemotherapy, surgical technique and knowledge of tumour biology have translated into marginal improvements in survival. Currently, only 15–20% of patients present with disease amenable to curative resection, of whom 20% are alive at 5 years.[190] The average 5-year OS for unresectable PDAC is 5%, with a median survival of 8–11 months for patients with metastatic disease receiving chemotherapy.[190,191] Due to the dismal prognosis in patients with localised resectable disease, surgery for metastatic PDAC has been contraindicated. Yamada et al.[192] examined the role of hepatectomy in non-neuroendocrine pancreatic cancer, including five patients with PDAC, one with adenosquamous carcinoma and one with cystadenocarcinoma. Patients were chosen for surgery if complete excision of hepatic disease was deemed feasible, reliable control of the primary disease was possible and the liver was the only site of spread. The 5-year OS in this cohort was 16.7%; however, five patients developed recurrence and subsequently died of their disease within 4–52 months. Prognostic factors appear to correlate with disease-free interval from primary to metastases and the presence of negative surgical margins at metastasectomy.[192] A study of 69 patients from six European centres evaluated synchronous pancreas and liver resections for patients with PDAC and isolated hepatic metastases. Outcomes were compared with 69 matched patients who did not undergo resection and median survival was greater in the resection group (14.5 months vs 7.5 months). Four patients were alive longer than 5 years in the resection group compared with none in the non-resection group.[193] Although these authors highlight the potential role of liver resection in metastatic PDAC, there is need for future studies to clarify the true benefit of this approach and identification of factors that can assist clinicians in selecting patients appropriately. A recent systematic review found 17 studies reporting resection for pancreatic liver metastases, with median survival ranging from 5.9 to 56 months.[194] In these studies, there is no pattern or consensus about patient selection for liver resection, regimens of chemotherapy or timing for liver resection. Furthermore, there is no consensus about which patients are most likely to benefit from resection. There is considerable variation on prognostic factors among different studies. The most relevant prognostic factors appear to be response to preoperative chemotherapy, oligometastatic disease and R0 resection. Molecular stratification biomarkers may prove useful in this rare setting.[195]

The available evidence for hepatectomy in the management of metastases from non-colorectal, non-neuroendocrine GI primaries is limited, and few meaningful statements can be made as to the utility of this treatment strategy. Gastric cancer specifically may be the exception to this with some encouraging reports from Asia of acceptable survival after liver resection from multiple centres. With improvements in safety of liver resection coupled with encouraging results from other malignancies metastasising to the liver, future prospective studies will shed light on the role of hepatic resection for non-colorectal, non-neuroendocrine GI cancers.

✔ The available evidence for hepatectomy in the management of metastases from non-colorectal, non-neuroendocrine GI primaries is limited, and few meaningful statements can be made as to the utility of this treatment strategy. There is emerging evidence from both Asia and Europe that acceptable results can be achieved for highly selected patients undergoing liver resection for gastric cancer metastases.

## TESTICULAR CANCER

Testicular cancer is the most common malignancy in young men between the ages of 15 and 35 years. Germ cell tumours (GCTs) can be seminomas or non-seminomas and account for approximately 95% of testicular malignancies. Non-seminomatous GCTs (NSGCTs) are less common but have more aggressive biology. The treatment consists of chemotherapy and surgery. Metastasectomy is well established in the management of disseminated non-seminomatous germ cell testicular carcinoma that does not completely

respond to chemotherapy, though isolated liver metastases are rare.[196] One series of 15 patients reported a 10-year OS of 62% after resection of hepatic metastases.[197]

A single-institution experience of 57 liver resections performed over the last two decades demonstrated that surgery for hepatic metastases from NSGCTs is safe and efficacious. In this series, 33% of the patients had active tumour. Based on the presence and histological type of tumour in the liver, 40–70% of patients remained disease-free at 20 months and the OS was 43%.[198,199] Negative prognostic indicators included viable tumour in the resected specimen, metastases > 3 cm in diameter and pure embryonal carcinoma in the primary lesion. The authors recommended liver resection in all patients with residual liver masses post chemotherapy except in those with elevated tumour markers. However, Copson et al.[200] identified 27 patients with GCT and liver metastases treated at a single centre. Of these, eight had a complete biochemical and radiological response to chemotherapy, and seven had residual radiological abnormalities in the liver with normal tumour markers. None of the seven patients underwent resection, and the median survival was 49 months, which was comparable with those in the surgical series. The authors suggested conservative management in patients with residual liver disease after initial treatment and surgical resection of liver metastasis only in cases of marker-negative relapse.

## UROTHELIAL CANCER

Urothelial carcinoma accounts for 90% of bladder cancers in North America. About 5–15% of patients have metastatic or unresectable disease at presentation.[201,202] The main treatment for advanced disease is chemotherapy with reported initial response rates of about 50%.[201,202] Approximately 20% of patients will have liver metastases with liver-only metastases in about 9%.[203] Data for metastasectomy in the management of disseminated urothelial cancer are sparse, and no studies specifically address the role of hepatectomy. Of those patients treated for primary urothelial cancer, 30% will recur, of which 75% will have distant spread. A 5-year survival of 28% has been reported following resection of lung, brain, adrenal, small bowel or lymph node metastases with variation in the use of adjuvant chemotherapy.[204] The experience with liver resection for metastatic bladder cancer is extremely limited. The conditions under which this operation might be considered are rare and include liver-only disease, minimal disease burden, ideally solitary lesion, good performance status and objective response to systemic chemotherapy. The decision to perform a liver resection for metastatic bladder cancer should include input from experts in urological oncology.

## LUNG CANCER

About 35% of the patients with small cell lung cancer will have liver metastases.[205] The management of metastatic lung cancer is largely restricted to radiation and chemotherapy. Although the surgical management of hepatic metastases remains controversial, most cases have been reviewed within the broader context of non-colorectal, non-neuroendocrine GI tumours. Hepatic metastases appear most commonly in right-sided non-small cell lung tumours with concomitant bone metastases. A small case series of highly selected patients with one or two liver lesions has shown that surgery may confer a marginal survival benefit.[206] Nevertheless, the role of surgery as well as other treatment modalities (RFA, TAE/TACE) cannot be definitively made with current evidence. Recent advances in targeted therapy and immunotherapy may guide decision-making in the future in this context.[207]

## ADRENOCORTICAL TUMOURS

Adrenocortical tumours with liver metastases are rare, and literature on the management of this disease scenario is mostly anecdotal. Case reports have provided no clear guidance regarding the role of surgical or ablative strategies, but disease control after resection of hepatic metastases has been reported.[208] Baur et al.[209] reported median survival of 76 months in patients following resection versus 10 months in patients who did not undergo resection. However, DFS after liver resection was only 9 months. Of note, patients with a time interval to the first metastasis/recurrence of greater than 12 months or solitary liver metastases showed significantly prolonged survival. Metachronous liver metastases with a disease-free interval > 1 year from primary to metastasis may derive benefit from metastectomy.[210]

## ENDOMETRIAL CANCER

Uterine cancer is the most common gynaecologic cancer in the United States with most patients diagnosed in an early stage of the disease. Only 10–15% of cases have advanced disease at the time of diagnosis. Metastatic endometrial cancer is usually multifocal and rarely managed operatively. However, complete cytoreduction of visible disease is associated with improved OS as well as PFS.[211–213] A single-centre report described the results of five patients who developed metastatic disease to the liver ranging from 11 months to 10 years after primary resection. All patients underwent hepatic surgery, with DFS of 8–66 months. Based on these results, the authors advocate referral to a hepatobiliary specialist with the intent of pursuing surgery.[214] A meta-analysis performed by Barlin et al.[215] reviewed the role of cytoreductive surgery in advanced or recurrent endometrial cancer and reported that complete cytoreduction and adjuvant radiation were both positively associated with survival, whereas adjuvant chemotherapy was associated with decreased survival. Furthermore, they showed that with each 10% increase in the proportion of patients undergoing complete cytoreduction, survival improved by 9.3 months. Other isolated reports of long-term survivors exist within the context of larger studies focused on NCRNNET hepatic metastases.

## CONCLUSION

The success of an aggressive surgical approach in the management of CRLM has, in part, provided the impetus for liver resection for non-CRLM. As experience with liver resection has increased, with an improved safety profile, enthusiasm for performing metastasectomy for non-colorectal primaries has also increased. Extrapolating surgical strategies from one malignancy to another is reasonable in some cases; however, fundamental biological differences between various neoplasms require thoughtful consideration of differences in the natural history and non-surgical treatment modalities that are available for each tumour site. Unfortunately, strong evidence-based data are lacking and it is therefore necessary for the treating surgeon to have a good working knowledge of the biology and management of various malignancies. In most cases, this is augmented by the multidisciplinary tumour board and a critical mass of subspecialists to assist in decision-making. Multidisciplinary review with experts in both hepatectomy and management of the primary tumour type should therefore be considered mandatory before performing liver resection for non-CRLM.

It is worth emphasising that, in most cases, liver metastasectomy should be performed with curative intent. The case for resection of breast cancer metastases is evolving, with some liver surgeons advocating resection in a selected patient population responsive to preoperative chemotherapy. There is no strong evidence that non-curative intent surgery is helpful for patients with liver metastases from GI tract primaries, with the possible exception of gastric cancer as discussed above.

The presence of extrahepatic disease is almost always a contraindication to liver resection, except within the context of a prospective trial or for specific malignancies such as ovarian cancer and NETs. The critical variables that usually predict cure after liver resection of secondary cancer of almost all types include prolonged disease-free interval from resection of the primary tumour, negative resection margins, additional complementary systemic treatment options and performance status.

Future efforts should be directed towards the conduct of randomised trials designed to test the role of liver surgery for the common non-colorectal malignancies, and the discovery of genetic signatures and other biomarkers.

> ## Key points
>
> - The majority of patients with non-CRLM have disseminated disease and are not candidates for hepatectomy.
> - Treatment decisions must take into account clinical surrogates of tumour biology. Patients with synchronous liver metastases, a short disease-free interval and extrahepatic disease are believed to have more aggressive tumours and are less likely to gain significant survival benefit from liver resection.
> - With few exceptions, liver resection for metastatic disease should be performed with curative intent. The ability to achieve negative resection margins is a significant prognostic factor.
> - Debulking surgery including liver resection has been shown to significantly improve survival in metastatic NETs. Aggressive cytoreduction, often using a multimodality approach, is indicated in most cases of metastatic NETs.
> - Cytoreduction including hepatectomy, followed by intraperitoneal chemotherapy, appears to improve survival in stage III/IV ovarian adenocarcinoma.
> - Patients with breast cancer liver metastases that respond to preoperative chemotherapy appear to gain a survival benefit from hepatectomy.
> - Level I and II evidence regarding hepatectomy for the treatment of non-CRLM is lacking, and the indications for surgery are evolving.
> - It behoves the surgical oncologist to keep abreast of the explosion of recent advances in systemic and biologic therapies, such as immunotherapy, to ensure proper selection of patients who will benefit from liver resection for non-traditional indications.

 References available at http://ebooks.health.elsevier.com/

# 9 Portal hypertension and liver transplantation

Chris J.C. Johnston | Gabriel C. Oniscu

## INTRODUCTION

Surgical management of portal hypertension with portosystemic vascular shunts has essentially been rendered obsolete by the success of less invasive endoscopic and radiological treatments. However, for patients who are suitable candidates, liver transplantation has become the treatment of choice with the unparalleled advantage of curing the underlying liver disease.

Acute variceal bleeding can also present to surgical teams either directly as an undifferentiated gastrointestinal haemorrhage or via referral from gastroenterology following failure of attempted endoscopic control. Therefore, all surgeons should have an understanding of portal hypertension pathophysiology and the management options for various presentations and complications. Pharmacotherapy, endoscopic band ligation (EBL) and radiological treatment with transjugular intrahepatic portosystemic shunts (TIPSS) are the most common treatment modalities for variceal bleeding. Liver transplantation is the definitive treatment for portal hypertension but is restricted to patients with chronic liver disease who fulfil specific criteria that reflect the severity of underlying liver pathology rather than the extent of portal hypertension itself.

This chapter provides an overview of the pathophysiology and management of portal hypertension and its complications with a specific focus on liver transplantation with the aim of bringing the non-specialist up-to-date with current practice and the evidence base.

## AETIOLOGY

Portal hypertension arises from a pathological increase in vascular resistance to blood flow within the portal system that leads to a sustained increase in portal blood pressure (normal pressure range 5–10 mmHg). The aetiology of portal hypertension is traditionally subdivided according to the anatomical location within the portal system where the resistance occurs: prehepatic (extrahepatic portal vein), intrahepatic (within the liver) or posthepatic (at the level of the hepatic venous outflow). This is undoubtedly an over-simplification of the pathophysiology (in that many liver conditions are associated with high portal pressure at more than one level); however it remains the most relevant from a surgical perspective and for consideration of treatment options.

Prehepatic causes of portal hypertension include thrombosis of the portal, mesenteric and splenic veins or extrinsic compression of the portal vein itself (e.g. by tumour or lymph nodes). Posthepatic causes of portal hypertension are rare and include thrombosis of the hepatic veins (Budd–Chiari syndrome) or inferior vena cava (IVC), as well as cardiac causes such as right heart failure and constrictive pericarditis.[1] Intrahepatic causes of portal hypertension are by far the most common. In the Western world, liver cirrhosis resulting in sinusoidal obstruction and increased vascular resistance is responsible for 90% of portal hypertension cases. Viral hepatitis and alcoholic liver disease (ALD) are the principal causes of liver cirrhosis, but other common causes include haemochromatosis, primary biliary cirrhosis (PBC) and primary sclerosing cholangitis (PSC).[2]

✔✔ The 2018 European Association for the Study of the Liver (EASL) Clinical Practice Guidelines for the management of patients with decompensated cirrhosis[2] provides comprehensive evidence-based guidance on the clinical management of complications of cirrhosis (including ascites, infection, bleeding and associated clinical syndromes).

## DEFINITION OF PORTAL HYPERTENSION

Portal hypertension is defined as a sustained increase in the pressure gradient between the portal and systemic venous circulation.[3] This difference can be measured as the 'hepatic venous pressure gradient' (HVPG), with a normal range of up to 5 mmHg in healthy adults. HVPG above 6 mmHg is pathological, and clinically significant complications begin to manifest when the pressure gradient rises above 10 mmHg. The incidence of complications from portal hypertension (e.g. ascites, variceal haemorrhage, encephalopathy), and indeed mortality, steadily increases as the portal pressure rises. Whilst HVPG is the gold standard measure for the assessment of portal hypertension, it is seldom used in clinical practice due to the need for invasive central venous catheters and inherent inter-operator variability. As a surrogate measure, non-invasive techniques such as hepatic ultrasound elastography (measuring liver stiffness) have consistently demonstrated a good correlation with cirrhosis and portal hypertension.[4]

✔✔ Transient elastography is a non-invasive technique with impressive accuracy for diagnosis of hepatic fibrosis (sensitivity of 91% and specificity of 75% with reference to liver biopsy[5]), and the severity of fibrosis detected correlates well with portal pressure.[4]

Cirrhosis can exist in a clinically silent, 'compensated' state for many years with an associated gradual increase in portal pressure. The development of clinical manifestations of acute decompensation occurs at a rate of up to 7% of patients per year and has a dramatic impact on overall median survival, from 12 years with compensated cirrhosis down to a median of 2 years.[6]

As the portal pressure rises, shunting of blood through portosystemic venous collaterals returns up to 90% of portal blood flow back to the heart.[7] Potentially troublesome collaterals develop at various watershed areas between the portal venous and systemic venous circulation. These areas include the oesophagus and cardia (between intrinsic and extrinsic gastro-oesophageal veins); the falciform ligament (through recanalised paraumbilical veins); and the anal canal (where the superior haemorrhoidal vein belonging to the portal system anastomoses with the middle and inferior haemorrhoidal veins which belong to the caval system).[1]

Of relevance to the surgeon, bleeding from gastro-oesophageal varices can be torrential and constitutes the leading cause of death in patients with cirrhosis. Periumbilical collaterals of enlarged veins in the falciform ligament ('caput medusae') may bleed during abdominal surgery. Stomal and parastomal varices can develop secondary to venous communications between the surgically relocated mesenteric veins of the bowel and the cutaneous veins that drain into the inferior epigastric veins. Finally, anorectal varices can be identified during the course of lower gastrointestinal investigations and although they rarely cause bleeding, can be life-threatening in severe cases.[8] At the time of diagnosis, varices are detected in 30% of patients with compensated cirrhosis, rising to 60% of patients presenting with decompensation and are associated with a corresponding risk of bleeding of 10–30% within 12 months.[9] Without treatment, up to 90% of patients with cirrhosis go on to develop varices and endoscopic surveillance from the time of diagnosis is therefore mandated by current guidelines.[2].

✔✔ Upon diagnosis of cirrhosis, endoscopic surveillance for gastro-oesophageal varices is recommended as a mandatory component of clinical care (EASL Clinical Practice Guidelines for the management of patients with decompensated cirrhosis, 2018).[2]

## PHARMACOLOGICAL THERAPY

The pathophysiology of portal hypertension is multifactorial: intrahepatic fibrosis leads to an increase in vascular resistance whilst metabolic changes lead to a hyperdynamic circulation with an increase in splanchnic blood flow in particular. Non-selective beta-blockers (NSBBs, e.g. propranolol) reduce the portal pressure via vasoconstriction of the splanchnic blood supply.

✔✔ NSBBs are generally well tolerated in patients with established cirrhosis, and several clinical trials have demonstrated a clear survival advantage.[10]

However, the systemic arterial blood pressure is also lowered and caution is therefore required in patients with cardiac failure or large volume ascites for whom development or exacerbation of hepato-renal syndrome can be a life-threatening adverse effect. Expert opinion is divided on the overall benefit of NSBBs in advanced cirrhosis with refractory ascites: there are some reports of poor survival rates,[11] whilst recent retrospective analyses demonstrate a higher mortality in patients who discontinued NSBBs.[12] This observation has been attributed to possible non-haemodynamic effects of NSBBs including a reduction in intestinal permeability and bacterial translocation.[13]

✔✔ The sixth international consensus meeting for stratifying risk and individualising care for portal hypertension in Baveno, Italy, recommended close monitoring in patients with refractory ascites and dose reduction or discontinuation of NSBBs only for those patients who develop hypotension (SBP < 90 mmHg), hyponatraemia or impaired renal function.[14]

For those patients who develop hypotension (SBP < 90 mmHg), hyponatraemia or impaired renal function, substitution of NSBBs with EBL of varices or TIPSS (discussed further below) is recommended for primary and secondary prevention of variceal bleeding, respectively.[14]

A further challenge with pharmacological therapy is variability in response to treatment: mortality is considerably reduced when a 20% reduction in portal pressure is achieved, but unfortunately up to 50% of patients do not respond to NSBB therapy.[10] Carvedilol is an NSBB that also acts as an alpha-1 receptor blocker, thereby vasodilating the intrahepatic vasculature and reducing the portal pressure further.[15,16] This additional mechanism is haemodynamically significant: one small randomised controlled trial (RCT) demonstrated an effective therapeutic reduction in portal pressure (HVPG) in 64% patients treated with carvedilol versus only 14% receiving standard therapy with propranolol.[17] Despite this, a recent Cochrane review of 10 RCTs failed to demonstrate a significant reduction in mortality or serious complications of cirrhosis with the use of carvedilol over traditional NSBBs, advising that further RCTs with longer-term follow-up are required to conclusively assess clinical outcomes.[16]

In the context of acute variceal haemorrhage, vasopressin analogues can be used to achieve a rapid reduction in splanchnic blood flow (and thereby portal pressure) without the hazard of reducing the cardiac output associated with beta-blockade.[18] Vasopressin does however carry a significant adverse-effect profile including hypertension and arrhythmia, such that it requires invasive monitoring and a continuous infusion. Terlipressin is a synthetic analogue of vasopressin with a more specific mechanism of action (V1 receptor) that allows it to be administered in bolus doses.

✔✔ A Cochrane review of seven studies comparing terlipressin with placebo (443 patients) demonstrated a 34% relative risk reduction in mortality and recommended terlipressin as the vasoactive drug of choice in acute variceal bleeding.[19]

EBL of varices is effective for controlling haemorrhage in the acute setting and electively for the eradication of varices as either primary or secondary prevention (i.e. after a variceal bleed). However, endoscopic banding only treats

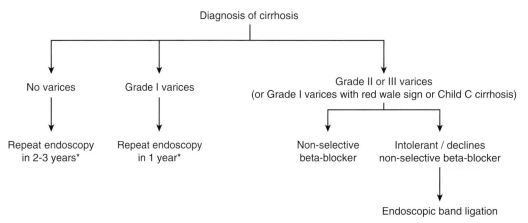

**Figure 9.1**    Algorithm for primary prevention of variceal bleeding. *Interval should be adjusted by the treating clinician if there is clear evidence of progression; endoscopy should also be offered at the time of decompensation. (Source: EASL Clinical Practice Guideline, 2018.)

the variceal manifestation of portal hypertension at a single site, without altering the underlying pathophysiology or portal pressure. EBL also requires endoscopic follow-up and presents a small risk of potentially life-threatening complications. It is therefore unsurprising that combination therapy with beta-blockers is associated with lower overall mortality than endoscopic banding alone, and treatment with NSBBs is generally preferred for primary prevention of variceal haemorrhage in the absence of individual patient contraindications.[2] A summary algorithm for the recommended approach for primary prevention of variceal bleeding in patients with cirrhosis is shown in Fig. 9.1.

It is becoming increasing clear that an underlying systemic inflammatory process (likely arising from abnormal bacterial translocation from the gut) may underpin the cardinal haemodynamic changes seen in cirrhosis.[20] Indeed, recent evidence suggests that statins may have an important additional role to play in lowering intrahepatic vascular resistance, contributing to a reduction in decompensation events and overall mortality.[21] As cirrhosis progresses and portal venous flow decreases, the risk of portal vein thrombosis steadily increases. This results in a sudden spike in portal pressure and decline in liver function as well as considerably adding to the operative risks of liver transplantation. Indeed, there is some evidence to suggest that anticoagulation in early cirrhosis is a safe and effective strategy for improving overall survival by reducing both the risk of portal vein thrombosis and the occurrence of episodes of decompensation overall.[22]

Development of ascites is often the first manifestation of decompensation (and accounts for approximately 80% of all causes of ascites in the Western world). An effective reduction of the circulating systemic blood volume secondary to splanchnic vasodilatation plays a key role in this process. Other features of portal hypertension are almost universally present at this stage of the disease process, but diagnostic paracentesis should always be performed at the time of first presentation to confirm the diagnosis and exclude spontaneous bacterial peritonitis.[2] The development of ascites marks a dramatic change in prognosis, with an overall predicted 1-year survival of 40%; in the absence of contraindications, referral for liver transplantation should be considered at this stage.[2]

## TRANSJUGULAR INTRAHEPATIC PORTOSYSTEMIC SHUNT

TIPSS (Fig. 9.2) is a procedure undertaken by interventional radiology whereby a stent is placed via the jugular vein, through a hepatic vein and into an intrahepatic portal vein branch, allowing the portal circulation to decompress directly into the systemic venous return to the heart. The effectiveness and comparatively low complication rate of this procedure has essentially rendered the (elegant but hazardous) repertoire of surgical portosystemic venous shunts for treating portal hypertension obsolete.

TIPSS can be employed in the elective setting for treating complications of portal hypertension including refractory ascites, hepatic hydrothorax and portal hypertensive gastropathy (PHG) after failure of medical therapy. It is also a very effective rescue therapy for treating active variceal bleeding when effective haemostasis cannot be achieved endoscopically (successful in 95% of cases with a re-bleeding rate of 18%).[23] Up to 90% of the portal blood flow can be diverted to the systemic circulation with TIPSS. This augments the venous return to the heart and can provide a substantial benefit to patients with perilous haemodynamic instability and renal function, such as those requiring recurrent large-volume paracentesis (LVP) for refractory ascites. However, shunting portal venous blood directly into the systemic circulation without any hepatic metabolism also underpins the foremost complication of TIPSS—the onset or exacerbation of encephalopathy (risk factors include age > 65 years, Child–Pugh score > 12 and previous history of encephalopathy). The incidence of post-TIPSS encephalopathy has been reported as high as 50%, but this rate has reduced considerably after the introduction of PTFE-covered metal stents and stents that can be dilated to variable diameters as required (e.g. 8–10 mm depending on indication and pressure gradient).[24] Additional procedural complications of TIPSS include intraperitoneal bleeding, biliary puncture, hepatic ischaemia and exacerbation of heart failure.

With regard to overall (transplant-free) survival, multiple meta-analyses of the six RCTs that compared TIPSS with recurrent LVP have provided conflicting results with no overall consensus.[2] However, the rate of complications from the covered stents in current standard clinical practice

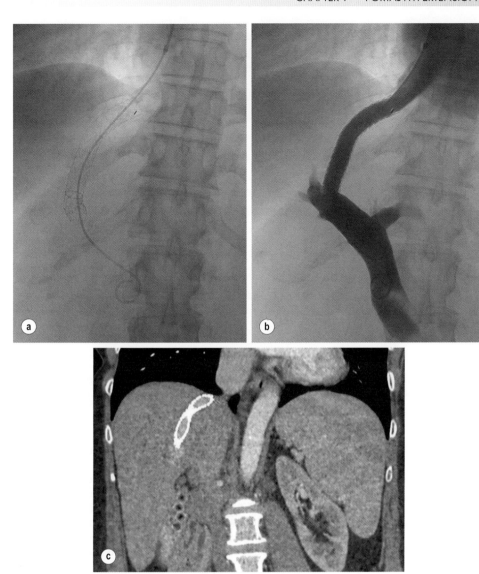

**Figure 9.2** Transjugular portosystemic shunt (TIPSS/TIPS). **(a)** Stent placement from hepatic vein, through liver parenchyma to portal vein. **(b)** Venogram confirming stent patency and diversion of portal venous blood flow. **(c)** Post-procedural CT scan.

**Table 9.1    Child–Pugh classification**

| Clinical/lab value | Points assigned | | |
|---|---|---|---|
| | **1** | **2** | **3** |
| Bilirubin (mmol/L) | < 34 | 34–50 | > 50 |
| Albumin (g/L) | > 35 | 28–35 | < 28 |
| Prothrombin time (seconds prolonged) | < 4 | 4–6 | > 6 |
| Encephalopathy | None | Mild | Marked |
| Ascites | None | Mild | Marked |

is dramatically lower (including the rate of stent thrombosis, leading to longer patency rates). Encouragingly, a recent RCT comparing covered stent TIPSS with LVP for recurrent ascites reported improved 1-year survival with TIPSS and no evidence of an increase in the rate of encephalopathy.[25] However, favourable outcomes remain confined to carefully selected patient groups.

The presence of varices increases progressively with the severity of cirrhosis (e.g. as classified by the Child–Pugh Classification, Table 9.1) from 42% of patients with Child's A cirrhosis, up to 72% of patients with Child's B or C cirrhosis.[26]

Untreated, variceal bleeding is the second most common manifestation of decompensation (after ascites) and presents an immediate threat to life with an overall mortality rate of up to 25% at 6 weeks.

## TREATMENT OF ACUTE VARICEAL HAEMORRHAGE

Balloon tamponade can be an effective temporising measure for uncontrolled massive haemorrhage from oesophago-gastric varices, until definitive treatment (either TIPSS or surgery) is available. A recent series reported effective haemostasis with oral-gastric tube placement in 79% of patients.[27] The Sengstaken–Blakemore tube (three-lumen tube) is the most commonly encountered oral-gastric tubes in clinical practice. Intubation and airway protection should be considered early in the management of any massive gastrointestinal haemorrhage but it is mandatory prior to oral-gastric tube insertion. Blind insertion of the tube is challenging (even with the assistance of a laryngoscope) and carries an inherent risk of fatal oesophageal rupture if the tube coils in the oesophagus prior to inflation of the gastric balloon. This can be largely prevented by railroading the tube over an endoscopically placed

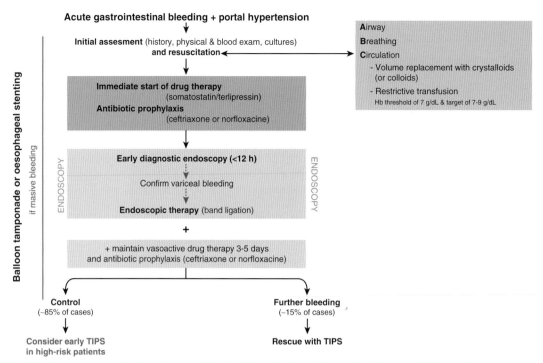

**Figure 9.3** Algorithm for management of acute gastrointestinal bleeding in patients with cirrhosis. *TIPS,* transjugular portosystemic shunt. (Source: Adapted from R. De Franchis, Baveno VI faculty Expanding consensus in portal hypertension: report of the BAVENO VI. Consensus Workshop: Stratifying risk and individualizing care for portal hypertension J Hepatol, 63 (2015), pp. 743-752.)

stiff guidewire (e.g. Amplatz®), although time and available resources do not always permit this approach.

The gastric balloon is inflated in the stomach (e.g. with 30 mL of water) and placed on gentle traction against the gastro-oesophageal junction. Even for oesophageal varices, inflation of gastric balloon alone achieves haemostasis in the majority of cases; inflation of the oesophageal balloon should be delayed and only undertaken if bleeding persists as there is an increased risk of necrosis at the gastro-oesophageal junction. The oesophageal balloon must be deflated every 12 hours to prevent necrosis, and for similar reasons the gastric balloon should not be inflated for more than 48 hours. Upon deflation of the balloons, re-bleeding occurs in 50% of patients with oesophago-gastric varices and re-bleeding is the rule for gastric varices unless more definitive control of bleeding is established.[28] Placement of an oro-gastric balloon is a high-risk intervention that requires appropriate expertise and timely availability of definitive treatment options. When endoscopy is immediately available, placement of (removable) covered self-expanding metal oesophageal stent appears to be an attractive novel alternative, with a recent RCT reporting superior haemostasis (85% vs 47%) with fewer serious adverse events (15% vs 47%).[29] A systematic approach to the management of acute variceal bleeding is summarised in Fig. 9.3.

## PORTAL HYPERTENSIVE GASTROPATHY

PHG is an abnormality of the gastric mucosa characterised endoscopically by a mosaic-like pattern resembling 'snake skin', with or without red spots. The overall prevalence of PHG in cirrhosis is roughly 80% and it is strongly correlated with the severity of cirrhosis.[30] The same pathology can arise in other

areas of the GI tract, albeit less commonly (portal hypertensive colopathy or intestinopathy). Clinically, the primary relevance of PHG is as a source of persistent occult bleeding leading to iron-deficiency anaemia; significant acute haemorrhage is rare. No effective endoscopic therapeutic options exist, so treatment revolves around lowering the portal pressure in the same way as for variceal bleeding (pharmacologically or with TIPSS), with consideration of liver transplantation if appropriate.

## SEGMENTAL PORTAL HYPERTENSION

Segmental portal hypertension resulting from splenic vein thrombosis should always be considered as the potential cause of bleeding gastric varices in patients with pancreatic pathology. Gastric varices have a variable appearance and are often covered with normal mucosa; caution (and/or endoscopic ultrasound assessment) is required before undertaking biopsy of any lesion of the gastric fundus or cardia, particularly in a patient with a history of pancreatic pathology. Patients with chronic pancreatitis who develop variceal bleeding as a result of thrombosis of the splenic vein should be considered for splenectomy (or splenic vein embolisation), which is often curative.[28]

## PORTAL VEIN THROMBOSIS

The aetiology of portal vein thrombosis can be categorised according to Virchow's triad: factors affecting the blood flow (including cirrhosis and extrinsic venous compression), hypercoagulable states (e.g. cancer, surgery, intra-abdominal infection, myeloproliferative conditions) and factors affecting endothelial integrity (e.g. surgery, adjacent invading tumour).

Often it is a combination of these factors that leads to thrombosis. The incidence of portal vein thrombosis is estimated to be 0.7 per 100 000 per year and, in the absence of underlying malignancy and cirrhosis, survival at 1 year and 5 years is 92% and 76%, respectively.[31] Portal vein thrombosis can present with an acute or chronic history, with the latter more likely to result in variceal bleeding due to portal hypertension.[32]

Treatment of portal vein thrombosis depends on the overall clinical picture and takes into consideration the presence of symptoms, the degree of reversibility of the precipitating causes, the presence of malignancy and/or cirrhosis. Medical management may involve observation with no active therapy (particularly if the patient is asymptomatic and has an obvious reversible precipitating cause such as abdominal infection or pancreatitis) or anticoagulation (with a low threshold in potential transplant candidates and when thrombosis extends into mesenteric veins or progresses on imaging without treatment). Conventional anticoagulant drugs such as low-molecular-weight heparin and warfarin may be used in cirrhotic patients with portal vein thrombosis, particularly in those eligible for liver transplantation as this may mitigate propagation of the clot, thus facilitating or even permitting transplantation. The presence of portal vein thrombosis is not an absolute contraindication to liver transplantation, but this may not be technically feasible if the thrombus extends into the entire portomesenteric system.[33]

Thrombectomy or thrombolysis may be considered if there is progressive abdominal pain suggestive of an emergency presentation with mesenteric ischaemia. Endovascular options in the setting of acute portal vein thrombosis include mechanical recanalisation, local targeted thrombolysis or a combination of these treatments. Acute portal vein thrombosis can also be treated by TIPSS combined with a combination of techniques for thrombolysis (e.g. clot disruption by balloon, suction embolectomy, basket extraction of clot and mechanical thrombectomy), but these carry the risk of vascular trauma.[32]

## LIVER TRANSPLANTATION

### BACKGROUND

The first successful liver transplant was undertaken by Dr Thomas Starzl in Denver, Colorado, in 1967.[34] Clinical outcomes for the first cohort of patients were universally dire, to the extent that Starzl self-imposed a moratorium on the liver transplant programme until further research yielded potential solutions to the then insurmountable problem of organ rejection resulting in inevitable graft loss. Roy Calne's introduction of ciclosporin in 1979 revolutionised the treatment of organ rejection, allowing liver transplantation to enter clinical practice with rapid expansion throughout the US and Europe in the 1980s.[35] Liver transplantation is now the treatment of choice for liver failure and related conditions; over 900 transplants are routinely performed in the UK annually, with an overall 1-year survival of 94%.[36] The current UK-wide median waiting time for an elective deceased donor adult liver transplant is 65 days.[37] One year after listing for transplantation (in 2017-18), 75% of patients underwent transplantation, 12% were still waiting, 9% died on the waiting list or were removed due to clinical deterioration that precluded safe transplantation and 4% were removed for other reasons (such as improvement in liver function).[37]

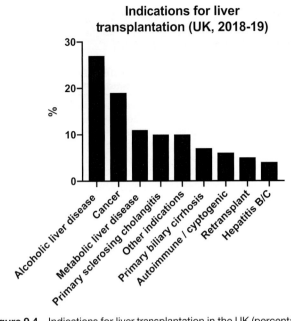

**Figure 9.4** Indications for liver transplantation in the UK (percentage of 996 nationwide adult transplants). (Based on data available from https://nhsbtdbe.blob.core.windows.net/umbraco-assets-corp/16782/nhsbt-liver-transplantation-annual-report-2018-19.pdf.)

## INDICATIONS FOR LIVER TRANSPLANTATION

End-stage liver failure secondary to chronic liver disease is the indication for liver transplantation in the majority (90%) of cases in the UK. The underlying aetiology of liver failure varies (e.g. ALD, viral hepatitis, autoimmune conditions as outlined in Fig. 9.4) and suitability for listing for transplantation is based on prognosis according to the degree of liver dysfunction. In the UK, this is assessed using the UK Model for End-Stage Liver Disease (UKELD) score which is a composite scoring system predicting prognosis taking into account international normalised ratio (INR), serum creatinine, serum bilirubin and serum sodium (discussed further in *organ allocation*, below). A UKELD score of 49, corresponds to a predicted survival without transplantation of less than 1 year and this is currently the minimum threshold for inclusion on the elective liver transplant waiting list as it indicates a survival advantage with liver transplantation over medical management. Aside from chronic liver failure, additional indications for consideration of liver transplantation include cancer, mainly hepatocellular carcinoma (HCC) and a small number of conditions that warrant transplantation on the basis of an unacceptable quality of life (such as intractable pruritis with PBC); these conditions are listed as 'variant syndromes' (Table 9.2) to facilitate donor liver allocation within the current system that determines priority largely according to liver function.

## ALCOHOLIC LIVER DISEASE

Cirrhosis secondary to ALD is consistently one of the commonest indications for liver transplantation in Europe. Outcomes in this group are excellent overall, comparable to patients with cirrhosis from other aetiologies, but individually contingent on avoidance of a return to alcohol.[38] A period of strict abstinence from alcohol is generally considered an essential requirement before listing for liver

**Table 9.2** 'Variant syndromes'—accepted non-liver failure indications for liver transplantation (in addition to hepatocellular carcinoma, UK)

| Accepted variant syndromes (non-liver failure) suitable for liver transplantation (UK) | |
| --- | --- |
| Hepatopulmonary syndrome | Hereditary haemorrhagic telangiectasia |
| Persistent and intractable pruritis | Ornithine transcarbamylase deficiency |
| Polycystic liver disease | Glycogen storage disease (symptomatic) |
| Familial hyperlipidaemia | Primary hyperoxaluria with renal impairment |
| Recurrent cholangitis | Porphyria |
| Hepatic epithelioid haemangioendothelioma | Maple syrup urine disease |
| Nodular regenerative hyperplasia | Portopulmonary hypertension |

transplantation. The minimum required duration of abstinence is usually 6 months. Liver function often improves during the first 3 months of abstinence, to the extent that many patients in this group may no longer require transplantation. Some studies have suggested that longer periods of abstinence correlate with lower rates of recidivism, but this has been strongly contested, with other factors such as patterns of drinking behaviour and current support networks having better predictive value.[33] Whilst recidivism after liver transplantation invokes a very negative public reaction that could affect the wider support for organ donation, insistence on long periods of abstinence carries a substantial risk of mortality for patients with end-stage liver disease who could potentially be assessed as presenting a very low risk of returning to alcohol at the time of transplant assessment. The option of early liver transplantation for severe acute alcoholic hepatitis was assessed in a multicentre prospective case control study by Mathurin et al.[39]: 26 patients who were assessed as having a low risk of recidivism were selected for early transplantation and compared with matched patients receiving best medical therapy. The survival advantage of early transplantation at 6 months was considerable (77% vs 23%, $P < 0.001$) and only 3 of the 26 transplanted patients returned to alcohol during 3 years of follow-up, but this was a highly selected group and the conclusions of the study have currently limited widespread support.

## NON-ALCOHOLIC FATTY LIVER DISEASE

Cirrhosis and end-stage liver failure secondary to non-alcoholic fatty liver disease (NAFLD), or more recently named metabolic-associated liver disease (MAFLD), is an increasingly frequent indication for liver transplantation worldwide.[40] Whilst most transplant units have no arbitrary upper limit of body mass index for transplant candidates, it is clear that obesity is associated with poorer outcomes after transplantation with increased risks of several complications (including cardiovascular events, wound infection and prolonged intensive care length of stay). Additionally, without specific intervention, weight gain and deterioration in control of associated diabetes is common after transplantation (secondary to immunosuppression and improved appetite).

Recent evidence suggests that bariatric surgery in the form of sleeve gastrectomy prior to (or at the time of) liver transplantation reduced the rate of post-transplant complications (diabetes, hypertension and recurrent NAFLD) compared with medically assisted weight loss.[41,42] However, the operative risks and limited physiological reserve to cope with complications of weight loss surgery in this group are a significant concern, such that this approach is not currently routine clinical practice.

## PRIMARY BILIARY CIRRHOSIS

PBC is a chronic cholestatic liver disease characterised by destruction of small intrahepatic bile ducts, leading to fibrosis and potentially cirrhosis.[43] PBC has a strong female preponderance (10:1) and is strongly associated with serum antimitochondrial antibody. The introduction of ursodeoxycholic acid (UDCA) has dramatically improved the medical management of PBC, increasing overall transplant-free survival.[44] However, up to 40% of patients do not respond to UDCA and as such, liver transplantation continues to play an important role in the management of this condition, both for end-stage liver failure secondary to cirrhosis and in the context of an intolerable quality of life (usually severe pruritis intractable to medical treatment). Unfortunately PBC can recur in up to 47% of patients after liver transplantation, requiring re-transplantation in a minority.[43]

## PRIMARY SCLEROSING CHOLANGITIS

PSC is another immune-mediated cholestatic disease characterised by inflammation, fibrosis and destruction of the bile ducts. In contrast to PBC, PSC affects larger ducts including the extra-hepatic biliary tree and no medical therapy (including UDCA, steroids or immunosuppression) has been shown to alter progression of the disease process.[45] PSC has a strong association with other immune-mediated conditions (particularly inflammatory bowel disease) but, unusually, affects male patients more than females with a ratio of 2:1. Whilst acute biliary obstruction secondary to 'dominant' focal biliary strictures may be amenable to treatment with endoscopic dilatation or stenting, typically the disease progresses towards cirrhosis and transplantation remains the only treatment that alters the underlying course of the disease. Development of cholangiocarcinoma is a particular risk with PSC (accounting for up to 58% of all patient deaths[46]), and accurate detection of cholangiocarcinoma before transplantation can be challenging, even with advanced endoscopic techniques such as SpyGlass® cholangioscopy, which has a reported sensitivity of around 60%.[47] Whilst overall outcomes of liver transplantation for PSC are excellent (comparable with other indications), PSC can recur after transplantation in up to 40% of patients.[48]

## HEPATOCELLULAR CARCINOMA

HCC represents 90% of all primary liver cancers; incidence increases with age (peak 70 years) and there is a strong male preponderance (2.5:1).[49] HCC is a major indication for liver transplantation worldwide (20% of the patients listed in the UK have HCC). The incidence of HCC varies widely geographically: the incidence of HCC has steadily increased in the US, and most of Europe over the last 10 years, but East Asia and Sub-Saharan Africa still account for more than 85% of cases worldwide.[49] Liver injury from viral hepatitis (primarily HBV or HCV) or established cirrhosis are major risk factors for the development of HCC. Cirrhosis has been shown to present an annual risk of developing HCC of 1–8%, amounting to a collective lifetime risk of 33%, with underlying HBV or HCV representing the highest risk groups.[50] Immunisation and, more recently, effective HCV antiviral therapy are effective strategies for the prevention of HCC,[51] although there is a 9- to 12-month time lag between virus eradication and the reduction of HCC risk. Ultrasound surveillance of patients at high risk of developing HCC that are amenable to treatment (i.e. Child's A or B cirrhosis, or Child's C cirrhosis awaiting liver transplantation) has proven beneficial and should be undertaken every 6 months.[52]

✔✔ The pathophysiology, diagnosis and multidisciplinary treatment options for HCC are discussed in further detail in Chapter 6, *Primary malignant tumours of the liver.*

Potentially curative treatment options for HCC confined to the liver include liver resection, radiofrequency ablation (RFA) and liver transplantation. Surgical resection is feasible in a fit patient with an otherwise healthy liver—up to 75% of the liver can be safely resected with an expected 5-year survival over 50%. However, in the UK setting, more than 80% of HCCs arise within the context of established cirrhosis. This presents two major problems for liver resection: first, the regenerative capacity of the liver is compromised, resulting in a higher risk of postoperative liver failure; second, there is a significant risk of recurrence from *de novo* tumour formation in the background cirrhotic liver. Established portal hypertension is considered a contraindication to resection. RFA involves placing a probe into the centre of a tumour (percutaneously or laparoscopically) and heating it to induce necrosis. RFA is a potentially curative treatment option for small tumours (< 4 cm) with a favourable location (i.e. not situated adjacent to major vessels or bile ducts), but

local recurrence rates are higher compared with surgical resection.[53] Therefore, RFA is generally restricted to patients who are not suitable for resection (in terms of fitness, liver function or anatomy) or those with very small tumours (< 2 cm) in anatomically favourable locations.

Transarterial chemoembolisation (TACE) encompasses catheter-directed instillation of chemotherapeutic agents (e.g. doxorubicin drug-eluting beads) directly into a tumour. TACE exploits the distinctive blood supply of HCC tumours, which arises from the hepatic arterial system alone (in contrast to the surrounding liver parenchyma for which 75% of the blood supply arises from the portal vein): catheterisation of arteries supplying the tumour therefore allows effective targeting of tumour cells with little 'collateral damage'. TACE is not curative, but it can significantly prolong patient survival by slowing tumour growth and progression, or as part of a combination therapy, reducing tumour size to facilitate RFA or liver transplantation.[50] Careful patient selection is required in the context of cirrhosis—TACE has the potential to precipitate decompensation (if liver function is precarious) or less commonly infarction (if co-incident portal vein thrombosis has developed).

Liver transplantation for HCC arising in a cirrhotic liver cures the end-stage liver disease and offers the potential for oncological clearance with a comparatively low risk of recurrence. Decision-making as to the most appropriate treatment strategy (e.g. resection, TACE, transplantation) can be guided by the Barcelona Clinic Liver Cancer (BCLC) staging system, the most widely endorsed HCC staging system worldwide that incorporates evidence-based prognostic features of tumour size, liver function and patient fitness (Fig. 9.5).

The Milan criteria are the most widely used criteria to define when liver transplantation should be considered for HCC and include a solitary HCC with a diameter < 5 cm, or up to three nodules each with a diameter < 3 cm and no evidence of extrahepatic spread or vascular invasion.[54] Recently, extended Milan criteria were implemented in the UK, allowing transplantation with up to five lesions < 3 cm, or a solitary 5–7 cm

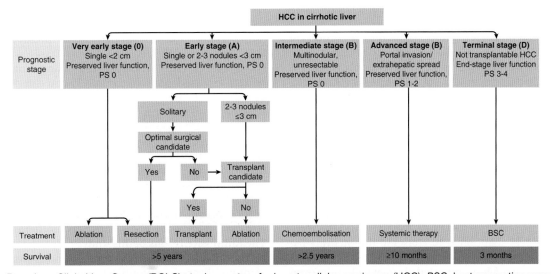

**Figure 9.5** Barcelona Clinic Liver Cancer (BCLC) staging system for hepatocellular carcinoma (HCC). *BSC,* best supportive care; *PS,* performance status (Eastern Co-operative Oncology Group: 0, no restriction on activity; 1, unable to carry out heavy physical work; 2, unable to work, active for more than half of the day; 3, confined to bed or chair for more than half of the day; 4, confined to bed or chair all day). (Reprinted with permission from Elsevier. A. Forner, M. Reig, J. Bruix. Hepatocellular carcinoma. Lancet (2018); Volume 391, Issue 10127: 1301-1314.)

| Duvoux Criteria for liver transplant eligibility (criteria for listing following downstaging treatment) | |
|---|---|
| **Variable** | **Points** |
| **Largest diameter** | |
| ≤3 | 0 |
| 3-6 | 1 |
| >6 | 4 |
| **Number of nodules** | |
| 1-3 | 0 |
| ≤4 | 2 |
| **AFP (ng/ml)** | |
| ≤100 | 0 |
| 100-1000 | 2 |
| >1000 | 3 |

Patients with a score of ≤2 points following treatment are eligible for listing.

Inclusion criteria:
- Interval of ≥6 months from downstaging treatment to imaging considered for listing

Specific exclusion criteria:
- Macrovascular invasion
- Extrahepatic or nodal metastases
- Ruptured HCC

**Figure 9.6** Duvoux criteria for hepatocellular carcinoma (HCC)—eligibility for liver transplantation after downstaging treatment (UK).

lesion downstaged with local therapy, provided there is < 20% growth and no new nodules appear over a 6-month follow-up period. The number of tumours is considered in conjunction with the AFP level, with a level > 1000 ng/mL considered to correlate with recurrence of HCC.[55] A score of ≤ 2 points following downstaging treatment is now used to determine eligibility for liver transplantation in the UK (Fig. 9.6).[55]

## OTHER ONCOLOGICAL INDICATIONS FOR LIVER TRANSPLANTATION

Globally, the number of patients that could potentially benefit from liver transplantation continues to considerably outstrip the supply of potentially suitable donor organs. Establishing equity of access to the life-saving resource of donated livers for patients with varied complex disease processes is challenging and remains imperfect. An arbitrary threshold of greater than 50% survival at 5 years post transplantation (approximated to the prognosis of transplantation for chronic liver disease) has been adopted by many healthcare systems.[56] Whilst this benchmark has been challenged, it does highlight the potential for expanding the list of suitable indications for liver transplantation to include non-HCC cancer as a routine component of a comprehensive oncology care pathway.

**Cholangiocarcinoma** encompasses a diverse group of tumours of the biliary tree that overall account for up to 20% of primary liver malignancies (second only to HCC). Perihilar cholangiocarcinoma (pCC, located between the cystic duct and the second-order intrahepatic bile ducts) continues to present a particularly dismal prognosis: only one-third of patients are suitable for surgical resection at the time of presentation and up to 50% of resection candidates are found to have unresectable disease at the time of surgery. Recurrence rates of up to 57% have been reported even after resections with microscopic oncological clearance (R0 resection).[57] Initial attempts at liver transplantation in this setting were disappointing due to very high rates of cancer recurrence (up to 84% at 2 years)[58] and the technique was largely abandoned to conserve donor livers for other transplant indications with much better prognoses. In 2000, the Mayo Clinic reported dramatically improved survival outcomes after transplantation for unresectable hilar cholangiocarcinoma in a highly selected group of patients who had managed to successfully complete a course of

aggressive neoadjuvant chemoradiotherapy.[59] This practice has been trialled in many centres around the world and a recent meta-analysis of 428 patients from 20 studies reported a 5-year survival after liver transplantation with neoadjuvant therapy for pCC of 65.1% compared with 31.6% after liver transplantation alone.[60] However, no RCT has yet been performed and the quality of study design and outcome reporting of the studies conducted to date is highly variable. In particular, a conclusive diagnosis of pCC (instead of a dominant stricture in PSC, for example) is a challenge, particularly after neoadjuvant systemic treatment, such that outcome data must be interpreted with caution.

**Colorectal cancer** is the third most common malignancy globally. Up to 50% of patients develop metastases, making colorectal liver metastases (CRLM) the most common liver tumour overall.[61] Metastasis to the liver via the portal circulation does not negate the possibility of complete oncological clearance, and the potential for long-term survival after liver resection was first established over 25 years ago.[62] Management of CRLM has advanced considerably since then with a multidisciplinary approach including surveillance and early detection, systemic chemotherapy, genetic tumour sequencing with targeted adjuvant therapy, parenchymal-sparing liver resection and staged liver resection for bilobar metastases. Despite these approaches, some patients remain 'unresectable' due to an inadequate predicted remnant liver volume, or the location of metastases adjacent to vital structures. Early studies of liver transplantation in this setting reported poor outcomes (5-year survival of up to 21%)[63] and the practice was abandoned. Following serial developments in liver transplantation and cancer care, in 2013 Hagness et al.[64] reported on a prospective pilot study of liver transplantation in 21 patients with unresectable CRLM with an overall survival at 5 years of 60%[64]. A follow-up prospective study with more stringent inclusion criteria including a clear response to systemic chemotherapy reported even better long-term outcomes with an overall 5-year survival of 83% (compared with a background expected median 5-year overall survival with palliative chemotherapy of 10%).[65] The impressive results of this study apply to a highly selected group of patients in the context of a more favourable ratio of donor livers to potential transplant recipients in Norway compared with most countries around the world. Two RCTs are in progress at the time of writing (TRANSMET - NCT02597348 and SECA III - NCT03494946) comparing liver transplantation to the current gold standard palliative chemotherapy regimens and could be transformative in extending the indication for liver transplantation to this large group of patients.

## ACUTE LIVER FAILURE

Acute liver failure (ALF) can be defined as the presence of hepatic decompensation (encephalopathy, jaundice, coagulopathy) in a patient without underlying chronic liver disease.[66] In the UK, the most common cause of ALF is paracetamol overdose, followed by non-A-E hepatitis, other drug-induced liver injuries and viral hepatitis. Clinical deterioration in this group of patients can be very rapid; early discussion with a liver transplant centre is advised with the aim of transferring severe cases prior to the onset of encephalopathy whenever possible. Once encephalopathy develops, management in an intensive care setting is required to mitigate against progression to multi-organ failure, cerebral oedema with raised intracranial pressure and the associated very high mortality rate. A number of artificial liver support systems (such as MARS® and Prometheus®) that act as a form of dialysis to remove toxins have been evaluated as a potential 'bridge' to transplantation; however, outcomes have been consistently disappointing and the quality of evidence to support their use in routine clinical practice remains low.[67]

✓✓ Systematic reviews incorporating 12 RCTs have failed to show any reduction in mortality using artificial liver support systems.[66]

Stem cell-derived hepatocyte transplantation has shown some promise in the setting of paediatric metabolic deficiencies,[68] but is some way off routine clinical practice and, as such, emergency liver transplantation remains the gold standard of care.

## ORGAN DONATION AND DONOR SURGERY

✓✓ Organ donation is discussed further in Core Topics in General & Emergency Surgery 7th Ed; Ch 10 Principles in Organ Donation & General Surgery in the Transplant Patient

Deceased donor organ retrieval surgery can be a challenging undertaking, requiring close co-operation between unfamiliar surgical teams working under time pressure, often at night in distant donor hospitals in what can be emotionally demanding circumstances.

In many countries around the world, liver transplantation is undertaken using livers donated from donors after brain death (DBD) and donors after circulatory death (DCD). Whilst the concept and definition of DBD is widely accepted, there remains large variability in the acceptance and practice of DCD. In general, a 5-minute 'stand-off/no-touch' period is required between declaration of death and the start of the retrieval procedure (although it can be as long as 30 minutes in some countries). Donation in this setting inevitably entails a period of organ ischaemia and this can particularly affect the liver, with higher rates of early allograft dysfunction, primary non-function and ischaemic cholangiopathy compared with DBD liver transplants.[69]

Organ retrieval arrangements vary widely, with many centres around the world still opting to send their own teams to retrieve the organs. In the UK, a National Organ Retrieval Service (NORS) provides an integrated abdominal and cardiothoracic retrieval service with 10 abdominal surgical teams and 6 cardiothoracic surgical teams that mobilise to the donor hospitals on a regional basis and organs dispatched to the receiving centre according to the organ-specific allocation policies. In the UK, 1942 potential organ donors were attended by NORS surgical teams in the 2019-20 financial year.[70]

## ORGAN RETRIEVAL PROCEDURE

After confirmation of suitability for donation and consent, DBD organ retrieval commences with a thorough laparotomy and thoracotomy to search for any occult tumours that might preclude donation and to identify any aberrant anatomy. Following brainstem death, spinal reflexes are usually intact, so muscle relaxant is required along with the assistance of an anaesthetic team for maintenance of mechanical ventilation and cardiovascular support, if required.

The 'warm phase' of the surgical procedure generally takes 60–90 minutes. Adhesions to the liver are taken down and the falciform and left triangular ligaments are divided. The liver is assessed for consistency, colour and sharpness of the edges, which can all give an indication about the quality of the graft and the degree of steatosis. The hepatogastric ligament is inspected for the presence of an accessory left hepatic artery whilst the presence of an accessory or replaced right hepatic artery is initially ascertained by palpation for arterial pulsation lateral and posterior to the portal vein. The common bile duct is divided above the duodenum, ligating the distal end. To minimise biliary injury from stagnant bile, the gallbladder is incised and irrigated until clear fluid drains from the cut end of the bile duct. The amount of dissection in the liver hilum depends on surgeon's experience, but in general identification and control of the gastroduodenal artery and splenic artery are sufficient in the warm phase. In co-ordination with the Specialist Nurse in Organ Donation (donor coordinator) and cardiothoracic retrieval team (if present), intravenous heparin is administered, the distal aorta is ligated and then the infra-renal aorta is cannulated in preparation for cold perfusion. Additional liver perfusion via the portal vein is useful particularly in DCD.

In DCD donation, time is critical as the combination of warm and cold ischemia is highly detrimental in particular to the liver function post-transplant. The duration of warm ischaemia generally accepted for liver donation is 30 minutes, but the definition of what constitutes warm ischaemic time is widely variable. 'Functional warm ischaemia time' is most commonly defined as the time between a fall in the donor systolic blood pressure below 50 mmHg and the commencement of *in situ* cold perfusion at organ retrieval, whilst the asystolic time is defined as the time between cessation of circulation and *in situ* cold perfusion. In the setting of DCD donation, there is no 'warm phase' dissection; when death is confirmed (5 minutes after asystole in most countries), the donor is transferred as quickly as possible to theatre and organs are usually retrieved with a 'super-rapid' technique, which involves a rapid thoraco-laparotomy with aortic cannulation and *in situ* cold perfusion.

The 'cold phase' dissection for DBD and DCD organ retrieval is essentially the same. The supraceliac or descending thoracic aorta is cross-clamped, venous drainage is achieved usually by venting the suprahepatic IVC in the chest and cold perfusion is commenced by rapid infusion of 5–6 L of cold organ preservation fluid (such as University of Wisconsin solution®) via a large aortic cannula. The entire abdominal cavity is packed with slush ice to allow rapid *in situ* cooling of the liver, including above the diaphragm in the costo-diaphragmatic angles. In view of the relatively prolonged warm ischaemic time compared with DBD donation, cold preservation fluid is also instilled via portal vein cannulation to enable a more rapid cooling of the liver *in situ*, prior to removal.

The cold phase dissection then proceeds with mobilisation of the colon followed by the small bowel (stapling the small bowel mesentery if the pancreas is retrieved). The renal veins are identified and the infrahepatic IVC is divided above their IVC insertion. In the porta hepatis, the gastroduodenal artery is divided (leaving a stump on the hepatic artery) and this exposes the portal vein, which is then divided approximately 1 cm above the duodenum (if the pancreas is retrieved). The common hepatic artery is followed towards the coeliac axis. The origin of the splenic artery is then divided leaving a 5-mm stump (longer if the pancreas is not being retrieved) to allow for arterial reconstruction if required. The coeliac trunk is taken with a small patch of aorta. The diaphragm is divided around the suprahepatic cava, starting on the left side of the IVC, continuing posteriorly and completing the division by taking a patch of the right hemidiaphragm around the right lobe of the liver. The right lobe is separated from the right adrenal gland and the right kidney, and the retroperitoneal tissue at the back of the IVC and the liver is removed.

Once removed, the liver is placed on ice before further *ex situ* cold perfusion of the portal vein, hepatic artery and bile duct on the back table at the donor centre. The liver should be kept at 4°C throughout the bench procedure by submerging it in cold preservation solution. The absence of arterial pulsation combined with a need for rapid removal of the organs contributes to a greater rate of organ injury during DCD retrieval. Therefore, an alternative approach is to remove the liver and pancreas *en bloc* from DCD donor, followed by *ex situ* separation of the liver and pancreas on ice on the back table to allow more time for careful identification of aberrant arterial anatomy. The liver is then checked for abnormalities or injuries, weighed and carefully packed in ice for transport to the recipient transplant centre.

Preparation for implantation is completed at the recipient centre. The vena cava is dissected free of adherent tissue and the phrenic and adrenal vein stumps are ligated to avoid bleeding on reperfusion. The portal vein is dissected down to its bifurcation. The hepatic artery is then dissected free of surrounding tissue, taking care to preserve an aberrant left hepatic artery arising from the left gastric artery. If an aberrant right hepatic artery is present, this is usually reconstructed by anastomosis onto the gastroduodenal artery stump.

## LIVER ALLOCATION

As patient outcomes continued to improve and liver transplant programmes flourished, the demand for donor livers dramatically increased. This led to the National Organ Transplant Act in the United States (1984), enshrining in law the concept of donor organs as national assets. Regional donor networks were established together with organ allocation algorithms, aiming to achieve the best possible outcomes for the waiting list population, within the limited resources available at any given time.

Several country-specific organ allocation systems have evolved round the world with the common considerations of equity (equal chance of receiving an organ for all patients who need one), need (to reduce mortality on the waiting list to the minimum possible), benefit (maximising post-transplant outcomes) and utility (maximising the overall life-years gained).[56,71] In 2002, the US (followed by many other countries) introduced an allocation system prioritising patients according to clinical need. This was quantified using the MELD score (Model for End-Stage Liver Disease, Fig. 9.7), which predicted mortality from liver disease based on patient's INR, serum bilirubin and serum creatinine. Amendments and score adjustments were later required for transplant indications other than liver failure (such as HCC or intolerable quality of life with pruritis). In 2018, the UK introduced a national liver offering scheme based on a transplant benefit score (quantifying the difference between a patient's expected survival with and without a transplant, calculated according to 21 recipient

---

**Model for End-stage Liver Disease (MELD)**

MELD is calculated for patients over the age of 12 years based on the following variables:
- Serum creatinine (mg/dL)
- Total bilirubin (mg/dL)
- INR (international normalised ratio)

The formula incorporates these variables as:

$$MELD = 3.78[Ln\ bilirubin(mg/dL)] + 11.2[Ln\ INR] + 9.57[Ln\ creatinine(mg/dL)] - 6.43$$

The following rules must be observed when using this formula:
- 1 is the minimum acceptable value for any of the three variables
- 4 is the maximum acceptable value for serum creatinine
- 40 is the maximum value of the MELD score (all higher calculated values are assigned a score of 40)
- If a patient has been dialysed twice within the last 7 days, the value used for serum creatinine should be 4

**Figure 9.7**  Model for End-stage Liver Disease (MELD) score.

parameters and 7 donor parameters).[72] Mathematical modelling of this scheme predicted that an additional 45 lives could be saved per year for patients on the waiting list,[36] but the full impact of the scheme is yet to be determined. Additional challenges are now on the horizon with the possibility of further expansion in the accepted indications for transplantation if current clinical trials confirm positive outcomes after transplantation for patients with CRLM[73] or cholangiocarcinoma.[60]

## NOVEL PERFUSION TECHNOLOGIES

The demand for liver transplantation continues to outstrip the supply of suitable deceased donor organs throughout the world.[33] This disparity is likely to increase, particularly if novel indications for liver transplantation gain acceptance. One effective strategy for addressing this issue is to increase the utilisation of marginal or 'extended criteria donor' organs (i.e. organs from older, obese and/or DCD donors). Novel perfusion technologies can play a key role in this approach by: 1) offering an opportunity for intervention to halt the ischaemic damage; and 2) providing vital additional information on liver function and injury and assisting the implanting surgeon to identify suitable organs for transplantation. Novel perfusion technologies for the liver can essentially be classified as *in situ* (normothermic regional perfusion [NRP]), or *ex situ* (normothermic machine perfusion [NMP] or hypothermic oxygenated perfusion [HOPE]).

NRP is a technique that utilises an extracorporeal membrane oxygenation (ECMO) device to re-establish an oxygenated blood flow to donor organs in a DCD donor after circulatory arrest. Arterial and venous cannulas are placed via the aorta and IVC (or femoral vessels) and the cerebral circulation is excluded by a cross-clamp on the descending thoracic aorta (for abdominal NRP) or ligation and division of the three aortic arch vessels (for the less commonly performed thoraco-abdominal NRP). Protocols vary internationally, but in the UK a regional oxygenated circulation is commenced as quickly as possible after asystole, then maintained for 2 hours before cold perfusion and organ retrieval in the standard fashion described earlier. The 2-hour period of NRP allows for a dynamic assessment of the perfused liver using serial blood and bile biochemistry tests. Multiple cohort studies have provided strong evidence for the benefits of NRP in terms of liver utilisation and clinical outcomes, to the extent that equipoise between NRP and standard DCD liver retrieval with static cold storage no longer exists. The largest cohort study from the UK (Edinburgh and Cambridge) compared outcomes from liver transplantation after NRP (44 patients) with standard DCD retrieval controls (185 patients)[74] and demonstrated a significant reduction in early allograft dysfunction (12% vs 32%, $P = 0.008$), a complete absence of ischaemic cholangiopathy compared with a rate of 27% in the control group ($P < 0.0001$). In contrast to *ex-situ* liver perfusion techniques, NRP offers the clear advantage of a simultaneous beneficial impact on the kidneys, pancreas and potentially heart for transplantation from the same donor.[75]

✔✔ The use of NRP for DCD retrieval is associated with a significant increase in DCD liver utilisation and a substantial reduction in the incidence of ischaemic cholangiopathy.[74,76]

*Ex situ* perfusion techniques may be further classified into warm or cold perfusion and can be initiated at the donor hospital or the recipient centre. NMP offers the advantages of dynamic organ assessment (e.g. lactate clearance, change in transaminases) and an ability to considerably extend safe organ storage times (up to an additional 24 hours), but adds an order of magnitude of complexity compared with cold storage approaches and the small but catastrophic risk of organ loss if oxygenated blood flow is interrupted (for example due to a twist in the hepatic artery or portal vein). A multicentre RCT comparing *ex situ* NMP initiated at the donor hospital ($n = 121$) to static cold storage ($n = 101$) of DBD and DCD livers has shown that NMP can safely prolong organ preservation times (714 vs 465 minutes), reduces organ discard rates (12% vs 24%, $P = 0.008$) and decreases the incidence of early allograft dysfunction (10% vs 49%, $P < 0.001$). However, no significant difference in ischaemic cholangiopathy was seen (11.1% vs 26.3%, $P = 0.18$) in the DCD subgroup. Separately, Mergental et al.[77] have shown that dynamic assessment of organ function with NMP can improve safe utilisation of marginal donor organs, reporting successful transplantation of 22 livers that had been declined by all UK centres with 100% 90-day patient and graft survival. However, notably, at a median follow-up of less than 2 years, 18% of the recipients of DCD livers developed ischaemic cholangiopathy requiring re-transplantation. Despite this, the evidence to date suggests that NMP has a clear role in increasing organ utilisation by facilitating the logistics of transplantation with longer organ storage times and reducing the discard rate of marginal organs through an in-depth functional assessment.

✔✔ *Ex situ* NMP safely extends the preservation time and increases the utilisation of extended criteria donor livers.[77,78]

Hypothermic *ex situ* liver perfusion is undertaken by circulating oxygenated cold preservation solution through the portal vein (HOPE) or with dual circulation through the portal vein and hepatic artery (D-HOPE). A recently published multicentre trial randomised 160 (conventionally retrieved) DCD livers to D-HOPE or static cold storage alone prior to transplantation.[79] The study involved 2 hours of D-HOPE at the recipient transplant centre after a period of static cold storage during transport and demonstrated a reduction in the rate of clinically relevant ischaemic cholangiopathy from 18% to 6%.

Novel organ perfusion technology is a rapidly evolving field and it is likely that the multiple approaches outlined above will emerge as complementary tools offering distinct capabilities for specific clinical scenarios (used alone or in combination).

## RECIPIENT HEPATECTOMY

The combination of thrombocytopenia, impaired synthetic liver function and portal hypertension with varices sets the scene for potentially catastrophic haemorrhage during hepatectomy. Close co-operation with an expert transplant anaesthetist is essential at every stage of the procedure.

Appropriate exposure is obtained with a Makuuchi or Mercedes incision. The falciform ligament is divided and a table-mounted retractor is placed for access. Dissection of the hepatoduodenal ligament proceeds with ligation and division of the bile duct, hepatic arteries and portal vein as high as possible to preserve length for subsequent anastomosis. A temporary porta-caval shunt (end-to-side anastomosis of portal vein to vena cava) can be created at this stage and improves the cardiac return, prevents venous congestion of the bowel and reduces blood loss during subsequent steps of the hepatectomy. The liver is then mobilised with division of peritoneal attachments and the right and left triangular ligaments.

The retro-hepatic vena cava can be resected en bloc with the liver or it can be preserved by careful ligation and division of the short hepatic veins and the hepatic veins. This latter approach allows for uninterrupted caval blood flow and negates the need for veno-venous bypass.

## IMPLANT

If the recipient vena cava has been preserved, the hepatic veins (either middle and left or all three) can be used to implant the liver using a 'piggy-back' technique whereby the suprahepatic IVC of the donor liver is anastomosed to the middle and left or all three recipient hepatic veins (Fig. 9.8). More recently, a 'modified piggy-back technique' which involves preservation of the native IVC and a side-to-side anastomosis with the donor's IVC has been favoured (Fig. 9.9). This offers the advantages of simplicity and excellent results, with a very low rate of venous outflow problems. If the native retro-hepatic cava has been removed, a 'classical' transplant is undertaken interposing the donor retrohepatic cava

with a suprahepatic and infrahepatic caval anastomosis (Fig. 9.10). The caval anastomosis is followed by reconstruction of the portal vein with an end-to-end anastomosis (after which the liver is reperfused) and then reconstruction of the hepatic artery with reconstruction of aberrant donor arteries on the back table beforehand if required. Biliary drainage is undertaken with an end-to-end anastomosis between the donor and recipient common bile duct or with a Roux-en-Y hepaticojejunostomy if the recipient bile duct is affected by PSC, or if a large size discrepancy exists.

## COMPLICATIONS OF LIVER TRANSPLANTATION

The risk of graft primary non-function is approximately 1% for DBD liver transplants and 2% for DCD liver transplants (without NRP). There is a relatively low incidence of hepatic artery thrombosis (1–7%, depending on the graft type) and this is considered an indication for super-urgent re-transplantation, particularly if it occurs within the first few weeks after transplant. Outflow obstruction caused by stenosis at the caval anastomosis is a rare but serious complication, with a reported incidence of 1–6%. Portal vein thrombosis occurs with an incidence of 2–26%.[33] Biliary complications include ischaemic cholangiopathy, as well as bile leak, bile duct necrosis, and anastomotic strictures requiring intervention or surgery. A previous meta-analysis included 25 studies with 62 184 liver transplant recipients (DCD = 2478 and DBD = 59 706) and reported that in comparison with DBD, there was a significant increase in biliary complications [OR = 2.4 (1.9, 3.1); $P < 0.00001$] and ischaemic cholangiopathy [OR = 10.5 (5.7, 19.5); $P < 0.00001$] following

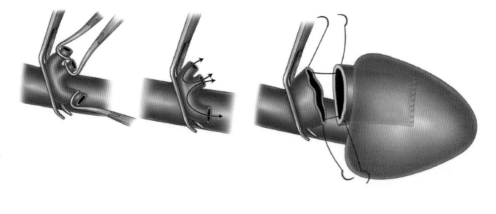

**Figure 9.8** 'Piggy-back' technique—preservation of the recipient vena cava with anastomosis of the recipient hepatic vein stump to donor vena cava.

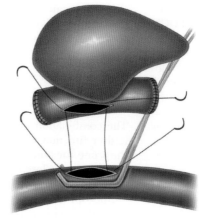
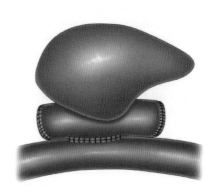

**Figure 9.9** Modified 'piggy-back' technique—preservation of the recipient vena cava with side-to-side anastomosis of the donor and recipient vena cavae.

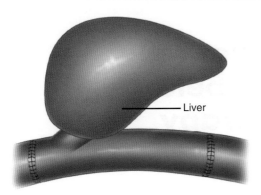

— Liver

**Figure 9.10** 'Classical' liver transplant with replacement of the recipient vena cava (effectively an interposition graft with two end-to-end anastomoses).

DCD liver transplantation. The overall incidence of biliary complications was 26% following DCD liver transplantation compared with 16% following DBD liver transplantation. The overall incidence of ischaemic cholangiopathy was 16% following DCD liver transplantation compared with 3% following DBD liver transplantation.[80] As discussed earlier, the risk of biliary complications from DCD donors is dramatically reduced with NRP,[74] to the extent that many transplant surgeons would now consider DCD grafts after NRP to be effectively equivalent to DBD grafts. Acute rejection can occur in as many as 40% of the patients during the first 3 months post-transplantation. Liver biopsy may be required to distinguish between rejection and viral infection. Intravenous corticosteroids, antithymocyte globulin, or other adaptions of the immunosuppressive regimen usually successfully treat episodes of acute rejection. Re-transplantation is the last option if medical therapy fails and hepatic failure ensues.

## RESULTS

According to the European Liver Transplant Registry, since 2000, survival at 1-, 3- and 6-months post-liver transplantation is 94%, 91% and 88%, respectively. When considering only patients who survive beyond 6 months, patient survival rates are excellent (96% at 1 year, 83% at 5 years, 71% at 10 years, 61% at 15 years and 52% at 20 years).[81] In the UK, the current patient survival rate after joining the transplant list (for an adult elective first liver transplant) is 85% at 1 year and 72% at 5 years post-registration, corresponding to a postoperative survival rate of 94% at 1 year and 84% at 5 years for those who make it to transplantation.[37]

### Key Points

- Effective treatment for portal hypertension include pharmacological therapy (beta-blockade, emergency terlipressin), transjugular intrahepatic portosystemic shunts (TIPSS) and liver transplantation. Surgical portosystemic venous shunts are now obsolete.
- 90% of liver transplants in the UK are performed for treatment of end-stage chronic liver disease (secondary to diseases including alcoholic liver disease, non-alcoholic fatty liver disease and autoimmune liver diseases). Liver transplantation is frequently used to treat hepatocellular carcinoma (within very specific criteria) and may be expanded to the treatment of other forms of cancer affecting the liver in the near future.
- The clinical need for liver transplantation continues to outstrip supply of suitable donor organs. Novel machine perfusion technologies are playing a key role in expanding the potential pool of donor organs that can be safely transplanted through overcoming logistical challenges (ischaemic times) and assisting objective assessment of 'marginal' organs.
- Liver transplantation is now a routine gold-standard treatment for management of several conditions, with excellent clinical outcomes (94% survival at 1 year post-transplant and 84% at 5 years).

 References available at http://ebooks.health.elsevier.com/

## ACKNOWLEDGEMENT

The authors are grateful to Mr Stephen O'Neill, consultant transplant surgeon, Belfast City Hospital, for his comprehensive contribution to a previous edition of this chapter.

# 10 Pancreas and islet cell transplantation: beta-cell replacement therapy

Andrew Sutherland | John Casey

## INTRODUCTION

The discovery of insulin by Banting and Best in the early part of the 20th century saw type I diabetes become a treatable chronic illness rather than a rapidly fatal diagnosis. Since then, patients with diabetes have been able to lead relatively normal lives, thanks to ongoing refinements in insulin therapy. Despite this, many patients suffer from the secondary complications of diabetes, including retinopathy, neuropathy, nephropathy and premature cardiovascular disease. The prognosis for a patient who has diabetic nephropathy is poor and the 10-year survival for a 45-year-old patient on dialysis is < 10%.[1] These patients can benefit from simultaneous pancreas and kidney (SPK) transplantation. This not only removes the need for dialysis but also results in normoglycaemia without the need for insulin in > 85% of patients.[2] Pancreas transplant alone (PTA) is reserved for patients in the absence of renal disease with life-threatening complications of diabetes, principally intractable impaired awareness of hypoglycaemia (IAH). For this set of patients, the risk of the surgery and life-long immunosuppression outweighs the risk associated with IAH and coma.

Unfortunately the morbidity and mortality associated with pancreas transplantation means that only a limited number of patients are deemed fit enough for surgery. An alternative treatment for these patients is islet transplantation. Many of the complications of whole pancreas transplantation are associated with the exocrine portion of the pancreas (pancreatitis, pancreatic fistula). The islets of Langerhans account for only 1% of pancreatic mass but contain the beta and alpha cells responsible for insulin and glucagon production necessary for glycaemic control. Islet cell isolation and transplantation has emerged over the last decade as an excellent treatment option for intractable hypoglycaemic awareness and offers a much lower risk alternative to PTA. Together pancreas transplant and islet transplant come under the banner of 'beta-cell replacement therapy'.

## BETA-CELL REPLACEMENT THERAPY

### HISTORY OF BETA-CELL REPLACEMENT THERAPY

The concept of extracting and transplanting islets is not new and was initially attempted in 1893 in Bristol when a fragmented sheep's pancreas was transplanted subcutaneously into a 15-year-old boy dying of ketoacidosis.[70] This early xenograft was, not surprisingly, unsuccessful but predated the discovery of insulin by nearly 30 years. The era of experimental islet research began in 1911, when Bensley stained islets within the guinea pig pancreas using a number of dyes, and was able to pick free the occasional islet for morphological study.[71] The average adult human pancreas weighs 70 g, contains an average of 1–2 million islets of average diameter 157 μm, constituting between 0.8% and 3.8% of the total mass of the gland.[72] Mass isolation of large numbers of viable islets from the human pancreas has proven to be a challenge ever since and it was almost 100 years later that Scharp et al.[73] reported insulin independence after islet transplantation in 1990. The first pancreas transplant was performed over 50 years ago in the University of Minnesota in 1966.[3] Early experience with pancreatic transplantation was disappointing and remained so for many years. Difficulties were related to the management of the exocrine secretions and septic complications, a high incidence of thrombosis, acute rejection and pancreatitis. For the first half of its 50-year history, less than 1200 pancreas transplants were performed worldwide. Even after the introduction of ciclosporin in 1983, 1-year patient and graft survival rates were only 75% and 37%, respectively. Understandably, in the 1970s and 1980s enthusiasm for pancreas transplantation was scarce; the predominant sentiment was scepticism. Throughout the 1990s significant changes occurred. These came about as a consequence of improvements in organ retrieval and preservation methods, refinements in surgical techniques, advances in immunosuppression, progress in the prophylaxis and treatment of infection, and the experience gained in donor and recipient selection. Success rates following pancreas transplantation are now comparable with other forms of organ transplantation. There have now been over 42 000 pancreas transplants performed worldwide.[4]

Interestingly, neither pancreas nor islet cell transplantation has ever been compared with insulin therapy in a prospective controlled trial and it is very unlikely that such a trial will ever be performed. However, considerable experience and a substantial body of evidence has accumulated, which now favours the viewpoint of the enthusiasts rather than of the sceptics.

### INDICATIONS FOR BETA-CELL REPLACEMENT

Both pancreas and islet cell transplantation aim to replace beta-cell function, reduce short- and long-term complications of diabetes and increase long-term survival. There are two main scenarios when transplantation is considered in diabetic patients:

## Box 10.1 Potential risks and benefits of simultaneous pancreas–kidney (SPK) transplantation

**Risks**
- Perioperative morbidity and mortality
- Potential for pancreas transplant to adversely affect kidney transplant outcome
- Consequences of higher immunosuppression

**Benefits**
- Improved quality of life, insulin independence
- Potential benefits on diabetic complications
- Improved life expectancy

## Box 10.2 Contraindications and risk factors for pancreas transplantation

- Inability to give informed consent
- Active drug abuse
- Major psychiatric illness or non-compliant behaviour
- Recent history of malignancy
- Active infection
- Recent myocardial infarction
- Evidence of significant uncorrectable ischaemic heart disease
- Insufficient cardiac reserve with poor ejection fraction
- Any other illness that significantly restricts life expectancy
- Age > 60 years
- Significant obesity (BMI > 30)
- Severe aortoiliac atherosclerosis

1. *Diabetic patients with renal failure:* SPK transplant is the treatment of choice in patients with type I diabetes and an estimated glomerular filtration rate of < 20 mL/min/1.73 m$^2$. Transplantation can also be considered in type II diabetics with renal failure who have a body mass index (BMI) of < 27. In patients who have already received a living or deceased kidney transplant, pancreas after kidney (PAK) transplant can be considered. In patients who are not deemed fit enough for SPK transplant, simultaneous islet kidney (SIK) transplant can be considered.

2. *Diabetic patients in the absence of renal failure:* Patients with diabetes complicated by frequent, severe metabolic complications despite optimum insulin therapy may be suitable for PTA. These patients are often at risk of IAH and coma, or severe hyperglycaemia that requires hospital admission. For patients with severe IAH, an alternative and lower risk option to PTA is islet transplantation. The risks and benefits of SPK transplant and contraindication and risks for transplant are summarised in Boxes 10.1 and 10.2. A treatment algorithm for beta-cell replacement is presented in Fig. 10.1.

## PANCREAS RETRIEVAL OPERATION

The pancreas is a close neighbour of the liver and shares important vascular structures. However, specific arterial anomalies of the blood supply to the liver that preclude successful liver or pancreas procurement for transplantation are very rare. Although a detailed description of the surgical procedure for pancreas retrieval is not given, several pertinent points are highlighted below.

University of Wisconsin (UW) solution was first developed as a pancreatic preservation solution[5] and remains the benchmark for pancreas preservation. The cold ischaemia tolerance of the pancreas is somewhere between that of the liver and the kidney. In pancreas allografts perfused with UW solution, 20 hours was thought to be the limit for successful preservation, beyond which a time-dependent deterioration in outcome occurred.[6] Although earlier data failed to demonstrate a clear benefit from a preservation time of < 20 hours, most surgeons intuitively aimed for shorter preservation times. More recent data now suggest that ischaemia time is of greater importance in recipients of suboptimal grafts. In such cases, ischaemia times > 12 hours are likely to be associated with poorer outcomes, and in the US median cold ischaemia time (CIT) for all pancreas transplants has been < 12 hours since 2006.[7,8]

The pressure gradient between mean arterial pressure and portal venous (PV) pressure that maintains blood flow through the pancreas can be significantly diminished during the perfusion of the abdominal organs in retrieval operations. Particular attention is required to maintain an adequate gradient if a cannula for perfusion is placed in the PV system as well as the aorta. Many transplant units perfuse abdominal organs with an aortic cannula only, and there is some evidence that supports the view that additional portal perfusion is unnecessary.[9] For the interests of the pancreatic allograft, aortic perfusion alone is the most 'physiological' state that allows satisfactory perfusion and adequate drainage of the effluent.

Some units flush the donor duodenum using a nasogastric tube with an antiseptic or antibiotic solution during the retrieval operation. No evidence exists to demonstrate the superiority of any solution used for duodenal decontamination, and povidone–iodine during cold storage may be toxic to duodenal mucosa.[10] Donor duodenal contents should be submitted for bacterial and fungal culture. The results may be important in guiding the management of infection in pancreas transplant recipients.[11]

Careful and minimal handling of the pancreas during retrieval is important. Removal of the spleen and the pancreatico-duodenal graft en bloc with the liver is the quickest and safest method for both organs. The organs are then easily and quickly separated on the back table at the retrieval centre.

Further back-table preparation of the pancreas, which takes place in the recipient centre, is a crucial part of the procedure and takes a minimum of 2 hours. The short stumps of the gastroduodenal artery (GDA) and the splenic artery should be marked with fine polypropylene sutures at the time of retrieval. Demonstration of good collateral circulation within the pancreatico-duodenal arcade (between the superior mesenteric artery [SMA] and the GDA) by flushing the arteries individually at the back table is reassuring. An iliac artery 'Y' graft of donor origin anastomosed to the SMA and the splenic artery is the most common method of reconstruction for the graft arterial inflow (Fig. 10.2). Meticulous dissection and ligation of the lymphatic tissue and

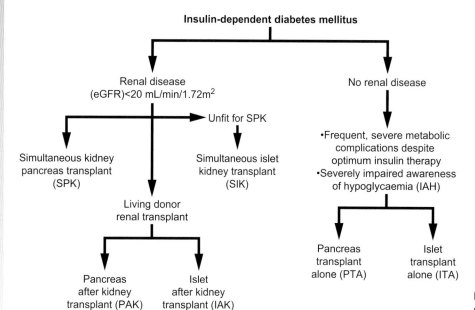

**Figure 10.1** Beta-cell replacement treatment algorithm.

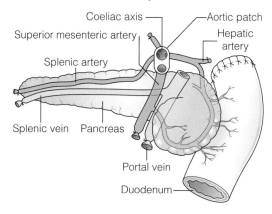

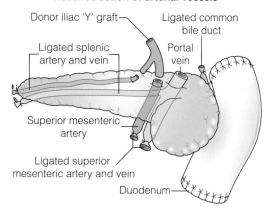

**Figure 10.2** Reverse view of the pancreas showing that the pancreatic graft reconstruction can be performed either using an aortic patch typically or in its absence using a donor iliac 'Y' graft.

small vessels around the pancreas is important to prevent haemorrhage upon reperfusion of the graft in the recipient. Particular attention should be paid to secure the duodenal segment staple lines by inversion with further sutures.

## THE PANCREAS TRANSPLANT OPERATION

### GENERAL CONSIDERATIONS

In SPK transplantation, pancreatic implantation is usually performed first because of the lower ischaemia tolerance of the pancreas. It is easier to implant the pancreatic graft on the right side. The renal allograft can also be placed intra-abdominally with anastomoses to the left iliac vessels. Alternatively, an extraperitoneal renal transplant on the left side can be performed using the same incision or through a separate left iliac fossa incision. A further alternative is to implant the renal graft ipsilaterally, using more caudal segments of the recipient right iliac vessels.

Severely atherosclerotic and calcified vessels in some diabetic recipients can be a challenge during pancreatic implantation. Iliac 'Y' grafts used for reconstruction offer greater flexibility in choosing a suitable arterial anastomotic site in the recipient vessels. The most common technique used for pancreas transplantation has been intra-abdominal implantation of the whole pancreas together with a donor duodenal segment. Currently the choices available to the surgeon are related to the management of the exocrine secretions and venous drainage, as discussed below.

### MANAGEMENT OF EXOCRINE SECRETIONS

Drainage of the exocrine secretions of pancreatic grafts into the recipient's bladder was the most common technique, accounting for 90% of US pancreas transplants during the 1980s and early 1990s. The popularity of this technique was due to its perceived safety, primarily less serious consequences of anastomotic leak (compared with enteric drainage) in the days of higher doses of corticosteroids and unrefined immunosuppression. The ability to monitor amylase levels in the urine has been considered an additional advantage of bladder drainage. However, the unphysiological diversion of pancreatic exocrine secretions into the urinary bladder causes frequent complications, often leading to chronic and disabling symptoms. As a consequence, conversion of the urinary diversion to enteric drainage is required in many patients. It is for this reason that enteric drainage has largely replaced bladder drainage as the method of choice for the management of exocrine secretions in the US and in most European centres.

Any part of the recipient's small bowel can be used for anastomosis with the allograft duodenum. No data exist to demonstrate the superiority of one particular site over another. Roux-en-Y loops, which were commonly used, are becoming rare and a simple side-to-side entero-enterostomy is preferred.[12]

Delayed endocrine function from the transplanted graft is uncommon and insulin infusion should be discontinued at the time of reperfusion. Recipients achieving insulin independence for the first time in many years is a gratifying consequence for the surgeon; however, patients can become hypoglycaemic at this stage. Blood sugar levels should be checked frequently and a low rate of dextrose infusion is often required.

## MANAGEMENT OF VENOUS DRAINAGE

Drainage of the venous outflow from pancreas grafts into the portal circulation was first described by Calne in 1984.[13] This complex surgical technique using a segmental graft and gastric exocrine diversion in a paratopic position has never gained popularity. Drainage of the venous outflow into the systemic circulation at the level of the lower inferior vena cava has now become the norm in pancreatic transplantation. However, some units still use PV drainage via the superior mesenteric vein (SMV).[14] Several studies, including prospective randomised comparisons, have shown that this offers at least equivalent outcome to that of systemic venous (SV) drainage, with no compromise in safety.[15–17] The impetus for PV drainage was to achieve a more physiological delivery of insulin. A theoretical benefit was considered to be avoidance of hyperinsulinaemia, which has been linked with atherogenesis.[18] However, none of the studies of metabolic function after PV drainage have shown a clear benefit in terms of glucose metabolism, lipid profiles or atherogenesis, but some studies have observed a reduction in acute rejection rates.[15–17]

## IMMUNOSUPPRESSION IN PANCREAS TRANSPLANTATION

Historically, there is ample evidence that the incidence of acute rejection is higher after pancreas transplantation than after kidney transplantation.[6,19] The reasons for this difference are not clear. Nevertheless, there has been general acknowledgement of the higher immunological risk of pancreas transplantation. This has resulted in the evolution of strategies that use more intense immunosuppressive protocols for pancreas transplantation than for kidney transplantation.

In Europe, immunosuppressive protocols in solid organ transplantation in general have been less aggressive compared with US protocols. In the evolution of immunosuppression for pancreas transplantation, tacrolimus has largely replaced ciclosporin and mycophenolate mofetil (MMF) has replaced azathioprine based on sound evidence from prospective randomised trials showing improved outcomes.[20–24]

Steroid withdrawal or avoidance has been a focus of study in the last decade. As yet, there is no evidence demonstrating a significant benefit from steroid avoidance or withdrawal, but experience reveals that it is feasible without adversely affecting outcome in pancreas transplant patients.[25,26]

Induction therapy with biological agents is part of the immunosuppressive protocol in nearly all pancreas transplants.[27] This is based on prospective multicentre trials that demonstrated a reduced incidence and severity of rejection episodes with biological induction therapy.[28–30] A comparison of different induction therapies (OKT3, ATG, basiliximab or daclizumab) compared with no induction showed a reduction in acute rejection with induction therapy, but no consistent pattern has emerged to demonstrate the superiority of any one specific biological agent when used in conjunction with tacrolimus-based immunosuppression.[31] More recent evidence from a single-centre randomised comparison suggests that alemtuzumab induction is associated with similar graft and patient survival rates compared with ATG induction, but results in a lower incidence of acute rejection and better safety profile, with a significantly lower incidence of cytomegalovirus (CMV) infection.[32]

## DIAGNOSIS AND MANAGEMENT OF ACUTE REJECTION FOLLOWING PANCREAS TRANSPLANTATION

One of the notable features about pancreas transplantation over the last 15 years has been the considerable reduction in the incidence of acute rejection. In 1992, 74% of SPK transplant recipients and 50% of PTA recipients (this probably underestimates the true incidence) were reported to have received antirejection therapy.[6,19] This had reduced to 19% and 17%, respectively, by 2000.[12]

An important feature of pancreatic graft rejection, for the purposes of patient management, is the lack of a reliable early marker. In SPK transplants, diagnosis of acute rejection almost completely relies on monitoring of renal allograft function by measuring serum creatinine levels and undertaking renal biopsy when indicated. Discordant rejection of allografts only occurs rarely following SPK transplantation, with isolated pancreas rejection in 5–10% of acute rejection episodes.[19] Monitoring for acute rejection and patient management in the early postoperative period is a particular challenge in patients following solitary pancreas transplantation.

Acute rejection of the pancreas affects the exocrine pancreas first. The inflammation may cause pain and a low-grade fever associated with a rise in serum amylase. These symptoms and signs are non-specific, can be subtle and do not distinguish between acute rejection and other causes of graft inflammation (such as ischaemia–reperfusion injury or allograft pancreatitis). Islets of Langerhans are scattered sparsely throughout the exocrine pancreas and beta cells have considerable functional reserve. Therefore, dysfunction of the majority of islets resulting in hyperglycaemia as a consequence of rejection occurs only very late in the course of pancreatic rejection. Imaging modalities such as computed tomography (CT) or magnetic resonance imaging (MRI) visualise the pancreas and are helpful to exclude other pathology (such as lack of perfusion which may be segmental, or intra-abdominal collections). There are no specific radiological signs of acute rejection. Detection of urinary amylase in bladder-drained grafts is a sensitive indicator of exocrine function. However, detection of hypoamylasuria lacks specificity. A > 25% reduction in urinary amylase correlates with acute rejection in no more than half of the cases when assessed by biopsy.[33] A stable urinary amylase may therefore be helpful in excluding acute rejection, but detection of hypoamylasuria is non-specific and unhelpful.

Pancreas allograft biopsy has recently become established as a reliable and safe technique, and is the gold standard in the diagnosis of acute rejection in solitary pancreas transplants. Percutaneous biopsy under ultrasound or CT guidance is the most common method. Histological criteria for the diagnosis and grading of rejection have been standardised.[34]

Histological examination of pancreas graft biopsies correlates with clinical and serological findings and has revealed two distinct pathways of rejection (similar to the more widely recognised pattern in kidney transplantation): T-cell-mediated rejection and antibody-mediated rejection.

✔ A recent article by Papadimitriou and Drachenberg[35] provides an authoritative and up-to-date review of the histological criteria for these two subtypes of acute pancreas allograft rejection, as well as mechanisms leading to graft injury and differential diagnosis.

The recognition of antibody-mediated rejection as a distinct entity in pancreas transplantation explains conflicting results in published data from earlier years, as some cases of treatment-resistant acute pancreas allograft rejection were thought to be cell-mediated rejection. It also partially explains the improved success rates in solitary pancreas transplantation as a consequence of liberal surveillance biopsies.[32] Finally, the increasing utilisation of pancreas allograft biopsies has cast doubt on the validity of the assumption that isolated rejection of the kidney or the pancreas graft in SPK recipients is uncommon. Monitoring of donor-specific antibodies (DSA) has become routine. In a multivariate analysis of 433 pancreas transplants at the Oxford Transplant Centre, development of de novo DSA emerged as a strong independent predictor of pancreas graft failure (hazard ratio 4.66, $P < 0.001$).[36]

Early or mild cell-mediated acute rejection of the pancreas allograft concurrent with kidney rejection can be successfully treated with high-dose corticosteroids. Recurrent acute rejection or moderate to severe rejection episodes require treatment with anti-T-cell agents. International Pancreas Transplant Registry (IPTR) data show that steroids were used in 85% of SPK and 80% of solitary pancreas transplant recipients diagnosed with acute rejection.[12] However, 48% of SPK transplant recipients and 80% of solitary pancreas transplant recipients with acute rejection were also given anti-T-cell agents, suggesting that many patients were treated with both. There are not enough data to make evidence-based recommendations on the optimum treatment for acute antibody-mediated rejection. Experience with the management of antibody-mediated rejection in kidney transplantation would suggest a potential role for plasma exchange with or without intravenous immunoglobulin and/or rituximab.

Acute rejection in pancreas allografts is not life-threatening and caution is advised against overimmunosuppression. If diagnosed before the onset of hyperglycaemia,

most rejection episodes are reversible. The United Network for Organ Sharing (UNOS) data for 4251 patients who received SPK transplants between 1988 and 1997 were analysed by Reddy et al.[37] in order to determine the influence of acute rejection on long-term outcome. Acute rejection of either graft increased the relative risk (RR) of pancreas and kidney graft failure at 5 years. The RRs, adjusted for other risk factors, were 1.32 and 1.53 for pancreas and kidney, respectively, if acute rejection occurred. The worst outcome was in patients who had both kidney and pancreas rejection.

## COMPLICATIONS OF PANCREAS TRANSPLANTATION

Pancreas transplantation is associated with a higher incidence and a greater range of complications than kidney transplantation. Furthermore, postoperative patient management constitutes a greater challenge (Box 10.3). Between a quarter and a third of patients require relaparotomy following pancreas transplantation to deal with complications. Part of the reason for the increased incidence of complications is the higher level of immunosuppression in a high-risk diabetic population who already exhibit impaired infection resistance, poor healing and a high prevalence of comorbidity. Other factors relate to the allograft, which unlike kidney or liver allografts is not sterile and uniquely possesses rich proteolytic enzymes, making it susceptible to specific complications such as secondary haemorrhage, pancreatitis, leaks and fistula formation. The blood flow to the pancreas is much lower than that to the kidney and this is a further risk factor, specifically for thrombotic complications. Finally, bladder drainage of the exocrine secretions is associated with a high incidence of complications unique to this unphysiological diversion. Increasing donor age, prolonged preservation time, recipient obesity and donor obesity are risk factors for complications and early graft loss.

---

### Box 10.3 Complications of pancreas transplantation

**Vascular complications**

- Thrombosis: allograft venous or arterial thrombosis
- Haemorrhage: early haemorrhage from allograft vessels and late haemorrhage (rupture of pseudoaneurysms)

**Infective complications**

- Systemic infection: opportunistic infections associated with immunosuppression
- Local infections: peritonitis, localised collections, enteric or pancreatic fistulas

**Allograft pancreatitis**

- Ischaemia–reperfusion injury or reflux pancreatitis (especially after bladder drainage)
- Complications specific to bladder drainage
- Chronic dehydration, acidosis, recurrent urinary tract infections, haematuria, chemical cystitis, urethral strictures or urethral disruption

## VASCULAR COMPLICATIONS

### Thrombosis

Allograft venous or arterial thrombosis occurs more commonly following pancreatic transplantation compared with kidney transplantation. Venous thrombosis is more common than arterial thrombosis by a factor of 2:1.[38] Graft thrombosis is by far the most common cause of early graft loss following pancreas transplantation. An analysis of US pancreas transplants performed until the end of 2008 revealed that 5% of SPK transplants and 7% of solitary pancreas transplants failed as a result of thrombosis[37] (Table 10.1). Among the recognised risk factors for thrombosis, donor-related factors have the greatest impact. These include donor age, donor BMI, cardiovascular and cerebrovascular cause of donor death, prolonged preservation time, excessive flush volumes and pressure, and the type of preservation solution. A technical factor predisposing to thrombosis could be the use of venous extension grafts for the portal vein anastomosis, which should be only very rarely required. Concern about a potentially higher incidence of thrombosis following PV drainage has not been borne out by clinical experience.

Graft thrombosis, once diagnosed, requires prompt laparotomy and graft pancreatectomy. There are reports of surgical, radiological and pharmacological interventions in small numbers of cases.[39–41] Virtually all of these refer to highly selected cases of segmental, incomplete thrombosis.

Routine use of heparin for prophylaxis against allograft vascular thrombosis is used by some but is not standard practice in many units and is associated with increased risk of haemorrhage.

Table 10.1 illustrates the relative prevalence of early complications of pancreas transplantation leading to graft loss from the IPTR database.

### Haemorrhage

Release of the vascular clamps and reperfusion of the pancreatic allograft during the recipient operation can be tricky, with potential for bleeding from multiple points on the allograft. The key to avoiding this is meticulous preparation of the allograft on the back table prior to implantation.

Haemorrhage in the early postoperative hours is often a result of the proteolytic and fibrinolytic activity of the pancreatic exocrine secretions leaking from the surface of the pancreas and coming into contact with thrombus-sealed small vessels or vascular anastomoses. Early postoperative bleeding is the most common indication for re-laparotomy after pancreas transplantation. Unlike graft thrombosis, however, bleeding has little impact on ultimate outcome and < 1% of pancreas grafts are lost to bleeding[42] (Table 10.1).

Late haemorrhage following pancreas transplantation is an uncommon but catastrophic complication, often due to the rupture of a pseudoaneurysm or direct erosion of one of the anastomoses secondary to a leak. Any unexplained fever, tachycardia, leucocytosis or abdominal pain in recipients of pancreas transplants should lead to investigation for a leak or intra-abdominal collection.

### Infective complications

Pancreas transplantation, in common with all transplant procedures that require immunosuppression, is associated

**Table 10.1  Causes of early graft loss after pancreas transplantation in the US primary deceased donor pancreas transplants (January 2004 to January 2009)**

| Causes of early graft loss | SPK | PAK | PTA |
|---|---|---|---|
| | $n = 4320$ | $n = 1148$ | $n = 494$ |
| Thrombosis | 5.1% | 7.4% | 6.6% |
| Infection | 0.6% | 0.8% | 0.4% |
| Pancreatitis | 0.6% | 0.4% | 0.4% |
| Anastomotic leak | 0.4% | 0.2% | 0.3% |
| Bleeding | 0.2% | 0.3% | 0.3% |
| Total graft loss | 6.9% | 9.1% | 7.9% |

*PAK*, pancreas after kidney transplants; *PTA*, pancreas transplantation alone; *SPK*, simultaneous pancreas–kidney transplants.

with an increased risk of mostly opportunistic infections. CMV disease is more common after pancreas transplantation than after kidney or liver transplantation. Antiviral prophylaxis in CMV-mismatched donor/recipient pairs is mandatory. Unique to pancreatic transplantation are intra-abdominal septic complications, which occur as a consequence of bacteria or fungi transmitted from the donor via the allograft, or as a consequence of an anastomotic leak. Patients on peritoneal dialysis at the time of transplantation have a higher rate of intra-abdominal infection compared with those on haemodialysis.[6]

### Allograft pancreatitis

Cold storage and ischaemia–reperfusion injury inevitably result in a degree of oedema of the pancreatic allograft. This is a commonly encountered finding if a re-laparotomy becomes necessary in the first few postoperative days, and it is not always associated with an elevation in serum amylase. There is no universally agreed definition of allograft pancreatitis. Bladder drainage (especially in the presence of autonomic neuropathy affecting bladder function and causing high intravesical pressures) can be associated with recurrent episodes of allograft pancreatitis due to reflux. Catheter drainage of the bladder for at least 7–10 days is usually adequate for the management of the acute episode, but ultimately enteric conversion may be required.

During the pancreas transplant operation, allograft exocrine function starts very promptly upon revascularisation and the duodenal segment quickly fills with pancreatic juice. Excessive distension of the stapled duodenal segment and consequent reflux may cause postoperative pancreatitis. Donor age, donor obesity and prolonged preservation times are other factors associated with allograft pancreatitis. The distinction between allograft pancreatitis and acute rejection in the presence of an oedematous pancreas, abdominal pain and a slightly raised serum amylase is a difficult clinical diagnosis.

### Complications specific to bladder drainage

The most common consequence of the diversion of the exocrine pancreatic secretions into the bladder is a chemical cystitis, which predisposes patients to infection, persistent haematuria and troublesome dysuria. Dysuria is more troublesome in men, with urethritis that can progress to urethral disruption. Failure of reabsorption of the exocrine secretions results in chronic dehydration and acidosis. Urinary tract infections are much more common than intestinal drainage. Persistent haematuria may necessitate repeated blood transfusions. As mentioned above, reflux allograft pancreatitis is another potential complication. As a consequence of one or more of these complications, enteric conversion of the exocrine drainage may become necessary. The enteric conversion rate in bladder-drained pancreas transplants increases with increasing follow-up and can be as high as 40% at 5 years.[19]

## OUTCOME FOLLOWING PANCREAS TRANSPLANTATION

Patient and graft survival rates following pancreas transplantation continue to improve. The most recent analysis of IPTR data reveals excellent short- and medium-term results, with 1-year and 3-year patient survival rates of 95% and 92%, respectively, in all three pancreas transplant categories.[43] The latest data from the UK shows that 1- and 3-year patient survival rates are now 99% and 96%, respectively, and graft survival rates are as high as 91% and 88%, respectively, for SPK transplants (NHSBT data, 2022).

### FACTORS INFLUENCING PANCREAS TRANSPLANTATION OUTCOME

#### Recipient age

Increasing recipient age is a small but significant risk factor in the outcome of pancreas transplantation. Historically, patient and graft survival rates have been higher in younger recipients. However, in recent years more careful patient selection has resulted in improved outcome in older recipients, to the extent that the short-term outcome following pancreas transplantation is no different for patients older than 45 years at the time of transplantation compared with younger patients.[44] Five-year patient survival after SPK transplantation is 86% for recipients aged 35–49 years at the time of transplantation compared with 81.7% for those aged 50–64 years.[44]

#### Re-transplantation

Re-transplantation appears as a consistent and significant risk factor for graft survival in all categories. One-year pancreas graft survival after re-transplantation in the SPK category is 70.8% (± 9.3%) compared with 85.4% (± 0.9%) in primary SPK transplants.[44]

#### HLA matching

Analyses of US registry data have inconsistently shown limited evidence for the influence of HLA matching on pancreas transplant outcome.[45] The effect of HLA matching, when present, has been small and seemed to affect different categories during different eras or was confined to different classes of HLA mismatches. The likely explanation is that HLA matching has negligible or no influence on the outcome of pancreas transplantation, as is suggested by the most recent analysis of the IPTR database.[43]

### Management of exocrine secretions and management of venous drainage

The surgical technique employed for exocrine diversion has no influence on outcome in pancreas transplantation. Pancreas graft survival rates at 1 year following SPK transplantation for the 2000–2004 cohort in the US were 87% and 85% for bladder-drained and enteric-drained grafts, respectively. More recent analyses confirm that the method of exocrine diversion has no influence on patient or graft survival rates.[27] Similarly, outcomes are similar comparing systemic and PV drainage.[44]

### Immunosuppression

Immunosuppressive therapy has a major influence on the outcome following pancreas transplantation. In the last decade, tacrolimus and MMF have been the basis of maintenance immunosuppression in the large majority of patients. Multivariate analyses reveal that the tacrolimus/MMF combination is associated with significant reductions in pancreas graft loss (RR = 0.74, $P = 0.08$ for SPK; RR = 0.51, $P = 0.001$ for PAK; and RR = 0.46, $P = 0.014$ for PTA). In a cohort of transplants undertaken between 2006 and 2010, antibody induction was associated with lower risk of pancreas graft failure following SPK, but not PAK or PTA, and only when depleting antibodies were used.[27]

### Donor factors

Donor age, donor obesity and donor cause of death have been linked with the outcome of pancreas transplantation. Whilst all of these variables may be independently associated with outcome, they are likely to be inter-related; for instance, younger donors are more likely to have died of trauma, whilst older and obese donors are more likely to have died of a cerebrovascular cause.

An analysis of all SPK transplants performed in the US during a 12-year period between 1994 and 2005 ($n = 8850$) has conclusively shown increasing donor age to be a risk factor in pancreas transplantation.[46] Pancreas and kidney graft survival and patient survival at 1 year were significantly inferior in the old donor group (> 45years) compared with the young donor group < 45 years (77% vs 85%, 89% vs 92% and 95% vs 93%, respectively). Five-year pancreas graft survival was 72% versus 60% for young versus old donor transplants, respectively.

Humar et al.[47] reported the outcome of 711 deceased donor pancreas transplants performed between 1994 and 2001. The outcomes were analysed for three groups based on donor BMI. Patients who received grafts from obese donors (BMI > 30) had a higher incidence of complications and inferior graft survival. The incidence of technical failure was 9.7% in the BMI < 25 group, 16.3% in the BMI 25–30 group and 21% in the BMI > 30 group ($P = 0.04$). More recently, the same group of authors published an analysis in a slightly larger cohort of pancreas transplant patients in order to determine risk factors for technical failure following pancreas transplantation.[48] Technical failure, defined as thrombosis, bleeding, leaks, infections or pancreatitis, was responsible for the loss of 13.1% of transplants (131 of 973). On multivariate analysis, the following were significant risk factors: recipient BMI > 30 (RR = 2.42, $P = 0.0003$), preservation time > 24 hours (RR = 1.87, $P = 0.04$) and cause of donor death other than trauma (RR = 1.58, $P = 0.04$). Donor obesity had borderline significance.

Pancreas grafts from paediatric donors (aged > 4 years) can be used with excellent results.[25] Organs from donation after circulatory/cardiac death (DCD) donors constitute an increasing proportion of the deceased donor pool. The University of Wisconsin experience and the pooled US data suggest that the outcome of pancreas transplantation using DCD grafts is equivalent to that achieved with donation after brain death (DBD) donor organs.[49,50] An analysis of data from Oxford, one of the world's largest pancreas transplant programmes, reveal a higher risk of pancreas graft failure with DCD grafts. The poorer outcome was, however, confined to solitary pancreas transplant recipients with prolonged preservation times.[7,8] Callaghan et al.[51] recently published data from over 2000 SPK transplants in the UK and again found equivalent outcomes in DCD donors when compared with DBD donors. However, it should be noted that DCD donors were generally younger, slimmer, less likely to have stroke as a cause of death, with lower terminal creatinine and shorter pancreas cold ischemic times than DBD donors. It is evident that donor selection has a major influence on the outcome of pancreas transplantation. Therefore, other risk factors such as preservation time, recipient BMI and comorbidity need to be considered when using suboptimal grafts for pancreas transplantation.

## LONG-TERM OUTLOOK FOLLOWING PANCREAS TRANSPLANTATION

### Pancreas transplantation and life expectancy

Clearly, one of the most important issues for patients considering pancreas transplantation is whether their life expectancy will be influenced by the transplant. Numerous studies and analyses of databases have consistently shown that successful pancreas transplantation is associated with improved survival prospects in diabetic patients. No prospective controlled study has ever been carried out that compares pancreas transplantation with insulin therapy and hence all available evidence is subject to selection bias.

Several studies have addressed the question of the impact of pancreas transplantation on long-term mortality in a number of different ways. The University of Wisconsin experience in 500 SPK transplant recipients published in 1998[51] simply quotes a 10-year patient survival rate of 70%. This is matched in their experience only by recipients of living-donor kidney (LKD) transplants. Unsurpassed as they are, these results were obtained in a highly selective group of young patients with a relatively short duration of diabetes and kidney failure and strict eligibility criteria excluding those with ischaemic heart disease.

A large US registry analysis published in 2001 looked at the outcome in 13 467 adults with type I diabetes registered on kidney and SPK transplant waiting lists between 1988 and 1997.[52] Adjusted 10-year patient survival was 67% for SPK transplant recipients, 65% for LKD transplant recipients and 46% for cadaveric kidney (CAD) transplant recipients. Taking the mortality of patients who remained on dialysis as a reference, the adjusted RR of 5-year mortality was 0.40, 0.45 and 0.74 for SPK, LKD and CAD recipients, respectively. Another large review of the UNOS database published in 2003 analysed long-term survival in 18 549 patients with type I diabetes transplanted between 1987 and 1996.[53] There was

a long-term survival advantage in favour of pancreas transplant recipients (8-year crude survival rates: 72% for SPK, 72% for LKD and 55% for CAD). This diminished but persisted after adjusting for donor and recipient variables and kidney graft function.

## INFLUENCE OF PANCREAS TRANSPLANTATION ON DIABETIC COMPLICATIONS

### Nephropathy

There is convincing evidence that successful pancreas transplantation can stop the progression of diabetic nephropathy and reverse associated histological changes. This evidence largely comes from studies that have assessed the course of diabetic nephropathy in kidney allografts in SPK or PAK transplant recipients.[54,55] Fioretto et al.[56] have shown that established lesions of diabetic nephropathy in native kidneys can be reversed with successful pancreas transplantation PTA. In the setting of clinical transplantation, the beneficial effect of the pancreas graft is counterbalanced by the nephrotoxicity of the immunosuppressive drugs.

### Retinopathy

Patients with type I diabetes often quote preservation of eyesight as one of the main reasons for considering pancreas transplantation. There is good evidence that better blood glucose control reduces the risk of progression of retinopathy.[57] However, in practice the large majority of patients undergoing pancreas transplantation will have advanced proliferative retinopathy. Hence, prevention of retinopathy is seldom a major factor in the consideration of the risks and benefits of pancreas transplantation.[58]

Retinopathy needs to be treated prior to transplantation with laser photocoagulation, which is an effective treatment. For the minority of patients who present with nonproliferative retinopathy or those who have recently undergone treatment for proliferative retinopathy, there is a risk of rapid progression of the retinopathy following transplantation. Such patients require close ophthalmic follow-up within the first 3 years of transplantation. Stabilisation of retinopathy after pancreas transplantation takes 3 years.[58–60] During this time, any patient who has an indication or develops an indication for laser treatment should undergo treatment.

Patients often report improved vision soon after pancreas transplantation. Improvement in macular oedema is demonstrable soon after transplantation and can result in early improvement of vision. It is unclear whether this is a consequence of euglycaemia or a consequence of the kidney transplant improving fluid balance. It is probable that euglycaemia offered by pancreas transplantation, over and above the benefits of the non-uraemic environment, results in better elimination of osmotic swelling of the lens, hence improving fluctuations in vision that patients with diabetes experience.[58]

### Neuropathy

Patients with end-stage renal failure and type I diabetes almost universally exhibit an autonomic and peripheral (somatic) diabetic polyneuropathy as well as uraemic neuropathy. Improvement in neuropathy following SPK transplantation using objective measures of nerve function has been demonstrated by several transplant centres.[61,62] For individuals with intractable and distressing symptoms of neuropathy, the clinical benefit may be considerable. Reversal of neuropathic symptoms takes many months and a clinically relevant benefit may not be evident for 6–12 months after transplantation. Obesity, smoking, the presence of advanced neuropathy and poor renal allograft function are predictors of poor recovery in nerve function after SPK transplantation.[63]

### Cardiovascular disease

Pancreas transplantation has demonstrable benefits on microangiopathy in diabetics.[64] Some of its effects on retinopathy, nephropathy and neuropathy may be mediated through this mechanism. It has been more difficult to demonstrate any improvement in macroangiopathy. The enhanced survival prospects after pancreas transplantation ought to be, at least in part, due to improvement in the cardiovascular risk profile. Evidence to support this is accumulating. Fiorina et al. demonstrated favourable influences of pancreas[65] and islet[66] transplantation on atherosclerotic risk factors, including plasma lipid profile, blood pressure, left ventricular function and endothelial function. This translates into reduced cardiovascular death rate.[67,68] Similar improvements occur in patients with early non-uraemic diabetes after PTA.[69]

## ISLET TRANSPLANTATION

Although Scharp et al.[73] reported insulin independence after islet transplantation in 1990, this was short-lived and difficult to reproduce. It was not until the Edmonton group in 2000 reported a series of seven consecutive patients that achieved insulin independence that islet transplantation became more widely adopted.[74] This remarkable outcome was achieved by transplanting at least two islet preparations from different donors and by using a novel steroid-free immunosuppression regimen of tacrolimus, sirolimus and induction with daclizumab.

✓✓ In 2000, the Edmonton group reported a series of seven consecutive patients in whom insulin independence was achieved after islet transplantation.[74]

This regimen has been termed 'the Edmonton protocol' and many units worldwide have attempted to replicate these outcomes, with variable success.[75,76] In the aftermath of the Edmonton protocol, islet transplantation is considered in many countries as 'standard of care' for a select group of patients with type I diabetes and is funded through the healthcare system in Canada and the NHS in the UK. The results of combined islet and kidney transplantation now match those of islet transplantation alone,[77,78] and recent data suggest that islets transplanted with a kidney may prolong the patient and kidney graft survival and protect against diabetic vascular complications.[79,80]

## PATIENT SELECTION AND ASSESSMENT

There are two principal indications for islet transplantation:

1. *Severely IAH despite optimum insulin therapy.* IAH occurs in 20–25% of patients with type I diabetes and is potentially life-threatening. These patients have a defective counter-regulatory hormonal response to hypoglycaemia, are unable to identify low blood sugars and therefore institute corrective measures.[81] Defective recognition of hypoglycaemia increases the risk of severe hypoglycaemic episodes that can result in coma and death. The impact on quality of life for these patients is substantial, and social activities and employment can be severely restricted; indeed, in the UK, patients with IAH cannot hold a UK driving licence.

2. *Patients with type I diabetes and a functioning kidney allograft who are unable to maintain their HbA1c below 7%.* In this patient group it is not necessary to demonstrate IAH as they are already taking immunosuppression and it has been shown that the improved glycaemic control after islet transplantation in this setting is associated with a reduction in long-term diabetic complications.

IAH can be assessed by patient history and by asking the patient to keep a diary of insulin usage, dietary intake and hypoglycaemic events, in particular those events requiring assistance from relatives or those requiring hospitalisation. The use of a continuous glucose monitoring sensor (CGMS) can be very useful in assessing daily glucose profiles pre- and post-islet transplantation (Fig. 10.3).[82] Scoring systems such as the Gold or Clark scores allow numerical documentation of the degree of IAH. The Gold score asks the question 'do you know when your hypos are commencing?' and the patient completes a linear scale from 1 to 7 (always aware to never aware). A score of 4 or above suggests IAH. The Clark method asks eight questions to document the patient's exposure and responses to moderate and severe hypoglycaemia, and again a score of 4 or more suggests IAH.[81] Ryan et al.[83] have described a composite HYPO score based on 4 weeks of glucose values. They suggest that this provides a more objective assessment of the metabolic instability of an individual patient and allows pre- and post-transplant comparison. Patients should be assessed by a multidisciplinary team consisting of a diabetologist, transplant surgeon, dietician and a diabetes nurse specialist. This will ensure an optimum insulin regimen and dietary compliance and that the patient is fully informed about the likely outcome of islet transplantation and the risks involved, principally post-transplant immunosuppression.

## ISLET ISOLATION

Donor factors contributing to successful islet isolation have been documented by Lakey et al. (Table 10.2).[84] This paper suggests that pancreases from older donors with a higher BMI should result in a significantly higher islet yield. O'Gorman et al.[85] have suggested a scoring system from 1 to 100 to give a numerical assessment of the likelihood of successful isolation from a specific donor pancreas. These studies, however, only predict successful isolation and do not take into consideration data that suggest that islets isolated from younger donors are functionally better.[86] In the UK, a sharing scheme was introduced in December 2010 where patients for SPK transplantation and islet transplantation are placed on a common waiting list and pancreases offered on a named patient basis. Multiple donor and recipient factors are taken into consideration, allowing islet and whole pancreas recipients equal access to suitable organs.

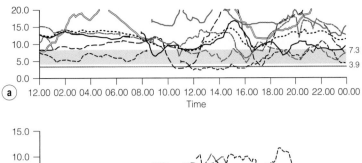

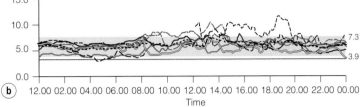

**Figure 10.3**   Continuous glucose monitoring sensor (CGMS) profiles before **(a)** and after **(b)** islet transplantation.

**Table 10.2   Donor-related variables predicting isolation success**

| Variable | P value | R value | Odds ratio |
|---|---|---|---|
| Donor age (yr) | < 0.05 | 0.18 | 1.10 |
| Body mass index | < 0.01 | 0.19 | 1.30 |
| Local vs distant procurement team | < 0.01 | 0.21 | 7.04 |
| Min. blood glucose | < 0.01 | −0.24 | 0.68 |
| Duration of cardiac arrest | < 0.01 | −0.17 | 0.81 |
| Duration of cold storage | < 0.05 | −0.13 | 0.86 |

Reproduced from Lakey JR, Warnock GL, Rajotte RV, et al. Variables in organ donors that affect the recovery of human islets of Langerhans. Transplantation 1996;61(7):1047–53. With permission from Lippincott, Williams & Wilkins.

Most of the outcome data on islet transplantation are based on organs from DBD donors; however, there is growing evidence that pancreases from DCD can produce transplantable preparations and good outcomes. Most of the early data on DCD islet transplantation came from the Kyoto group and although long-term graft survival is obtained, insulin independence is less common.[87–90] The Leiden group recently published their results with DCD islet transplantation. Although islet yields were lower from DCD donors, clinical outcomes in terms of stimulated c-peptides and Igls scores were equivalent at 1 and 2 years post-transplant.[91]

It is critical that the pancreas for islet isolation is retrieved with the same care as that for whole pancreas transplantation and that CIT is minimised, ideally to under 8 hours.[92] Pancreases should be transported rapidly and the staff in the isolation laboratory should be ready to begin the isolation immediately. It has been demonstrated that suspending the explanted pancreas in a bilayer of oxygenated perfluorocarbon (PFC) and UW solution during or after transport allows satisfactory islet preparations to be obtained from suboptimal pancreases and may even increase yields from pancreases with long ischaemia times.[93,94] PFC-based preservation may also help expand the donor pool by improving islet isolation from DCD pancreases and older donors.[95]

The semi-automated process for islet isolation that is used in most laboratories was described by Ricordi et al. in 1989.[96] This involves digestion of the pancreas using a combination of collagenase enzyme and mechanical dissociation of the pancreas in the Ricordi chamber (Fig. 10.4). A number of new enzyme blends have been developed for human isolation, including collagenase NB1 (Serva), Liberase MTF (Roche) and C1 collagenase HA (Vitacyte). Each of these differs slightly in the enzyme blend and manufacturing process but promises to deliver more consistent, better-quality islet yields. The preparation is then purified on a continuous density gradient using a COBE 2991 cell separator, resulting in a packed cell volume of only 1–2 mL (Fig. 10.5).[97] Although unpurified preparations can be used (particularly in autotransplants), the risk of portal vein thrombosis, portal hypertension and disseminated intravascular coagulation (DIC) is increased.[98–101]

After isolation and purification, it is now standard practice to place the islet preparation in culture for 12–48 hours. There are compelling data that this does not adversely affect islet graft function and does in fact increase purity of the preparation.[102] Extended culture up to 48 hours can also be used to assess the viability of an islet graft, particularly after DCD isolation.

The number of islets in the preparation is documented in terms of islet equivalents (IEQ). This counting method adjusts for the fact that islets vary greatly in size, and cell viability stains such as fluorescein diacetate/propidium iodide and SYTOGreen/ethidium bromide are used to determine the viable beta-cell mass.[103]

The minimum release criteria in the UK for an islet preparation are:

- > 200 000 islet equivalents
- > 70% viability
- > 30% purity
- Gram stain negative
- Endotoxin negative

It is accepted that these criteria are subjective and open to observer variation and error. Some assessment of the 'quality' of the preparation should also be made. Experienced islet laboratory staff can comment on the morphology of the cells, the integrity of the islets and whether or not there is evidence of central necrosis within the islets. Islet oxygen

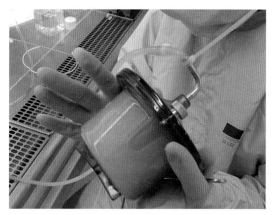

**Figure 10.4**   Ricordi chamber.

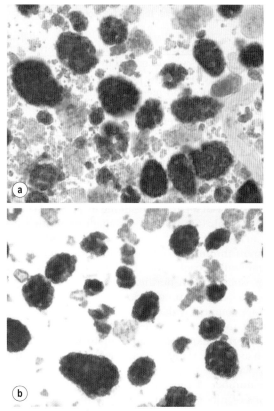

**Figure 10.5**   Islets stained red with dithizone before **(a)** and after **(b)** purification.

consumption rate and beta-cell ATP content show good correlation between product testing and in vivo islet function in animal studies, and may be useful in the future, but are time-consuming and expensive. The Minnesota group has demonstrated good correlation between marginal mass islet transplants in diabetic nude mice and outcome of human islet transplants from the same donor.[104]

Modern islet isolation facilities must comply with current good manufacturing practice (cGMP). The facility must be purpose-built to comply with regulatory authorities, which in the UK comprise the Human Tissue Authority (HTA) and the Medicines and Healthcare products Regulatory Authority (MHRA). These regulations are designed to ensure that each laboratory produces a safe, consistent and traceable

product, by influencing the structural design of the laboratory, the documentation of standard operating procedures and of individual isolations, and training of members of the isolation team. Modern islet isolation is therefore expensive and requires a large number of staff to cover a 24/7 on-call rota. In the UK, a hub-and-spoke model exists, whereby three isolation facilities provide islets for transplantation in seven centres.

## THE ISLET TRANSPLANT

In the original Edmonton protocol, > 11 000 IEQ/kg were required to achieve insulin independence and therefore at least two islet infusions are normally required.[74] Islet preparations are blood group matched with the potential recipient, but the need for close tissue matching is not clear. There is no evidence that closely matched preparations have a better outcome; however, it is likely to be beneficial to avoid repeated common mismatches as recipients may, in the event of graft rejection, become sensitised to multiple common alloantigens.

The islets are normally infused into the portal vein of the recipient under local anaesthetic and sedation in the radiology suite.[105] A 4-Fr cannula is introduced under ultrasound and videofluoroscopy into the main portal vein and the islet preparation infused under gravity feed over a period of 15–20 minutes (Fig. 10.6). PV pressures are measured during the infusion process and if there is a significant rise, the infusion should be stopped until the portal pressure falls. The islet preparation is heparinised (35 U/kg patient body weight) to reduce the risk of portal vein thrombosis. This should ideally be done by experienced interventional radiologists and the track of the cannula occluded on withdrawal to reduce the risk of bleeding. The infusion into the portal vein can also be carried out by surgical cannulation of an omental vessel or the umbilical vein. The intraportal site for islet embolisation was recognised to be the most efficient location for islet implantation in the rodent, with the benefit of high vascularity, proximity to islet-specific nutrient factors and physiological first-pass insulin delivery to the liver.[106] While many different sites have been tried for islet implantation, the optimal site appears to be through PV embolisation. Attempts to embolise the spleen have led to significant life-threatening complications of splenic infarction, rupture and even gastric perforation.[107,108] More recently, reports of experimental implantation of islets into the gastric submucosa have shown improved vascularisation of the graft.[109] Recent developments in encapsulation technology have stimulated interest in using alternative sites. Encapsulation devices protect the islets from immunological attack while allowing insulin to be secreted.[110] Such devices have been implanted subcutaneously, intramuscularly and into the omentum, but with limited clinical application to date.

After infusion into the liver, the islets undergo a process of angiogenesis, which takes 14–21 days. Interestingly, this is often reflected in the reduced need for insulin in islet graft recipients around 3–4 weeks post-transplant.

## IMMUNOSUPPRESSION AND OUTCOMES

All seven patients in the original Edmonton experience were insulin-independent at 1 year post-transplant; however,

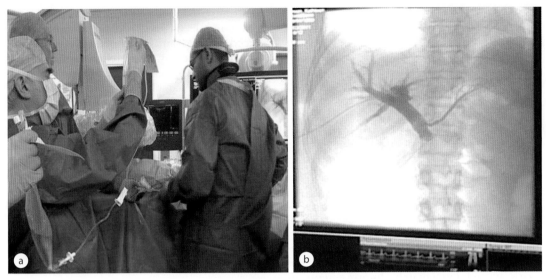

**Figure 10.6** Islet infusion into the portal vein.

follow-up of this cohort revealed that only 10% remained free of insulin at 5 years.[111] Alternative immunosuppression strategies have been reported in an attempt to improve these long-term outcomes. T-cell-depleting agents such as antithymocyte globulin (ATG), anti-CD3 and alemtuzumab (campath/anti-CD52) have been used as alternative induction therapy and combined with agents such as etanercept/tumour necrosis factor (TNF)-α or MMF/tacrolimus as maintenance therapy.[112] Barton et al.[113] have published data from the Collaborative Islet Transplant Registry on 677 patients receiving 1375 islet infusions between 1999 and 2010. These data demonstrated a significant improvement in long-term insulin independence in the 2007–2010 era compared with earlier years (Fig. 10.7), with 3-year insulin independence approaching 50%. This report also documented that patients who received T-cell-depleting agents combined with TNF-α inhibition had better 3- to 5-year insulin independence rates (62% vs 43%). More recently, data from the UK and the US clearly demonstrate that islet transplantation provides protection from severe hypoglycaemic episodes, restores awareness of hypoglycaemia and improves glycaemic control.[114,115] A recent analysis of the UK islet cell transplant programme demonstrated 94% 1-year graft survival in recipients of two transplants. Furthermore, 64% of those with uninterrupted graft function at 1 year sustained graft function at 6 years.[116]

Serious adverse events after islet transplantation are either related to the infusion procedure or the immunosuppression. The more serious procedure-related complications of segmental portal vein thrombosis and bleeding have been reported in 4% and 10%, respectively.[117,118] The risk of portal vein thrombosis can be minimised by heparinisation of the recipient and by using only low-volume, high-purity preparations. Bleeding from the liver puncture can be avoided by using a fine-bore cannula and by ablating the track in the liver using coils, thrombostatic agents or a coagulative laser.[105] Leukopenia, neutropenia and sepsis have all been described after islet transplantation.[119] A reduction in estimated glomerular filtration rate has been described in islet transplant recipients in the long-term post-transplantation, but reports of clinically significant renal impairment are rare.[113]

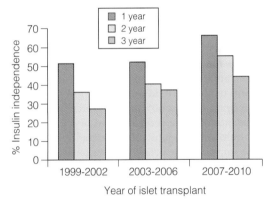

**Figure 10.7** Improvement in long-term insulin independence after islet transplantation from 1999 to 2010.[113]

One of the biggest challenges in islet transplantation is monitoring the graft. No reliable investigations exist to monitor graft function or detect acute rejection. Experimental studies in rats suggest that islets labelled with superparamagnetic iron oxide (SPIO) nanoparticles can be monitored using MRI scanning and that loss of the islet-related MRI spots correlates with rejection.[120] Metabolic studies such as the C-peptide response to a glucose challenge may give an indirect indication of ongoing graft mass but as yet cannot aid in predicting acute rejection.[121]

## BARRIERS TO LONG-TERM FUNCTION

Figure 10.8 illustrates the multiple factors that contribute to islet death and subsequent graft failure. The organ retrieval process and subsequent CIT have a significant negative impact on the outcome of islet isolation. The increasing use of pancreases from DCD donors where there have not been physiological changes associated with brain death may be beneficial for islet isolation, and techniques such as using extracorporeal membrane oxygenation (ECMO) circuits in the donor may result in islets that are protected from ischaemic change. There is no doubt that minimising the time between cross-clamp in the donor and beginning the isolation process in the laboratory improves the islet

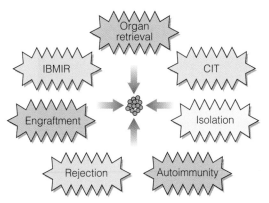

**Figure 10.8** Barriers to long-term islet graft function. *CIT,* cold ischaemia time; *IBMIR,* immediate blood-mediated inflammatory reaction.

yield and long-term graft function, requiring that pancreases must be transported rapidly to the laboratory and the isolation process started immediately. Improvements in isolation techniques have seen an increase in the average number of islets that can be produced per isolation with resultant improvements in graft survival.

There is an immediate blood-mediated inflammatory reaction (IBMIR) to the islet graft as soon as the islets are infused into the portal vein. Platelets bind to the surface of the islets and leucocytes infiltrate the graft. This contributes largely to the early loss of islets post-transplantation, which can be as high as 60% of the graft.[122] Strategies such as heparinisation of the recipient and ongoing insulin therapy may help to abrogate this process.[123] Little is known about the engraftment process of human islets within the liver. Transient elevation of liver enzymes is very common post-islet transplantation and it is interesting that the use of anti-inflammatory agents such as TNF-α blockers appears to improve graft survival.

## ISLETS AS A CELL THERAPY

The shortage of organ donors coupled with the increased demand for islets has led to much research into alternative sources of insulin-producing cells that would be renewable and not depend solely on the availability of human cadaveric donors. The use of foetal or adult porcine islets for human xenotransplants has been explored; however, the high levels of immunosuppression required and the risk of transmission of porcine endogenous infections means that xenotransplantation is still some way in the future.

Stem cells are capable of both self-renewal and multilineage differentiation. They have the potential to proliferate and differentiate into any type of cell and to be genetically modified in vitro, thus providing a renewable source of cells for transplantation. Several potential strategies exist for developing a replenishable supply of beta cells. One of these is through directed differentiation of human embryonic stem cells (hESCs).[124] Functioning beta cells have been produced using this technology, but concerns have been raised around the reproducibility of these processes and the potential for these cells to develop into teratomas. In 2006, Takahashi and Yamanaka described a technique whereby adult somatic cells could be de-differentiated and then induced to develop into different cell types.[125] They used a cocktail of

four transcription factors to produce these induced pluripotent stem cells (iPS cells), and many groups have now reproduced this work and developed cells of multiple lineages using this technology. The Melton group demonstrated that, in vivo, three transcription factors are required for beta-cell development, namely Ngn3, Pdx1 and MafA.[126] These are encouraging steps forward in the development of stem cell-derived islets, but there are still issues around upscaling of cell numbers and the potential for residual de-differentiated cells to produce tumours in the recipient. Recent developments in large-scale beta-cell production in vivo are grounds for optimism, and an exciting prospect is the potential existence of stem cells within the pancreas that could develop into new beta cells or with the potential to transdifferentiate non-endocrine tissue into functioning islets.[127–129]

## Key points

- As of the end of 2010, over 35 000 pancreas transplants have been performed worldwide. In the US alone, there are more than 100 000 patients with functioning transplants; around 10 000 of these are pancreas allografts.
- The outcome following pancreas transplantation has improved considerably in the last 10–15 years. It is now comparable to the outcome for other solid-organ transplants.
- The number of pancreas transplants reached a peak in 2004. Activity has been declining in the US since then in all three categories. An overall decrease of 20% was observed in 2010, compared with 2004. The largest decrease was observed in the PAK category (55%), followed by PTA (30%) and SPK (8%).
- Pancreas transplantation activity in the UK has followed a different pattern, with a much sharper increase in activity between 2000 and 2007, followed by a more modest decline since then.
- Despite the reduction in activity, pancreas transplant outcomes have remained at least as good in the last decade.
- Induction immunosuppression with biological agents is used in pancreas transplantation more often than any other solid-organ transplant. Tacrolimus/MMF combination is the basis of the most commonly used maintenance immunosuppression protocols. Steroid minimisation or avoidance is gaining momentum.
- Over the last 15 years, enteric drainage has gradually replaced bladder drainage as the preferred technique for the management of exocrine secretions in pancreas transplantation.
- Portal venous drainage, introduced in the mid-1990s, has not gained increasing popularity. It is used in just under a fifth of SPK and PAK transplants, and in 10% of PTA transplants.
- Evidence regarding the influence of pancreas transplantation on diabetic complications and life expectancy is not available from prospective controlled trials. Nevertheless, accumulating evidence from many studies strongly suggests that successful pancreas transplantation has a favourable influence on diabetic complications and survival prospects for patients.
- Islet transplantation is now considered as 'standard of care' for patients with type I diabetes and severely impaired awareness of hypoglycaemia.
- The long-term outcomes of islet transplantation have improved significantly over the last 10 years, with insulin independence at 3 years approaching that of whole pancreas transplantation.
- Immunosuppression with T-cell-depleting agents appears to give the best long-term graft survival.

 References available at http://ebooks.health.elsevier.com/

## ▶ RECOMMENDED VIDEO

- Pancreas and islet cell transplant – https://youtu.be/z_mb9_FHdgI

## KEY REFERENCES

[35] Papadimitriou JC, Drachenberg CB. Distinctive morphological features of antibody mediated and T-cell mediated acute rejection in pancreas allograft biopsies. Curr Opin Organ Transplant 2012;17:93–9. PMID: 22227719.

*This publication provides an authorative review of the histological criteria for acute pancreas allograft rejection and the mechanisms leading to graft injury.*

[36] Mittal S, Page SL, Friend PJ, et al. De novo donor-specific HLA antibodies: biomarkers of pancreas transplant failure. Am J Transplant 2014;14(7):1664–71. PMID: 24866735.

*In a multivariate analysis of 433 pancreas transplants at the Oxford Transplant Centre, development of de novo donor-specific antibodies (DSA) emerged as a strong independent predictor of pancreas graft failure (hazard ratio 4.66, P < 0.001).*

[57] The Diabetes Control and Complications Trial Research Group. The effect of intensive treatment of diabetes on the development and progression of long-term complications in insulin dependent diabetes mellitus. N Engl J Med 1993;329:977–86. PMID: 8366922.

*This paper provides good evidence that better blood glucose control reduces the risk of progression of retinopathy.*

[74] Shapiro AM, Lakey JR, Ryan EA, et al. Islet transplantation in seven patients with type 1 diabetes mellitus using a glucocorticoid-free immunosuppressive regimen. N Engl J Med 2000;343(4):230–8. PMID: 10911004.

*This publication from the Edmonton group demonstrated that long-term insulin independence can be achieved with islet transplantation and paved the way for the modern era of islet transplantation.*

[96] Ricordi C, Lacy PE, Scharp DW. Automated islet isolation from human pancreas. Diabetes 1989;38(Suppl. 1):140–2. PMID: 2642838.

*This paper was the first to describe the semi-automated technique of human islet isolation – a technique that is still used by islet laboratories worldwide.*

[113] Barton FB, Rickels MR, Alejandro R, et al. Improvement in outcomes of clinical islet transplantation: 1999–2010. Diabetes Care 2012;35(7):1436–45. PMID: 22723582.

*Data from the CITR is presented in this paper that demonstrates improved outcomes after islet transplantation over three eras, with a 3-year insulin independence rate after islet transplantation of > 40% in the current era.*

# 11 The spleen and adrenal glands

Brendan Visser | Geoffrey W. Krampitz | Garrison Carlos

## INTRODUCTION

The spleen is a little understood organ largely mystifying early physicians since antiquity. It was not until the latter half of the 20th century that the spleen's four main functions are better understood: antibody presentation and production, foetal haematopoiesis, sequestration of formed blood elements, and phagocytosis for recycling of blood cells, iron and particulate matter. Though splenic primary and secondary malignancies are rare, the differential diagnosis and indications for surgical splenectomy remain broad. Indications include traumatic rupture, autoimmune disorders, red blood cell dyscrasias, vascular abnormalities, lymphomas or myeloproliferative disorders, adjacent organ resection, hypersplenism/cytopenias or abscesses/cysts. Given the immunological consequences of asplenism—notably overwhelming post-splenectomy infection syndrome (OPSI)—the indications for complete surgical resection have evolved, giving rise to splenic conservation in trauma and left upper quadrant operations.

## ANATOMY AND EMBRYOLOGY

The spleen is the largest reticuloendothelial organ, defined by monocyte progenitors participating in phagocytosis and antigen presentation, approximately the size of a clenched fist measuring 10 to 12 cm in length and normally weighting 150–250 g.[1] The spleen has two surfaces, the diaphragmatic surface that is smooth and convex and is in contact with the diaphragm, and the visceral surface that is irregular and concave and has impressions contacting the fundus of the stomach, left kidney, splenic flexure of the colon and tail of the pancreas. The spleen is invested by two fibrous capsules, the outer tunica serosa that is derived contiguous with the peritoneum and invests the organ except at the hilum, where the peritoneum reflects into the phrenicocolic and gastrosplenic ligaments, and the tunica albuginea that invests the entire organ and at the hilum is reflected inward along the vessels to form sheaths from which the trabecular framework of the spleen emanates. The spleen is an intraperitoneal organ that is suspended by multiple ligamentous folds of peritoneum, namely, the gastrosplenic connecting the hilum of the spleen with the greater curvature of the stomach, the splenorenal connecting the hilum of the spleen to the left kidney and containing the splenic vessels and tail of the pancreas, and the phrenicocolic connecting the left colic flexure and diaphragm to the diaphragmatic

surface of the spleen.[2] The spleen forms from the cephalic aspect of the lateral plate mesoderm during the 5th week of gestation. Multiple aggregations of mesodermal cells condense to form a single organ. In up to 11% of individuals, one or more of these aggregates of splenic tissue fails to condense, and instead forms an accessory spleen, or splenules.[3]

The spleen derives its major blood supply from the splenic artery, which emanates from the abdominal aorta as a branch of the coeliac trunk, traverses a tortuous course along the superior border of the pancreas, giving rise to the left gastroepiploic artery and short gastric arteries before dividing into multiple branches that enter the hilum of spleen. The arteries ramify throughout the organ radially into splenic arterioles that branch into penicillar arterioles that ultimately terminate in splenic cords. Here, the reticuloendothelial cells and splenic macrophages come in intimate contact with blood and its contents as it percolates through the splenic cords and across walls of the splenic sinuses. Owing to the large amount of infiltrating blood, the red pulp is a principal site of blood filtration, where ageing blood cells are destroyed via programmed cell removal.[4] Scattered throughout the red pulp are local expansions of lymphocytes that appear as white pulp (Fig. 11.1). White pulp is closely associated with central arterioles that are surrounded by periarterial lymphatic sheaths containing T lymphocytes. Surrounding the T lymphocytes are follicles that contain B lymphocytes. In response to antigen presentation, these B lymphocytes become activated and produce antibodies that play a significant role in opsonisation of extracellular organisms including encapsulated bacteria. Between the red and white pulps is a marginal zone that contains antigen-presenting cells crucial for initiating lymphocyte activation. The association of lymphoid and myeloid cells in the red and white pulp makes the spleen a principal site of intersection between the innate and adaptive immune systems.[1] The major vascular outflow from the spleen occurs via coalescence of the open sinuses via reticular trabeculae into the splenic vein, which exits via the hilum of the spleen and courses medially to converge with the superior and inferior mesenteric veins to form the portal vein.

## MANAGEMENT OF SURGICAL ASPLENIA

Splenectomy decreases innate and adaptive immune responses which can manifest in OPSI. OPSI is the development of a fulminant, rapidly fatal bacterial infection following splenectomy. OPSI is the most feared complication after removal of the spleen. All patients undergoing splenectomy

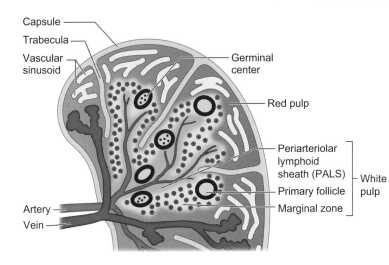

**Figure 11.1** Microscopic anatomical features of the spleen. The red pulp of the spleen is the principal site of blood filtration where reticuloendothelial cells and splenic macrophages come into intimate contact with the blood and its contents as it percolates through the splenic cords and across walls of the splenic sinuses. The white pulp of the spleen is local expansions of lymphocytes scattered throughout the red pulp. White pulp is closely associated with central arterioles and their surrounding periarterial lymphatic sheaths that contain T lymphocytes, which are surrounded by clusters of B lymphocytes. Between the red and white pulps is a marginal zone that contains antigen-presenting cells crucial for initiating lymphocyte activation.

or at high risk for splenectomy should receive vaccinations for the encapsulated bacteria *Streptococcus pneumoniae*, *Haemophilus influenzae* type b and *Neisseria meningitidis*. Administration is recommended 14 days after emergent splenectomy or prior to discharge from the hospital if patient follow-up is tenuous. For elective splenectomy, vaccinations should be given at least 14 days prior but ideally 10 to 12 weeks in advance; however, early vaccination is difficult to realise in practice.[4]

✔✔ Patients undergoing splenectomy should have appropriate vaccinations, prior to procedure when possible.

Depending on the country of practice and vaccinations available, providers should anticipate multiple temporally spaced doses for optimal response against meningococcal and pneumococcal serotypes. All other recommended vaccinations, such as seasonal influenza, should be administered. In high-risk patients, daily penicillin-based prophylactic regimens may be preferred with clarithromycin being an acceptable alternative in highly allergic patients unable to be desensitised. High risk applies to children withing the first year of splenectomy or younger then 5 years of age. Additionally, any patient, regardless of age, with a concurrent immunocompromising condition is considered high risk. The risk of OPSI does depend on the indication behind the resection. When trauma is the indication, OPSI is nearly five times less likely to occur when compared with haematological malignancies. Left upper quadrant solid tumour resections with simultaneous splenectomy also appear to have a lower incidence of OPSI and are generally not prescribed daily prophylactic antibiotics.[5]

## INDICATIONS FOR SPLENECTOMY

Traumatic splenic injury was previously the most common indication for splenectomy and routinely performed through celiotomy during exploratory surgery; however, medical indications are overtaking indications for splenectomies performed worldwide.[6] Haematologic diseases, like immune thrombocytopenia (ITP), are now among the most

common indications. Elective splenectomy allows for preoperative planning, appropriate vaccinations and use of minimally invasive approaches.

## TRAUMA

The spleen's juxtaposition in the left upper abdomen to the 9th, 10th and 11th ribs renders some protection posteriorly, though the spleen remains at risk of injury during blunt or penetrating trauma. Haemodynamically unstable patients should undergo emergency celiotomy and splenectomy without delay. The use of focused assessment with sonography for trauma (FAST) is particularly useful in cases of patient instability where an abdominal source of extravasation is not certain. FAST allows rapid diagnosis and preparation for abdominal exploration if free fluid or a large perisplenic anechoic band is seen. Patients who are haemodynamically stable should undergo abdominal computed tomography (CT) with intravenous contrast and delayed phases to evaluate the extent of splenic injury. The most widely used grading criteria for traumatic splenic injuries is shown in Table 11.1.[7] Non-operative management (NOM) has become the standard of care for haemodynamically stable patients with low to moderate-grade injuries (grade I–III) in the absence of peritonitis or active extravasation on initial contrast-enhanced CT. Contrast blush on CT imaging by itself is not an indication for selective angioembolisation (SAE) or operative intervention and may not be seen on subsequent angiography, especially in paediatrics.[8,9] Failure of NOM, defined as hypotension or evidence of ongoing haemorrhage requiring operative intervention, is associated with hypotension on presentation, grade III injury with contrast blush, or grade IV/V injuries.[10] Furthermore, 95% of NOM failures occur within 72 hours of injury.[11] Increasingly, spleen-preserving SAE is performed as an adjunct to prevent NOM failure in patients with grade IV or V injuries or following failure of NOM. Angiography is reasonable in patients with evidence of ongoing bleeding or contrast blush as well as moderate haemoperitoneum.[12] Success rates vary widely depending on the institution and protocols used, but centres that perform angioembolisation frequently have reduced splenectomy rates.[13,14]

**Table 11.1   Spleen organ injury scale (2018 revision)**

| AAST grade | AIS severity | Imaging criteria (CT findings) | Operative/Pathologic criteria |
|---|---|---|---|
| I | 2 | - Subcapsular haematoma < 10% surface area<br>- Parenchymal laceration < 1 cm depth<br>- Capsular tear | Identical to CT findings |
| II | 2 | - Subcapsular haematoma 10–50% surface area; intraparenchymal haematoma < 5 cm<br>- Parenchymal laceration 1–3 cm | Identical to CT findings |
| III | 3 | - Subcapsular haematoma > 50% surface area; ruptured subcapsular or intraparenchymal haematoma > 5 cm<br>Parenchymal laceration > 3 cm depth | Identical to CT findings |
| IV | 4 | - Any injury in the presence of splenic vascular injury or active bleeding confined within splenic capsule<br>- Parenchymal laceration involving segmental or hilar vessels producing > 25% devascularisation | - Parenchymal laceration involving segmental or hilar vessels producing > 25% devascularisation |
| V | 5 | - Any injury in the presence of splenic vascular injury with active bleeding extending beyond the spleen into the peritoneum.<br>- Shattered spleen | - Hilar vascular injury which devascularises the spleen<br>- Shattered spleen |

Vascular injury is defined as a pseudoaneurysm or arteriovenous fistula and appears as a focal collection of vascular contrast that decreases in attenuation with delayed imaging. Active bleeding from a vascular injury presents as vascular contrast, focal or diffuse, that increases in size or attenuation in delayed phase. Vascular thrombosis can lead to organ infarction. Grade based on highest grade assessment made on imaging, at operation or on pathologic specimen. More than one grade of splenic injury may be present and should be classified by the higher grade of injury. Advance one grade for multiple injuries up to a grade III.
From Kozar RA, Crandall M, Shanmuganathan K, et al. Organ injury scaling 2018 update: Spleen, liver, and kidney. J Trauma Acute Care Surg 2018;85(6):1119–1122.

✓✓ Selective angioembolisation should be considered in grade IV and V splenic injuries. There is evidence of retained splenic function following SAE, although significant complications including pain, fever, hyposplenism, splenic abscess, splenic infarction, contrast-induced renal insufficiency or pancreatitis do occur (Fig. 11.2).[15,16]

## HAEMATOLOGICAL

## THROMBOCYTOPENIC DISORDERS

### IMMUNE THROMBOCYTOPENIA AND THROMBOTIC THROMBOCYTOPENIC PURPURA

The most common indication for splenectomy is in patients with ITP. ITP, previously known as idiopathic thrombocytopenic purpura, is an autoimmune disorder characterised by both antibody-induced platelet destruction and decreased antibody production while clinically absent splenomegaly. ITP has an incidence rate of 3.3 per 100,000 adults and 1.9–6.4 per 100,000 children per year.[17] Children are more likely to achieve remission, whereas adults are at higher risk of developing chronic ITP defined by greater than 12 months of ongoing disease. ITP is nearly always initially treated with glucocorticoids. Splenectomy was previously indicated for steroid refractory ITP.[18] Now, rituximab and thrombopoietin-receptor agonists (TPO-RA), such as romiplostim, are mainstays of the traditional armamentarium and recommended prior to undergoing splenectomy. Splenectomy is superior to TPO-RA and rituximab in achieving durable responses (86.7%, 65.7%, and 62.1%, respectively); however, splenectomy is generally postponed until after at least a year of diagnosis due to the higher chance of spontaneous remission or medical cure.[19,20] Laparoscopic approach achieved equal remission rates as open splenectomy.[21]

✓✓ Laparoscopic splenectomy should be performed in refractory ITP following failure of steroid and TPO-RA therapy (Fig. 11.3).

## THROMBOTIC THROMBOCYTOPENIC PURPURA

Once uniformly fatal, thrombotic thrombocytopenic purpura (TTP) is an autoimmune disorder caused by antibodies to ADAMTS13 that results in altered von Willebrand factor homeostasis leading to thrombotic microangiopathy. TTP classically has been defined as the pentad of fever, thrombocytopenia, microangiopathic haemolytic anaemia, renal dysfunction and neurologic symptoms, although presentation of these symptoms is highly variable. Acutely, TTP is treated with plasmapheresis, which results in remission in more than 80% of cases. Patients who are refractory to plasmapheresis or who develop recurrence of disease require splenectomy.[22] The majority of patients undergoing splenectomy experience complete disease remission.[23]

## ERYTHROCYTE DISORDERS

### HEREDITARY SPHEROCYTOSIS AND PYRUVATE KINASE DEFICIENCY

Hereditary spherocytosis (HS) is an autosomal dominant or recessive abnormality of erythrocytes caused by mutations in membrane structural proteins. These mutations lead to cytoskeletal instability resulting in alteration of the normal biconcave erythrocytes into pathognomonic spherocytes that are osmotically fragile and prone to rupture. Cells with these dysfunctional proteins are degraded in the spleen leading to anaemia, jaundice and splenomegaly. A common complication of HS is cholelithiasis from pigmented stones. Splenectomy is curative, and

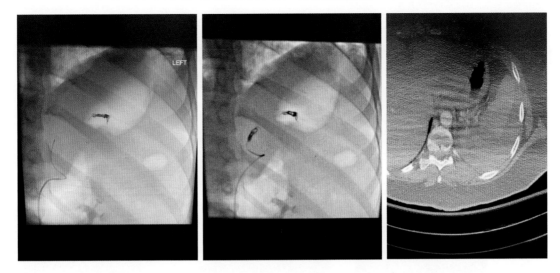

**Figure 11.2** Angiogram during selective angioembolisation of active splenic haemorrhage. A 25-year-old female presenting as major trauma following motor vehicle collision with grade IV splenic laceration and contrast blush. Initial haematocrit remained stable and interventional radiology performed expectant selective embolisation at redemonstrated contrast blush. First coil migrated distally and second coil was placed. She experienced no complications and was discharged after receiving appropriate vaccinations.

concurrent cholecystectomy should be performed if indicated. Similarly, pyruvate kinase deficiency is an autosomal recessive mutation that causes decreased conversion of phosphoenolpyruvate to pyruvate, thereby leading to decreased ability to form ATP and increasing oxidative injury to erythrocytes. Subsequently, the spleen, removes the damaged erythrocytes leading to severe anaemia which can be fatal in utero. The disease represents the most common cause of hereditary non-spherocytic haemolytic anaemia at a rate of nearly 5:100 000.[24] Splenectomy leads to increased haemoglobin levels but does not eliminate ongoing haemolysis. Patients undergoing splenectomy should also be evaluated for cholecystectomy.

## SICKLE CELL ANAEMIA AND THALASSAEMIA

Other disorders of erythrocyte structure include sickle cell anaemia (SCA) and thalassaemia. SCA is an autosomal recessive disease caused by mutations in haemoglobin subunit beta-globin, which leads to reductions of the elasticity of the protein under conditions of low oxygen tension that result in deforming of the erythrocyte into a sickle shape. A major feature of SCA is painful episodes of sickle cell crisis complicated by vaso-occlusion, aplastic or haemolytic anaemia, as well as splenic sequestration. Splenic sequestration can lead to hypersplenism and ultimately splenic infarction. Treatments include blood transfusion and hydroxycarbamide with splenectomy for refractory cases.[25] Thalassaemia comprise a group of genetic disorders that lead to abnormal ratios or absence of haemoglobin subunits. Beta-thalassaemia results in an excess of alpha-globin that forms insoluble tetramers which precipitate within the erythrocyte interfering with erythropoiesis, cell maturation and function, leading to anaemia. Alpha-thalassaemia results in an excess of beta-globin that also forms tetramers, which, under conditions of stress, precipitate leading to anaemia. Treatment of thalassaemia includes blood transfusion and iron chelation therapy.[26] Splenectomy is indicated in high transfusion-dependent patients with hypersplenism.

## FELTY SYNDROME AND AUTOIMMUNE HAEMOLYTIC ANAEMIA

Autoimmune haemolytic anaemia (AIHA) is a heterogenous group of disorders caused by antibodies directed against erythrocytes leading to Fc or complement-mediated haemolysis in the spleen. Patients can present with severely low haemoglobin levels below 6 g/dL and will have a positive Coombs test unless drug-induced. AIHA can be primary, idiopathic or secondary to another underlying illness (lymphoproliferative disorders and other autoimmune disorders) or drug reactions. Treatment includes immunosuppressive therapies (corticosteroids, rituximab, azathioprine) and splenectomy in refractory cases. Individuals most likely to benefit from splenectomy are patients with warm AIHA antibodies or antibodies secondary to a splenic marginal zone lymphoma. Overall, the efficacy of splenectomy is nearly 75% which is comparable with glucocorticoid treatment. When planning surgery, note that 30% of patients may have splenomegaly.[27]

Felty syndrome comprises a triad of rheumatoid arthritis, splenomegaly and neutropenia. Approximately 1–3% of all patients with rheumatoid arthritis are affected by Felty syndrome. Increased mortality is associated with recurrent infections due to neutropenia secondary to decreased granulogenesis and increased peripheral destruction of granulocytes. Although the exact cause of Felty syndrome is unknown, it is thought to be an autoimmune disorder associated with HLA-DR4, rheumatoid factor and antinuclear antibody. Neutropenia can be effectively treated with disease-modifying anti-rheumatic drugs. Splenectomy results in immediate improvement of neutropenia in 80% of patients and is only indicated in patients with severe or recurrent neutropenia and infections.[28]

## NEOPLASTIC

A number of neoplasms may require splenectomy including Hodgkin's lymphoma, non-Hodgkin's lymphoma (NHL), chronic myelogenous leukaemia (CML), chronic lymphocytic

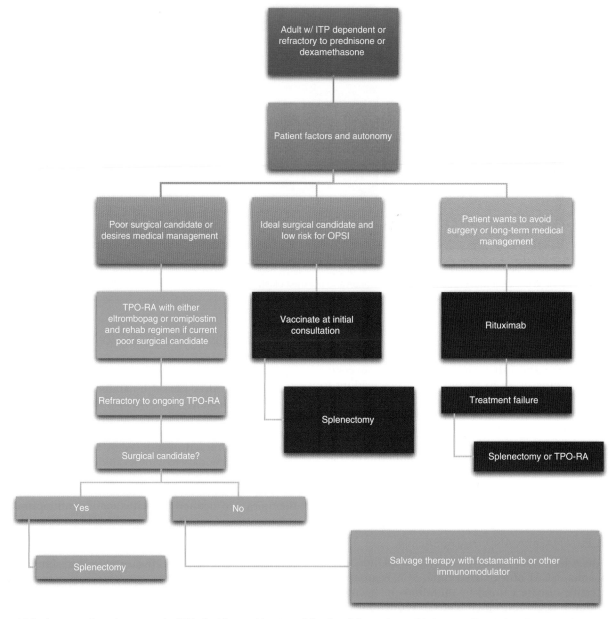

**Figure 11.3** Immune thrombocytopenia (ITP) decision-making tree following failure of steroid therapy. Three-tiered approach to treatment of ITP following steroid therapy. *ITP,* immune thrombocytopenia; *OPSI,* overwhelming post-splenectomy infection; *TPO-RA,* thrombopoietin-receptor agonist.

leukaemia (CLL), hairy cell leukaemia (HCL), littoral cell angiomas, haemangiosarcomas, hamartomas, primary myelofibrosis or splenic lymphomas. Another important indication for splenectomy is adjacent abdominal neoplasms in which the splenic artery cannot be preserved for oncologic resection. Overall, the indications for splenectomy have greatly decreased due to more efficacious, anti-neoplastic medications, radiographic staging and image-guided biopsies.

## HODGKIN'S LYMPHOMA AND LEUKAEMIA

Representing the minority of lymphomas, Hodgkin's lymphoma is a neoplastic proliferation of large B cells with multilobed nuclei termed Reed–Sternberg cells which nearly always stain positive for CD15 and CD30. The disease classically presents with systemic symptoms such as fever, chills, weight loss, and enlarging cervical or mediastinal lymph nodes. Traditionally,

Hodgkin's lymphoma was staged by laparotomy and splenectomy, although this is no longer necessary. Following the Ann Arbor Staging Classification, only patients with early stage I or II disease and uncertain radiographic findings should be considered for surgical staging. Since favourable stage I and II disease is routinely managed solely with involved field radiation, a negative splenectomy would spare the need for systemic chemotherapy. However, recent evidence suggests improved outcomes in combination with chemoradiation even in limited disease resulting in overall survival rates nearing 99% at 4 years. Involvement of the spleen mandates stage III disease and systemic chemotherapy in addition to radiation therapy—not splenectomy.[29–31]

Haematological malignancies such as HCL, CML and CLL may present with symptomatic splenomegaly and pancytopenia that may require splenectomy in selected patients.[32] Splenectomy does not improve survival for these patients but is rather palliative for cytopenias or abdominal distention. Primary splenic angiosarcoma is a rare and aggressive malignant neoplasm arising from splenic vascular endothelium. It is associated with a very poor prognosis, and splenectomy is the only chance of cure.[33] Littoral cell angioma are a rare primary vascular neoplasm from littoral cells which line the red pulp. Littoral cell angiomas are associated with other malignancies or Crohn's disease and have newly identified malignant potential; therefore, splenectomy is indicated.[34]

The most common primary sources of splenic metastasis are the breast, lung, colorectal, ovarian and melanoma. Splenectomy may be indicated in the event of oligometastatic disease. Although metastases to the spleen are usually asymptomatic, they may occasionally lead to splenomegaly or spontaneous rupture.

## INFECTIOUS

Infectious diseases involving the spleen may require splenectomy. Hydatid disease caused by *Echinococcus granulosus* in the spleen has been reported. Hydatidosis is treated with albendazole and en bloc resection of the parasitic cysts. Splenectomy must be performed without rupturing the cyst to avoid disseminated disease and potential anaphylactic reaction. Albendazole is an effective adjuvant therapy in the treatment of hydatid cyst.[35] Drug resistance is an increasingly common problem for common parasitic infections including trypanosomiasis, malaria and leishmaniasis. In the case of visceral leishmaniasis, termed kala-azar, splenectomy may be required for source control as untreated cases are nearly universally fatal. Until the recent development of miltefosine, resistance and progression of disease was unacceptably high. Common in sub-Saharan Africa, limited access to medical therapy of kala-azar makes splenectomy a necessary consideration. Bacterial splenic abscesses that are multiloculated, not amenable to percutaneous drainage, or that have failed to resolve with percutaneous drainage and antibiotics may require splenectomy. The spleen is a common site of septic embolism and abscesses commonly develop in patients with endocarditis, pneumonia, or perforation of gastrointestinal tract (Table 11.2).

## SPLENECTOMY

### OPEN

Open splenectomy is preferred in patients with splenomegaly and sinusoidal hypertension, although laparoscopic splenectomy for splenomegaly as large as 1500 g has been demonstrated safe with low conversion rates.[36] The procedure can be performed with the patient in the supine position with arms extended and using a midline or left subcostal incision depending on the indication. Packs are placed behind the spleen to elevate and bring it towards the midline. The colon is retracted inferiorly and the stomach is retracted superiorly to expose the gastrocolic ligament. The gastrocolic ligament is divided in the avascular plane to open the lesser sac and expose the splenic artery coursing along the superior border of the pancreas. The gastrosplenic ligament containing the short gastric arteries and the phrenicocolic ligament are divided to mobilise the spleen medially and allow elevation to expose the splenorenal ligament. Ligation and division of the splenic artery and vein using clamps and ties or a vascular linear stapling device is performed. Once the specimen is removed, the abdomen is inspected for accessory spleens, which are removed if found.

### LAPAROSCOPIC

Laparoscopic splenectomy has become the standard approach for removal of the spleen for most indications. The patient is positioned in the right lateral decubitus position flexed at the hip, which allows for maximum exposure of the left hypochondrium and gravity, to reveal the ligamentous attachments. The right arm is extended and the left arm suspended. Video monitors are positioned at the head of the bed. Four trocars are generally placed below the left costal margin once pneumoperitoneum is achieved. Alternatively, a supraumbilical midline incision for the creation of hand-assist port allows for a hand-assisted approach allowing laparoscopic resection of massive splenomegaly over 3000 g.[36] The optical trocar is usually inserted in the anterior axillary line below the left costal margin. Lateral working ports at the mid-axillary line and posterior-axillary line, as well as a medial working port at the mid-clavicular line below the left

**Table 11.2  Common pathophysiologies associated with splenic disease and relative benefit of splenectomy**

| Common indications | Rare indications | Contraindications |
|---|---|---|
| Required for oncologic resection of adjacent tumour (pancreatic) | Chronic lymphocytic leukaemia | Thrombocytopenia in hepatic cirrhosis |
| Warm autoimmune haemolytic anaemia (AIHA) | Splenic infarction | Cold agglutinin disease |
| Splenic abscesses | Primary myelofibrosis | Paroxysmal cold haemoglobinuria |
| Immune thrombocytopenia | Thrombotic thrombocytopenic purpura | Autoimmune lymphoproliferative syndrome (ALPS) |
| Hereditary spherocytosis | Gaucher's disease | |
| Felty syndrome | Hairy cell leukaemia | |
| Pyruvate kinase deficiency | Sickle cell disease sequestration crisis | |
| Massive splenomegaly | Thalassaemia | |
| Splenic marginal zone lymphoma | Hodgkin's lymphoma | |

costal margin are placed under direct vision. A medial to lateral dissection is the preferred technique. The lesser sac is entered through division of the gastrosplenic ligament and short gastric vessels, which mobilises the stomach medially to reveal the hilum of the spleen and splenorenal ligament containing the splenic artery and vein. In cases of splenomegaly, the arterial pedicle is taken first to limit inflow and decrease the spleen's size and potential blood loss. The vessels can be taken at this point followed by dissection of remaining peritoneal attachments. Care is taken when dividing the vascular hilum in order to protect the pancreas. The freed specimen is placed in a bag, morcellated and removed. Once the specimen is removed, the abdomen is inspected for accessory spleens, which are removed if found.

## ROBOTIC

Since the introduction of the Da Vinci robotic system, numerous surgical approaches have been tailored to the new technology. Robotic splenectomy is an appropriate choice for difficult dissections owing to the greater surgical range of motion; however, most study outcomes did not demonstrate significant benefit against the laparoscopic approach.[37–39] The robotic approach is associated with increased costs; however, there is evidence that in the appropriate hands, this may be the technique of choice in difficult dissections, subtotal splenectomies, splenic tumours or advanced cirrhosis with associated decreased operative time and decreased blood loss. To perform the robotic approach, the patient may be positioned in right lateral decubitus position or supine. Docking the robot should follow standard protocol with the left hypochondrium as the target. The dissection remains the same as the laparoscopic approach. Port placement is surgeon dependent and should follow established principals of port spacing.

## PARTIAL SPLENECTOMY

Partial splenectomy may be done open or laparoscopically, although a minimally invasive technique either robotically or laparoscopically is usually the preferred method.[40] The indications for partial splenectomy include benign tumours (hamartoma, epidermoid cyst, or localised lymphangioma or haemangioma) and haematologic conditions leading to hypersplenism. Partial splenectomy may not be performed for tumours that are centrally located due to the terminal blood supply of the spleen. Depending on the location of the tumour, the vessels terminating in the pole or region containing the abnormality are isolated. Placing a temporary clamp will create an area of demarcation to confirm the appropriate selection. The artery and vein are then divided in sequence (if the upper pole is selected, the short gastric vessels will be divided as well). The line of demarcation is then used to guide the transection along the surface of the parenchyma. The parenchyma is then cauterised and divided. The omentum can be placed in contact with the cut section of the spleen. The remainder of the procedure is similar to the laparoscopic approach.

## ADRENAL

### INTRODUCTION

The adrenal glands are robust bilateral neuroendocrine organs that are situated superiorly in relation to the kidneys. The word adrenal originated from the Latin *ad renalis*, meaning 'of the kidneys'. The modernisation of treatment for adrenal pathology stems from improvements in biochemical testing, understanding indications, and minimally invasive techniques for performing adrenalectomy with focus placed on preventative medicine.

### ANATOMY AND EMBRYOLOGY

The adrenal glands are retroperitoneal endocrine organs situated above and slightly medial to the kidneys within the renal fascia on both sides of the abdomen (Fig. 11.4). The

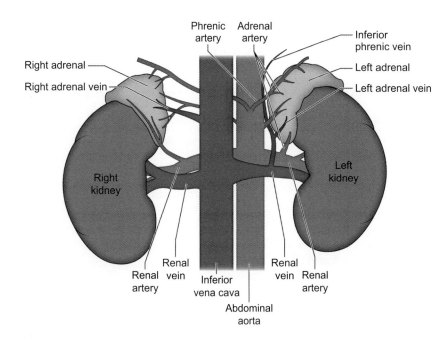

**Figure 11.4** Gross anatomical features of the adrenals. The adrenal glands are retroperitoneal endocrine organs situated above and slightly medial to the kidneys, which receive their blood supply from the superior, middle and inferior adrenal arteries. The right adrenal drains via a shorter right adrenal vein directly into the inferior vena cava, while the left adrenal gland drains via a longer left adrenal vein that is often joined by the left inferior phrenic vein before emptying into the left renal vein.

right adrenal gland has a pyramidal shape, whereas the left adrenal gland is semilunar. The left adrenal gland is bounded anteriorly by the peritoneum, tail of the pancreas and splenic artery, posteriorly by the left crus of the diaphragm and kidney, and medially by the left inferior phrenic artery and left gastric arteries. The right adrenal gland is bounded anteriorly by the inferomedial angle of the bare area of the liver, posteriorly by the diaphragm and superior pole of the right kidney, and medially by the inferior phrenic artery and vena cava. The adrenal glands are composed of two heterogenous types of tissue that are arranged into distinct components. The cortex is the outermost component of the adrenal gland and is derived from intermediate mesoderm. The cortex is subdivided into different layers, namely the zona glomerulosa, zona fasciculata and zona reticularis (Fig. 11.5). The medulla is the innermost component of the adrenal gland and is derived from neural crest cells (Fig. 11.5). The adrenal glands are highly vascular organs that receive their blood supply from the superior adrenal artery (a branch of the inferior phrenic artery), the middle adrenal artery (a direct branch from the aorta), and inferior adrenal artery (a branch of the ipsilateral renal artery) (Fig. 11.4). Venous drainage is different for the right and left adrenal glands. The right adrenal drains via a shorter right adrenal vein directly into the inferior vena cava, while the left adrenal gland drains via a longer left adrenal vein that is often joined by the left inferior phrenic vein before emptying into the left renal vein. Lymphatic drainage from the adrenal glands flows directly into the adjacent periaortic and paracaval nodes.

## PHYSIOLOGY

Two separate endocrine organs, namely the cortex and medulla, comprise the adrenal gland. The adrenal cortex metabolises cholesterol to produce different steroid hormones in each zone (Fig. 11.5). In all three zones, the rate-limiting step is the conversion of cholesterol to pregnenolone by cholesterol desmolase, which is directly regulated by adrenocorticotropic hormone (ACTH) from the pituitary, which in turn is regulated by corticotropin-releasing hormone (CRH) from the hypothalamus. The zona glomerulosa is the main site for the production of mineralocorticoids that regulate salt balance and blood volume. Aldosterone is the principal mineralocorticoid that acts by binding nuclear receptors in cells of the distal convoluted tubules and collecting duct of the kidneys and drives transcription of genes that activate basolateral Na/K pumps to increase reabsorption of sodium and excretion of potassium and acid. The zona fasciculata is the main site for production of glucocorticoids that have many effects on metabolism. The major glucocorticoid in humans, cortisol, is secreted directly into the circulation immediately upon its synthesis and circulates in both bound and free unbound state. The free form passes into target cells by diffusion and binds to cytosolic receptors found in virtually all cells in the body. Once bound to its receptor, cortisol not only has glucose-regulating properties but also exerts a myriad of effects on gluconeogenesis, glycogenesis, protein synthesis, lipolysis, mineral homeostasis, vascular tone, immunosuppression and wound healing. The zona reticularis is the principal site for androgen production. A series of hydroxylase and dehydrogenase enzymes convert pregnenolone to androstenedione and testosterone. These androgens can be modified by aromatases resulting in oestrone and oestradiol, and by 5-alpha-reductase to produce dihydrotestosterone, resulting in male characteristics during development.

There are a number of enzyme defects that can lead to adrenal dysfunction and congenital adrenal hyperplasia. The most common form of congenital adrenal hyperplasia is caused by a 21-hydroxylase deficiency that leads to excess androgen and mineralocorticoid, and deficient glucocorticoid resulting in salt-wasting dehydration and ambiguous genitalia or virilisation.

Like the peripheral sympathetic ganglia, the adrenal medulla is embryologically derived from neural crest cells. The medullary chromaffin cells have rudimentary nerve fibres and the ability to synthesise, store and secrete

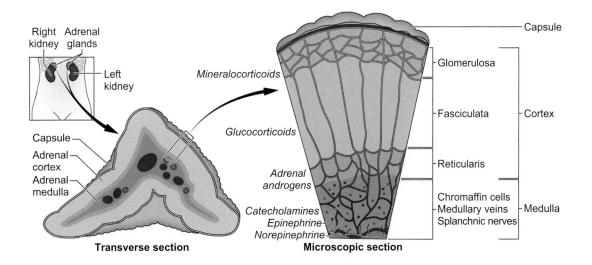

**Figure 11.5** Microscopic anatomical features of the adrenals. The adrenal glands are composed of an inner medulla and outer cortex. The adrenal medulla produces catecholamines. The adrenal cortex is divided into the zona glomerulosa, where mineralocorticoids are produced; zona fasciculata, where glucocorticoids are produced; and the zona reticularis, where androgens are produced.

catecholamines, primarily epinephrine.[41] The rate-limiting step is the formation of dopa from tyrosine via the enzyme tyrosine hydroxylase, which is principally regulated by ACTH. Although peripheral nerve terminals and the adrenal medulla both have the ability to produce norepinephrine, only the adrenal medulla contains the enzyme phenylethanolamine-N-methyltransferase (PNMT) that converts norepinephrine to epinephrine, which constitutes 80–85% of the adrenal medulla secretion. Catecholamines released by the adrenal medulla bind a large family of transmembrane-signalling adrenoreceptors to exert a variety of effects associated with acute stress responses, including tachycardia, hypertension, increased peripheral vascular resistance, gastrointestinal inactivation, bronchodilatation and increased metabolism.[42]

## INDICATIONS FOR ADRENALECTOMY

Adrenal masses may be benign or malignant and functional or non-functional. The systematic work-up of any suspected adrenal pathology should begin with a thorough history and physical examination investigating the possibility of functional symptoms and assessment for the rare possibility of a genetic syndrome. The history and physical examination should query for poorly controlled hypertension, diabetes, oedema, palpitations, diaphoresis, central obesity, weakness, striae, dorsocervical lipodystrophy, headaches, flushing or ecchymosis.

## DISORDERS OF ADRENAL HOMEOSTASIS

### PRIMARY HYPERALDOSTERONISM

Primary hyperaldosteronism is a small group of disorders defined by hypertension secondary to the overproduction of aldosterone with simultaneously suppressed plasma renin. The signs and symptoms of primary hyperaldosteronism are non-specific and include resistant hypertension and hypokalaemia, although a majority of patients present with normal potassium levels.[43] The incidence of hyperaldosteronism has increased by 5- to 15-fold in response to widespread adoption of screening via obtaining plasma aldosterone to plasma renin ratios in normokalaemic patients. Primary hyperaldosteronism is now recognised as the most common treatable form of hypertension representing up to 6% of patients with hypertension. The risk of underlying primary hyperaldosteronism increases in relation to the degree of hypertension such that severe hypertension has autonomous aldosterone secretion in up to 13% of cases.[44] Excess aldosterone, even in the absence of hypertension, is associated with excess risk for development of diastolic dysfunction, left ventricular hypertrophy, cerebrovascular complications and metabolic syndrome, highlighting the benefit of accurate identification and resection.[45]

The most common causes of primary aldosteronism are solitary aldosterone-producing adenomas (APA) or aldosteronomas and bilateral adrenal hyperplasia (BAH). Less common causes are familial hyperaldosteronism syndrome (some resolve with glucocorticoid administration) and aldosterone-producing adrenocortical carcinoma (ACC). Following a positive screening test via the aldosterone-to-renin ratio (ARR), confirmatory testing

and localisation of the disease is necessary—except in severe cases defined by undetectable renin, hypokalaemia, and significantly elevated plasma aldosterone.[46] Confirmatory testing can be done via captopril challenge, intravenous or oral saline loading and fludrocortisone suppression. Each method carries unique considerations and may not be appropriate depending on the patient's comorbidities—e.g. salt loading in congestive heart failure. Following a positive confirmatory test, adrenal protocol CT is performed to look for concerning masses (large adrenal cortical carcinomas producing aldosterone) or potential localising findings. Adrenal vein sampling (AVS) should be conducted in all patients except under strict criteria even in the setting of a potential localising lesion. Nearly 50% of imaging is found to be discordant with the true causative aldosteronoma after AVS.[47] Only in patients younger than 35 years with characteristic appearing adrenal adenomas should AVS be considered optional. If unilateral disease is confirmed, patient should undergo laparoscopic adrenalectomy. If bilateral disease is present, medical management with a mineralocorticoid receptor antagonist is the standard of care.

### CUSHING SYNDROME

Cushing syndrome results from prolonged exposure to elevated glucocorticoid levels. Adrenal Cushing disease represents nearly 10% of overt Cushing syndrome. The most common non-iatrogenic cause of this syndrome is Cushing disease, caused by an ACTH-producing pituitary adenoma. The pituitary adenomas of Cushing disease secrete excessive amounts of ACTH while retaining negative feedback responsiveness to high-dose glucocorticoids. In contrast, ectopic ACTH-producing tumours can also cause the syndrome but are insensitive to negative feedback by high doses of glucocorticoids allowing biochemical differentiation based on response to steroid administration. The major cause of ACTH-independent Cushing syndrome is a glucocorticoid-producing adrenal adenoma. Because these tumours secrete excessive cortisol, production of ACTH is suppressed in an otherwise normal hypothalamus–pituitary–adrenal axis. The initial step in the diagnosis of Cushing syndrome is to confirm the presence of elevated cortisol levels by measuring night time serum or salivary cortisol, 24-hour urinary cortisol and/or undertaking an overnight low-dose dexamethasone suppression test. The next step is to determine whether the cause of hypercortisolaemia is an ACTH-dependent or -independent process. If serum ACTH levels are suppressed, an ACTH-independent process originating from the adrenal glands is the likely cause of the syndrome. If serum ACTH levels are elevated, a high-dose dexamethasone suppression test is required. If ACTH levels are suppressed with high-dose dexamethasone, the likely aetiology is a pituitary tumour. However, if ACTH levels are unaffected by high-dose dexamethasone, an ectopic source of ACTH is the likely cause as commonly seen in paraneoplastic syndromes (frequently small cell lung cancer). Recent data suggest that testing for the presence of a low serum dehydroepiandrosterone sulphate (DHEAS) is as sensitive and more specific than the current gold standard of dexamethasone suppression test for diagnosing subclinical adrenal Cushing disease. DHEAS has a relatively long half-life compared with cortisol's diurnal pattern, allowing for better interpretation of results. In the setting of low ACTH or DHEAS, an adrenal CT should be performed to localise the tumour.[48] Adrenal adenomas are generally lipid rich with lower attenuation ( < 10 Hounsfield [HU] units) and are characterised by rapid enhancement and washout. Malignant lesions demonstrate slower washout and lower lipid content making CT preferable to magnetic resonance imaging (MRI) for identification. As is the case with aldosterone-producing adenomas, localisation should be confirmed by AVS. However, AVS may not always be diagnostic even when sampling is calibrated as a ratio of cosecretion with plasma aldosterone or plasma metanephrines. Nuclear imaging has also been used to localise lesions when AVS is non-diagnostic. Patients with unilateral and bilateral adrenal Cushing disease should undergo laparoscopic resection to remove involved glands (Table 11.3).

## NEOPLASTIC

### Pheochromocytoma

Pheochromocytoma is a catecholamine-secreting typically benign tumour that arises from the neuroectodermally derived chromaffin cells of the adrenal medulla. Paragangliomas are related tumours that arise from similar cells of the sympathetic ganglia. These tumours are rare, occurring in < 0.2% of patients with hypertension.[49] The majority of pheochromocytomas are benign, solitary and unilateral, and occur in adults. Pheochromocytomas are usually sporadic, although they can accompany genetic syndromes including multiple endocrine neoplasia (MEN) 2a and 2b caused by a number of somatic mutations in the gene *RET* that encodes a transmembrane receptor tyrosine kinase involved in a number of signalling pathways,[50] von Recklinghausen's syndrome caused by mutations in the *NF1* gene that encodes neurofibrin

1, a negative regulator of the ras signal transduction pathway, and von Hippel–Lindau syndrome caused by a mutation in the tumour suppressor *VHL* gene. Patients typically present with refractory hypertension, palpitations, headaches and diaphoresis. Symptoms are usually episodic with variable frequency and duration. The diagnosis of pheochromocytoma is dependent on demonstrating elevated catecholamines in the plasma or urine. Initially, plasma metanephrine and normetanephrine levels should be obtained. In addition, 24-hour urine vanillylmandelic acid, metanephrines and fractionated catecholamines may be obtained. Once a biochemical diagnosis has been made, the tumour can be localised by CT, MRI or [123]I meta-iodobenzylguanidine (MIBG) scan.

Patients with pheochromocytoma have chronic hypersecretion of catecholamines that causes volume contraction as well as haemodynamic and glycaemic instability. Thus, they must be premedicated with a selective alpha-adrenergic receptor blocker (phenoxybenzamine) for several weeks before proceeding to adrenalectomy. Postoperatively, patients are susceptible to vasoplegia and hypoglycaemia, and should be monitored closely.

## PRIMARY ADRENOCORTICAL CARCINOMA

ACCs are rare tumours that can be non-functional or in 60% of cases produce hyperaldosteronism, hypercortisolism and/or virilisation/feminisation. Androgen-secreting tumours—and to a greater degree oestrogen-secreting tumours—are usually malignant; however, hypercortisolism is the most frequent derangement encountered in nearly half of functional ACCs. ACCs are commonly diagnosed after producing clinical syndromes of hormonal excess, often developing rapidly, followed by clinically apparent abdominal mass or as an incidental finding on cross-axial imaging. Most ACCs are sporadic, but some occur as part of several hereditary cancer syndromes, including Li–Fraumeni syndrome caused by

**Table 11.3 Differentiating causes of hypercortisolism**

| Cause of Cushing disease | Cortisol level | Low-dose dexamethasone | DHEAS | ACTH | High-dose dexamethasone | Pathology | Treatment |
|---|---|---|---|---|---|---|---|
| Exogenous glucocorticoids | Increased | n/a | Low | Low | n/a (already low) | Bilateral adrenal atrophy | Reduction of exogenous steroids as able |
| Ectopic ACTH secretion | Increased | No suppression | Elevated | Elevated | No suppression | Bilateral adrenal hyperplasia | Standard of treatment for cause; e.g. chemotherapy for small cell lung cancer |
| Functional adenoma | Increased | No suppression | Low | Low | n/a (already low) | Incidentaloma or nodular hyperplasia | Unilateral adrenalectomy |
| ACTH-secreting pituitary adenoma | Increased | No suppression | Elevated | Elevated | Suppression | Bilateral adrenal hyperplasia | Transsphenoidal resection* |

*Cushing disease refractory to transsphenoidal resection may require bilateral adrenalectomy.
Biochemical changes associated with different causes of hypercortisolism.
*ACTH,* Adrenocorticotropic hormone.

inactivating mutations of the *TP53* tumour suppressor gene, Beckwith–Wiedemann syndrome caused by a mutation in the insulin-like growth factor 2 (*IGF2*) gene, and MEN1 caused by inactivating mutations of the *MEN1* tumour suppressor gene.[51]

In patients with suspected ACC, a significant number have distant metastases at presentation, usually to liver, lungs, lymph nodes and bone. Initially, a biochemical workup similar to those described above must be pursued and can provide medical treatment options even in unresectable disease. Additionally, fluorodeoxyglucose (FDG)/positron emission tomography (PET)/CT is also useful for determining distant sites of disease and can accurately distinguish between benign and malignant adrenal tumors.[52] Complete workup should include CT of the chest, abdomen and pelvis. MRI can be used for precise surgical planning allowing consideration of local invasion, vascular involvement, or tumour thrombosis within the inferior vena cava. If the ACC is determined to be localised disease, open adrenalectomy should be performed with consideration for mitotane and external beam radiation if high risk for local reoccurrence based on operative findings. High-risk features include positive final margins, gross tumour invasion, Ki-67 > 10%, rupture of capsule, large size or high-grade features. The 5-year disease-specific survival rate remains low in advanced stages. Complete surgical resection is the only potentially curative treatment for ACC, although mitotane, an adrenocorticolytic drug, is routinely used in the adjuvant setting or for unresectable or recurrent disease.[53–55]

## INCIDENTALOMA

Adrenal incidentalomas are tumours incidentally discovered on imaging performed during the workup of unrelated conditions. Due to increasing use of cross-axial imaging, studies suggest an increasing incidence of clinically unapparent adrenal masses of 1–9%, which increases with age.[56] The workup of adrenal incidentalomas must address functionality and malignant potential of the mass that will guide treatment or observational approaches. Biochemical evaluations as described above should be performed to rule out aldosterone, cortisol or catecholamine-producing adrenal masses. Although most adrenal incidentalomas are non-functional, approximately 10–15% secrete excess adrenal hormones.[57] Risk of malignancy is rare as fewer than 5% of adrenal incidentalomas are primary ACC or non-adrenal metastases.[58] The size and imaging characteristics are useful in determining whether an adrenal mass is benign or malignant. PET/CT can also be used in cases where imaging is equivocal and tissue diagnosis by fine-needle aspiration (FNA) should be generally avoided, except for metastases and only after pheochromocytoma has been ruled out. Adrenalectomy is recommended for functional lesions, masses > 4 cm or tumours with imaging characteristics concerning for malignancy.[58] For masses with benign appearances (< 10 HU, washout > 50%), small (< 4 cm) and completely non-functional, imaging and biochemical surveillance between 3 and 12 months is reasonable; however, in patients younger than 40, closer follow-up is recommended as incidentaloma are rare.

| Differential diagnosis | Diagnostic likelihood based on large surgical series |
| --- | --- |
| Non-functional adenoma | 70% |
| Pheochromocytoma | 7% |
| Myelolipoma | 8% |
| Cortisol-producing adenoma | 10% |
| Adrenocortical carcinoma | 8% |
| Adrenal cyst | 5% |
| Ganglioneuroma | 4% |
| Aldosteronoma | 6% |
| Metastasis | 5% |

\*\*Total percentage is greater than 100% as data is reported as median percentage drawing from multiple studies. The average percentages should be viewed in the context of a selection bias causing overestimation as only patients who eventually underwent surgery or autopsy were able to provide pathological specimen.

## SECONDARY ADRENAL METASTASES

Metastases should be suspected in patients with adrenal masses and a history of extra-adrenal malignancy. Renal cell carcinoma, melanoma, non-small cell lung cancer, breast cancer, colorectal cancer and lymphoma have a predilection for spread to the adrenal glands. Most adrenal metastases are asymptomatic and are discovered on surveillance imaging for cancer. They are usually unilateral, although a significant percentage may be bilateral. Although chemotherapy is usually the treatment for disseminated cancer, open or laparoscopic adrenalectomy may be performed in patients with otherwise well-controlled disease with either synchronous or metachronous oligometastases to the adrenal gland.[59]

## ADRENALECTOMY

Adrenalectomy can be safely performed via a variety of approaches. The open anterior, open posterior, open thorcoabdominal, laparoscopic and robotic approaches all have relative indications for different pathologies and patient populations. Regardless of approach, adrenalectomy requires special consideration to postoperative hormonal and subsequent physiological changes that occur after resection. Patients with pheochromocytoma are best managed by an operative team experienced with the characteristic haemodynamic changes and should have close haemodynamic monitoring for intraoperative hypertensive emergency and postoperative hypotension due to alpha blockage and volume constriction. Patients undergoing resection for primary hyperaldosteronism should have potassium tested before and after surgery to avoid hypokalaemia and hyperkalaemia, respectively. Stress steroids should be administered to patients undergoing resection for adrenal Cushing disease followed by 6 months of supplementation until evidence of endogenous ACTH has returned. In subclinical Cushing disease, cosyntropin stimulation test may be necessary to determine if steroid supplementation is required. Regardless of indication, intravenous hydrocortisone should be given perioperatively before transitioning to oral hydrocortisone and fludrocortisone 0.1 mg qD after bilateral adrenalectomy. Open surgery should be performed in cases of suspected ACC for ideal oncologic resection.

## OPEN

### Left

The patient is placed in a slight right lateral decubitus position. The abdomen is accessed via an extended subcostal incision. The splenic flexure of the colon is mobilised and the omental attachments along the transverse colon are divided allowing access to the lesser sac. The splenorenal, splenophrenic and retroperitoneal attachments of the spleen are divided and the tail of the pancreas is rotated medially, exposing the adrenal gland in the retroperitoneum. Gerota's fascia and the upper border of the left kidney are identified and divided. The left renal hilum is dissected to reveal the left renal vein and its confluence with the left adrenal vein, which is ligated and divided just cephalad to its confluence with the inferior phrenic vein. The retroperitoneal fat and suprarenal tissue are elevated and dissected off the superior pole of the left kidney, lateral abdominal wall and left quadratus lumborum muscle. The three main arterial branches from the left renal artery, aorta and left phrenic artery are ligated during the dissection. The medial dissection is carried as far as necessary to obtain a negative margin. For oncologic adrenalectomy, para-aortic lymph nodes are dissected and removed en bloc with the specimen. The pitfalls of left adrenalectomy are injury to the spleen, pancreas or diaphragm, rupture of the capsule of the gland and misidentification of the vascular anatomy.

### Right

The patient is placed in a slight left lateral decubitus position. The abdomen is accessed via an extended subcostal incision. The liver is mobilised medially by dividing the triangular ligament to allow exposure of the inferior vena cava and the right adrenal gland. The right border of the vena cava is dissected caudally to the diaphragm to allow the right adrenal vein to be identified, ligated and divided. The right border of the vena cava is dissected rostrally to reveal the right renal hilum. Gerota's fascia and the upper border of the right kidney are identified and divided. The retroperitoneal fat and suprarenal tissue are elevated and dissected off the superior pole of the right kidney, lateral abdominal wall and right quadratus lumborum muscle. The three main arterial branches from the right renal artery, aorta and right phrenic artery are ligated during dissection of the right suprarenal tissues. If performed for oncological purposes, an en bloc dissection of the associated lymph nodes is also performed as part of the medial extent of the dissection of the suprarenal tissue. The major pitfalls of a right adrenalectomy are tumour rupture, injury to the vena cava and right diaphragmatic injury.

## LAPAROSCOPIC

### Left

The patient is placed in a right lateral decubitus position flexed at the hip. The right arm is extended and the left arm suspended. The surgeon faces the patient and the assistant is behind the patient. Video monitors are positioned at the head of the bed. Four trocars are generally placed along a linear curve situated below the left costal margin once pneumoperitoneum is achieved using the Hasson technique. After exploration of the abdomen, the spleen is mobilised by dividing the splenorenal ligament starting at the inferior pole and extending up to the left crus of the diaphragm. The medial reflection of the spleen and pancreas is dissected along the splenic vein exposing the left renal and adrenal veins. The left adrenal vein is dissected cephalad to reveal its convergence with the inferior phrenic vein, where it is ligated and divided. Next, the inferior, middle and superior adrenal arteries are ligated and divided. The superior, posterior and lateral aspects of the gland are dissected free. Cephalad retraction allows dissection of the gland along its inferior adrenal pedicle, which frees it from the superior pole of the kidney. The gland is then placed in a plastic bag and removed.

### Right

The patient is placed in a left lateral decubitus position flexed at the hip. The left arm is extended and the right arm suspended. The surgeon faces the patient and the assistant is behind the patient. Video monitors are positioned at the head of the bed. Four trocars are generally placed along a linear curve situated below the right costal margin once pneumoperitoneum is achieved using the Hasson technique. The right adrenal gland is situated behind the liver, necessitating its medial mobilisation by dividing the triangular ligament. An atraumatic liver retractor is introduced through the lateral port to hold the liver out of the way. Mobilisation of the liver allows for identification of the vena cava, which is the main anatomical landmark for identifying and dissecting the right adrenal gland. The right border of the vena cava is dissected caudally to expose the renal vein, which constitutes the inferior landmark of the operating field. The vena cava is then dissected cephalad to the diaphragm, to expose the main adrenal vein and, if present, the accessory adrenal vein. Both are ligated and divided. The arterial blood supply is then identified, ligated and divided. The gland is then freed from its fatty and inferior ligamentous attachments along the superior pole of the kidney. The gland is then placed in a plastic bag and removed.

---

## Key points

- Splenectomy remains an important procedure for the repertoire of the General Surgeon in treatment of traumatic and refractory haematologic disease.
- Elective management of splenic pathology is moving towards minimally invasive approaches.
- Traumatic splenic injuries can be safely managed with arterial embolisation with acceptable risks.
- Hyperaldosteronism remains an underdiagnosed chronic medical condition amenable to surgical correction
- Incidentalomas request special diagnostic consideration; though the rates of adrenal cortical carcinoma are low, complete surgical excision remains the only chance at a lasting cure.

 References available at http://ebooks.health.elsevier.com/

## KEY REFERENCES

[5] Edgren G, Almqvist R, Hartman M, Utter GH. Splenectomy and the risk of sepsis: a population-based cohort study. Ann Surg 2014;260(6):1081–7

*Retrospective cohort study evaluating standardised incidence of OPSI based on indication of splenectomy.*

[13] Rosenberg GM, Weiser TG, Maggio PM, et al. The association between angioembolization and splenic salvage for isolated splenic injuries. J Surg Res 2018;229:150–5

*Large nationwide retrospective study analysing success of SAE in traumatic splenic injury.*

[19] Neunert C, Terrell DR, Arnold DM, et al. American Society of Hematology 2019 guidelines for immune thrombocytopenia [published correction appears in Blood Adv. 2020;4(2):252. Blood Adv 2019;3(23):3829–66

*American Society of Hematology's position statement on the treatment of ITP.*

[44] Yang Y, Reincke M, Williams TA. Prevalence, diagnosis and outcomes of treatment for primary aldosteronism. In: Best practice and research: clinical endocrinology and metabolism, vol. 34. Bailliere Tindall Ltd; 2020. p. 101365. https://doi.org/10.1016/j.beem.2019.101365. Issue 2

*Expert review of prevalence, diagnosis, and treatment standards of primary hyperaldosteronism.*

[48] Dennedy MC, Annamalai AK, Prankerd-Smith O, et al. Low DHEAS: a sensitive and specific test for the detection of subclinical hypercortisolism in adrenal incidentalomas. J Clin Endocrinol Metab 2017;102(3):786–92

*Diagnostic study comparing diagnosis of Cushing disease via DHEAS showing with high sensitivity and specificity when compared with current gold standard testing via dexamethasone suppression testing.*

[55] Delozier OM, Stiles ZE, Deschner BW, et al. Implications of conversion during attempted minimally invasive adrenalectomy for adrenocortical carcinoma. Ann Surg Oncol 2021;28(1):492–501

*Retrospective analysis of National Cancer database in which overall survival was superior in patients with planned open resection.*

[58] Kebebew E. Adrenal incidentaloma. N Engl J Med 2021;384(16):1542–51

*Review of current guidelines and management of incidentaloma by expert opinion.*

# Gallstones 12

Ian Beckingham

## INTRODUCTION

The gallbladder serves as a reservoir to hold bile and release it in a bolus when fat is ingested (Fig. 12.1). Fat in the stomach results in the release of cholecystokinin (CCK) which causes contraction and emptying of the gallbladder as food enters the duodenum. Bile helps to emulsify fat within the small bowel and aid its absorption. Whilst in the gallbladder, bile is concentrated by the absorption of up to 70% of the water content.

Many animals do not have gallbladders—all members of the deer family (except the musk deer), all of the equine family, camels, giraffes, elephants, rhinoceroses, whales, some birds (such as doves, pigeons and parrots), rats and some fish. It is thought that the presence of a gallbladder is related to the interval of food intake. Thus animals, like humans, cats and dogs, which take in food at intervals, require a larger amount of bile acids to aid digestion of fats arriving in a bolus, rather than in a more constant stream.

In some societies, the gallbladder is attributed with more than just physical properties. In Korea, the flighty nature of deer is blamed on its lack of a gallbladder, and when a person acts eccentrically or irrationally Koreans say the person lacks a gallbladder. Conversely, when someone is brave, bold and daring, they say the person has a big gallbladder.[1] The Chinese proclaim the calming influence of bile and use powdered bovine gallstones in their traditional medicines as an antipyretic and to aid sleep and cure diseases of the liver and epilepsy. Ox gallstones are also used as an aphrodisiac and bovine gallstones can fetch up to $14 000/kg on the commercial market.

## PATHOGENESIS OF GALLSTONES

Bile is composed of a complex solution of bilirubin (the byproduct of effete red blood cells), cholesterol, fatty acids and various minerals. If one or more of the major components is present in excess, then the solution becomes supersaturated and cholesterol crystals form within the bile (Fig. 12.2). These eventually coalesce to form cholesterol or 'mixed' (cholesterol/bilirubin) gallstones. Cholesterol supersaturation can result from either excessive hepatic secretion of cholesterol, or decreased hepatic secretion of bile salts or phospholipids with relatively normal cholesterol secretion. In > 90% of patients, supersaturation results from altered hepatic cholesterol metabolism.[2,3] For stones to form, there is a need for a nidus. Mucin secreted by the gallbladder wall may serve as a nidus and act as a pronucleating (crystallisation-promoting) protein. Variations in mucin composition and decreased degradation of mucin by lysosomal enzymes are associated with a higher incidence of stone formation.[4]

Loss of gallbladder motility and excessive sphincteric contraction are also associated with gallstone formation (Fig. 12.3). Hypomotility leads to prolonged bile stasis (delayed gallbladder emptying) and decreased reservoir function. If the situation persists for long enough, crystals coalesce, with formation of biliary sludge and subsequently stones.[5]

Patients with Crohn's disease, or who have undergone intestinal resection or total colectomy, are also more prone to develop cholesterol stones. This is due to impaired enterohepatic circulation leading to reduced hepatic secretion of bile salts in the bile (Fig. 12.4). This results in higher concentration and decreased solubilisation of cholesterol and its precipitation as crystals, with eventual stone formation.

## RISK FACTORS

As with most diseases, the development of gallstones is caused by a mixture of genetic and environmental factors. Patients with cholelithiasis often have a strong family history, with gallstones occurring three times more frequently in first-degree relatives than in spouses or unrelated controls.[6] It has been estimated that genetic factors account for approximately 25% of gallstones.[7] Gallstones are most common in White European and American populations and least common in Black Africans (Fig. 12.5). Intermediate rates are found in Asian populations. The highest prevalence is seen in native American populations with a prevalence of 60% in the Pima Indian population of Southern Arizona.

Female sex (10:1 female-to-male ratio), previous pregnancy and a family history of gallstone disease are highly correlated with cholelithiasis (Box 12.1).[8] Oestrogen increases cholesterol secretion and diminishes bile salt secretion, increasing the cholesterol saturation within bile. Diminished gallbladder motility is commonly seen during pregnancy, with a 10–15 times higher incidence of cholelithiasis seen in women who have had children.[8] Biliary sludge is found in 5–30% of pregnant women and definitive gallstones become established in 5%.[9]

A number of disease processes can result in the supersaturation of cholesterol in bile, including rapid weight loss in the morbidly obese patient (due to excess cholesterol within

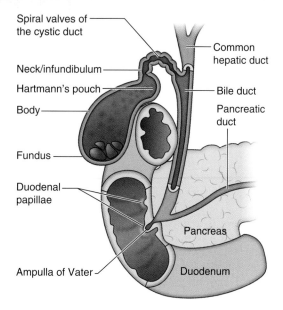

**Figure 12.1**    Anatomy of the gallbladder and bile ducts.

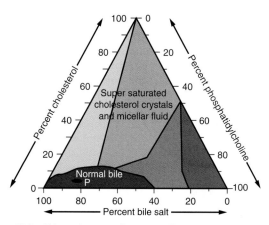

**Figure 12.2**    Triangular coordinate equilibrium phase diagram of the cholesterol–phospholipid–bile salt system in the gallbladder. Bile composition at point P (normal, non-lithogenic bile); bile salts (80%); phospholipids acids (15%); cholesterol 5%.

the bile), total parenteral nutrition (which induces gallbladder hypomotility in the presence of high lipid levels), and drugs that promote cholesterol secretion into the bile, e.g. fibrates.

Other risk factors include a high dietary intake of fats and carbohydrates, a sedentary lifestyle, type 2 diabetes mellitus and dyslipidaemia (increased triglycerides and low high-density lipoprotein). A diet high in fats and carbohydrates predisposes a patient to obesity, which increases cholesterol synthesis, biliary secretion of cholesterol, and cholesterol supersaturation. Individuals with a BMI > 45 have a sevenfold higher incidence of gallstones than non-obese females.[10] However, a direct correlation between high dietary intake of fats and cholelithiasis has not been established.

## PIGMENT STONES

Black pigment stones account for approximately 10% of gallstones. They are formed when there is an excess of

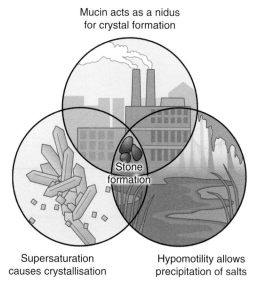

**Figure 12.3**    Components required for gallstone formation.

unconjugated bile as a result of increased enterohepatic circulation of bilirubin caused by excessive breakdown of red blood cells. The increased bilirubin concentration within the bile results in precipitation of calcium bilirubinate to form black pigmented stones. These stones are most frequently seen in patients with chronic haemolytic anaemias (e.g. hereditary spherocytosis, sickle cell disease, B thalassaemia), ineffective erythropoiesis (e.g. pernicious anaemia) and liver cirrhosis.

Patients with ileal disease (e.g. Crohn's disease) who have undergone extended ileal resections or total colectomy have impairment of intestinal bile salt absorption and an increased incidence of gallstones. These may be cholesterol stones due to loss of specific bile salt transporters in the terminal ileum resulting in excessive bile salt excretion in faeces and a diminished bile salt pool. However, in some patients these changes may also lead to formation of pigment gallstones because increased bile salt delivery to the colon enhances solubilisation of unconjugated bilirubin, thereby increasing bilirubin concentrations in bile (Fig. 12.4). Patients with cystic fibrosis also have bile acid malabsorption and approximately 20–30% of patients will develop gallstones.

Brown pigment stones differ from other types of gallstone in that they predominate within the other areas of the biliary tract, particularly the intrahepatic ducts, as well as within the gallbladder. They are mostly seen in South-East Asian populations and are usually associated with parasite infestation and *Escherichia coli* infection (see later section: Intrahepatic stone disease).

## PRESENTATION

Gallstones are very common, with an incidence of 10–15% in the adult population.[11] The majority of people with gallstones are asymptomatic and therefore unaware of their presence. In post-mortem studies, approximately 90% of people with gallstones had no attributable symptoms during their lifetime.

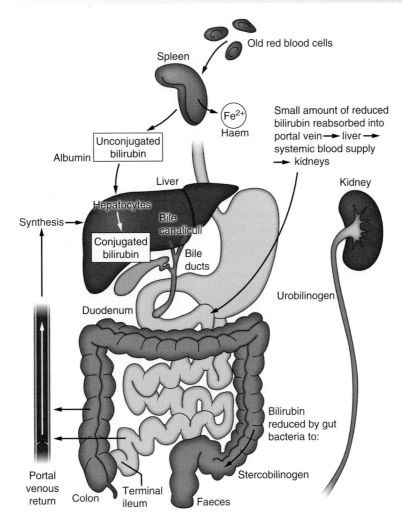

**Figure 12.4** Enterohepatic bile circulation.

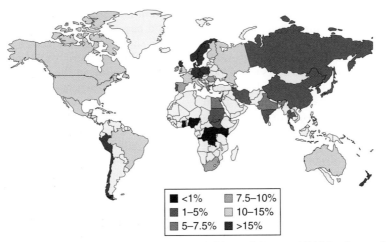

**Figure 12.5** Geographical prevalence of gallstones. (Adapted from Figge A, Matern S, Lammert F. Molecular genetics of cholesterol cholelithiasis: identification of human and murine gallstone genes. Z Gastroenterol 2002;40(6):425–32.)

## BILIARY PAIN

Gallstones cause symptoms when the cystic duct is occluded during the attempted expulsion of bile from the gallbladder. The resulting contraction of the gallbladder smooth muscle results in activation of visceral nerve fibres in the gallbladder wall and the sensation of referred pain in the associated dermatome (T9) in the epigastrium and radiation round or

through to the back. Viscerally innervated pain is often poorly localised and may be accompanied by nausea or vomiting. Local cytokine release can cause irritation of the adjacent parietal peritoneum resulting in pain in the right upper quadrant (RUQ). The pain lasts for a significant period of time (typically 30 minutes to several hours) and may be related in part to ischaemia within the gallbladder wall as a result of muscular occlusion of the gallbladder microcirculation. The severity of

## Table 12.1    Typical features of biliary pain

| | |
|---|---|
| Location | Epigastric/right upper quadrant |
| Duration | > 30 minutes |
| Radiation | Round or through to back (band-like) |
| Severity | Severe (inhibits daily activity) |
| Periodicity | Intermittent |
| Less strongly associated | Nocturnal onset |
| | Post fatty meal |

the pain is sufficient to interfere with performance of daily activities. It is frequently very severe and often described by women as 'worse than childbirth'. The popular term 'biliary colic' is a misnomer since the pain is constant and unrelenting and not colicky in nature. It is therefore more accurately referred to as biliary pain. Similarly, use of the term 'chronic cholecystitis' should be avoided since it implies the presence of a chronic inflammatory infiltrate that may or may not be present. The number of stones, their size and the thickness of the gallbladder wall do not correlate well with the presence or absence, or severity of biliary symptoms. In many patients with significant biliary pain, the gallbladder looks quite normal at the time of surgery.

The importance of clarifying what constitutes true biliary pain is to better predict relief following surgery (Table 12.1).[12] Cholecystectomy fails to relieve 'biliary pain' in 10–30% of patients with documented gallstones.[13,14] It is observed that patients who have had cholecystectomy for biliary pain often have improvement in other symptoms, such as belching and low-grade epigastric discomfort ('biliary dyspepsia'). Some patients may be offered surgery for these symptoms alone. However, these vague symptoms are probably vagal nerve-mediated and also frequently associated with other functional gut disorders such as irritable bowel syndrome or gastro-oesophageal reflux disease. Thus, results for cholecystectomy in patients with 'biliary dyspepsia' alone have worse outcomes than in patients who have more classic bouts of acute biliary pain, and should only be undertaken after appropriate exclusion of other causes where possible and with clear counselling that benefits are less likely.

Once patients have started to develop symptoms from their gallstones, the likelihood of having further episodes is approximately 38–50% per annum[15,16]; however, approximately 30% of patients will never have further symptoms. The risk of developing complications of gallstones is higher in patients with symptomatic gallstones than in asymptomatic patients and is approximately 1–2% per annum.[17]

## ACUTE CHOLECYSTITIS

When biliary pain persists for more than a few hours and is accompanied by localised RUQ discomfort, it is termed acute cholecystitis. Pathophysiologically, prolonged obstruction of the cystic duct causes release of prostaglandins within the gallbladder mucosa resulting in fluid secretion producing a cycle of increased distension and further mucosal damage and inflammation. The inflammatory process results in irritation of the parietal peritoneum. Palpation of the RUQ is tender, and inspiration with the examiner's hand in this region results in pain as the inflamed gallbladder pushes against it (Murphy's sign), which can similarly be confirmed with the ultrasound probe. Inflammatory markers (WCC/ESR/CRP) may be elevated. Liver function tests (LFTs) are often deranged as a result of localised inflammation within the adjacent liver parenchyma or due to compression of the common bile duct (CBD) from the inflamed gallbladder. Secondary infection can develop in this setting but is rarely the primary event.

The condition may evolve and can result in a variety of complications (Fig. 12.6):

- Obstruction of the cystic duct, usually by a large stone in Hartmann's pouch, can cause a tense tender gallbladder due to mucus (mucocoele).
- If the obstructed gallbladder becomes infected, it may fill with pus (empyema), presenting classically with high swinging fevers, rising white cell count and a significantly elevated C-reactive protein (> 50).
- Emphysematous cholecystitis may develop when secondary infection in the gallbladder wall occurs with gas-forming bacteria, such as *Clostridium welchii*, *E. coli* or anaerobic streptococci. Imaging may reveal the presence of gas within the gallbladder wall. It is most commonly seen in elderly men with diabetes.
- The inflamed gallbladder may become adherent to an adjacent loop of bowel (duodenum, jejunum or colon) and eventually rupture into it, discharging its contents. Rarely a large stone passes through the gallbladder wall into the small bowel and causes obstruction (gallstone ileus) (Fig. 12.7). Gastric outlet obstruction due to impaction of a gallstone in the duodenum is known as Bouveret's syndrome. Discharge into the colon only rarely causes obstruction due to the larger diameter of the colon but can be encountered at cholecystectomy as a cholecysto-colic fistula.
- The gallbladder may rupture into the peritoneal cavity resulting in free pus and generalised peritonitis (1%), or may become walled off by adjacent bowel and omentum and form a localised pericholecystic abscess.

## COMMON BILE DUCT STONES

Approximately 8–16% of patients with symptomatic gallbladder stones will have simultaneous CBD stones. With the exception of brown pigment stones, the vast majority (if not all) of these stones originate from the gallbladder and pass from there through the cystic duct into the CBD. The natural history of these CBD stones is unknown, but there is evidence that many do not cause symptoms. Faecal sampling of patients with multiple gallbladder stones confirms that stones often pass freely into the gut without symptoms. Furthermore, studies of patients with known CBD stones

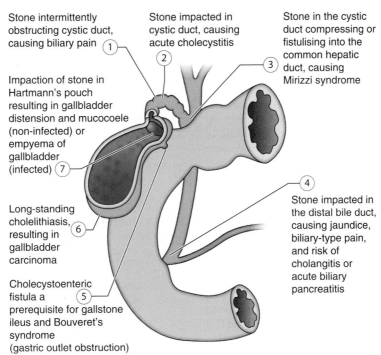

Stone intermittently obstructing cystic duct, causing biliary pain (1)

Stone impacted in cystic duct, causing acute cholecystitis (2)

Stone in the cystic duct compressing or fistulising into the common hepatic duct, causing Mirizzi syndrome (3)

Impaction of stone in Hartmann's pouch resulting in gallbladder distension and mucocoele (non-infected) or empyema of gallbladder (infected) (7)

Long-standing cholelithiasis, resulting in gallbladder carcinoma (6)

Cholecystoenteric fistula a prerequisite for gallstone ileus and Bouveret's syndrome (gastric outlet obstruction) (5)

Stone impacted in the distal bile duct, causing jaundice, biliary-type pain, and risk of cholangitis or acute biliary pancreatitis (4)

**Figure 12.6**  Potential complications of gallstones.

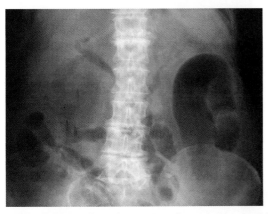

**Figure 12.7**  Gallstone ileus. Large stone impacted in small bowel causing obstruction. Note pneumobilia from the cholecysto-jejunal fistula.

awaiting or having had cholecystectomy and who are then re-imaged often show passage of the stones from the CBD.[18,19] Incidental (asymptomatic) CBD stones are also identified in patients undergoing imaging for unrelated non-biliary conditions. Thus, it would appear that many CBD stones may never cause any problems at all. However, because of the uncertainty in their natural history, once CBD stones are discovered, most clinicians would advise patients to have them removed, even if they are asymptomatic.

When stones enter the CBD and cause partial or complete obstruction, patients present with obstructive jaundice with an elevated bilirubin (conjugated), alkaline phosphatase (ALP) and gamma-glutamyl transferase (GGT). The transaminases (AST/ALT) may also be elevated ('a mixed pattern') as a result of secondary inflammation of the hepatocytes. Classically, obstructive jaundice is accompanied by pale stools due to lack of the brown pigment stercobilin (which requires the presence of bilirubin in the gut) and

dark urine (due to increased bilirubin in the urine). These clinical features are not always present, particularly in the early phases of obstruction or with incomplete biliary obstruction. Obstructive jaundice resulting from CBD stones is often associated with biliary pain. This contrasts with jaundice associated with malignant obstruction which is usually painless, but the distinction is not absolute. As obstruction progresses, dilatation of the biliary tract occurs which is evident on ultrasound or cross-sectional imaging (e.g. magnetic resonance imaging [MRI], computed tomography [CT]).

CBD stones, when present, are only occasionally identified with ultrasound because the lower part of the bile duct lies behind the gas-filled duodenum preventing visualisation. The presence of a dilated CBD or intrahepatic ducts with deranged LFTs raises the suspicion of CBD stones, which are best visualised by magnetic resonance cholangiopancreatography (MRCP) or endoscopic ultrasound (EUS). A recent meta-analysis has shown that EUS and MRCP are equally good at identifying CBD stones, with similar sensitivity and specificity.[20] However, EUS is more costly, less widely available and more invasive than MRCP. These techniques have replaced the use of endoscopic retrograde cholangiopancreatography (ERCP) (with its attendant risks) as a diagnostic tool.

If infection develops in an obstructed bile duct, jaundice is invariably accompanied by high temperatures and RUQ pain (Charcot's triad) and is termed cholangitis. Fevers are typically fluctuating, with high temperatures of 39–40°C punctuated by chills and shaking bouts (rigors). Cholangitis is caused by secondary infection within the biliary tract, usually caused by enteric bacteria from the duodenum (most commonly Gram-negative spp.—*E. coli* [25–50%], *Klebsiella* spp. [15–20%], *Enterobacter* spp. [5–10%] or less commonly, Gram-positive bacteria, *Enterococcus* spp. [10–20%]).[21] Early management with intravenous antibiotics (broad-spectrum cephalosporin or ciprofloxacin) followed by early biliary decompression by stone removal or stenting is essential.

Failure to treat this condition frequently results in septicaemia, which can be fatal.

## ACUTE PANCREATITIS

CBD stones (usually small) may pass out of the papilla at the lower end of the bile duct and in some cases result in acute pancreatitis. The most popular theory for the pathogenesis of gallstone pancreatitis is that an impacted gallstone in the distal bile duct obstructs the pancreatic duct, increasing pancreatic pressure, thereby damaging ductal and acinar cells (see Chapter 15).

## MIRIZZI SYNDROME

First described by Argentinian surgeon Pablo Mirizzi in 1948, the term is used to describe the situation where a stone impacted in Hartmann's pouch produces an inflammatory process that results in adherence of Hartmann's pouch to the CBD with loss of the space between the two structures (i.e. obliteration of Calot's triangle). The result is a partial obstruction of the common hepatic duct (CHD) with deranged LFTs. The most useful subclassification is into type I, where there is no fistula present, and type II, where the stone has eroded into the bile duct itself resulting in a cholecysto-choledochal fistula (Fig. 12.8).

## INTRAHEPATIC STONE DISEASE

In certain parts of the world, primary bile duct stones (synonyms include intrahepatic stone disease [IHSD], oriental hepatolithiasis, cholangiohepatitis, recurrent pyogenic cholangitis, Hong Kong disease) form by a very different pathogenesis to cholesterol and black pigment stones, and

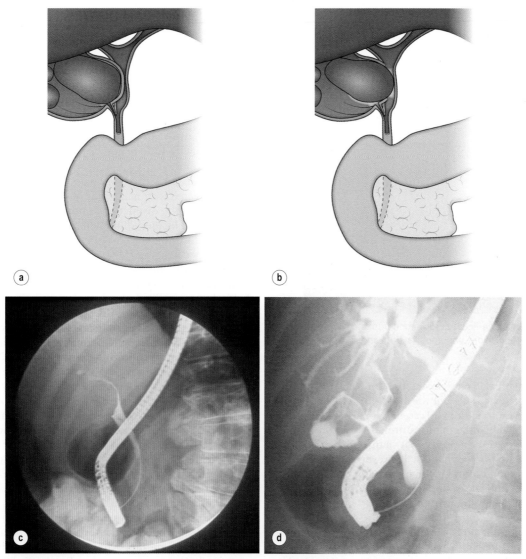

**Figure 12.8**   Mirizzi syndrome. **(a)** Type 1 Mirizzi (pressure from stone in gallbladder on common bile duct). **(b)** Type 2 Mirizzi (stone eroded through gallbladder wall into common bile duct— a cholecysto-choledochal fistula). **(c)** Type 1 Mirizzi (no contrast seen in gallbladder on ERCP). **(d)** Type 2 Mirizzi (contrast seen with in gallbladder via the cholecysto-choledochal fistula on ERCP).

present with a different clinical picture. The highest prevalence of this disease is seen in South-East Asia where it has been associated with the liver fluke *Clonorchis sinensis*. However, it also exists in other areas of the world, most notably South Africa, Pakistan and Colombia in the absence of *Clonorchis*, where the main linked epidemiological factor is severe poverty. In these communities, there may be an association with the round worm *Ascaris lumbricoides* infestation.

Stones formed in this disease are very different from cholesterol- and bilirubin-rich stones and are brown, soft and friable. The stones form in any part of the biliary tract as a result of anaerobic bacteria secreting enzymes that hydrolyse ester and amide linkages in biliary lipids as insoluble anions or calcium salts. These precipitates deposit on obstructing elements such as small cholesterol crystals, black stones from the gallbladder, parasite eggs and dead worms or flukes.[22]

Patients with IHSD present with sepsis and RUQ pain, and initial management is with antibiotics. Symptoms are far more commonly related to ductal stones, and infective and inflammatory processes around the stones result in strictures and proximal dilatation of the ducts. Simple cases caught early can be managed by decompression of pus from the CBD with a plastic stent. Subsequent definitive surgical management aims to clear the biliary tract of stones, provide adequate biliary drainage and, where necessary, provide adequate access to the biliary duct. When there is an extrahepatic or hilar duct stricture, hepaticojejunostomy (HJ) is performed leaving the afferent loop long and fixing it to the abdominal wall as an 'access loop' which permits subsequent percutaneous or endoscopic management of recurrent stones and strictures.[23] A proportion of patients require resection of an atrophied portion of the liver containing multiple stones. The disease more frequently affects the left lobe than the right. Patients with IHSD have a 10% risk of developing cholangiocarcinoma.[24]

## MANAGEMENT OF GALLSTONES

### CONSERVATIVE

Patients with gallstones without symptoms do not require treatment. The risk of people with asymptomatic cholelithiasis developing symptoms (biliary pain) is low, averaging 2–3% per year, or approximately 10% by 5 years.[25] Major complications related to gallstones are very rare in asymptomatic patients.[26] Expectant management is therefore an appropriate choice for silent gallstones in the general population.

✓ Asymptomatic gallstones in the gallbladder do not require further investigation or management. Patients with symptomatic gallbladder stones should be offered laparoscopic cholecystectomy unless medically unfit for surgery.

### NON-OPERATIVE MANAGEMENT

Even in the laboratory, gallstones are difficult to dissolve and most chemicals that successfully dissolve gallstones are too toxic to ingest or inject into the gallbladder (e.g. methyl tetra butyl ether [MTBE], monooctanoin, carbon tetrachloride). During the 1970–80s, there were many attempts to develop strategies to achieve non-medical management of gallstones by oral dissolution, injection of solvents into the biliary tract and extracorporeal shock wave lithotripsy (ESWL). However, none achieved significant reliable dissolution of the stones, even in highly selected study groups, and all required long-term bile salt therapy (with a high incidence of abdominal cramps and diarrhoea) to prevent recurrent stone formation.[27] With the development of laparoscopic cholecystectomy (LC) in the late 1980s with its low morbidity and ability to definitively remove the 'stone factory', research in this area has dwindled.

Alternative treatments such as the 'gallbladder flush' (essentially consisting of giving purgative agents such as Epsom salts, olive oil and lemon juice) have been popularised by the Internet, but there is no evidence of any efficacy, although they do result in the production of small pellet-like faeces which can be mistaken by enthusiasts of the procedures as stones![28]

## CHOLECYSTECTOMY

Patients with biliary pain should be offered cholecystectomy as definitive treatment for their disease. Up until the early 1990s, the operation was usually performed through an incision in the RUQ (Kocher's incision). The cholecystectomy procedure consists of detaching the gallbladder from the biliary tract by division of the cystic duct, division of the cystic artery and subsequent removal of the gallbladder from its attachments to the gallbladder fossa of segments 4 and 5 of the liver.

The first LC was performed on 12 September 1985 by Erich Muhe in Boblingen, Germany.[29] Within a few years, the 'open' procedure was superseded by the laparoscopic procedure, and in 2016 more than 98% of cholecystectomies were performed laparoscopically in England (HES data). Although never subjected to large-scale randomised trial, improved clinical outcomes led to rapid adoption. Smaller incisions result in less tissue damage, less pain and a faster recovery. The average length of stay following cholecystectomy reduced from approximately 5 days to 1 day. This has progressed further to widespread realisation that the procedure can be carried out as a day case procedure. In 2020, over 70% of LCs in England were performed as day case procedures (HES data). Patients are now routinely discharged within a few hours of their operation.

The major disadvantage following the widespread introduction of LC has been cited as a rise in the incidence of bile duct injury. The true incidence of major bile duct injury (defined as injury affecting > 25% circumference of the CBD) in the open cholecystectomy era was poorly documented, but was in the order of 0.1–0.5%.[30,31] Initial results from small series of LC demonstrated an increase in these rates,[32,33] but subsequent large multicentre and single-centre prospective studies show that bile duct injury rates are similar to the open era at approximately 0.2–0.3%.[34,35] A number of studies have shown that the incidence of bile duct injury is related to the surgeons' inexperience with the technique,[36,37] but even experienced surgeons can cause an injury. When bile duct injury does occur with LC, it is frequently more proximal and more extensive than with open cholecystectomy (i.e. complete transection or excision of the bile duct).

The technique for a routine elective LC consists of gaining entry to the abdominal cavity under general anaesthesia, usually by an open 'Hasson' technique around the umbilical area, followed by insufflation of the cavity with carbon dioxide gas at a pressure of 12 mmHg. Classically, three additional ports are inserted in the RUQ and epigastrium, the fundus of the gallbladder is grasped and pushed cephalad to expose the porta hepatis. Careful dissection of the peritoneum overlying the structures in Calot's triangle (Fig. 12.9) permits identification of the cystic artery and cystic duct. Once clearly confirmed, these two structures are clipped and divided, and the gallbladder is dissected free from its attachments to the undersurface of the liver. Following inspection of the gallbladder fossa to ensure no bleeding or bile leak, and that the clips on the cystic duct and artery remain intact, the gallbladder is removed, usually within a bag to reduce contamination of the port sites. The gas is emptied from the abdominal cavity and the port sites are closed. Antibiotics are not routinely given. The patient is fed within a few hours of the procedure and typically is discharged home the same day with an expectation of return to full normal function and activities over the following 2–4 weeks.

There are variations in the number and size of the ports (5 mm/12 mm) used to perform the laparoscopic procedure.

Newer even less invasive techniques have been developed: single-incision laparoscopic surgery (SILS) involves a single larger incision at the umbilicus to further reduce scarring[38]; natural orifice transluminal endoscopic surgery (NOTES) allows scarless abdominal surgery using a flexible endoscope inserted via the mouth or vagina to remove the gallbladder.[39] Whilst feasibly possible, these techniques have failed to convince the majority of surgeons and patients that the elimination of three or four small incisions offers a significant benefit to patient recovery sufficient to justify the longer operative times, greater costs, greater technical challenges in more difficult cases, and increased additional potentially serious risks of these procedures. The standard four-port laparoscopic technique remains the gold standard allowing better triangulation of Calot's triangle and reducing the potential error of excessive cephalad traction and misidentification of the CBD for the cystic duct.

There are very few true contraindications to the laparoscopic approach and most of the former contraindications, including acute cholecystitis, obesity, respiratory disease and pregnancy (middle trimester ideally when necessary), are now the preferred options compared with 'open' surgery. Multiple previous laparotomies and RUQ stomas remain a relative indication for open surgery.

✅✅ Laparoscopic cholecystectomy is the only recommended treatment for symptomatic gallbladder stones.

## INTRAOPERATIVE BILE DUCT IMAGING AND PREVENTION OF BILE DUCT INJURY

Intraoperative cholangiography (IOC) is an essential skill for all surgeons performing cholecystectomy. It enables identification of CBD stones and the biliary tract anatomy. Routine use of IOC is considered by some as important in reducing the incidence of bile duct injury[40]; however, there are many series that have shown no difference in incidence, nor in the number of bile duct injuries missed during surgery.[41] Other series have shown that more than 50% of injuries revealed on the cholangiograms were missed by the operating surgeon. In the UK, selective cholangiography appears to be the favoured approach, with IOC performed in < 10% of LCs (HES data).

Laparoscopic ultrasound (LUS) is a fast and reliable technique to identify CBD stones and with the addition of colour Doppler can aid in identification of anatomical structures (vessels and ducts) within the porta hepatis. It is not widely available but has been shown to be superior to IOC in identification of CBD stones.[42]

Recently indocyanine green (ICG) given intravenously 15 minutes before surgery has been shown to facilitate identification of the biliary anatomy in LC. ICG is concentrated in the liver and excreted from the biliary tract and with the aid of a near infrared (NIR) filter on the laparoscope, the ICG within the ducts fluoresces and can be clearly seen. The sensitivity of ICG in the recognition of the cystic duct and CBD was 100% irrespective of the presence of fat or inflammation in Calot's triangle.[43] It has also been shown to be useful in identifying the origin of bile leaks at surgery although the specialist equipment required is not widely available at present.

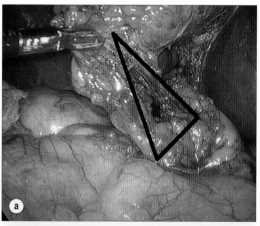
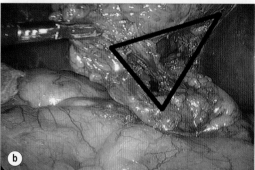

**Figure 12.9** Calot's triangle and the cystohepatic triangle. (a) Calot's original description bounded by the cystic duct, cystic artery and common hepatic duct. (b) The cystohepatic triangle bounded by the gallbladder wall, cystic duct and common hepatic duct, with the cystic artery lying within the space. Although technically incorrect, the term Calot's triangle is widely used in surgical texts to refer to the cystohepatic triangle.

Safe cholecystectomy and prevention of bile duct injuries require clear visualisation of the anatomy which itself demands proper exposure of the critical structures. Avoiding these injuries requires use of caudal and lateral traction on Hartmann's pouch to counter-tract the cephalad retraction of the fundus, and always dissecting as close to the gallbladder wall as possible. No structure should be clipped or divided unless its identity is certain, and an intraoperative cholangiogram should be performed if any uncertainty exists. Conversion to open surgery should not be seen as a failure and should be considered if doubts persist.

Several methods have been proposed to reduce the incidence of bile duct injury—e.g. identification of Rouviere's sulcus, the flag technique, the infundibular technique and the critical view of safety (CVS). The CVS (Fig. 12.10) has become the most widely used technique and is the method recommended and taught by the Society of American Gastroenterological and Endoscopic Surgeons (SAGES). The CVS requires demonstration of three criteria—Calot's triangle is cleared of fat and fibrous tissue; the lower third of the gallbladder is separated from the liver to expose the cystic plate; demonstration of two (and only two) structures to be seen entering the gallbladder.[44] Its usage has been shown to reduce the incidence of bile duct injury in several large studies.[45,46]

When the anatomy in Calot's triangle is unclear as a result of inflammation and fibrosis, subtotal cholecystectomy is a safe technique avoiding the need to dissect in the hostile area of Calot's triangle. Subtotal cholecystectomy is with division of the gallbladder at the level of Hartmann's pouch, removal of the stone(s) with or without complete removal of the posterior wall of the gallbladder and securing Hartmann's pouch with an endoloop, suture or stapler as appropriate. Occasionally the cystic duct cannot be secured at all due to friable tissues and a drain can be left, with the majority of leaks settling without further intervention. Further surgery is rarely required following subtotal cholecystectomy as long as all the stones are removed at the original procedure. In a review of over 1000 cases following subtotal cholecystectomy, further surgery was required in < 2% of cases.[47] If

the whole area is 'frozen' with dense adhesions, cholecystostomy (insertion of a drain directly into the gallbladder) offers a safe alternative allowing transfer to a specialist unit if required.

It is widely held that the majority of bile duct injuries are preventable and result from inadequate training, poor surgical technique or misidentification of the normal anatomy (Box 12.2). Perhaps surprisingly, unusual amounts of bleeding, severe inflammation and emergency operations are typically involved in < 25% of injuries,[48] and it is noteworthy that in this extensive Swedish review, the patients most at risk of bile duct injury were young, slim females who had not undergone previous surgery. Similar studies have suggested that 84% of injuries were in non-complicated LCs and 97% were due to perceptual errors.[49]

## ACUTE CHOLECYSTITIS

Patients with acute cholecystitis generally require admission for analgesia and intravenous fluid rehydration. Non-steroidal anti-inflammatory agents such as diclofenac or indomethacin have been shown to reduce inflammation and speed recovery.[50] Broad-spectrum antibiotics, such as a second-generation cephalosporin, are recommended to prevent secondary bacterial infection.

The approach to the management of acute cholecystitis has changed radically over the last 20 years. Optimal management has shifted from leaving the cholecystectomy for 6 weeks in an effort to reduce inflammation and facilitate easier dissection following a realisation that this practice

| Box 12.2 | Bile duct injuries—risk factors |
|---|---|
| Dangerous anatomy | 7% |
| Dangerous pathology | 9% |
| Dangerous surgery | 84% |

Adapted from Johnson GW. Iatrogenic bile duct injury: an avoidable surgical hazard. Br J Surg 1986;73:246–7.

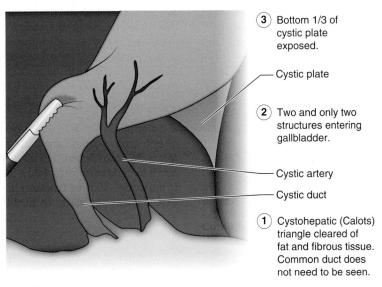

③ Bottom 1/3 of cystic plate exposed.

Cystic plate

② Two and only two structures entering gallbladder.

Cystic artery

Cystic duct

① Cystohepatic (Calots) triangle cleared of fat and fibrous tissue. Common duct does not need to be seen.

**Figure 12.10**  The critical view of safety.

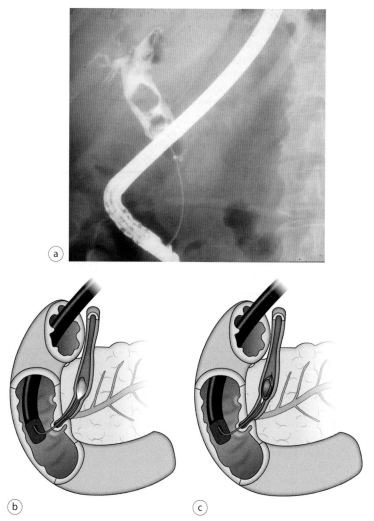

**Figure 12.11**   Endoscopic retrograde cholangiopancreatography techniques for common bile duct stone removal: (a) balloon extraction; (b) SpyGlass cholangioscopy with contact lithotripsy; (c) basket removal.

resulted in a 20% need for urgent surgery, 20% readmission rates, as well as prolonged and unnecessary pain, discomfort and inactivity. It is now recognised that surgery should ideally be undertaken within 48 hours of the onset of symptoms when the inflammatory process is still acute and before the development of more difficult fibrosis sets in. Benefits are still evident up to 10 days from onset of symptoms.[51,52] These cholecystectomy procedures can be challenging and there remains a significant conversion to open surgery (10–30%). Surgeons operating on this group of patients must have the full repertoire of techniques and equipment (e.g. cholangiography and choledochoscopy) and be prepared to perform a subtotal cholecystectomy or cholecystostomy.

✔✔ Patients with acute presentation of cholecystitis or gallstone pancreatitis should undergo early cholecystectomy, preferably on the same admission unless there are contraindications to surgery.

## PROPHYLACTIC CHOLECYSTECTOMY

There have been arguments made for certain patient groups to undergo prophylactic cholecystectomy—patients with diabetes mellitus (falsely assumed to have a higher incidence of acute cholecystitis and infective gallbladder complications); patients undergoing weight loss surgery (high incidence of postoperative gallstones); patients with hereditary spherocytosis undergoing splenectomy for their disease (high incidence of black pigment stones); patients awaiting heart transplant (higher incidence of post-transplant gallbladder problems)—however, the evidence in all these groups seems to suggest that complications of gallstones are not sufficiently frequent to warrant prophylactic cholecystectomy and that patients can be safely managed if symptoms develop.

## BILE DUCT STONES

There are two main approaches to the removal of CBD stones—ERCP or surgical bile duct exploration.

### ENDOSCOPIC RETROGRADE CHOLANGIOPANCREATOGRAPHY

The most common approach to the management of CBD stones is by ERCP (Fig. 12.11). This procedure involves insertion of a side-viewing endoscope (a duodenoscope) through the mouth into the duodenum. The papilla is cannulated with a fine cannula to enter the bile duct. The papilla can be cut using a sphincterotome, which uses diathermy to divide the sphincter of Oddi, and stones can be extracted with baskets or balloons. Larger stones can be crushed with a mechanical lithotripter. Large, impacted or multiple stones that cannot be removed can be managed by insertion of a plastic stent left within the bile duct to prevent the stone obstructing. These stones might be suitable for extraction using an ultrathin endoscope that passes down the working channel of the duodenoscope (e.g. SpyGlass endoscope). This ultrathin scope can pass up the CBD and enables direct visualisation of the stone to permit piezoelectric or laser contact lithotripsy. ERCP is performed under sedation and carries a risk of acute pancreatitis due to manipulation of the papilla (approximately 5%), bleeding or perforation (approximately 1%) and death (0.1%).

## SURGICAL BILE DUCT EXPLORATION

Bile duct exploration was originally performed via laparotomy, but increasingly the procedure is performed laparoscopically. At open surgery, the bile duct is opened longitudinally in the mid part of the anterior wall (choledochotomy) and stones are removed with Desjardins forceps, flushing and the use of a flexible choledochoscope. Prior to the development of flexible choledochoscopes, retention of CBD stones was high (10–15%) and a T-tube was inserted into the choledochotomy to prevent inadvertent leakage, potential stone impaction or swelling due to the traumatic stone extraction. With optical magnification, direct visualisation and more delicate instrumentation, trauma to the bile duct was reduced, missed CBD stones were rarer and primary duct closure became more common.

Laparoscopic bile duct exploration (LBDE) can be performed either via the cystic duct (transcystic) or directly through a choledochotomy (transductal). Small stones (< 5 mm) can be removed by a transcystic approach with a 3-mm choledochoscope or caught in a basket under fluoroscopy and retrieved via the cystic duct, or can be pushed through the papilla. A balloon to occlude the proximal duct whilst giving a smooth muscle relaxant, such as buscopan or glucagon, and then flushing through the balloon catheter can also be used to clear small distal duct stones. The transcystic approach is limited to stones small enough to be retrieved through the cystic duct (typically stones < 5 mm) and it is not usually possible to access the proximal hepatic duct due to inability to retroflex the choledochoscope and other instruments.

Larger stones can be managed by a transductal approach by making a choledochotomy (a longitudinal incision in the anterior surface of the bile duct) and extracting stones by a combination of manipulation of the duct, Dormia basket and balloon extraction with a 5-mm flexible choledochoscope. Large and impacted stones can be removed by shattering under direct vision using piezoelectric or laser lithotripsy. Most bile ducts are primarily closed with an absorbable suture. Bile can leak through the choledochotomy suture line and a drain is usually left for 24 hours or so post procedure. Where the duct is inflamed and friable (e.g. after recent cholangitis), in the presence of pus or multiple small stones a T-tube can be left within the choledochotomy to be removed after a period of at least 2 weeks, to permit safe drainage and reduce the risk of peritoneal bile leakage. Post-procedural acute pancreatitis is rare unless there has been traumatisation of the papilla.[53] Regardless of exact technique, the high rates of duct clearance reported with LBDE[54,55] can be increased to near 100% with the availability of intraductal lithotripsy.[56] Long-term results also appear favourable.[57,58]

## MANAGEMENT OF CBD STONES IN PATIENTS WITHOUT ACCESS TO THE PYLORUS, OR AFTER BILE DUCT RECONSTRUCTION

Around 6000 bariatric operations are performed each year in the UK (BOMSS data) and with successful rapid weight loss more than half will develop gallstones. Roux-en-Y gastric bypass (RYGB) accounts for approximately half of all bariatric procedures which, because of the detachment of the proximal stomach and attachment of a roux limb, prevents a standard ERCP approach to the bile duct if CBD stones develop. Similar loss of access to the papilla occurs in patients who have undergone Billroth II gastrectomy or gastric bypass surgery for benign or malignant diseases. Access is also lost in patients who have had bile duct excision or reconstruction (e.g. for bile duct injury) with reconstruction by Roux-en-Y HJ.

In some cases, if the afferent limb of the bypass is relatively short, then ERCP may still be possible. It is a complex procedure and may require double-balloon endoscopy to traverse the afferent limb particularly when long.[59] Even if the papilla is accessed, sphincterotomy (with a specially designed S-shaped sphincterotome) and duct clearance is highly challenging and the procedure, equipment and skills are not widely available.

If the pylorus is still patent (as in gastric bypass surgery for obesity), laparoscopic-assisted ERCP can be performed. This can be done either by inserting a port directly into the stomach at laparoscopy, or via a mini-laparotomy locating the stomach and inserting a purse string suture. The duodenoscope is then placed directly into the stomach to perform a 'regular' ERCP under general anaesthetic.[60]

If the bile ducts are dilated and in patients with a previous HJ, a percutaneous approach via the liver into the dilated intrahepatic ducts can be used. Smaller stones can be removed with a radiological basket[61] by dilating the strictured HJ and pushing stones through into the roux limb. More recently, this technique has been largely superseded by inserting a SpyGlass or choledochoscope over the previously inserted percutaneous wire directly into the intrahepatic ducts, using lithotripsy to the stone and flushing the debris through the roux limb. Additional balloon dilatation of any strictures can be undertaken at the same procedure.[62]

## APPROACHES TO THE MANAGEMENT OF SIMULTANEOUS CBD AND GALLBLADDER STONES

Preoperative identification of CBD stones in the presence of gallbladder stones offers two principal management options: a two-stage preoperative clearance of the CBD followed by LC, or a single-stage LBDE and cholecystectomy. Several trials have shown that there is no significant difference in clinical outcomes between the two approaches.[63–65] However, most studies show that single-stage LBDE is associated with a reduction in overall hospital stay when compared with the two-stage approach and has a lower overall cost.[63,66] Furthermore, the complications of surgical duct exploration are predominantly related to choledochotomy (bile leak) and T-tube use (bile leakage, tube displacement) that has largely been replaced with primary bile duct closure, resulting in shorter operative time, reduced hospital length of stay and faster return to work of approximately 8 days.[65] The UK national guidelines currently recommend that both approaches are considered equally valid treatment options and that training of surgeons in LBDE is to be encouraged.[67]

LBDE is largely replacing open BDE, with approximately 80% of BDE now performed laparoscopically in England (HES data). However, for preoperatively identified stones, a US survey reported that 86% of surgeons would choose preoperative ERCP over BDE, and for intraoperatively discovered CBD stones, only 30% would choose LBDE, citing availability of ERCP, lack of equipment and lack of skill performing LBDE.[68]

A third option that has been used in a few centres is the use of intraoperative ERCP at the time of LC.[69] Although feasible and with low morbidity, its use is not widespread due to the logistic difficulties of requiring ERCP equipment and staffing.

✔✔ Bile duct stones should be removed either by simultaneous bile duct exploration or perioperative ERCP depending on local resources and skills.

## APPROACHES TO ABNORMAL LFTS PRIOR TO LC

The decision and desire of surgeons to identify the presence of stones in the CBD prior to LC is highly variable. There are now several different preoperative diagnostic techniques (MRCP and EUS) and intraoperative techniques for imaging (IOC and LUS), and several options to manage any CBD stones identified (pre-, intra-, or postoperative ERCP, open or laparoscopic BDE). At present, there are no studies to support one or other approach and it is therefore important to develop an individual strategy for the preoperative and operative management of patients with gallstones dependent upon the local availability of techniques and skills.

The financial and logistic implications of preoperative imaging of all patients undergoing LC would inflict a significant cost and strain on resources with currently around 100 000 procedures performed per annum in the UK and 600 000 in the USA, and would be of questionable benefit.

Therefore, most clinicians will attempt to stratify patients in some way according to the probability of bile duct stones being present. Patients with normal LFTs, non-dilated bile ducts on ultrasound and no history of jaundice will have a < 1.5% chance of having a CBD stone.[70] This low-risk group can undergo LC without the need for further preoperative imaging or IOC, with an incidence of retained CBD stones of < 1% and a very low risk of significant problems from retained stones.[71,72]

Patients who are at highest risk of bile duct stones are those with jaundice at the time of surgery and those with preoperative US visualisation of a stone in the CBD (positive predictive value [PPV] of 0.86 and 0.74, respectively, at subsequent IOC). Another study found that patients with persistently abnormal LFTs, tested prior to MRCP with the presence of at least two of bilirubin > 110 μmol/L, ALP > 400 IU/L or ALT > 750 IU/L together with a dilated CBD (> 8 mm) or dilated intrahepatic ducts, had a PPV of 87% for stones (compared with only 32% if the bile ducts were not dilated), and even less correlation with the presence of subsequently confirmed CBD stones when only the incident LFTs were used for prediction.[73]

The combination of US duct dilatation and abnormal LFTs yields the next highest incidence of CBD stones preoperatively, e.g. the presence of two or more of: presentation with jaundice/bilirubin > 20 mmol (2 g/dL), ALP > 150 mmol, CBD > 10 mm and/or a CBD stone seen on US, yielded a PPV for CBD stones of 56%. Similar findings were reported in patients with a history of jaundice and dilated ducts on preoperative US, with a PPV of 56%.[71] Thus, these criteria might be used to identify patients at intermediate risk of CBD stones to select for preoperative MRCP prior to preoperative ERCP, or for selection of patients for referral to a surgeon who performs single-stage LBDE. However, in a significant number of patients identified preoperatively with definite stones, at least 25% had passed stones spontaneously without problems by the time of surgery.[71]

Less marked or singly elevated LFTs, particularly with non-dilated biliary ducts, have very poor sensitivity and specificity for predicting CBD stones, with an incidence in these groups of approximately 15–16% (Table 12.2).[74] This is only slightly higher than the incidence of CBD stones in the overall population of patients with symptomatic gallstones (9–13%).[75] The choice between the various strategies in this low-risk group of patients at present depends largely

### Table 12.2  Risk stratification for likelihood of common bile duct (CBD) stones

|  | Criteria | Relative risk of CBD stones |
|---|---|---|
| High risk | Preoperative US showing CBD stone | 0.74–0.86 |
|  | Jaundice at the time of procedure |  |
| Intermediate risk | At presentation, two of: | 0.56 |
|  | Bilirubin > 20 mmol/L |  |
|  | ALP or AST/ALT > 2–3 × normal |  |
|  | Dilated CBD (> 8 mm) |  |
|  | History of jaundice + dilated ducts |  |
| Low risk | Single elevated ALP or AST/ALT | 0.15 |
|  | History of acute gallstone pancreatitis |  |
| Minimal risk | Normal LFTs | 0.01 |

ALP, alkaline phosphatase; ALT, alanine transaminase; AST, aspartate transaminase; LFTs, liver function tests; US, ultrasound.

upon the quality of the surgical and endoscopic therapies available, but ERCP should not be performed without prior demonstration of stones in this group.

There are three possible approaches to management of patients undergoing cholecystectomy with regard to the dilemma of the CBD and possible CBD stones:

1. Identification of CBD stones prior to LC in order to remove them by ERCP prior to surgery. This approach sets a threshold at which to perform MRCP based on abnormalities of LFTs ± ultrasound findings. If stones are found at MRCP, then ERCP can be performed and CBD stones removed. Most surgeons would then avoid intraoperative IOC. The disadvantage of this approach is a very high level of unnecessary MRCPs (around 85% depending on the threshold) and exposure to the risks of ERCP in the positive MRCP group.
2. Using preoperative stratification to perform selective IOC (or LUS) or alternatively performing routine IOC (or LUS) on all patients. If CBD stones are identified, then the options are:
   (a) Exploration of the bile duct with removal of the CBD stones intraoperatively by transcystic removal or choledochotomy.
   (b) Secure closure of the cystic duct and perform postoperative ERCP.
   The potential disadvantage of this approach is the risk of failure of ERCP to remove the CBD stones, although in practical terms this is < 5%. Some surgeons place an antegrade stent at LC to further reduce this risk.

3. Not performing any pre- or intraoperative imaging and assessing patients on symptoms, or persistence of abnormal LFTs to select for postoperative CBD imaging.

It is clear that a small proportion of patients undergoing LC regardless of pre- or intraoperative investigations will thus have 'missed' CBD stones. The *potential* risks posed by these CBD stones are of subsequent acute gallstone pancreatitis, and postoperative bile leak due to CBD stone impaction and raised intrabiliary pressure causing clip failure in the first few days before the cystic duct has sealed. A study of 10 000 LC procedures in Switzerland identified that the immediate risk of acute postoperative pancreatitis was 0.34% and was due to CBD stones in only four patients (0.0004%).[76] The incidence of CBD stones in patients with cystic duct stump leaks is only 3–5%,[77,78] and thus neither of these concerns is significant.

Furthermore, several studies have shown that the incidence of symptoms relating to retained CBD stones is itself low and in fact not significantly different to the incidence of symptoms in patients who had undergone IOC with supposedly clear ducts.[79,80] The complication rate in these groups of patients with retained stones was very low.[76,77]

The author's favoured approach is the use of preoperative imaging (MRCP) in the small group of patients presenting with gallbladder stones and obstructive jaundice (where the presence of CBD stones is > 50%) and selective IOC in patients with acute gallstone pancreatitis or deranged LFTs. If stones are found on IOC, the favoured approach would be to proceed with LBDE for large stones if the CBD is > 8 mm, or post-LC ERCP for small stones/small ducts (Fig. 12.12).

With so many options available, and with differences in availability of resources, this area requires further research

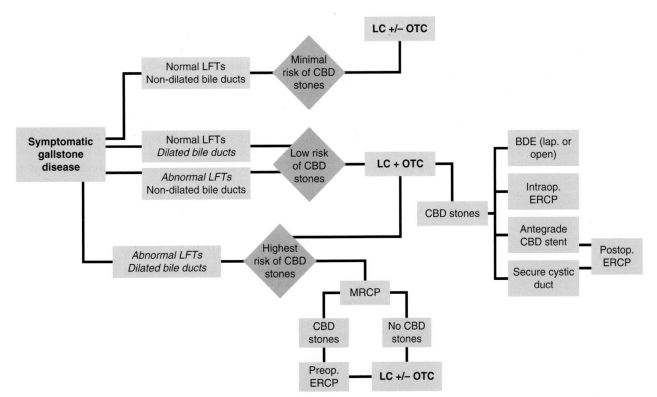

**Figure 12.12** Management algorithm for management of cholelithiasis. *BDE,* bile duct exploration; *CBD,* common bile duct; *ERCP,* endoscopic retrograde cholangiopancreatography; *LC,* laparoscopic cholecystectomy; *LFT,* live function test; *MRCP,* magnetic resonance cholangiopancreatography; *OTC,* on-table cholangiography.

to establish the best and most cost-effective approach. A large multicentre study in the UK is in progress (the Sunflower study).

✓ Patients with mild or moderately elevated LFTs can safely undergo laparoscopic cholecystectomy with intraoperative bile duct imaging or postoperative investigation of ongoing biliary symptoms, reducing the high number of unnecessary preoperative MRCPs.

## MANAGEMENT OF SPECIFIC SCENARIOS

### GALLSTONE ILEUS

Gallstone ileus (another misnomer) is not a dysfunction of motility but is a mechanical obstruction of the bowel caused by an impacted gallstone. It occurs as the result of an acutely inflamed gallbladder becoming adherent to a segment of bowel with subsequent inflammation and erosion of the stone through the bowel wall. The median age of affected patients is 70 years. It represents 1% of small bowel obstructions in patients aged < 70 years, but 5% in those aged > 70 years.[81] Presentation is with vomiting and abdominal distension and only rarely with acute cholecystitis. Half will have a preceding history of symptomatic gallstone disease. The stones are invariably large (> 2.5 cm) and obstruction is most frequently at the level of the terminal ileum. Management following resuscitation is to remove the stone via a small enterotomy with primary closure of the bowel usually possible. Bowel resection is only necessary in the presence of perforation or ischaemia. Removal of the gallbladder is fraught with hazard due to the presence of the inflammation and cholecysto-enteric fistula. In most cases the stones have passed and the fistula closes spontaneously. Elective cholecystectomy and closure of the fistula is rarely necessary.[82]

### MIRIZZI SYNDROME

Type I Mirizzi syndrome can be managed by subtotal cholecystectomy with removal of the majority of the gallbladder leaving the posterior wall where it is adherent to the bile duct, and ligation of the cystic duct if identified and still patent. Sometimes no cystic duct is found and a drain is simply left in the gallbladder fossa in case a later leak does occur. Type II Mirizzi is defined by the presence of a fistula between the gallbladder and the bile duct due to erosion of the impacted gallbladder stone in Hartmann's pouch. There is usually a large amount of chronic inflammation present and primary closure and T-tube insertion rarely works. Typically, the CBD will need to be reconstructed with a Roux-en-Y HJ (see Chapter 13).

## POSTCHOLECYSTECTOMY COMPLICATIONS: IDENTIFICATION AND MANAGEMENT

### EARLY PRESENTATION

With the majority of LCs performed as day case procedures, surgeons need to have a high index of suspicion for complications, and patients deviating from the normal pathway of early and rapid return to normal function within the first few hours or days of an elective cholecystectomy should be reviewed by an experienced surgeon.

Excessive pain in the early postoperative period may be an indicator of intraperitoneal leakage of bile or bowel contents. Significant hypotension and pain may be an indicator of bleeding. Early re-laparoscopy, to identify and correct these problems, is preferred to diagnostic imaging, which is likely to add delay and may be inconclusive.

Common sites of bleeding are from a slipped cystic artery clip or missed cystic artery, damage to the middle hepatic vein within the gallbladder bed of the liver, or damage to the superior epigastric vessels from port insertion. Bile leaks may be from slipped cystic duct clips, damage to the cystic duct during IOC, a duct of Luschka injury or injury to the main bile duct.

The duct of Luschka is a subvesical duct which lies within the gallbladder bed of the liver close to the surface and can be damaged during removal of the posterior gallbladder wall. These ducts are small and away from the porta hepatis. When a leak is identified, it should be clipped or sutured to seal it and prevent ongoing leakage (Fig. 12.13). Failure to identify the exact source of a small bile leak should be managed by insertion of a drain. Most low-volume leaks from a duct of Luschka will resolve with simple drainage. In prolonged drainage (> 5 days), resolution may be expedited by ERCP and stent insertion. Persistent leakage requires formal identification of the damaged duct and suturing, or rarely, resection of a segment of liver and should be dealt with in a specialist hepatopancreaticobiliary (HPB) unit.

Cystic duct stump leak requires further clip application or suturing. Clips used to hold a cholangiogram catheter in place can cause a small hole when removed and caution should be used to ensure that the lower most definitive clip is placed below the IOC cannula clip to prevent this.

Identification of a bile leak from the porta hepatis should be managed by insertion of a drain to the gallbladder fossa area, with discussion and early transfer to an HPB unit for investigation. The algorithm for investigation of a potential bile duct injury will depend on the timing postcholecystectomy, the presence or absence of sepsis and physiological well-being of the patient (see below).

✓ Patients who do not follow the normal pattern of straightforward recovery within the first 48 hours following cholecystectomy should be suspected of having a biliary leak until proven otherwise.

### DELAYED PRESENTATION

Patients who have been discharged home and re-present with ongoing or new onset of abdominal pain following LC should be investigated with assessment of full blood count and LFTs, and consideration of CT. Ultrasound is rarely helpful in this setting due to the presence of RUQ tenderness and intra-abdominal gas. A small amount of gas and fluid in the gallbladder bed may be normal, but collections of fluid or gas elsewhere may represent a bile leak. If haemostatic agents (e.g. Surgicel) have been used to control bleeding in the gallbladder bed, there may be gas containing foreign material seen on US or CT. Elevated abnormal LFTs also raise suspicion of a bile leak or retained CBD stone. MRCP or ERCP

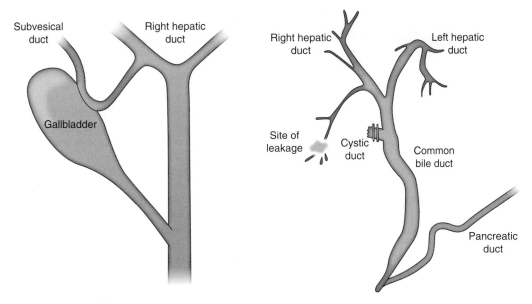

**Figure 12.13**  Anatomy of the duct of Luschka injury.

will be diagnostic and the exact approach is dictated by the initial findings and clinical suspicion, the patient's condition and clinical urgency, and local availability and expertise. Concerns over MRI and dislodgement of cystic duct or artery clips in the immediate postoperative period are unfounded since virtually all metallic clips in current usage are non-ferrous.[83] The presence of bile collections or dilated intrahepatic ducts raises the suspicion of a bile duct injury and warrants early discussion and transfer to a specialist HPB unit.

Visualisation of a fluid collection in the presence of excessive pain, sepsis and/or abnormal LFTs should be evaluated with a percutaneous radiologically sited drain (or alternatively, the patient should be taken back to theatre for re-laparoscopy). If bile is drained, an MRCP should be arranged to look for bile leakage or CBD stones with progression to ERCP if either is identified. If neither is identified and the patient is not septic, then it is likely that the leak is small and will settle without further intervention and the drain can be removed once dry.

Retained CBD stones identified by MRCP in the postoperative period are best dealt with by ERCP. Success rates in most centres exceed 95% and recent developments of ultrathin cholangioscopy (e.g. SpyGlass) permitting break-up of stones under direct vision using either electrohydraulic or laser lithotripsy are likely to increase this rate further.[84] LBDE can be performed in those where ERCP is not possible, e.g. large duodenal diverticulum, previous gastric bypass surgery.

✓ Patients re-presenting following cholecystectomy should undergo CT to look for a collection. In the presence of sepsis or significant abdominal pain, needle aspiration and subsequent drainage is mandated to look for a bile leak.

## BILE DUCT INJURY

It is widely held that the incidence of bile duct injuries increased twofold following the introduction of laparoscopic surgery to around 0.4%.[85] Increasing recognition and the development and promulgation of techniques to prevent

bile duct injury have reduced the rates to approximately 0.2–0.3%; however, this disguises the fact that there has been a significant incidence in more severe injuries in the laparoscopic group and a recognition that injury to the right hepatic artery is also present in approximately 25% of patients with a major bile duct injury.[86]

Davidoff et al.[87] described the mechanisms and errors involved in the causation of a 'classical' bile duct injury in the laparoscopic era. In this injury, there is misidentification of the common duct for the cystic duct with subsequent ligation and division of the CBD, often with ligation of the right hepatic artery. This injury results in complete excision of a segment of the bile duct (Fig. 12.14). The classification of bile duct injuries and their management is further discussed in Chapter 13.

## POSTOPERATIVE PROBLEMS (CHRONIC)

Postoperative pain resolution following cholecystectomy is dependent upon case selection. Postcholecystectomy pain is invariably the result of precholecystectomy symptoms/other diagnoses and there is no evidence that the procedure of LC in itself results in the development of abdominal pain.

A proportion of patients (approximately 5%) develop looser bowel habit or urgency of defaecation, although this is usually in patients who had some degree of symptoms (e.g. irritable bowel syndrome) pre-LC. Severe high-volume diarrhoea is fortunately extremely rare.[88,89] Loose stools may be due to the more constant flow of bile entering a relatively empty bowel resulting in irritation of the bowel rather than a bolus of bile delivered by contraction of the gallbladder in response to CCK into a small bowel containing fat. In half of these patients, a degree of adaptation appears to occur with resolution of symptoms over a period of 3–6 months. Patients who continue to be troubled with diarrhoea may benefit from loperamide to control urgency and/or a bile-binding agent such as cholestyramine.[90]

Gallstones which are dropped at the time of cholecystectomy as a result of perforation of the gallbladder are

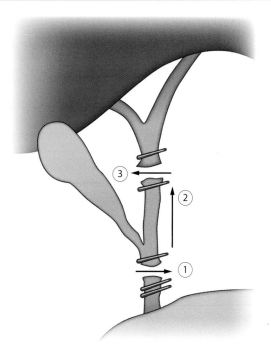

**Figure 12.14** The 'classical' bile duct injury. Excessive cephalad retraction of the gallbladder leads to dissection of the common bile duct low down (1). Subsequent mobilisation of the bile duct occurs (2). Removal of the gallbladder specimen requires further division of the bile duct (3) and, in around 25% of cases, division of the right hepatic artery (RHA) as well. (Adapted from Davidoff AM, Pappas TN, Murray EA, et al. Mechanisms of major biliary injury during laparoscopic cholecystectomy. Ann Surg 1992;215(3):196–202.)

quite commonly seen with an estimated incidence of spilled stones in approximately 7% of LCs, and of stones definitely left within the peritoneal cavity of approximately 2%.[91] Complications of dropped stones are, however, uncommon. The commonest complication of dropped stones is the development of an intra-abdominal abscess which occurs in 0.1–2.9% of patients with dropped stones, presenting on average 14 months after surgery.[92] Some of these present with subphrenic abscess formation requiring repeat laparoscopy or laparotomy to drain the pus and find the causative stone(s). The stones themselves may be very small but can usually be identified on CT. Attempts should therefore be made to remove all spilled stones where possible, although conversion to laparotomy is not considered advisory to achieve complete clearance.

## GALLSTONES AND CANCER

A number of studies purported to show both positive and negative associations between gallstones or cholecystectomy and various non-biliary tract cancers, in particular with the development of gastrointestinal tract cancers. A large population-based study in the US suggests that there may be a slight increase in liver, pancreatic and gastro-oesophageal cancers but a decrease in colorectal cancers. Whether these increases are true or occur by chance, the risk ratios are small and insufficient to advise a change of practice either way.[93]

There is an association between gallstones and the development of gallbladder cancers, with a relative risk of 4.9.[94] The relative risk is further increased from 2.4 in patients

with stones < 3 cm, to 10 with stones > 3 cm. However, there is no justification for removal of the gallbladder based solely on concerns over the risk of developing gallbladder cancer.

## PORCELAIN GALLBLADDER

Extensive calcium encrustation of the gallbladder wall is referred to as porcelain gallbladder. The incidence of porcelain gallbladder is reported to be 0.6–0.8%, with a male-to-female ratio of 1:5. Most porcelain gallbladders (90%) are associated with gallstones.[95,96] Patients with a porcelain gallbladder are asymptomatic, and the condition is usually found incidentally on plain abdominal radiographs, US or CT imaging. Surgical treatment of porcelain gallbladder is based on results from studies performed between1931 and 1973, which demonstrated a very high frequency (22–68%) of adenocarcinoma in porcelain gallbladder.[97]

However, the causal relationship between porcelain gallbladder and malignancy has not been established and the very high rates of carcinoma originally quoted seem, for whatever reason, to be less high than previously recorded in more recent case series (i.e. dating from 2001 to 2011) that show incidences ranging from 2.3% to 7%.[98,99] Current guidance is that patients found to have porcelain gallbladder should undergo LC to prevent the risk of developing gallbladder cancer.

## OTHER DISEASES OF THE GALLBLADDER

## ACUTE ACALCULOUS CHOLECYSTITIS

Acute acalculous cholecystitis is a life-threatening condition that occurs in critically ill patients. It is an uncommon problem encountered largely in patients in intensive care or in cardiac patients as a result of poor perfusion. The cystic artery is an end-organ artery with no collateral circulation and poor perfusion can result in gallbladder ischaemia with resultant pain and tenderness. The diagnosis is often elusive and the condition is associated with significant mortality (up to 50%). Risk factors include severe trauma or burns, major surgery such as cardiopulmonary bypass, prolonged fasting, total parenteral nutrition, sepsis, diabetes mellitus, atherosclerotic disease, systemic vasculitis, acute renal failure and acquired immunodeficiency syndrome (AIDS). The condition is thought to be caused by microvascular occlusion of end arteries within the gallbladder wall resulting in ischaemia and, in up to 60% of cases, in gangrene.[100] Over 70% of patients have atherosclerotic disease, which might explain the higher prevalence of the condition in elderly men.[101]

The diagnosis of acute acalculous cholecystitis is often hindered by obtundation of the patient, the presence of pre-existing diseases or recent abdominal surgery, and requires a high index of suspicion. Ultrasound confirms the diagnosis within the intensive care unit and allows immediate percutaneous cholecystostomy which reduces the tension on the gallbladder wall and has become the preferred alternative to cholecystectomy in the treatment of the condition in severely ill patients.[102] Early cholecystectomy may still be appropriate depending on the patient's clinical condition and if cholecystostomy fails to improve the patient's condition, as gangrene can develop with subsequent perforation of the gallbladder.

## PRIMARY INFECTIONS OF THE GALLBLADDER

Primary infective cholecystitis is rare and is more commonly seen in immunocompromised patients. Typical causative organisms include *Salmonella typhi*, *Campylobacter jejuni* and *Vibrio cholera*. The presentation is similar to patients with acute acalculous cholecystitis, but there is often an antecedent history of a gastroenteritis-like illness.

AIDS patients are susceptible to opportunistic gastrointestinal infections including acute cholecystitis and cholangitis, especially when the CD4 count falls below 200. In half the cases, there are no associated gallstones within the biliary tract. The most common infecting agents are cytomegalovirus and cryptosporidium, and less commonly *Candida*, fungi and *Mycobacterium tuberculosis*. The 30-day mortality in AIDS patients with acute cholecystitis is 20%.

Treatment is by appropriate intravenous antibiotics followed by LC.

## CHRONIC ACALCULOUS CHOLECYSTITIS

Chronic acalculous cholecystitis is a poorly understood condition. The term is used to describe patients with biliary pain but without cholelithiasis. In some cases, biliary sludge may be responsible for a localised inflammatory response in the gallbladder with pain and tenderness typical of low-grade biliary pain. Occasionally a tiny stone within the spiral valve of the cystic duct is found at cholecystectomy which was missed preoperatively.

In patients with typical biliary pain, cholecystectomy may be justifiable in the absence of other disease processes and treatment options. Informed consent with an understanding of at best a 50% likelihood of pain resolution must be emphasised.

Isotope scans with HIDA or DISIDA (cholescintigraphy) have been used to improve outcomes in this group by selecting patients with a non-functioning gallbladder (failure to take up isotope within 4 hours of injection) or poorly functioning gallbladder. The gallbladder ejection fraction (GBEF) is used to calculate gallbladder function by giving a CCK analogue or fatty meal following uptake of the isotope by the gallbladder. These stimulate emptying of the gallbladder, allowing an ejection fraction to be calculated. Administration of CCK may also recreate the pain. Normal GBEF is around 75% and LC in patients with low GBEFs (< 40%) achieves long-term symptom relief in 65–80% of cases.[103,104]

## GALLBLADDER DISEASE IN CHILDHOOD

Underlying conditions are identified in 60% of children presenting with gallstones. These include haemolytic anaemias, congenital anomalies (choledochal cyst, prematurity, necrotising enterocolitis), genetic disorders (Down syndrome, cystic fibrosis), Crohn's disease and ileal resection, liver disease and cirrhosis, cancer or leukaemia therapy.[105] Obesity is becoming an increasingly important risk factor in development of childhood cholelithiasis. Overall, the risk of gallstones in children is 0.13% (0.27% in females). Management is similar to that of adults, with LC.[106] CBD stones are the commonest cause of obstructive jaundice in children.

Acalculous cholecystitis in children may follow burns and trauma and may also be seen as a postoperative complication of abdominal surgery. It occurs at any age from 1 month to 15 years[107] and is frequently misdiagnosed as appendicitis. Cholecystostomy is the treatment of choice.

## ADENOMYOMATOSIS

Adenomyomatosis of the gallbladder is an acquired, hyperplastic lesion characterised by excessive proliferation of the gallbladder mucosa with invaginations into the muscle layer to produce deep clefts (Rokitansky–Aschoff sinuses). It may be generalised or localised to one area (adenomyoma). The involved gallbladder wall is thickened to 10 mm or greater. Gallstones are found in 60% of cases. It is usually an incidental radiological or pathological finding and simple adenomyomatosis is not considered a premalignant condition.

In the absence of biliary tract symptoms, adenomyomatosis requires no treatment. If the patient has biliary pain and evidence of adenomyomatosis with calculi, a cholecystectomy is indicated. The benefit of LC in patients with biliary pain and adenomyomatosis but no gallstones is more difficult to predict but the likelihood of benefit from surgery increases the more extensive or severe the adenomyomatosis.[108]

---

### Key points

- Biliary pain is typically epigastric/right upper quadrant pain, radiating around or through to the back, lasting > 20 minutes, often occurring at night or associated with eating fatty foods.
- People with gallstones but without symptoms do not require further management or follow-up.
- People with gallstones and biliary pain should be offered laparoscopic cholecystectomy as definitive treatment to prevent further episodes of pain and development of complications.
- Laparoscopic cholecystectomy is one of the commonest general surgical procedures in the UK, with around 100 000 procedure performed per annum.
- Current advice is to remove all CBD stones, which can be done most cost-effectively by simultaneous laparoscopic bile duct exploration but is still most frequently done by ERCP.
- Following cholecystectomy, patients presenting with abdominal pain in the first 48 hours should be investigated quickly to identify potential biliary leaks/bile duct injury.

---

 References available at http://ebooks.health.elsevier.com/

### KEY REFERENCES

[29] Reynolds W. The first laparoscopic cholecystectomy. J Soc Laparoend Surg 2001;5:89–94.
   *Good review of the early history of laparoscopic cholecystectomy.*
[44] Strasberg SM, Brunt LM. Rationale and use of the critical view of safety in laparoscopic cholecystectomy. J Am Coll Surg 2010;211:132–8. PMID: 20610259.
   *Essential reading for rationale and technique of safe cholecystectomy avoiding bile duct injury.*
[67] Williams EJ, Green J, Beckingham I, et al. Updated guidelines on the management of common bile duct stones (CBDS). Gut 2017;66(5):765–82. PMID: 28122906.
   *Definitive guidelines on current diagnosis and management of CBD stones.*
[87] Davidoff AM, Pappas TN, Murray EA, et al. Mechanisms of major biliary injury during laparoscopic cholecystectomy. Ann Surg 1992;215(3):196–202. PMID: 1531913.
   *Analysis of causes of bile duct injury during laparoscopic cholecystectomy.*

# 13 Benign biliary tract diseases

Benjamin N.J. Thomson

## INTRODUCTION

Apart from those disorders related to choledocholithiasis, benign diseases of the biliary tree are relatively uncommon (Box 13.1). The most challenging patients are those who present with symptoms associated with biliary strictures, which arise more commonly following iatrogenic injury during cholecystectomy. Congenital abnormalities such as biliary atresia and choledochal cysts are usually in the domain of the paediatric surgeon, although later presentation of cysts may occur after missed diagnosis or when revisional surgery is required. Most of the published literature regarding benign non-gallstone biliary disease is retrospective or at best prospectively gathered, non-randomised data, but clear guidelines can be followed based upon this experience.

## CONGENITAL ANOMALIES

### BILIARY ATRESIA

Biliary atresia occurs in approximately 1 per 10 000 live births, but its aetiology remains unclear. There is experimental evidence for a primary perinatal viral infection as well as cellular and humoral autoimmunity. An inflammatory process before birth may result in failure of the biliary lumen to develop in all or part of the extrahepatic biliary tree. Several clinical variants are thought to originate during intrauterine development with different outcomes from surgical hepatic portoenterostomy. Around 80% have an isolated form which includes a cytomegalovirus variant. A congenital malformation accounts for 10–20% and this includes a biliary atresia malformation syndrome (BASM) and cystic biliary atresia (CBA).[1]

Presentation is usually in the early neonatal period with prolongation of neonatal jaundice. Most patients are treated in specialist neonatal surgical units; however, occasionally patients may be referred to adult units for assessment for liver transplantation following previous unsuccessful treatment. Management in the neonate is by surgical porto-enterostomy (Kasai procedure), which involves anastomosis of a Roux limb of jejunum to the tissue of the hilum. Restoration of bile flow has been reported in 86% of infants treated before 8 weeks of age, but only 36% in older children.[2] The 4-year survival rate is dependent on the timing of surgery. Of 349 North American children with biliary atresia, 210 (60%) required later liver transplantation, with a 4-year

transplantation survival of 82%.[3] A properly performed Kasai porto-enterostomy can postpone the need for liver transplantation and improve outcome. Better outcomes are also seen following maternal living donor-related liver transplantation, potentially due to tolerance to non-inherited maternal antigens.[4]

## CHOLEDOCHAL CYSTS

Presentation is usually in childhood, with jaundice, fever or an abdominal mass. Around 25% are diagnosed in the first year, although prenatal diagnosis is usually possible with improvements in antenatal ultrasonography. Adult centres treat a small proportion of those presenting with late symptoms or complications from previous cyst surgery.

The incidence of choledochal cysts in Western countries is around 1 in 200 000 live births, but it is much higher in Asia. There is frequent association with other hepatobiliary disease such as hepatic fibrosis, as well as an aberrant pancreaticobiliary duct junction. Magnetic resonance cholangiopancreatography (MRCP) is the non-invasive imaging investigation of choice (Fig.13.1).

### CLASSIFICATION

The modified Todani classification is employed to describe the various forms of choledochal cyst[5] (Fig. 13.2). Type I, the most common, represents a solitary cyst characterised by fusiform dilatation of the common bile duct (CBD). Type II comprises a diverticulum of the CBD, whilst type III cysts are choledochocoeles. Type IV is the second most common, with extension of cysts into the intrahepatic ducts. Lastly, type V involves intrahepatic cystic disease with no choledochal cyst, which merges into the syndrome of Caroli disease.

### RISK OF MALIGNANCY

In the Western literature, the incidence of cholangiocarcinoma (Fig. 13.1) is reported to be approximately 12%,[6] but is higher in Japanese reports. Sastry et al.[7] reported 434 cancers in 5780 patients with a choledochal cyst from 78 studies. Cholangiocarcinoma occurred in 70.4% and gallbladder cancer in 23.5%, but cancer occurring before the age of 18 years was rare. Cyst drainage without cyst excision does not prevent later malignant change, and there is continuing debate regarding the precise ongoing risk following cyst resection with reports of remnant biliary tract malignancy developing as long as 30 years post resection. In a report of 180 patients who underwent primary surgery, synchronous malignancy was found in 36 patients (20%), with only one of the remaining patients developing malignancy during follow-up.[8] At present there are no guidelines for the follow-up of patients post resection, but given the risk of malignancy magnetic resonance imaging (MRI) allows effective surveillance imaging.

## MANAGEMENT

Surgical resection of types I, II and IV choledochal cysts is required to prevent recurrent episodes of sepsis and pain, to prevent the risk of pancreatitis from passage of debris and calculi, and because of the association with cholangiocarcinoma. Complete cyst excision with preservation of the pancreatic duct is required, with hepaticojejunostomy for reconstruction. Some authors advocate liver resection for type IV cysts with intrahepatic extension for complete removal of the cyst, although the advantage is debatable. For those patients with Caroli disease, resection may be feasible if the biliary involvement is localised to one part of the liver. For other patients, endoscopic or radiological techniques may be required to address biliary sepsis

by improving biliary drainage, while others may need to be considered for hepatic replacement if liver failure develops.

Cyst-enterostomy, or drainage of the cyst into the duodenum, should no longer be performed for extrahepatic cysts as the cyst epithelium remains unstable and malignant potential exists. If previous drainage has been performed, symptoms of cholangitis generally persist and conversion to a Roux-en-Y hepaticojejunostomy is advisable.

## SPECIAL OPERATIVE TECHNIQUES

During operative exposure, intraoperative ultrasound is very useful to identify the biliary confluence, the intrahepatic extension of the cyst and the relationship to the right hepatic artery above and to the pancreatic duct below (Fig. 13.3). Small aberrant hepatic ducts may enter the cyst below the biliary confluence and these are missed frequently on preoperative imaging. Such aberrant ducts are usually identified once the cyst has been opened. The uncomplicated cyst is normally best excised in its entirety and this is facilitated by opening it along its anterior length. This aids identification of the vessels from which the cyst is fed. Early identification of the biliary confluence aids the surgeon in planning the incorporation of any segmental duct into the eventual hepaticojejunal Roux-en-Y anastomosis. Dissection into the head of the pancreas is made easier by use of bipolar scissors and the CUSA™ (ultrasonic surgical aspiration system, ValleyLab, Boulder, CO) if the plane of dissection is obscured by fibrosis or inflammation. It may be necessary to leave a small oversewn lower CBD stump to avoid compromise to the pancreatic duct lumen; however, recurrent pancreatitis and possible malignant transformation remain possible complications. Pancreaticoduodenectomy is difficult to justify in the uncomplicated case when dealing with the residual lower bile duct. Laparoscopic and robotic resection and reconstruction have been described; Senthilnathan et al.[9] reported 110 adults and children successfully managed, with three adults requiring conversion, a re-exploration rate of 1.8% and one death. Cholangitis occurred in three patients, with three requiring intervention for anastomotic strictures on the short-term follow-up. (See recommended video at the end of chapter.)

✓✓ There is an accepted association between choledochal cyst and cholangiocarcinoma. The cyst should be excised and the biliary tree reconstructed by means of a Roux-en-Y hepaticojejunostomy.

---

### Box 13.1  Benign causes of biliary strictures

**Strictures of the extrahepatic biliary tree**

*Iatrogenic biliary injury*

Post cholecystectomy
Trauma
Other

*Gallstone-related*

Mirizzi syndrome

*Inflammatory*

Recurrent pyogenic cholangitis
Parasitic infestation
    *Clonorchis sinensis*
    *Opisthorchis viverrini*
    *Echinococcus*
    *Ascaris*
HIV/AIDS cholangiopathy
Primary sclerosing cholangitis
Benign strictures imitating malignancy
Pancreatitis
IgG4-related disease
    Autoimmune pancreatitis
    IgG4-related cholangiopathy
    Inflammatory pseudotumour

---

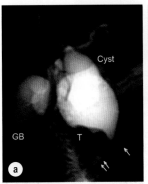
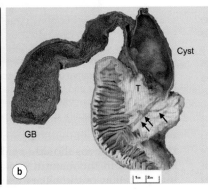

**Figure 13.1** Magnetic resonance cholangiopancreatography **(a)** and macroscopic photograph **(b)** demonstrating a type I choledochal cyst with a distal cholangiocarcinoma in a 42-year-old White woman requiring a pancreatico-duodenectomy. Gallbladder *(GB)*, tumour *(T)*, pancreatic duct *(single arrow)* and aberrant common channel *(double arrow)* are shown. (Courtesy of Professor Prithi S. Bhathal, Pathology Department, University of Melbourne, Australia.)

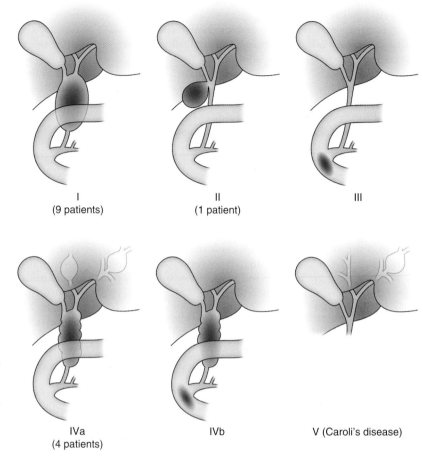

I
(9 patients)

II
(1 patient)

III

IVa
(4 patients)

IVb

V (Caroli's disease)

**Figure 13.2** Modified Todani classification for choledochal cysts.[9] (Reproduced from Todani T, Watanabe Y, Narusue M et al. Congenital bile duct cysts: classification, operative procedures, and review of thirty-seven cases including cancer arising from choledochal cyst. Am J Surg 1977;134:263–9. With permission from Elsevier.)

## IATROGENIC BILIARY INJURY

The commonest cause of an injury to the extrahepatic biliary tree is as a result of an iatrogenic injury at the time of cholecystectomy. Although it is recognised that injury may also occur during other gastric or pancreatic procedures, this is much less common with the reduction in ulcer surgery and increasing specialisation in pancreaticobiliary surgery. Rarely, the injury may be related to abdominal trauma,[10] injection of scolicidal agents in the management of hydatid cyst, ablation of hepatic tumours or radiotherapy. The true incidence of biliary injury following laparoscopic cholecystectomy remains obscure, but there has been a slight increase since its introduction, with a reported incidence of 0.3–0.7%.[11] Despite the expectation that the rate of injury would decrease with experience, the Swedish quality register reported a rate of 0.3% in 55 134 cholecystectomies performed from 2007 to 2011.[12] Recent variations in technique such as single-incision laparoscopic surgery (SILS) cholecystectomy are not immune to biliary injury, with a rate of 0.72% reported in 2626 patients undergoing SILS.[13]

## AETIOLOGY

Previous reports of injury during laparoscopic cholecystectomy suggested that injury was more likely to occur when performed for pancreatitis, cholangitis or acute cholecystitis.[14]

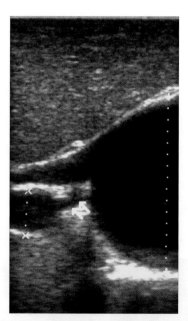

**Figure 13.3** Operative ultrasound scan of a type I choledochal cyst. The junction of the undilated proximal biliary tree with the cyst (long dotted line) is demonstrated. The right hepatic artery is posterior (two arrows), as is the right branch of the portal vein (short dotted line).

However, surgeons should remain vigilant regardless of the indication. In the majority of patients the problem is misinterpretation of the biliary anatomy, with the CBD being confused with the cystic duct. Associated injury to the right hepatic artery often occurs as it is mistaken for the cystic artery. Partial injury may occur to the CBD after a diathermy burn or due to rigorous traction on the cystic duct, leading to its avulsion from the bile duct.

## TECHNIQUES TO AVOID INJURY

Many techniques have been described to decrease the risk of injury to the CBD during cholecystectomy. The main risk factors are thought to be inexperience, aberrant anatomy and inflammation.[14,15] However, in an analysis of 252 laparoscopic bile duct injuries, the authors suggested that the primary cause of error was a visual perceptual illusion often resulting in loss of situational awareness in 97% of cases, whilst faults in technical skill were thought to have been present in only 3% of injuries.[16]

Correct identification of the biliary anatomy is essential in avoiding injury to the extrahepatic bile duct. Dissection of Hartmann's pouch should start at the junction of the gallbladder and cystic duct and continue lateral to the cystic lymph node, thus staying as close as possible to the gallbladder. The biliary tree and hepatic arterial anatomy is highly variable and therefore great care must be taken in identifying all structures within Calot's triangle before ligation. In Couinaud's published study of biliary anatomy, 25% had drainage of a right sectoral duct directly into the common hepatic duct.[17] Sometimes this structure may follow a prolonged extrahepatic course, where it can be at greater risk from cholecystectomy (Figs. 13.4 and 13.5). The right hepatic artery may also course through this area. All structures should be traced into the gallbladder to minimise the risk of injury.

Calot's original description of gallbladder anatomy described a triangle formed by the cystic duct, common hepatic duct and superior border of the cystic artery. For satisfactory visualisation of the structures, dissection should also extend above the cystic artery to the liver. Extensive dissection should be avoided in Calot's triangle as diathermy injury may occur to the lateral wall of the common hepatic duct. Furthermore, arterial bleeding in this area should not be cauterised or clipped blindly. Most bleeding can be controlled with several minutes of direct pressure with a laparoscopic forceps compressing Hartmann's pouch on to the bleed point. During the era of open cholecystectomy, many advocated complete excision of the cystic duct to its insertion into the CBD to avoid a cystic duct stump syndrome. However, extensive dissection around the CBD with or without diathermy may cause an ischaemic stricture due to damage to the intricate blood supply of the common hepatic duct.

Strasberg described the 'critical view of safety' with complete dissection of Calot's triangle by mobilisation of the gallbladder neck from the gallbladder bed of the liver before transecting the cystic artery and duct.[15] More recently, Connor et al.[18] suggested a five-point checklist to limit the occurrence of biliary injury at laparoscopic cholecystectomy. The five steps are: '(i) confirm the gallbladder lies in the hepatic principal plane and is retracted to the 10 o'clock position; (ii) confirm Hartmann's pouch is lifted up and towards the segment IV pedicle; (iii) identify Rouviere's sulcus; (iv) confirm the release of the posterior leaf of the peritoneum covering the hepatobiliary triangle; and (v) confirm the critical view with or without intraoperative cholangiography'.

Many authors argue that operative cholangiography is essential to avoid biliary injury.[11,14] Fletcher et al.[14] reported an overall twofold reduction in biliary injuries with the use of operative cholangiography, with an eightfold decrease in complex cases. Flum et al.[11] analysed retrospectively the Medicare database in the USA and identified 7911

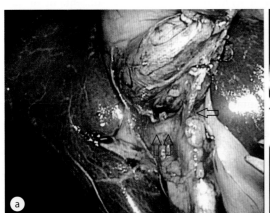 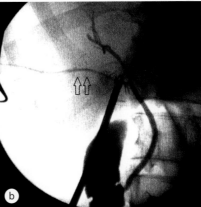

**Figure 13.4** Aberrant biliary anatomy. The normal biliary anatomy is a trifurcation of the right sectoral and left hepatic ducts forming the common hepatic duct which receives the cystic duct after a variable distance. Operative photograph **(a)** and a cholangiogram **(b)** of a short cystic duct (*single arrow*) draining into the right posterior sectoral duct (*double arrow*), which has a long extrahepatic course.

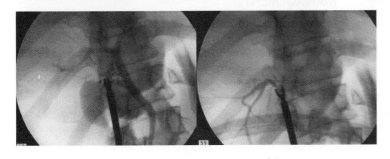

**Figure 13.5** Operative cholangiography of an aberrant right sectoral duct. The injury was recognised after division of the duct following cholangiography. The cholangiogram catheter was used to obtain a cholangiogram of the aberrant duct. The surgeon obtained advice by telephone and a decision was made to ligate the duct. The patient remains asymptomatic.

CBD injuries following cholecystectomy. After adjusting for patient-level factors and surgeon-level factors, the relative risk was 1.49 when intraoperative cholangiography was not used. In a recent meta-analysis of 2 million cholecystectomy patients, 9000 bile duct injuries were included. The rates of bile duct injury were 0.36% when cholangiography was used routinely and 0.53% when used selectively.[19]

When the use of intraoperative cholangiography has undergone cost analysis, routine cholangiography has been found to be most cost-effective during high-risk operations when employed by less experienced surgeons.[20]

Unfortunately, many operative cholangiograms are interpreted incorrectly and injuries are missed. Although this event should be less frequent with the use of modern C-arm imaging, in reported series of biliary injuries only 6–33% of operative cholangiograms are interpreted correctly. For correct anatomical interpretation of the proximal biliary tree, both right sectoral/sectional ducts and the left hepatic duct should be visualised. In the presence of an endoscopic sphincterotomy, contrast will preferentially flow into the duodenum and the patient may need to be placed in a head-down position to fill the intrahepatic ducts. If the anatomy is unclear, no proximal clip should be placed on what is presumed to be the cystic duct, to avoid a crush injury to what may be the common hepatic duct.

Retrograde cholecystectomy has been described previously as a safe technique when inflammation around Calot's triangle makes identification of the anatomy difficult. Nonetheless, care still needs to be exercised during dissection to avoid injury to the right hepatic artery and common hepatic duct, which may be adherent to an inflamed gallbladder. Eight such vasculobiliary injuries were described by Strasberg and Gouma.[21] If identification remains impossible, then the gallbladder can be opened to facilitate identification of the cystic duct. A subtotal cholecystectomy should be considered if a safe plane of dissection cannot be established, thus avoiding injury to the common hepatic or left hepatic ducts. Originally described for open cholecystectomy, these techniques have now also been performed laparoscopically.

✓✓ Bile duct injury can be avoided by careful identification of the biliary anatomy, dissection close to the gallbladder and avoidance of diathermy in Calot's triangle. The use of operative cholangiography and its correct interpretation is associated with a reduced incidence of bile duct injury.

## CLASSIFICATION

Injury to the distal biliary tree is less technically demanding to repair than involvement of the biliary confluence. The success of reconstruction depends on the type of injury and the anatomical location.[22] Bismuth[23] first described a classification system for biliary strictures reflecting the relationship of the injury to the biliary confluence (Table 13.1). Strasberg et al.[24] further proposed a broader classification to include a number of biliary complications, including cystic stump leaks, biliary leaks and partial injuries to the biliary tree (Fig. 13.6). Recently the European Association for Endoscopic Surgery (EAES) has proposed the ATOM (anatomic, time of detection, mechanism) classification to facilitate epidemiologic and comparative studies.[25]

**Table 13.1 Bismuth classification of biliary strictures**

| Bismuth classification | Definition |
| --- | --- |
| Bismuth 1 | Low common hepatic duct stricture—hepatic duct stump > 2 cm |
| Bismuth 2 | Proximal common hepatic duct stricture—hepatic duct stump < 2 cm |
| Bismuth 3 | Hilar stricture with no residual common hepatic duct—hepatic duct confluence intact |
| Bismuth 4 | Destruction of hepatic duct confluence—right and left hepatic ducts separated |
| Bismuth 5 | Involvement of aberrant right sectoral hepatic duct alone or with concomitant stricture of the common hepatic duct |

## PRESENTATION

It is preferable that injuries are recognised at the time of surgery to allow the best chance of repair, but this occurs in less than a third of patients. An unrecognised injury may present early with a postoperative biliary fistula, symptoms of biliary peritonitis or jaundice. Early symptoms or signs may be lacking, but ductal injury should be suspected in the patient whose recovery is not immediate or is complicated by symptoms of peritoneal or diaphragmatic irritation and/or associated with deranged liver function tests in the first 24–48 hours of surgery. Signs may range from localised abdominal tenderness through to generalised peritonitis with overwhelming sepsis. Ligation of the bile duct will present early with jaundice; however, later presentation may occur as a result of stricture formation from a partial injury, localised inflammation or ischaemic insult.

Ligation of sectoral ducts may cause subsequent or late atrophy of the drained liver segments. Occasionally liver resection or transplantation may be required for unilobar hepatic necrosis or fulminant hepatic failure secondary to combined biliary and vascular injuries.[26] More commonly, liver failure presents late with liver failure due to secondary biliary cirrhosis as a result of the injury, and may require liver transplantation.[26]

In many patients there is a delay in referral despite suspicion or evidence of a biliary injury. In a report by Mirza et al.,[27] the median interval until referral was 26 days. This delay is not inconsequential as the opportunity for an early repair is lost and may result in the liver sustaining further damage.

## MANAGEMENT

### INTRAOPERATIVE RECOGNITION

In a review by Carroll et al.,[28] only 27% of patients underwent a successful repair by the primary surgeon responsible for the injury, whilst 79% of repairs performed following referral had a successful outcome. If experienced help is not at hand, an attempt should not be made to remedy the situation since this may compromise subsequent successful management. Advice should be sought immediately and a T-tube or similar drain should be placed to the biliary injury and drains left in

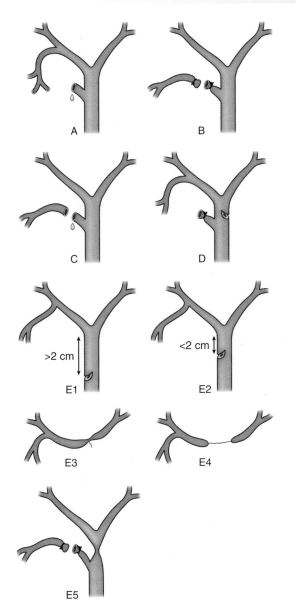

**Figure 13.6** Strasberg classification. Type A injuries include leakage from the cystic duct or subvesical ducts. Type B involves occlusion of part of the biliary tree, most usually an aberrant right hepatic duct. If the former injury involves transection without ligation, this is termed a type C injury. A lateral injury to the biliary tree is a type D injury. Type E injuries are those described by Bismuth and subdivided into his classification (Table 13.1). (Adapted from Strasberg SM, Hertl M, Soper NJ, et al. An analysis of the problem of biliary injury during laparoscopic cholecystectomy. J Am Coll Surg 1995;180:102–25. With permission from the American College of Surgeons.)

the subhepatic space, followed by referral to a specialist centre. Some specialist units may offer a surgeon with expertise in biliary reconstruction who can travel to the site of referral to expedite immediate repair. No attempt should be made to repair a transection or excision of the bile duct.

A partial injury to the bile duct may sometimes be managed by direct closure with placement of a T-tube through a separate choledochotomy. Primary repair with or without a T-tube for complete transection of the CBD is nearly always unsuccessful. This may result from unappreciated loss

of common duct, an associated arterial injury, or result from local diathermy injury or devascularisation of the duct from overzealous dissection of the CBD (Fig. 13.7a and b). Successful endoscopic treatment is possible for failed primary repair; however, as many as 32% of patients will require subsequent hepaticojejunostomy.[29]

✓✓ If an injury to the biliary tree is suspected during cholecystectomy, help must be sought from an experienced hepatobiliary surgeon. A successful repair by the surgeon who has caused the injury is far less likely than one performed by a surgeon experienced in performing a biliary reconstruction.

## POSTOPERATIVE RECOGNITION: BILIARY FISTULA

Any patient who is not fit for discharge at 24 hours due to ongoing abdominal pain, vomiting, fever or bile in an abdominal drain should be considered to have a biliary leak. The lack of bile in an abdominal drain does not exclude the possibility of a biliary leak, particularly if there is liver function test derangement. Symptoms and signs vary widely, and widespread soiling of the abdominal cavity may be present with few signs in the early period following cholecystectomy.

Initial investigation should include full blood examination and determination of serum levels of urea, electrolytes, creatinine and liver function tests. Ultrasound is usually the initial investigation, but it cannot readily differentiate bile and blood from a residual fluid collection following uneventful cholecystectomy. It may provide important information about the presence of intra-abdominal or pelvic fluid, biliary dilatation or retained stones within the bile duct. Computed tomography (CT) is normally preferred since it provides more objective information and allows assessment of the liver vasculature.

If there is evidence of significant peritoneal irritation from widespread biliary peritonitis, laparoscopy allows confirmation of this and provides an opportunity for abdominal lavage. The porta hepatis can be inspected to determine the cause of the bile leak. Whilst dislodged clips from the cystic duct can be managed by application of further clips or suture, any other form of bile leak should lead to specialist referral. Drains can be placed to the subhepatic space as well as the subdiaphragmatic space and pelvis if required. No attempt should be made to repair an injury at laparoscopy. If laparotomy is required, this should be considered in conjunction with specialist assistance if bile duct injury is suspected.

Further assessment depends on the clinical situation. The majority of biliary fistulas are due to leaks from the cystic duct stump or subvesical ducts, and endoscopic retrograde cholangiopancreatography (ERCP) allows anatomical definition, endoscopic sphincterotomy or stent placement when abdominal contamination has been controlled. As complete transection of the bile duct precludes ERCP, computed tomography intravenous cholangiography (CT-IVC) or MRCP can determine continuity of the biliary tree prior to endoscopy. Occasionally, persistent bile drainage is associated with choledocholithiasis requiring endoscopic sphincterotomy and stone extraction. Most simple cystic duct stump leaks are resolved by endoscopic stenting if cannulation is possible at ERCP and occasionally side

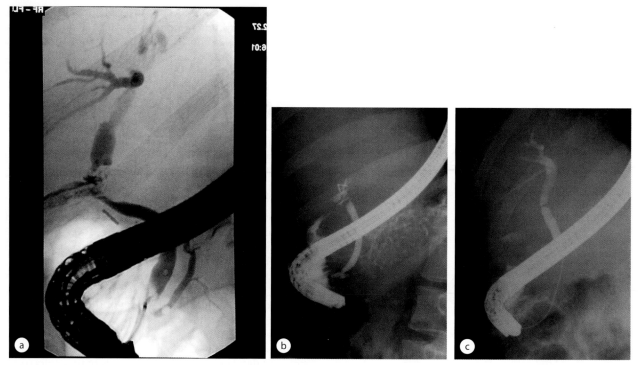

**Figure 13.7    (a)** Failure of primary repair with T-tube. Primary repair was performed for an injury to the common bile duct presenting with biliary peritonitis. A T-tube was inserted through the anastomosis, and this was removed at 4 weeks. An anastomotic stricture developed and the patient required a hepaticojejunostomy 2 months later. **(b)** Failure of primary repair for ligation of the common bile duct. A complete transection of the common bile duct identified at postoperative endoscopic retrograde cholangiopancreatography (ERCP). Immediate repair was performed with a direct duct-to-duct repair. **(c)** A tight anastomotic stricture is demonstrated at a later ERCP.

injury to the biliary tree can be controlled with endoscopic stent placement.

If ERCP is unsuccessful or the bile duct is ligated or occluded by clips, percutaneous transhepatic cholangiography (PTC) may facilitate biliary decompression but it is less frequently employed for diagnosis or delineation of the biliary anatomy. Occasionally, both sides of the liver may need to be externally drained to gain control of a biliary fistula, especially with Strasberg E4 injuries (Fig. 13.6) to the biliary confluence. However, injury to the biliary tree detected in this way may allow surgical repair to be considered within the first week of injury in the stable non-septic patient, and again such further investigation or management decisions should only be considered following specialist referral.

Where the diagnosis of bile duct injury has been delayed, the aim should be to control the biliary fistula with external drainage using surgical or radiologically placed drains. Further control may be required with endoscopic stenting or external biliary drainage. Delayed repair can be considered subsequently once sepsis and intra-abdominal soiling have resolved, as a planned elective procedure in a specialist unit, usually 2–3 months following injury. Such an initial conservative approach renders a potentially difficult operation into a repair that will be considerably easier.

✓✓ Diagnosis of a bile duct injury in the postoperative period should lead to immediate referral to a specialist centre since inappropriate attempts to manage this outside a specialist centre will compromise the outcome.

## POSTOPERATIVE RECOGNITION: BILIARY OBSTRUCTION

Ligation or inadvertent clipping of the biliary tree presents early in the postoperative period with jaundice. Later, stricture formation may occur as a result of direct trauma during dissection, clips placed inadvertently on the cystic duct but compromising the bile duct, or from damage to the intricate vascular supply of the bile duct by extensive mobilisation or diathermy. Initial investigation should include haematology, assessment of coagulation by estimation of prothrombin time, and liver function tests. Ultrasound may indicate the level of obstruction or exclude the presence of a correctable cause of obstructive jaundice, such as a retained stone in the CBD.

ERCP will identify a stricture or complete transection of the bile duct; however, identification of complete transection with MRCP will avoid the risks of an unnecessary ERCP. CT-IVC is not indicated as the contrast agent (Biliscopin) will not be excreted. Overzealous instillation of contrast at ERCP should be avoided due to the potential to introduce infection above the stricture. Placement of an endoscopic stent should be considered only after consultation with a specialist unit since this may introduce sepsis into the biliary tree and compromise further management. Furthermore, an undrained biliary tree may allow proximal biliary dilatation, thereby facilitating later reconstruction.

Although some have reported satisfactory resolution of biliary strictures with endoscopic stenting alone, the follow-up has usually been short and frequently patients require later surgery. Partial occlusion of the duct by a clip may be remedied by balloon dilatation with or without placement of a stent; however, delay in diagnosis may result in subsequent recurrent stricture formation. Nonetheless, de Reuver et al.[30] reported 110 patients with bile duct strictures following cholecystectomy who were treated with endoscopic stenting, 48 (44%) of which had already undergone attempted surgical repair. At a mean follow-up of 7.6 years, 74% of patients had a successful outcome. Parlak et al.[31] recently reported 156 partial biliary strictures following cholecystectomy with only 11% requiring further intervention at 7.5 years median follow-up post stent removal. The technique of placing multiple, increasing numbers of stents every 3–4 months was associated with a better outcome than single stent replacement. The development of removable endoscopic expandable metal stents has recently been described,[32] although long-term results and large series are not yet available. Furthermore, stent migration can complicate treatment.

✔ If repair needs to be delayed in the setting of biliary obstruction, stent placement may still be avoidable and a decision will generally be made based on the individual patient circumstances. Suspicion or evidence of arterial injury may influence the management decision.

✔ For strictures that declare late, appropriate indications for stent placement are the presence of sepsis, severe itch resistant to medical therapy or significant hepatic dysfunction.

## THE TIMING OF REPAIR

### Early repair

When an injury is recognised in the early postoperative period and there is minimal peritoneal contamination or sepsis, a definitive repair by an experienced surgeon can be successful (Fig. 13.8). In our series of 123 patients referred with injury to the biliary tree, 22 patients underwent primary biliary repair in the first 2 weeks following injury and 3 patients had revision of a failed biliary repair. Between 2 weeks and 6 months, a further 22 injuries were repaired selectively. Successful repair was possible in 22 of 25 early repairs compared with 20 of 22 delayed repairs.[33] Kirks et al.[34] compared immediate repair (< 48 hours) with delayed repair (> 48 hours) and found equivalent outcomes in 61 patients when managed by an experienced team. Dominguez-Rosado

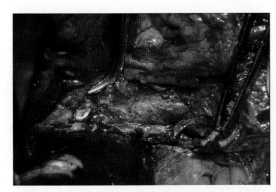

**Figure 13.8** Operative picture of an early repair of an E4 injury. A right-angle forceps is placed in the opening of the left hepatic duct, whilst the open right hepatic duct is visible below. The portal vein is skeletonised with ligation and excision of both the extrahepatic biliary tree and right hepatic artery (held by forceps).

et al.[35] reviewed 614 bile duct injuries and found that the intermediate group (repair between 8 days and 6 weeks) had a higher risk of complications than early or delayed repair groups. Overall decisions about the timing of surgery will depend upon the type of injury, associated sepsis, vascular injury, patient comorbidities and local surgical expertise.

### Delayed repair

Many injuries continue to be unrecognised or referral delayed, including patients with generalised peritonitis. Controlling the biliary injury and associated sepsis is the first treatment aim, which may require endoscopic or percutaneous biliary decompression, allowing jaundice to settle or biliary sepsis to be drained. Intra-abdominal collections may be drained percutaneously, or in the early postoperative period this may be better achieved by laparoscopic means. It is accepted, however, that bile collections are frequently loculated and difficult to eradicate in patients with intra-abdominal sepsis or widespread biliary contamination or peritonitis. The most effective treatment may be laparotomy with extensive lavage and the placement of large intra-abdominal drains. Definitive repair should not be contemplated if there is severe peritoneal soiling since injudicious attempts to repair the injury may aggravate the injury and result in a poor outcome.

Once these objectives have been met, the patient should be allowed to recover from the combined insult of surgery and sepsis. A period of rehabilitation at home is generally required before repair is contemplated in these compromised patients. Abdominal and biliary drainage can be managed on an outpatient basis with community nursing support. Nutritional supplementation may be required, particularly in those who have required a prolonged admission to the intensive care unit and hospital. Attention should be paid to the consequences of prolonged external biliary drainage and consideration given to recycling of bile.

✔ If the diagnosis of ductal obstruction is made early within the first week after surgery, the bilirubin level is only moderately elevated and there is no coexisting coagulopathy or sepsis; immediate repair offers the best chance of a successful outcome.

## ASSOCIATED VASCULAR INJURY

In patients with a delayed diagnosis, abdominal CT is required to ensure resolution of intra-abdominal collections and before repair to exclude the presence of liver atrophy. Atrophy can occur from prolonged obstruction to the segmental, sectional or hepatic ducts but is generally associated with the presence of a vascular injury, most usually of the right hepatic artery. Liver resection may occasionally be needed at the time of definitive repair to remove a source of ongoing sepsis, or if satisfactory reconstruction to the left or right duct is not possible.

Buell et al.[36] identified associated vascular injury as an independent predictor of mortality, with 38% of patients dying compared with 3% ($P < 0.001$) where no arterial injury was present. Some authors advocate arteriography before repair to identify such associated vascular injury as a repair is less likely to be successful, or for consideration of hepatic arterial reconstruction at the time of hepaticojejunostomy.[37] However, Pulitano et al.[38] were unable to demonstrate any difference in outcome between patients with and without hepatic arterial injury. Alves et al.[39] described 55 patients with post-cholecystectomy strictures who underwent surgical reconstruction with a left duct approach and preoperative coeliac axis and superior mesenteric artery angiography. Twenty-six patients (47%) had an associated vascular injury, of which 20 (36%) were of the right hepatic artery. In this series, only one patient in each group (vascular injury vs no injury) developed a recurrent stricture after repair.[39] A proximal anastomosis may offer a better blood supply, minimising the risk of anastomotic stricturing (Fig. 13.9). In support of this theory, Mercado et al.[40] demonstrated that an anastomosis fashioned below the biliary confluence was more likely to require revisional surgery (16%) compared with an anastomosis performed at the biliary confluence (0%; $P < 0.05$). MRI and spiral CT technology now provide impressive arterial and venous anatomical reconstructions, which should negate the need for invasive arteriography.

Injury to the hepatic arterial supply (usually the right hepatic artery) may present with haemobilia or intra-abdominal haemorrhage from a false aneurysm, usually associated with ongoing subhepatic sepsis. If suspected, urgent angiography is required (Fig. 13.10). Haemorrhage may be controlled by embolisation of the feeding vessel, although re-bleeding can occur and necessitate further embolisation. However, in our experience, further bleeding in the presence of ongoing sepsis usually requires laparotomy for control of bleeding and drainage of any subhepatic collection.

Rarely, combined injury to the hepatic artery and portal vein can occur with resultant infarction of the affected hepatic parenchyma, usually the right liver. Such injuries may require urgent hepatic resection or transplantation.[26]

### FURTHER IMAGING

For patients with injury to the biliary confluence (E3 and E4), preoperative imaging will help in the planning of future repair. In the presence of a biliary stricture, invasive cholangiography by ERCP or PTC risks introducing sepsis. However, if PTC is required for external biliary drainage, an adequate cholangiogram may be obtained at this time. With ongoing improvements in MRI technology, detailed biliary anatomical reconstructions can be produced, thereby negating the need for more invasive imaging.

### OPERATIVE TECHNIQUES

Biliary reconstruction should be performed under optimal circumstances at the time of injury or soon thereafter. Once this opportunity has been lost, repair should only be considered when the patient has been optimised, in the absence of intra-abdominal sepsis, and when sufficient time has elapsed to allow for maturation of adhesions and the tissues at the porta hepatis.

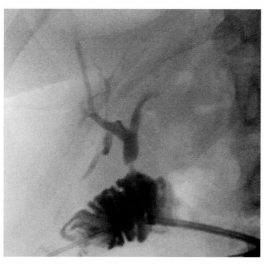

**Figure 13.9** Anastomotic stricture following repair of biliary injury. Percutaneous transjejunal cholangiogram (PTJC) of a Bismuth 1 injury repaired by hepaticojejunostomy at the level of the transection of the common bile duct (not to the left hepatic duct). Three months later, the patient required reconstruction of the anastomotic stricture.

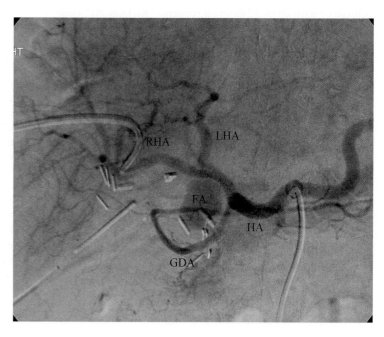

**Figure 13.10** Digital subtraction angiogram demonstrating a false aneurysm of the common hepatic artery. Embolisation was required for control. The patient has undergone a primary repair for a complete transection of the common bile duct. *FA*, false aneurysm; *GDA*, gastroduodenal artery; *HA*, common hepatic artery; *LHA*, left hepatic artery; *RHA*, right hepatic artery.

A right subcostal incision is used for access, which can be extended across the midline if required. Retraction is provided with an upper abdominal (Omni-tract®, Omni-tract surgical, St Paul, MN) mechanical retractor. Laparotomy is undertaken to assess the liver and to allow adhesiolysis, thereby freeing the small bowel for reconstruction. Frequently the omentum, hepatic flexure, duodenum and hepatoduodenal ligament are involved in a dense inflammatory mass, and occasionally an unsuspected fistula between bile duct and duodenum or colon is identified. Dissection is often easier if commenced laterally and then directed towards the biliary structures. The CBD can be difficult to identify, particularly in the presence of extensive fibrosis, and intraoperative ultrasound is a useful tool in allowing its location and relationship to vessels to be determined.

For injuries that involve the biliary confluence, lowering of the hilar plate allows easier identification of the left and right hepatic ducts. This may be aided by the use of an ultrasonic dissector (CUSA), which is also employed to break down the contracted fibrotic tissue in the gallbladder bed and to facilitate the division of any bridge of liver tissue between segments III and IV. Opening these two planes on the right and left sides facilitates identification of and access to the biliary confluence.

Since the blood supply to the bile duct is often damaged at the time of injury, the common hepatic duct should be opened as proximally as possible, although frequently there has been retraction of the fibrotic remnant superiorly. Extension of the incision into the left hepatic duct allows a wide anastomosis to be fashioned with adequate views of the left- and right-sided ducts. Care should be taken since there may be a small superficial arterial branch crossing the left duct anteriorly and running above to segment IV. For injuries involving separation of the confluence, the right and left hepatic ducts can be anastomosed together before formation of a hepaticojejunostomy, allowing a single biliary anastomosis. If possible, injuries to an isolated right sectoral duct are best repaired or drained into a Roux limb of jejunum (Fig. 13.5). Simple ligation will lead to atrophy of the drained segments, which may become a nidus for sepsis. However, enteric drainage of a small sectoral duct may also lead to sepsis if an anastomotic stricture occurs.

Repair should be effected by a hepaticojejunostomy with a 70-cm Roux limb of jejunum, thereby minimising the risk of enteric reflux and chronic damage to the biliary tree. Moraca et al.[41] advocate hepatico-duodenostomy for biliary injury on the basis that it is more physiological, quicker to perform and allows later ERCP for imaging and intervention. They found no difference in outcome following hepatico-duodenostomy when compared with hepaticojejunostomy, although median follow-up was only 54 months. Hepatico-duodenostomy has largely been abandoned in the treatment of other benign biliary disease due to ongoing enteric reflux. There have been anecdotal reports of the late development of cholangiocarcinoma,[42] as well as the need to undertake liver transplantation in patients so managed when secondary biliary cirrhosis due to enteric reflux has resulted. In my opinion, hepatico-duodenostomy has no role in the management of bile duct injury.

Fine absorbable interrupted sutures of 4/0 or 5/0 polydioxanone sulphate (PDS II) should be used to fashion an end-to-side hepaticojejunostomy, with care being taken to produce good mucosal apposition. Some authors advocate the use of an access limb, particularly for E3 and E4 injuries, to allow subsequent radiological intervention for dilatation of recurrent strictures.[43] However, others believe that advances in percutaneous transhepatic techniques have made this unnecessary and have achieved satisfactory results without using this surgical approach. Regardless, formation of an access limb by fixation of the small bowel to the anterior abdominal wall and marked with Ligaclips is a straight-forward surgical procedure with minimal risk.

Rarely, there may be no recognisable bile ducts visible in the porta hepatis. In such cases, a variation of porto-enterostomy (Kasai procedure) can be considered with the Roux limb sutured to the fibrous structure of the hilar plate (S.W. Banting, personal communication).

Partial injury to the biliary tree can be repaired with fine interrupted sutures, although when resulting from diathermy dissection, formal hepaticojejunostomy may be necessary as conduction of the thermal injury may cause later stricture formation. If a T-tube is placed to protect a primary duct repair, this should be placed through a separate choledochotomy. Laparoscopic repair has also been described with a recent report of 29 cases. The majority were managed with a primary repair with eight hepaticojejunostomies and the longest follow-up of only 36 months.[44] At present laparoscopic or robotic repair offers little benefit over open biliary reconstruction and that primary repair is an inferior treatment modality.

## MANAGEMENT OF COMPLICATIONS RELATED TO REPAIR

### Revisional surgery

Many patients with biliary injury continue to suffer from complications despite reconstruction. Factors such as the experience of the surgeon performing the initial repair, the level of injury, associated sepsis and/or liver atrophy all affect the chance of an unsuccessful repair. Following primary repair of a ductal tear or laceration, further stricture formation may result if there has been extensive dissection around the common hepatic duct. In such instances, surgical revision with the formation of a Roux-en-Y hepaticojejunostomy is indicated.

The majority of patients requiring revisional surgery will have undergone a previous biliary enteric drainage procedure. Anastomotic stricturing will require revision of the anastomosis, with extension of the choledochotomy into the left hepatic duct (Fig. 13.9). There is very little literature to guide decisions about the management of anastomotic stricture formation following reconstruction of the bile duct with a Roux-en-Y hepaticojejunostomy, but surgical revision remains the gold standard.

### Liver resection and transplantation

In the acute setting of bile duct injury, long-term damage to the hepatic parenchyma is difficult to predict. Major vascular injury or unrecognised segmental biliary obstruction may lead to atrophy of the liver, chronic intrahepatic infection, abscess formation or secondary biliary cirrhosis. In such patients, careful operative assessment is required; CT should be performed to identify areas of associated liver atrophy and to exclude portal vein thrombosis.

In our experience, the majority of patients requiring liver resection are those with ongoing sepsis in an obstructed segment or those where drainage of the extrahepatic biliary tree is not possible due to sectoral duct damage or fibrosis.[26] Truant

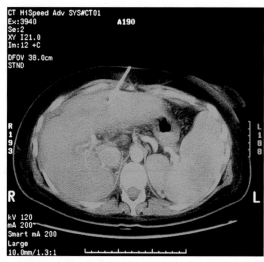

**Figure 13.11** Contrast-enhanced computed tomography (CT) of the liver after unsuccessful revisional hepaticojejunostomy. The surgeon who performed the laparoscopic cholecystectomy performed the hepaticojejunostomy for an E4 injury. A revisional hepaticojejunostomy was performed before referral, which was complicated by an anastomotic stricture and portal vein thrombosis. The CT shows evidence of right lobe atrophy and splenomegaly as well as a percutaneous biliary drain.

et al.[45] identified 99 patients (5.6%) requiring hepatectomy among 1756 patients with post-cholecystectomy bile duct injury, with combined arterial and Strasberg E4 and E5 injuries more likely to require hepatic resection. Occasionally, early hepatic resection is required for combined arterial, portal venous and biliary injury, although results are poor.[21] Very rarely, resection may be needed to gain access to the biliary tree, especially when the injury involves the biliary confluence (E4), although some authors routinely advocate resection of segments IVb and V for access to the right hepatic ducts.[46] The right lobe is most commonly affected by sepsis and atrophy as the right-sided sectoral ducts and arterial supply are more likely to be damaged during cholecystectomy, although both left- and right-sided hepatic resections have been reported in patients with severe biliary injury. Resection of the right liver can be performed, for example at the time of delayed reconstruction if there is any doubt regarding the integrity of the anastomosis to the right sectoral or hepatic duct and when a satisfactory anastomosis can be achieved to the long extrahepatic left duct.

Failed reconstruction and persistent cholangitis may lead to end-stage liver failure within a few years and this may require liver transplantation (Fig. 13.11).[26] A long interval between injury and referral is known to be associated with end-stage liver disease. Rarely, liver transplantation may be needed when the combined biliary and vascular injury is so severe as to preclude attempted reconstruction, although the results are universally poor.[26]

## PROGNOSIS

### Success of repair

Successful repair has been well described and can be achieved in 90% of patients in a specialised unit.[33,47] As for laparoscopic cholecystectomy, a learning curve for biliary repair has also been described for tertiary centres managing bile duct injury. Over a 20-year period, Mercado et al.[48] reported an improvement with experience and a reduction of post-repair strictures

from 13% to 5%. Stilling et al.[49] recently reported 139 bile duct injuries repaired with a hepaticojejunostomy in one of the five Danish HPB centres with only a 70% successful primary repair. Forty-two patients (30%) developed an anastomotic stricture, with 19 managed with redo-hepaticojejunostomy and the remainder with percutaneous transhepatic dilatation. As well as anastomotic strictures, liver atrophy and cirrhosis may also occur many years following repair. Predictors of a poor outcome include involvement of the biliary confluence,[22] repair by the injuring surgeon,[28,50,51] three or more previous attempted repairs[22] and recent active inflammation.[51]

### Survival

Mortality following injury to the biliary tree is significant. Death may follow the acute injury itself, following the biliary repair, or occur later as a result of biliary sepsis or cirrhosis. In a report of a nationwide analysis of survival following biliary injury after cholecystectomy, Flum et al.[50] identified 7911 (0.5%) injuries from 1 570 361 cholecystectomies. Within the first year after cholecystectomy, the mortality rate was 6.6% in the uninjured group and 26.1% in those with injury to the CBD. The adjusted hazard ratio for death during follow-up was higher for those with an injury (2.79; 95% CI 2.71–2.88). The risk of death increased significantly with advancing age and comorbidities. If the initial repair was performed by the injuring surgeon, then the adjusted hazard of death increased by 11%.

### Quality of life

Boerma et al.[52] first undertook an assessment of quality of life in patients who had sustained biliary injury or leak that required additional intervention. Five years after injury, quality of life in the physical and mental domains was significantly worse than controls, despite a successful outcome in 84% of treated patients and regardless of the type of treatment or severity of injury. However, the length of treatment was an independent predictor of a poor mental quality of life. Melton et al.[53] report that quality of life in 89 patients who had undergone biliary repair following laparoscopic cholecystectomy showed no difference in the physical or social domains when compared with controls. However, in the psychological domain, patients were significantly worse, particularly in the 31% of patients who sought legal recourse for their injury.

### Associated malignancy

A small number of reports exist about the development of cholangiocarcinoma at the site of anastomosis 20–30 years following repair.[43] Enteric reflux into the biliary tree with sepsis and the production of mutagenic secondary bile salts may be responsible. Furthermore, hepatocellular carcinoma may develop due to secondary biliary cirrhosis (Fig. 13.12).[54]

## BENIGN BILIARY STRICTURES

## MIRIZZI SYNDROME (see Chapter 12)
## HEPATOLITHIASIS (see Chapter 12)
## PARASITIC INFESTATION CAUSING JAUNDICE

### LIVER FLUKES (TREMATODES)

Infestation with liver flukes is caused through consuming inadequately cooked, pickled or salted infected fish. The immature

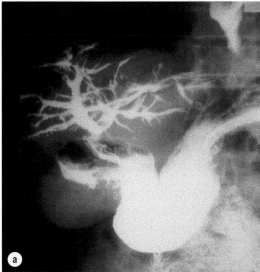

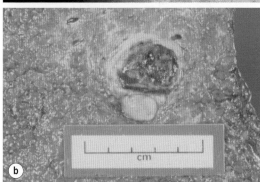

**Figure 13.12**  Hepatocellular carcinoma as a consequence of biliary injury. This patient required a liver transplant for secondary biliary cirrhosis, which developed following hepatico-duodenostomy for a biliary injury **(a)**. At pathological examination, a hepatocellular carcinoma was detected in the explanted liver **(b)**.

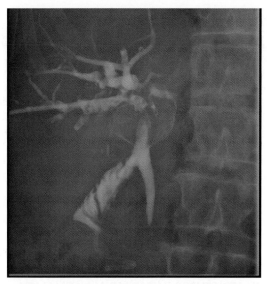

**Figure 13.13**  Complicated hilar stricture secondary to a central hydatid cyst previously ruptured into the left hepatic duct. The patient required a hepaticojejunostomy with access loop and percutaneous biliary drain when intrahepatic stones were unable to be removed endoscopically.

fluke passes into the biliary tree, where it grows to maturity. Ova are passed into the gastrointestinal tract and subsequently to water supplies, infecting molluscs and fish. Infection with *Clonorchis sinensis* occurs in China, Japan and South-East Asia, whilst *Opisthorchis viverrini* is found in parts of Eastern Europe and Siberia. Infection may be asymptomatic or the patient may present with an acute febrile illness or chronic symptoms. Chronic infestation results in hepatolithiasis.

Diagnosis is possible by the detection of ova within the stool or in duodenal aspirates, and an eosinophilia may also be present on blood film. ERCP may demonstrate slender filling defects within the bile duct as well as associated changes of fibrosis and calculus formation. Treatment is with praziquantel or albendazole.

## ECHINOCOCCUS

Hydatid cysts involving the liver remain endemic in parts of the Mediterranean and Far East, as well as sheep farming areas of Australia, New Zealand, South America and South Africa. Infection is from *Echinococcus granulosus*, and less commonly *Echinococcus multilocularis* in Central Europe.

Biliary obstruction can occur due to local compression of the common hepatic duct by the expanding cyst, or when

daughter cysts pass down the common hepatic duct following rupture of the cyst into intrahepatic radicles. Erosion into the biliary tree is usually associated with death of the cyst contents due to toxicity of the bile. Secondary sclerosing cholangitis has been described following inappropriate injection of scolicidal agents into the hepatic cyst when there is communication with the biliary tree.[55]

### Treatment

Preoperative endoscopic cholangiography may identify debris within the biliary tree, and endoscopic sphincterotomy may prevent further episodes of biliary obstruction. Endoscopic stenting may also allow resolution of obstruction secondary to a large intrahepatic cyst.

The secondary sclerosing cholangitis produced by inappropriate instillation of a scolicidal agent into the biliary tree will often only be amenable to hepatic replacement. Surgical bypass may be possible for localised strictures or Roux-en-Y hepaticojejunostomy and access loop formation for ongoing percutaneous radiological procedures (Fig. 13.13).

## ASCARIS LUMBRICOIDES

The roundworm *Ascaris lumbricoides* is the commonest worm to infect humans. Rarely, an infected patient can present with obstructive jaundice due to migration of the worm into the biliary tree and this is difficult to distinguish from stone disease. The more frequent presentation is from cholangitis due to the worm traversing the ampulla. *Ascaris* has also been associated with recurrent pyogenic cholangitis.

Ultrasound sometimes identifies a long, linear filling defect within the biliary tree. Identification may occur at the time of ERCP where endoscopic extraction may be possible. Medical treatment exists with the anthelmintics mebendazole or albendazole, which are often curative. The late complication of papillary stenosis can be treated with endoscopic sphincterotomy.

## HIV/AIDS-ASSOCIATED CHOLANGIOPATHY

HIV- or AIDS-associated cholangiopathy is thought to be secondary to opportunistic infection of the biliary tree by cytomegalovirus, *Cryptosporidium* and other organisms. The usual presentation is with right upper quadrant pain and abnormal liver function tests, although jaundice is unusual. MRCP demonstrates the characteristic ductal abnormalities of multiple intrahepatic strictures, papillary stenosis and long segmental extrahepatic strictures.[56] Endoscopic retrograde cholangiography is the gold standard for diagnosis and provides symptomatic relief following endoscopic sphincterotomy for papillary stenosis.[57] Antiretroviral therapy has been associated with regression of cholangiographic abnormalities,[58] but endoscopic interventions have not been associated with improvements in prognosis.[57]

## BILIARY STRICTURES IMITATING MALIGNANCY

It is not unusual for benign biliary pathology to be found in resected specimens of the pancreatic head that had been thought to be malignant. Prior to the routine use of endoscopic ultrasound and fine-needle aspirate cytology (EUS-FNA), approximately 10% of panreaticoduodenectomy resections for malignancy were found to have benign pathology. Most commonly, the pathology is chronic pancreatitis related to alcohol or gallstone disease. However, other confounding pathologies include IgG4-related disease, primary sclerosing cholangitis and choledocholithiasis.

Up to 14% of patients undergoing surgery for presumed malignant hilar obstruction are found to have a benign fibrotic stricture of the bile duct.[59] Feng et al. recently reported that 18 (6.2%) of 289 patients who underwent radical biliary resection for presumed malignancy had IgG4-related disease.[60] It is usually impossible to differentiate them from malignancy preoperatively and thus resection is often attempted and nearly always feasible. Successful treatment has been described with the use of steroids in particular for IgG4-related diseases.

## PRIMARY SCLEROSING CHOLANGITIS

### AETIOLOGY

Primary sclerosing cholangitis is a rare condition, and although the precise cause has yet to be determined there is increasing evidence of an immunological basis as well as an overall increase in the incidence.[61] Between 60% and 80% of patients will have ulcerative colitis, or more rarely Crohn's disease. There is a strong association with a number of human leucocyte antigens.[62]

### PRESENTATION

Primary sclerosing cholangitis is a progressive obliterative fibrosis of the intrahepatic and extrahepatic biliary tree with a wide clinical spectrum and frequent remissions and relapses. In the early stages of disease, most patients are asymptomatic but later in the disease process patients may have pruritus, ill-defined pain, fever, jaundice and weight loss. Many asymptomatic patients are diagnosed by detection of abnormal liver function tests during the investigation of inflammatory bowel disease. Although some patients may present at an advanced stage, signs of liver failure develop over a period of time. Sudden deterioration may suggest the development of cholangiocarcinoma, with which there is a strong association.

### INVESTIGATION

Liver biochemistry demonstrates a cholestatic picture. Although antineutrophil cytoplasmic antibodies are present in the majority of patients, testing for autoantibodies is usually performed to exclude primary biliary cirrhosis, a condition from which it can be difficult to differentiate.

The mainstay of investigation is cholangiography, which usually demonstrates a diffuse picture of stricturing and attenuated intrahepatic bile ducts. As well as providing anatomical details of the biliary tree, ERCP enables endoscopic therapy and the opportunity for brush cytology if malignancy is suspected. MRCP however is highly sensitive, with a diagnostic accuracy comparable to ERCP, and is now preferred as a means of both diagnosing and assessing the extent of disease to avoid the introduction of bacteria causing severe biliary sepsis. CT-IVC also provides a good alternative when MRCP is contraindicated.

### MANAGEMENT

The prognosis of primary sclerosing cholangitis is poor, with a median survival of only 9.6 years from diagnosis to death or liver transplantation.[63] Survival may improve with earlier diagnosis and liver transplantation; however, subsequent development of cholangiocarcinoma and colorectal cancer has now become the leading cause of death.[64] The use of ursodeoxycholic acid has not been demonstrated to be of benefit following randomised studies,[65] and there is little benefit from immunosuppression or antibiotics.[66] Episodes of cholangitis can be treated with antibiotics covering biliary pathogens. There is no evidence that colectomy for inflammatory bowel disease alters disease progression.

Endoscopic or transhepatic dilatation of short dominant strictures with or without endoscopic stenting has been described as effective, safe and well tolerated, although no randomised trials have been performed. More recently, covered endoscopic removable metal stents have been used but again without strong evidence. Dilatation achieves palliation at 1 and 3 years in 80% and 60% of patients, respectively.[67] In those patients without cirrhosis but with jaundice secondary to a dominant stricture, surgical drainage with an access limb has been described.

Liver transplantation is necessary to treat end-stage liver disease and is the fifth commonest reason for liver transplantation in the USA.[68] However, it is now more usual for patients to be considered if there is persistent jaundice, intractable pruritus, recurrent cholangitis, malnutrition or fatigue. Many patients undergo transplantation before liver failure supervenes or when cholangiocarcinoma is suspected, with survival rates of 80–92% at 5 years.[69,70] Recurrence rates of 15–25% in the transplanted liver have been reported.[71]

## EXCLUSION OF ASSOCIATED MALIGNANT STRICTURE

Cholangiocarcinoma and gallbladder cancer complicate 10–36% of patients with primary sclerosing cholangitis[63] and need to be excluded before liver transplantation.

In the majority of patients, concern regarding occult cholangiocarcinoma is small, and liver transplantation is undertaken in the absence of a dominant stricture. Serum carbohydrate antigen (CA) 19-9 has been used in an attempt to identify cases with an occult biliary malignancy. Patients with a sudden rapid deterioration in their clinical state or with a dominant stricture must be considered to have a cholangiocarcinoma and be investigated extensively. Brush cytology at ERCP may provide the diagnosis if a malignant smear is obtained, but ERCP-based cholangioscopy with targeted biopsies appears to be the most accurate.[72] CT or MRI may demonstrate a mass lesion in association with the biliary tree, although the usual appearance is of a stricture indistinguishable from a benign disease. EUS-FNA of dominant strictures has been used, but evidence remains lacking. Positron emission tomography (PET) is superior to conventional radiological investigations to differentiate primary sclerosing cholangitis and cholangiocarcinoma.[73]

Laparoscopy identifies the majority of patients with unresectable biliary tract cancer,[74] and may be of use in assessing those considered for transplantation in whom a cholangiocarcinoma is suspected since tumour dissemination often occurs early. Laparoscopic ultrasound may further aid assessment, and occasionally laparotomy may be required if there is diagnostic doubt regarding cholangiocarcinoma.

## IMMUNOGLOBULIN G4 (IgG4)-RELATED DISEASE

IgG4-related disease is an immune-mediated condition that mimics many malignant, infectious and inflammatory disorders, but the aetiology remains obscure. Autoimmune pancreatitis was the first condition to be associated with high serum IgG4.[75] It is also known as lymphoplasmacytic sclerosing pancreatitis.

Other IgG4 diseases include IgG4 sclerosing cholangitis, retroperitoneal fibrosis, periaortitis, sclerosing mesenteritis, inflammatory pseudotumour and multifocal fibrosclerosis as well as other extra-abdominal diseases such as Riedel's thyroiditis.[76] Tissue is the gold standard for diagnosis, with demonstration of a high number of IgG4-positive plasma cells.[76] Several clinical entities can cause biliary strictures, which include autoimmune pancreatitis, IgG4-related sclerosing cholangitis and inflammatory pseudotumours. Adequate biopsy material from these disorders can be difficult to obtain at endoscopic ultrasound and biopsy.

### AUTOIMMUNE PANCREATITIS

Two types of autoimmune pancreatitis are reported, with type I associated with IgG4 disease. Although only accounting for about 2.4% of pancreatic resections, the condition is important since a proportion of patients will develop either biliary anastomotic strictures or intrahepatic strictures following resection. In a series of 31 patients, 8 (28%) went on to develop recurrent jaundice after resection.[77] Often the diagnosis is radiological, with an enlarged pancreatic head mass with delayed enhancement without pancreatic duct dilatation. EUS-FNA cytology may be helpful if plasma cells are detected, but usually the diagnosis remains indeterminate.

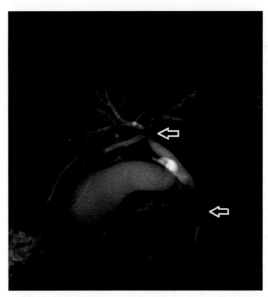

**Figure 13.14** IgG4-related cholangiopathy in a 70-year-old man presenting with jaundice and a recent history of retroperitoneal fibrosis. His jaundice resolved within 2 weeks after treatment with prednisolone without endoscopic stenting. The *arrows* point to benign biliary strictures at the hilum of the liver and intrapancreatic bile duct.

### IgG4-RELATED SCLEROSING CHOLANGITIS

IgG4-related sclerosing cholangitis is commonly associated with type I autoimmune pancreatitis and can be difficult to differentiate from cholangiocarcinoma.

### TREATMENT

Glucocorticoids are the mainstay of treatment,[78] but no randomised studies have been performed. In patients with jaundice, treatment with steroids should lead to resolution within 1–2 weeks so avoidance of endoscopic stenting may be beneficial to aid in the diagnostic process (Fig. 13.14). In the absence of biochemical or histological proof of IgG4 disease but typical radiological appearance, treatment with high-dose glucocorticoids usually leads to prompt resolution of jaundice and imaging findings. FDG PET CT response can also be useful in the assessment of treatment response.[79]

## FUNCTIONAL BILIARY DISORDERS

Most patients who present for investigation of sphincter of Oddi dysfunction have already undergone cholecystectomy for presumed gallbladder pain. However, 39–90% of patients with idiopathic recurrent pancreatitis may also have sphincter of Oddi dysfunction.[80] In those patients with postcholecystectomy pain, the presentation and investigation identifies three types:[81]

- Type 1 – Abdominal pain, obstructive liver function tests, biliary dilatation and delayed emptying of contrast at ERCP
- Type 2 – Pain with only one or two of the above-mentioned criteria
- Type 3 – Recurrent biliary pain only

Between 65% and 95% of group 1 patients will be found on biliary manometry to have sphincter of Oddi dysfunction compared with only 12–28% of type 3.[80] Diagnosis is usually by exclusion of other causes of abdominal pain such as peptic ulcer disease and irritable bowel syndrome. Liver function tests, abdominal ultrasonography, CT, endoscopy and MRCP have often already been performed. Morphine–neostigmine and secretin provocation MRCP studies may also be of diagnostic value. Development of pain on taking codeine is almost pathopneumonic of sphincter of Oddi dysfunction.

At ERCP, biliary manometry is not required if there is delayed drainage of contrast in type 1 or 2 patients. This investigation should be reserved for those patients in whom the diagnosis remains unclear.

Medical therapy with calcium channel blockers, nitrates and botulinum toxin is available, but long-term results are unknown. Avoidance of opiate analgesia, particularly over-the-counter preparations containing codeine, may prevent the onset of pain in the majority. The development of severe abdominal pain with codeine is almost diagnostic. Endoscopic sphincterotomy is a potential treatment; however, 5–16% of patients will develop postprocedural pancreatitis[82] and good or excellent responses are reported in only 69% of patients at long-term follow-up.[83] Surgical sphincterotomy is now indicated rarely due to the lower cost and lower morbidity of endoscopic sphincterotomy, but it may be required if the endoscopic approach has been unsuccessful. Avoidance of codeine and reassurance about the benign nature of the condition is the safest path.

## Key points

- Choledochal cysts should be treated with complete cyst excision and hepaticojejunostomy due to the risk of malignancy in the remaining biliary epithelium.
- Identification of the biliary anatomy and minimisation of diathermy near the CBD are essential during laparoscopic cholecystectomy to avoid biliary injury.
- Operative cholangiography is useful for delineating the biliary anatomy during cholecystectomy; however, many cholangiograms are not interpreted correctly at the time of biliary injury.
- Following laparoscopic cholecystectomy, any patient who is not fit for discharge at 24 hours due to ongoing abdominal pain, vomiting, fever or bile in an abdominal drain should be considered to have a biliary leak.
- Diagnosis of a bile duct injury in the postoperative period should lead to immediate referral to a specialist centre since inappropriate attempts to manage this with a specialist centre will compromise the outcome.
- In the absence of sepsis, repair of injuries to the biliary tree can be performed successfully within the first week.

References available at http://ebooks.health.elsevier.com/

## ▶ RECOMMENDED VIDEOS

- **Excision of a choledochal cyst:**

Although not the authors' recommended technique, this video offers excellent vision of the dissection: Laparoscopic excision of a choledochal cyst from SAGES 2015 – https://www.youtube.com/watch?v=gZRw8rf3l2Y

[Comment: Decision not to excise the upper hepatic bile duct/CBD may increase risk of stricture formation given consideration of blood supply to the bile duct.]

## KEY REFERENCES

[11] Flum DR, Dellinger EP, Cheadle A, et al. Intraoperative cholangiography and risk of common bile duct injury during cholecystectomy. JAMA 2003;289(13):1639–44. PMID: 12672731
    *A retrospective analysis of more than 1.5 million cholecystectomies detailing the risk of injury and the decreased risk if operative cholangiography is used.*

[14] Fletcher DR, Hobbs MS, Tan P, et al. Complications of cholecystectomy: risks of the laparoscopic app¬roach and protective effects of operative cholan-giography: a population-based study. Ann Surg 1999;229(4):449–57. PMID: 10203075
    *A retrospective audit of biliary injury in Western Australia that identified the increased risk of biliary injury after laparoscopic cholecystectomy compared with open cholecystectomy. This study also identified a significantly reduced risk of injury if operative cholangiography was performed.*

[16] Way LW, Stewart L, Gantert W, et al. Causes and prevention of laparoscopic bile duct injuries: analysis of 252 cases from a human factors and cognitive psychology perspective. Ann Surg 2003;237(4):460–9. PMID: 12677139
    *Analysis of 252 bile duct injuries according to the principles of the cognitive science of visual perception judgment and human error showing that the majority of errors result from misperception, not errors of skill, knowledge or judgement.*

[24] Strasberg SM, Hertl M, Soper NJ. An analysis of the problem of biliary injury during lapa¬roscopic cholecystectomy. J Am Coll Surg 1995;180(1):101–25. PMID: 8000648
    *This paper describes a very useful classification system for biliary injury that includes the Bismuth classification as well as other less major injuries.*

[50] Flum DR, Cheadle A, Prela C, et al. Bile duct injury during cholecystectomy and survival in medicare beneficiaries. JAMA 2003;290(16):2168–73. PMID: 14570952
    *A retrospective analysis of survival following bile duct injury among Medicare beneficiaries in the USA. This study demonstrates the increased hazard ratio of death following injury in comparison with a control group of routine cholecystectomy patients.*

[52] Boerma D, Rauws EA, Keulemans YC, et al. Impaired quality of life 5 years after bile duct injury during laparoscopic cholecystectomy: a prospective analysis. Ann Surg 2001;234(6):750–7. PMID: 11729381
    *A prospective analysis of quality of life that demonstrated a poor outcome at 5 years, despite successful repair.*

[53] Melton GB, Lillemoe KD, Cameron JL, et al. Major bile duct injuries associated with laparoscopic cholecystectomy: effect of surgical repair on quality of life. Ann Surg 2002;235(6):888–95. PMID: 12035047
    *A study of the impact of biliary injury on quality of life that demonstrated a significantly worse psychological domain, especially in those pursuing legal action.*

[78] Kamisawa T, Shimosegawa T, Okazaki K, et al. Standard steroid treatment for autoimmune pancreatitis. Gut 2009;58(11):1504–7. PMID: 19398440
    *An excellent and comprehensive review article for IgG4 disease.*

# Malignant lesions of the biliary tract

14

Caitlin A. McIntyre | William R. Jarnagin

## INTRODUCTION

Malignant lesions of the biliary tract, including the gallbladder, are uncommon and account for approximately 15% of hepatobiliary neoplasms and 3% of gastrointestinal (GI) malignancies overall. Biliary tract cancers are prevalent in certain regions, such as Thailand, Chile and India, while rare in most Western countries. It was estimated that there would be 11 980 new cases, and 4310 deaths from a gallbladder or biliary cancer within the USA in 2021.[1] While the incidence of biliary tract malignancies is increasing, the mortality is decreasing.[2]

Cholangiocarcinoma is divided into intrahepatic (ICC) and extrahepatic (ECC) subtypes, with the latter further subdivided into hilar, mid-duct and distal bile duct cancer. These distinctions are based purely on anatomic location and the operation required for resection; as such they are arbitrary. The vast majority of these tumours are either hilar or distal in origin, with mid-duct tumours very uncommon. Gallbladder carcinoma is a distinct clinical entity and represents the most common site of malignancy in the biliary tract. Each of these neoplasms displays distinct clinical, pathologic and genomic features.

The diagnosis of a biliary malignancy requires the integration of objective data, radiological evaluation and clinical experience. Surgery remains the mainstay of treatment as it provides the best option for prolonged disease-specific survival (DSS) and the only chance for cure. However, the majority of patients present with locally advanced or metastatic disease, and many of those who undergo resection will recur. While advances have been made in both the understanding and treatment of biliary neoplasms, 5-year overall survival (OS) remains low at 10–20%. Herein, we discuss the epidemiology, work-up, management and outcomes of patients with biliary adenocarcinoma, including cholangiocarcinoma (hilar, intrahepatic and extrahepatic) and gallbladder carcinoma.

## CHOLANGIOCARCINOMA

### EPIDEMIOLOGY

Cholangiocarcinoma accounts for 3% of all GI malignancies, with an incidence of approximately 8000 new cases per year in the USA.[3] ICC is the second most common primary liver tumour accounting for about 15% of primary liver cancers, and is now the leading cause of primary liver tumour–related death.[4] Approximately 10% of cholangiocarcinomas are intrahepatic, while the remaining 90% are extrahepatic, the most common of which is perihilar that accounts for 50–60% of cholangiocarcinoma.[5] Overall, men are affected 1.5 times as often as women, and the majority of patients are older than 65 years at the time of diagnosis, with the peak incidence in the eighth decade of life. Cholangiocarcinoma has a higher prevalence in Hispanics and Asians than their White and Black counterparts.[6] The incidence of ICC has increased over the last several decades, while ECC has decreased both in the USA and worldwide.[2,7]

## RISK FACTORS

The majority of patients with cholangiocarcinoma have no known risk factors and present with sporadic disease. However, there are several well-established entities that increase the risk of developing cholangiocarcinoma, many of which are associated with chronic inflammation. Certain risk factors are unique for a specific subtype of cholangiocarcinoma or associated with particular geographic regions.

### PRIMARY SCLEROSING CHOLANGITIS

The most common risk factor for cholangiocarcinoma is primary sclerosing cholangitis (PSC). PSC is also strongly associated with inflammatory bowel disease which is present in 70–80% of patients with PSC; however, only a minority of patients with inflammatory bowel disease develop PSC.[8] Unlike sporadic cases of cholangiocarcinoma, the age at presentation in patients with PSC is younger and typically occurs between 30 and 50 years. The natural history of PSC is variable, and the true incidence of cholangiocarcinoma in this population varies between studies. In a Swedish series of 305 patients, 8% of patients developed cancer with a median follow-up of 63 months. On the other hand, occult cholangiocarcinoma has been reported in up to 40% of autopsy specimens and in up to 36% of liver explants from patients with PSC.[8] Additional studies have noted that the relative risk of developing cholangiocarcinoma in patients with PSC ranges more than 200-fold compared with patients without PSC.[9,10] Unfortunately, the subset of patients with PSC-associated cholangiocarcinoma are not candidates for resection because of multifocal disease or severe underlying hepatic dysfunction. Additionally, these patients are often disqualified from transplantation because of the cancer diagnosis.

181

## CONGENITAL CYSTS

Congenital biliary tree abnormalities (choledochal cysts and Caroli's disease) are associated with an increased risk of developing cholangiocarcinoma, with the estimated risk ranging 3–20%.[6,11,12] Soares et al.[11] published a multi-institutional study of 354 adults and children undergoing resection for choledochal cysts. The authors demonstrated that a concomitant cholangiocarcinoma was diagnosed in 2.5% of patients, and during a median follow-up of 28 months 3.3% of patients were diagnosed with cholangiocarcinoma. Additionally, in a series of 119 patients undergoing transduodenal sphincteroplasty, Hakamada et al.[13] found a 7.4% incidence of cholangiocarcinoma over a follow-up period of 18 years. Although the cause is unknown, the belief is that the abnormal pancreaticobiliary duct junction found in this patient population predisposes the patients to reflux of pancreatic secretions into the biliary tree, resulting in chronic inflammation and bacterial contamination, ultimately leading to malignant transformation.[14]

## HEPATOLITHIASIS

Hepatolithiasis is a well-established risk factor for the development of cholangiocarcinoma. In Japan and parts of South-East Asia, up to 10% of patients with hepatolithiasis will develop cholangiocarcinoma. This association has also been demonstrated in Western countries.[15,16] The pathophysiology is thought to be secondary to a recurrent inflammatory state. Chronic portal bacteraemia and portal phlebitis lead to intrahepatic pigment stone formation, obstruction of intrahepatic ducts and recurrent episodes of cholangitis and stricture formation.[17,18]

## PARASITIC INFECTION

The literature has suggested a pathogenic association between liver fluke infestation (*Opisthorchis viverrini*, *Clonorchis sinensis*) and the development of cholangiocarcinoma.[19] Although exceedingly rare in the USA, these organisms are endemic in South-East Asia.

## VIRAL HEPATITIS AND CIRRHOSIS

Hepatitis B, hepatitis C infection and cirrhosis have been linked to the development of cholangiocarcinoma.[16] In a prospective study from Japan, the risk of developing cholangiocarcinoma in patients infected with hepatitis C virus was 3.5% at 10 years compared with their non-infected counterparts who harboured a rate 1000 times less.[20] Moreover, the fact that cholangiocytes and hepatocytes arise from the same progenitor cell and that the hepatitis C virus has been found within cholangiocarcinoma tumour specimens allude to a strong probable pathogenic association.[6]

## METABOLIC RISK FACTORS

The incidence of metabolic syndrome and associated comorbidities has been increasing in the USA and worldwide. Studies have demonstrated that type 2 diabetes, hyperlipidaemia, obesity and non-alcoholic fatty liver disease are associated with an increased risk of both intrahepatic and ECC.[16,21]

## CHEMICAL EXPOSURE

Tobacco use and smoking are well-established risk factors for many cancers, including cholangiocarcinoma.[16] Several chemical agents have been implicated in the development of cholangiocarcinoma. Exposure to Thorotrast (a radiological agent used in the 1960s) is associated with a 300-fold increase in the development of biliary malignancy.[22] Additional environmental toxins, such as dioxin and vinyl chloride, have also been associated with an increased risk of developing cholangiocarcinoma.[22]

## CLASSIFICATION

### HISTOPATHOLOGY

Cholangiocarcinoma is classified according to the site of origin within the biliary tree—hilar, intrahepatic and extrahepatic. Malignancies arising from the biliary confluence are classified as hilar cholangiocarcinoma and are the most common type of cholangiocarcinoma (approximately 60% of all cases), while those that originate within the extrahepatic bile duct account for 20–30% of cases, and the remaining 10% arise from the intrahepatic biliary tree.[23] Of note, patients can present with multifocal or diffuse involvement of the biliary tree, although this is quite rare.[24] The vast majority of ICC, ECC and hilar cholangiocarcinoma are adenocarcinoma, whereas other histologic variants comprise approximately 5% of tumours.[6] These include different patterns with focal areas of papillary carcinoma with mucous production, signet-ring cells, squamous cell, mucoepidermoid and spindle cell variants.[25]

ICC is divided into three morphologic subtypes based on the classification established by the Liver Cancer Study Group of Japan: (1) mass-forming type; (2) periductal infiltrating type; and (3) intraductal growth type.[4,25] Each subtype is characterised by a different growth pattern. The mass-forming subtype is characterised by discrete mass formation within the liver, which is in comparison with the periductal infiltrating subtype which grows along the biliary tree, resulting in fibrosis of periductal tissues and annular bile duct thickening.[6,25,26] The intraductal subtype is characterised by growth within the lumen of the bile duct, resulting in papillary-like projections.[25,26]

ECC can be further classified based on both macroscopic appearance and location within the extrahepatic biliary tree. Three macroscopic subtypes of ECC are described: sclerosing, nodular and papillary, of which the first two are often combined into one (i.e. nodular-sclerosing) since features of both types are often seen together.[27] Papillary tumours represent a less common variant, accounting for approximately 10% of ECCs, and are more common in the lower bile duct than at the hilum.[27,28] Papillary tumours are characterised by a mass that expands rather than contracts the duct, and may be associated with little transmural invasion. They may grow to significant size, yet they often arise from a well-defined stalk, with the majority of tumour being mobile within the ductal lumen. While less common, recognition of this entity is important since they are more often resectable and have a more favourable overall prognosis than other histologic subtypes. ECCs, primarily tumours of the mid- and distal bile duct, can be classified according to their anatomical location, although there may be overlap. Mid-bile duct tumours arise between the upper border of the duodenum and the cystic duct, while distal bile duct tumours arise from the duodenum to the ampulla of Vater. Tumours of the distal bile duct represent approximately 5–10% of all periampullary tumours,[23] while true mid-duct tumours are uncommon.

## GENOMICS

With advances in technology and next-generation sequencing over the last two decades, there has been an increased understanding of the molecular underpinning of biliary tract malignancies, including distinct genomic differences between subtypes (Fig. 14.1).[29] Furthermore, this has led to an increase in available treatment options through targeted sequencing.

The genomic landscape of ICC and ECC are distinctly different, indicating that these represent different disease processes. The mutational spectrums of these cancers differ, and therefore, the potential molecular targets do as well. There are several similarities between subtypes of biliary malignancies. For example, *TP53*, *KRAS* and chromatin modifiers (i.e. *ARID1A*) are frequently altered in all three cancer types. However, *IDH1/2*, *FGFR2* and *BAP1* mutations are more common in ICC, while *EELF3* and *ARID1B* as well as *PRKACA-PRKACB* fusions are more likely to be seen in ECC.[4,29]

## CLINICAL PRESENTATION

The clinical presentation of cholangiocarcinoma is determined by the location of the primary tumour and the level of biliary involvement. Patients with ECC may present earlier due to outflow obstruction of the biliary tree, and may demonstrate classic signs and symptoms of hyperbilirubinaemia (painless jaundice, pruritus, pale stool and dark urine). Patients with papillary tumours may give a history of intermittent jaundice, perhaps due to small fragments of tumour having passed into the common bile duct or the ball-valve effect of a pedunculated mass within the lumen.

In contrast, patients with ICC are typically asymptomatic. In the majority of cases, early symptoms are nebulous (weight loss, abdominal discomfort) and many tumours are identified incidentally on cross-sectional imaging or following work-up for abnormal liver function tests. In patients with no previous biliary intervention, cholangitis is rare at initial presentation. Occasionally, patients with long-standing biliary obstruction and/or portal vein involvement may present with symptoms related to portal hypertension. Additionally, in those with PSC, distal ductal or periductal lesions can be difficult to differentiate from benign biliary strictures.[6]

## DIAGNOSIS AND WORK-UP

Preoperative imaging should assess the extent of local disease as well as evaluate for the presence of distant metastases. Work-up should focus on resectability of the primary

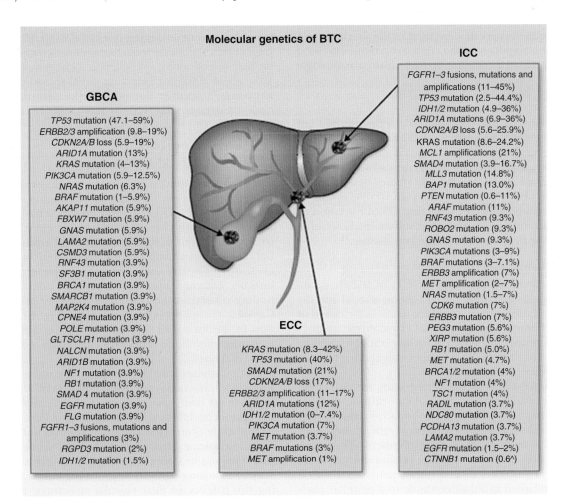

**Figure 14.1** Biliary tract cancers *(BTC)*, intrahepatic cholangiocarcinoma *(ICC)*, extrahepatic (hilar and distal) cholangiocarcinoma *(ECC)* and gallbladder adenocarcinoma *(GBCA)* are characterised by different genomic profiles. (Reproduced with permission from Valle et al., Cancer Discovery, 2017.[182])

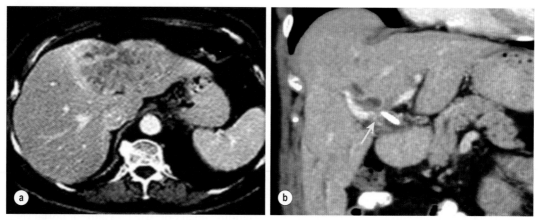

**Figure 14.2** Characteristic appearance of intrahepatic cholangiocarcinoma on CT, demonstrating heterogeneous enhancement of the primary tumour **(a)**, and hilar cholangiocarcinoma **(b)** *(arrow)*.

tumour, including predicted functional liver remnant (FLR) following surgical resection.

Cross-sectional, contrast-enhanced imaging is the mainstay of investigation. Imaging should include thin cuts to elucidate detailed relationships between the tumour and porta hepatis structures. It is preferred that initial imaging studies be performed prior to biliary stenting (if necessary), as stenting will cause local inflammation, making assessment of tumour extent difficult. Additionally, there are several more invasive modalities that are used in the diagnosis and staging of cholangiocarcinoma, and are commonly used for a more detailed evaluation or to confirm a pathologic diagnosis.

## ULTRASONOGRAPHY

Ultrasonography of the abdomen is a non-invasive, but operator-dependent, imaging modality that is often used early in the course of work-up. Characteristic appearance of ICC includes a hypoechoic, heterogeneous liver mass with minimal internal blood flow.[30] Early studies demonstrated that Doppler ultrasonography had comparable results as other imaging modalities for detecting tumour invasion of the portal vein and extent of biliary involvement; however, it is limited in the detection of extrahepatic disease.[31]

## COMPUTED TOMOGRAPHY

Multiphasic computed tomography (CT) of the chest, abdomen and pelvis including portal venous, arterial and delayed phases, is the modality of choice to assess for extent of the primary tumour and metastasis. Characteristic findings of ICC on contrast-enhanced CT include variable rim-like enhancement on arterial phase images with gradual centripetal enhancement on delayed phase.

Cross-sectional CT is an important study for evaluating patients with biliary obstruction and can provide valuable information regarding the level of obstruction, vascular involvement and liver atrophy. CT offers excellent assessment of the radial extent of soft-tissue involvement, direct liver invasion of perihilar lesions and the relationship to portal structures. For instance, dilated intrahepatic ducts with a normal or collapsed gallbladder allude to a perihilar cholangiocarcinoma, particularly if there is any evidence of a soft-tissue mass. This is in comparison to a distended gallbladder with normal intrahepatic ducts which alludes to

either stone disease or tumour obstructing the cystic duct, and a distended gallbladder with dilated intra- and extrahepatic ducts that suggests either choledocholithiasis or a distal biliary malignancy.[6] Segmental or lobar atrophy may be evident on CT that would suggest portal venous occlusion or long-standing biliary obstruction in the absence of portal venous involvement (Fig. 14.2).[32]

CT has been found to identify cholangiocarcinoma in 94–100% of patients and the positive and negative predictive values for determining resectability are 92% and 85%, respectively.[33–35] Reported accuracy for detecting the longitudinal spread along bile ducts is 81% compared with an accuracy of 100% for detecting radial spread into adjacent structures.[36] Another limitation is the detection of lymph node metastases since CT has a documented sensitivity of 35–65%.[36]

## MAGNETIC RESONANCE IMAGING/ CHOLANGIOPANCREATOGRAPHY

Cholangiocarcinoma is hypointense on T1-weighted images and hyperintense on T2-weighted imaging on magnetic resonance imaging (MRI).[6] These tumours demonstrate initial rim enhancement characterised by progressive and concentric enhancement post administration of contrast material, but the lesions usually do not completely enhance post-contrast. ICCs may only enhance completely on delayed imaging obtained hours after contrast administration—a finding related to the desmoplastic nature of the tumour. Capsular retraction may also be seen (Fig. 14.3).[37,38] A lesion in the liver with this morphology on MRI evaluation is pathognomonic for cholangiocarcinoma, even without a tissue diagnosis.

Several studies have demonstrated the utility of magnetic resonance cholangiopancreatography (MRCP) in evaluating patients with biliary obstruction.[39,40] MRCP identifies the tumour and the level of biliary obstruction, and can also demonstrate obstructed and isolated ducts not appreciated at endoscopic or percutaneous study. By virtue of being an axial imaging modality, MRCP has further advantages over standard cholangiography by providing information regarding the patency of hilar vascular structures, the presence of nodal or distant metastases, the presence of lobar atrophy and with its high tissue contrast helps to detect hepatic parenchymal involvement or metastatic hepatic disease.

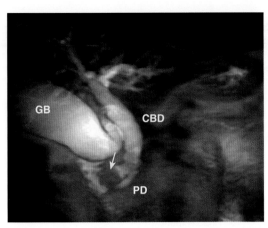

**Figure 14.3** Cross-sectional magnetic resonance cholangiopancreatography from a patient with distal cholangiocarcinoma *(arrow)*. The common bile duct *(CBD)* and pancreatic duct *(PD)* appear white. *GB*, gallbladder.

Compared with invasive cholangiopancreatography, MRCP has comparable rates of detecting the location and extent of tumour within the biliary tree, yet is associated with decreased infectious complications compared with standard cholangiography as it does not require biliary intubation.[33,41] Furthermore, as MRCP images the biliary tree both below and above the level of obstruction, MRCP can more accurately evaluate biliary ducts proximal to a lesion that may not be adequately filled with contrast during endoscopic retrograde cholangiopancreatography (ERCP).[6] Reported accuracy in determining the extent of bile duct involvement is 71–96%.[42,43] Limitations of MRCP include understaging up to 20% of perihilar cases, overstaging patients with indwelling biliary stents and can be limited by motion artifact.[6]

## POSITRON EMISSION TOMOGRAPHY

The utility of fluorodeoxyglucose positron emission tomography (FDG-PET) imaging is not routinely used in all centres in the work-up of cholangiocarcinoma, although can be used in select cases, particularly those where there is concern for metastatic disease. The possibility of false positives with the use of PET-CT should be considered, especially in patients with other causes of inflammation or indwelling biliary stents.

Several studies have demonstrated that the addition of PET-CT to CT alone does not improve the diagnostic accuracy or resectability of the primary tumour,[44,45] but it can aid in the detection of distant metastases. Identification of regional lymphadenopathy varies based on the study, with some demonstrating poor detection of lymph nodes,[46] and others demonstrating improved diagnosis compared with CT alone.[45,47,48] For example, Kim et al.[48] demonstrated that PET-CT improved the diagnostic accuracy of regional lymph node metastases compared with CT alone (76% vs 61%, $P = 0.004$). The use of PET-CT has been shown to improve the accuracy of diagnosis of distant metastases. A meta-analysis that included 2125 patients from 47 studies demonstrated that the overall sensitivity and specificity for distant metastases was 85% and 90%, respectively.[49]

Studies have demonstrated that there is an association between maximum standardised uptake value (SUVmax)

and outcomes following resection. For example, Ma et al.[50] demonstrated that an SUVmax of greater than 8 was associated with worse OS (3-year, 29% vs 74%, $P = 0.048$) and recurrence-free survival (RFS) (3-year, 21% vs 63%, $P = 0.004$) following resection in patients with resectable cholangiocarcinoma. Ultimately, PET-CT changes surgical management in 20–30% of cases,[51–54] and therefore, should be used in select cases where there is uncertainty regarding the presence of metastatic disease.

## INVASIVE MODALITIES

### Direct cholangiography

Percutaneous transhepatic cholangiography (PTC) evaluates the intrahepatic bile ducts more reliably, and may be required in patients with an obstructive perihilar lesion. Unlike diagnostic radiographic imaging modalities, PTC offers the ability to obtain tissue for sampling (brushing, biopsy) and also to place a biliary stent to relieve symptoms of obstructive jaundice.

### Endoscopy

Endoscopic modalities, including endoscopic ultrasound and ERCP, offer the ability to further characterised indeterminate biliary strictures and assess for the presence of a biliary ductal mass, especially in cases of biliary dilatation without an obvious lesion seen on cross-sectional imaging. It can also be used to identify and biopsy lymphadenopathy for staging and perform biliary stenting for decompression of the biliary tree.

Endoscopic choledochoscopy utilises a narrow-calibre fibreoptic choledochoscope passed through the working channel of a standard duodenoscope. It can be used to directly visualise luminal filling abnormalities noted on MRCP or direct cholangiography. Malignant biliary strictures are characterised by the presence of dilated or tortuous vessels, mucosal ulceration, polypoid or nodular masses, or villous mucosal morphology.[55,56] Endoscopic choledochoscopy combined with ERCP and tissue sampling increases the sensitivity for the detection of malignancy in patients with indeterminate biliary strictures from 58% to 100% compared with ERCP and biopsy alone.[57]

SpyGlass may overcome some limitations of conventional cholangioscopy. In an analysis of a cohort of patients with indeterminate biliary lesions, 52 patients underwent SpyGlass and targeted biopsies with a definite diagnosis made in 94% of cases. The sensitivity, specificity, and positive and negative predictive values were 88%, 94%, 96% and 85%, respectively. Overall, SpyGlass allowed adequate biopsy sampling and definite diagnosis in the vast majority of patients with indeterminate biliary lesions.[58]

## SERUM MARKERS

Cancer antigen (CA) 19-9 and carcinoembryonic antigen (CEA) levels may be elevated in patients with cholangiocarcinoma, although they are non-specific. These markers can also be elevated in patients with benign conditions, such as cholestasis, hepatic parenchymal injury and benign biliary obstruction, or in other malignancies, including gastric, pancreatic and colorectal cancers. Alpha-fetoprotein (AFP) can also be obtained to rule out hepatocellular carcinoma.

The overall sensitivity and specificity of CA 19-9 and CEA varies between studies and may be beneficial in certain circumstances. For example, CA 19-9 levels > 100 U/mL have a sensitivity of 53% in diagnosing cholangiocarcinoma in patients without PSC, yet there is a wider range in patients with PSC.[59] Although the diagnostic accuracy of CA 19-9 in patients with cholangiocarcinoma is variable, a very elevated level may be indicative of unresectable or metastatic disease.

While serum CA 19-9 has been shown to have a low sensitivity and specificity, some studies have demonstrated that it has prognostic value following resection. Prior data has shown that patients who have elevated CA 19-9 preoperatively that does not normalise postoperatively have worse OS than patients who have normalisation of their CA 19-9.[60,61] For example, in a study of 317 patients who underwent curative resection with biliary tract cancers, patients with normal CA 19-9 at the time of resection and those with normalisation of CA 19-9 following resection demonstrated an improved OS compared with those with a CA 19-9 that did not normalise (70% and 73% vs 31%, $P < 0.001$).[61]

## STAGING

### INTRAHEPATIC CHOLANGIOCARCINOMA

The 8th edition American Joint Committee on Cancer (AJCC) is the staging system that is currently used for ICC.[62] This most recent edition includes separation of tumour size, vascular invasion and multifocal tumours. Stratification based on T1a, T1b and T2 has been shown to be associated with survival based on National Cancer Database (NCDB) data ($P < 0.001$).

### HILAR CHOLANGIOCARCINOMA

The modified Bismuth–Corlette classification is a widely used staging system for hilar cholangiocarcinoma, and stratifies patients solely based on the extent of biliary duct involvement by tumour with no consideration of other disease-related variables.[63] Type I tumours involve the common hepatic duct below the biliary confluence, type II involve the biliary confluence, type IIIa/b involve the biliary confluence extending into the right and left hepatic ducts, respectively, and type IV involve the confluence and extend into both the left and right hepatic ducts. However, this staging system does not fully account for all of the tumour-related variables that influence resectability, including extent of involvement of the biliary tree, lobar atrophy and vascular involvement, nor does it demonstrate association with survival outcomes.

The 8th edition AJCC staging system for hilar cholangiocarcinoma was updated in 2017.[64] Early versions of this system were largely based on pathologic criteria and had little applicability for preoperative staging; however, the MSKCC staging system was incorporated in the 7th edition (2009) of the AJCC staging system for hilar cholangiocarcinoma.

The Blumgart clinical staging system stratifies the extent of disease based on four factors: (1) involvement of the biliary confluence; (2) second-order biliary radical involvement; (3) portal vein involvement; and (4) hepatic lobar atrophy (Table 14.1, Fig. 14.4). A clinical T-stage is determined based on a combination of these factors.[65–67] For example, a tumour with unilateral extension into second-order bile ducts that is associated with ipsilateral portal vein involvement and/or lobar atrophy would still be considered

**Table 14.1    Proposed MSKCC T-stage criteria for hilar cholangiocarcinoma**

| Stage | Criteria |
|---|---|
| T1 | Tumour involving biliary confluence ± unilateral extension to second-order biliary radicles |
| T2 | Tumour involving biliary confluence ± unilateral extension to second-order biliary radicles AND *ipsilateral* portal vein involvement ± *ipsilateral* hepatic lobar atrophy |
| T3 | Tumour involving biliary confluence + bilateral extension to second-order biliary radicles OR unilateral extension to second-order biliary radicles with *contralateral* portal vein involvement OR unilateral extension to second-order biliary radicles with *contralateral* hepatic lobar atrophy OR main or bilateral portal venous involvement |

Reproduced with permission from Jarnagin WR, Fong Y, DeMatteo RP, et al. Staging, resectability, and outcome in 225 patients with hilar cholangiocarcinoma. Ann Surg 2001;234:507–19.[65]

potentially resectable, while such involvement on the contralateral side would preclude resection. The primary strength of this staging system is to better assesses resectability as it evaluates both portal venous involvement and lobar atrophy, which is important when evaluating for hepatectomy. T-stage based on the aforementioned criteria correlates with resectability, likelihood of achieving an R0 resection, distant metastases and OS based on three independent series (Table 14.2).[66,68,69] The authors' criteria for unresectability are detailed in Box 14.1.

✔✔ The Blumgart clinical staging system for hilar cholangiocarcinoma is based on four factors: (1) involvement of the biliary confluence; (2) second-order biliary radical involvement; (3) portal vein involvement; and (4) hepatic lobar atrophy. This staging system has been shown to correlate with resectability, metastatic disease and OS.[66,68]

### EXTRAHEPATIC CHOLANGIOCARCINOMA

Carcinomas of the distal common bile duct are staged according to the 8th edition AJCC System, for tumours of the extrahepatic bile ducts.[70] In this edition, T-stage is now based on tumour depth, compared with the 7th edition AJCC, in which distal cholangiocarcinomas were staged based on the extent of invasion within or through the bile duct wall. The 7th edition T-stage did not adequately predict survival, and instead depth of the primary tumour has been shown to correlate with OS, and thus has been adopted by the AJCC 8th edition.[71–74] The main limitation of the AJCC staging system is that it does not define resectability of the primary tumour, similar to the weaknesses of the AJCC staging system used for hilar cholangiocarcinoma.

## MANAGEMENT

### PREOPERATIVE TISSUE DIAGNOSIS

A pathologic diagnosis is not warranted prior to surgical resection but is required in cases of advanced disease in which

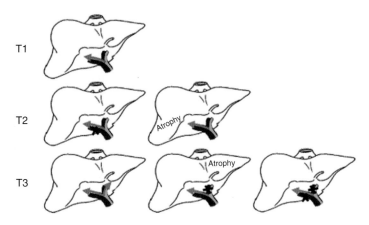

T1

T2

Atrophy

T3

Atrophy

**Figure 14.4** The Blumgart staging system for hilar cholangiocarcinoma. (Reproduced with permission from Matsuo et al., JACS, 2012.[66])

**Table 14.2** Resectability, incidence of metastatic disease and survival stratified by T-stage for patients with hilar cholangiocarcinoma

| T-stage | n | Explored with curative intent | Resected | Negative margins | Hepatic resection | Portal vein resection | Metastatic disease | Median survival (months) |
|---------|-----|----------|----------|----------|----------|----------|----------|----------|
| 1 | 87 | 73 (84%) | 51 (59%) | 38 | 33 | 2 | 18 (21%) | 20 |
| 2 | 95 | 79 (83%) | 29 (31%) | 24 | 29 | 7 | 40 (43%) | 13 |
| 3 | 37 | 8 (22%) | 0 | 0 | 0 | 0 | 15 (41%) | 8 |
| Total | 219 | 160 (71%) | 80 (37%) | 62 | 62 | 9 | 73 (33%) | 16 |

Reproduced with permission from Jarnagin WR, Fong Y, DeMatteo RP et al. Staging, resectability, and outcome in 225 patients with hilar cholangiocarcinoma. Ann Surg 2001;234:507–19.[65]

---

**Box 14.1    Criteria for unresectability of hilar cholangiocarcinoma**

*Patient factors*
• Medically unfit or unable to tolerate a major operation
• Cirrhosis

**Local tumour-related factors**
• Tumour extension to secondary biliary radicles bilaterally
• Encasement or occlusion of the main portal vein proximal to its bifurcation
• Atrophy of one hepatic lobe with contralateral portal vein branch encasement or occlusion
• Atrophy of one hepatic lobe with contralateral tumour extension to secondary biliary radicles
• Unilateral tumour extension to secondary biliary radicles with contralateral portal vein branch encasement or occlusion

*Metastatic disease*
• Histologically proven metastases to distant lymph node basins*
• Lung, liver or peritoneal metastases

---

\* Includes peripancreatic, periduodenal, coeliac, superior mesenteric or posterior pancreaticoduodenal lymph nodes.
Reproduced with permission from Jarnagin WR, Fong Y, DeMatteo RP, et al. Staging, resectability, and outcome in 225 patients with hilar cholangiocarcinoma. Ann Surg 2001;234:507–19.

---

patients will receive systemic or locoregional therapy.[75,76] The finding of a biliary stricture combined with the appropriate clinical presentation is sufficient for a presumptive diagnosis of cholangiocarcinoma, and surgical intervention

can be planned in such cases. Sensitivities for brush cytology during PTC or endoscopy range from 30% to 60%,[77] and therefore negative results in the setting of a suspicious clinical picture and radiographic appearance should be interpreted with caution.

Additionally, it should be noted that the histologic findings of ICC can be similar to those of metastatic tumours to the liver. Immunohistochemical markers have the ability to differentiate ICC from liver metastases; however, it is important that a thorough work-up is done to rule out the presence of an extrahepatic primary tumour.[76]

## PREOPERATIVE BILIARY DRAINAGE

The use of routine preoperative biliary drainage in patients with cholangiocarcinoma remains controversial. The need for preoperative drainage varies based on location of the primary tumour, as ICC often does not result in biliary obstruction, whereas ECC and hilar cholangiocarcinoma do so more frequently. Routine preoperative biliary drainage had been recommended as it was thought that the sequela of hyperbilirubinemia were associated with poor postoperative outcomes, specifically increased risk of postoperative liver failure following resection of hilar cholangiocarcinoma. Indeed, resection for hilar cholangiocarcinoma has historically been associated with high morbidity and mortality, largely due to the large sacrifice of liver parenchyma in the setting of an impaired future liver remnant (secondary to biliary obstruction). In an effort to mitigate the risk of resection, routine drainage of the liver remnant combined with preoperative portal vein embolisation (PVE; vide infra) have been advocated; however, a more selective approach to these procedures has been adopted in recent years.

Several studies have demonstrated that preoperative biliary drainage is associated with improved perioperative outcomes, yet results are mixed. Proponents of biliary drainage believe that stent placement improves hepatic function and nutritional status, and reduces the risk of cholangitis and postoperative liver failure. Data supports the use of biliary drainage in patients with a predicted FLR of < 30%. In a study of 60 patients, those with FLR < 30% had worse outcomes if they did not undergo preoperative biliary drainage compared with those who did.[78] Similarly, on an assessment of 287 consecutive patients undergoing major liver resection for perihilar cholangiocarcinoma, incomplete drainage of the future liver remnant in patients with FLR < 50% predicted postoperative mortality.[79] However, in a multicentre, retrospective study, preoperative biliary drainage did not result in improved postoperative outcomes in patients undergoing major surgical resection for perihilar cholangiocarcinoma, although on subset analysis in patients requiring right hepatectomy, there was an association with decreased mortality due to liver failure.[80]

Risks associated with preoperative biliary drainage include tumour seeding, cholangitis, bile leakage and perioperative infectious complications. Several studies have demonstrated that patients who undergo preoperative biliary drainage have an increased risk of postoperative infection. In an analysis of 71 patients who underwent either resection or palliative biliary bypass for proximal cholangiocarcinoma, all patients stented endoscopically and 62% of those stented percutaneously had bacterobilia. Moreover, postoperative infectious complications were doubled in those patients stented before operation compared with their non-stented counterparts.[81]

Hilar tumours present unique challenges and frequently involve multiple major ducts, and thus may require two or more stents for adequate drainage. A randomised clinical trial assessed bilateral versus unilateral stent placement and found unilateral stenting to be associated with higher rates of successful drainage (87% vs 77%, $P = 0.041$), fewer complications (19% vs 27%, $P = 0.026$) and lower rates of cholangitis (9% vs 17%, $P = 0.013$), yet there was no significant difference between the two groups with regard to procedure-related mortality, 30-day mortality, complications or median survival.[82]

✔ Biliary decompression of an atrophic lobe does not typically provide significant benefit in terms of lowering serum bilirubin or improving hepatic function and should only be performed if necessary to treat cholangitis.

Preoperative biliary drainage can be done either percutaneously or endoscopically. Both methods of stenting have been associated with increased morbidity and mortality following surgical resection for hilar cholangiocarcinoma. There were two recent trials comparing percutaneous versus endoscopic biliary drainage in hilar cholangiocarcinoma, both of which were terminated early. The INTERCEPT study was stopped early due to slow accrual,[83–85] whereas the DRAINAGE trial was terminated secondary to increased mortality in the percutaneous biliary drainage group.[86] One of the most important considerations is drainage of the remaining lobe. Decompression of an atrophic lobe usually does not provide significant benefit in terms of

hepatic function, and should only be done when the patient is cholangitic.

## PORTAL VEIN EMBOLISATION

Assessment of FLR is necessary prior to determining resectability. As previously identified by our group, FLR < 30% in patients undergoing liver resection for hilar cholangiocarcinoma was associated with increased risk for hepatic insufficiency and death.[78] Furthermore, in a series of 287 consecutive perihilar cholangiocarcinoma patients who underwent resection, postoperative mortality at 90 days was independently associated with FLR < 30%.[79] PVE is considered in patients who have an estimated/anticipated FLR < 30% of the total liver volume in the context of a normal liver; however, in patients with underlying liver dysfunction or those who have been heavily pre-treated with systemic chemotherapy, FLR < 40% may be used as the cut-off to consider PVE.[6] Traditionally, it has been used more often in the setting of an extended right hepatectomy, since the left lateral sector often does not comprise sufficient volume to support an extended resection.

PVE results in liver hypertrophy of the non-embolised segments secondary to altered portal blood flow. Contraindications to PVE include portal hypertension as well tumour thrombus in the ipsilateral portal vein. On average, up to a 15% increase in the total volume of the FLR can be expected within 4–6 weeks, although up to 25–40% of patients fail to undergo resection either due to inadequate hypertrophy or disease progression.[6] To date, numerous studies have reported the safety and efficacy of PVE in increasing the remnant liver volume before extended hepatectomy.[87–89] Furthermore, PVE has been shown to be associated with a decreased rate of postoperative liver failure and mortality following major hepatectomy for hilar cholangiocarcinoma.[90]

✔✔ PVE can reduce the risk of postoperative hepatic dysfunction by inducing preoperative compensatory hypertrophy of the non-embolised lobe.

## GENERAL OPERATIVE PRINCIPLES

Cholangiocarcinoma is an aggressive malignancy; complete resection of the primary tumour is definitive management, and is the only chance in achieving cure. Perhaps only 50% of patients diagnosed with cholangiocarcinoma have resectable disease at the time of diagnosis, with 20–40% unresectable at the time of operation secondary to locally advanced or metastatic disease. Contraindications to resection include metastatic disease, extensive lymphadenopathy, and predicted inadequate postoperative FLR. Surgical resection often involves a major hepatectomy for ICC and hilar cholangiocarcinoma, or resection of the extrahepatic biliary tree and pancreatoduodenectomy for distal bile duct tumours. Principles of operative resection include achieving an R0 resection, maintaining an adequate liver remnant, and portal lymphadenectomy.

## DIAGNOSTIC LAPAROSCOPY

Diagnostic laparoscopy is recommended for staging, especially in patients who are at an increased risk of metastatic disease based on preoperative work-up. This includes patients with elevated CA 19-9, possible vascular invasion or suspicion for peritoneal disease.[76] While there have been improvements in preoperative imaging, 15–40% of patients are still found to have unresectable disease at the time of staging laparoscopy depending on the location of the primary tumour.[91–95]

Multiple studies evaluating patients with biliary cancer have shown that staging laparoscopy can identify a significant proportion of patients with radiographically occult metastases, the yield of which is greatest in locally advanced tumours. For hilar cholangiocarcinoma, approximately 25–30% of patients are found to have advanced disease precluding resection.[65,94] Weber et al. evaluated 56 patients with potentially resectable hilar cholangiocarcinoma, 25% of whom were noted to have unresectable disease on laparoscopy. In patients with locally advanced disease (T2/T3), the yield of diagnostic laparoscopy was higher than those with T1 disease (36% vs 9%).[94] Similarly, staging laparoscopy identified unresectable disease in 25–38% of patients with ICC, and 13% of patients with distal cholangiocarcioma.[91–93,95]

✔ Even when thought to be resectable by imaging, up to 30–40% of patients with cholangiocarcinoma will be deemed unresectable at the time of exploration. Therefore, diagnostic laparoscopy is recommended for patients at increased risk of metastatic disease based on preoperative work-up.

## MARGIN-NEGATIVE RESECTION

The overall goal of surgical treatment is to resect all gross and microscopic disease to achieve an R0 resection. Prior data has demonstrated that an R0 resection is associated with improved perioperative outcomes in ICC, ECC and hilar cholangiocarcinoma. The extent of resection should be dictated by what is necessary to achieve a negative margin and this may require an extended resection, and is dependent on the location of the tumour.

Prior studies have demonstrated that an R0 resection is associated with improved OS in ICC, although results have been mixed.[7,84,85] In a multi-institutional study of 583 patients, those who underwent an R1 resection had an increased risk of recurrence (HR: 1.86, 95% CI: 1.54–2.25, $P$ < 0.001) and worse OS (HR: 1.86, 95% CI: 1.54–2.25, $P$ < 0.001) compared with those who had a margin-negative resection. Furthermore, Li et al.[85] performed a meta-analysis of 21 studies that included 3201 patients, which demonstrated that patients who had a positive surgical margin following resection had lower OS (HR: 1.86, 95% CI: 1.54–2.25, $P$ < 0.001) and lower RFS (HR: 2.03, 95% CI: 1.03–4.01, $P$ = 0.041) than patients who underwent an R0 resection. The increased utilisation of hepatic resection has been responsible for the increased percentage of R0 resections and the observed improvement in postoperative survival. This point is emphasised by a reported series of 269 patients over a 20-year period demonstrating a progressive increase in the proportion of patients subjected to partial hepatectomy, with a corresponding increase in the incidence of negative histological margins and in turn, improved survival.[96] This is similar for hilar and distal cholangiocarcinoma, in which an R1 resection is associated with worse OS.[28,97] For distal cholangiocarcinoma, simple excision of the extrahepatic biliary tree is generally avoided, as this approach is associated with a high probability of R1/R2 resections and inferior OS,[98] and instead, formal resection including a pancreatoduodenectomy for distal cholangiocarcinoma should be performed.

✔✔ The achievement of pathologically negative margins (R0 resection) is the most predictive factor of oncologic outcome for ICC and ECC. R0 resection has been shown to be associated with improved clinical outcomes.

Intraoperative frozen section should be obtained to ensure an R0 resection; if positive, more extended resections should be considered to obtain pathologically negative margins. Of course, whether or not this is feasible technically will be dictated by the location of the tumour. For ECC, bile duct excision alone (combined with porta hepatis lymphadenectomy) may be feasible in some cases; however, frozen section should be obtained on the proximal and distal bile duct margins and, if positive, hepatectomy or pancreaticoduodenectomy should ensue. For most extrahepatic biliary cancers, extended hepatectomy or pancreaticoduodenectomy are necessary for complete resection. In an MSKCC analysis of ECC, 82% of proximal lesions required a combined hepatectomy, whereas 92% of distal lesions required a pancreaticoduodenectomy.[99] Rarely, tumour extent is such that only a combination of hepatectomy and pancreaticoduodenectomy can achieve an R0 resection. While these very extended resections may be appropriate in a few highly selected patients, morbidity and mortality rates are substantial, and the decision to proceed must be carefully weighed against the high risk of recurrence and the survival benefit.

It must be recognised that intraoperative frozen section is associated with some degree of inaccuracy. In one study, the false-negative rate was 9% for the proximal bile duct margin.[100] Resection to a negative margin (R0) has been shown to be associated with improved survival similar to an R0 resection, compared with an R1 resection in both hilar and distal cholangiocarcinoma.[101–104] However, it has also been shown to be associated with an increased risk of complications, so morbidity of additional resection must be taken into consideration.[101] In a series of 215 patients undergoing resection for hilar cholangiocarcinoma, a secondary R0 resection (that obtained following an initial positive margin on frozen section) was associated with comparable OS as that of an R0 resection (HR: 0.9, 95% CI: 0.4–2.3, $P$ = 0.829), whereas an R1 resection was associated with worse OS (HR: 1.3, 95% CI: 1.0–1.7, $P$ = 0.027).[104] Similar results were demonstrated in distal cholangiocarcinoma, in which a retrospective study evaluating 107 patients demonstrated that additional resection of the proximal bile duct margin during a pancreaticoduodenectomy was associated with increased R0 resection, which translated to improved OS.[103]

## VASCULAR RESECTION

Vascular resection is at times warranted in patients with cholangiocarcinoma with macrovascular invasion, and should be considered in selected patients. Venous resection can include resection of the portal vein and/or inferior vena cava (IVC), and data has demonstrated that these resections can be completed with reasonable morbidity and survival outcomes.[105–111] For example, in a study of 95 patients with hilar cholangiocarcinoma, 42 required resection of the portal vein. Patients who underwent portal vein resection had perioperative mortality and morbidity similar to those who did not. The 5-year OS was 43%. Negative margins were achieved in 84% of cases and were associated with improved survival ($P < 0.01$); on multivariate analysis, the only predictor of survival was negative margin status.[105]

En bloc IVC resection and hepatectomy can be completed in certain circumstances, and studies have demonstrated appropriate safety, oncologic and survival outcomes.[106,111] For example, Hemmings et al.[106] reported data on 60 patients who underwent IVC resection for a hepatic malignancy, 26 of whom had ICC. The authors demonstrated an R0 resection rate of 92%, 43% overall morbidity and an actuarial 1-year and 5-year OS of 89% and 35%, respectively. Ultimately, venous involvement does not preclude resection, and venous resection in conjunction with hepatectomy in selected patients to achieve a negative margin can result in good oncologic outcomes and meaningful survival.

The role of arterial resection and reconstruction is more controversial, since many studies have shown arterial resection and reconstruction to be associated with significantly increased morbidity and mortality without long-term survival benefit.[109]

✔ Portal vein involvement and the need for vascular resection/reconstruction should not be considered a contraindication to resection. Although series have reported potentially higher postoperative morbidity and mortality, hepatectomy combined with portal vein resection has been demonstrated to be associated with improved survival.

## PORTAL LYMPHADENECTOMY

Lymphadenectomy is routinely recommended for patients with cholangiocarcinoma.[112] Lymphadenectomy provides prognostic information, yet whether it provides any therapeutic benefit is unclear. An international study group for ICC initially advocated routine portal lymph node dissection at the time of resection, as approximately 30% of patients who underwent evaluation were found to have lymph node involvement,[113] and now lymphadenectomy is recommended for all patients with cholangiocarcinoma undergoing resection.

Metastatic disease to the regional lymph nodes has been shown to be associated with poor outcomes following resection in ICC, hilar and distal cholangiocarcinoma.[99,113–116] In one study evaluating 749 patients with ICC, 36% were found to have lymph node-positive disease. This group of patients had a significantly increased risk of death compared with those who were lymph node-negative (HR: 2.42, 95% CI: 1.98–2.95, $P < 0.001$).[114] This has also been shown in distal cholangiocarcinoma. Fong et al.[115] found that lymph node status was the only independent predictor of long-term survival after complete resection, with positive nodes conferring a 6.7 times greater likelihood of recurrence and death. Similarly, Allen et al.[99] reported lymph node positivity to be an independent predictor of 5-year DSS (node-negative 42% vs node-positive 22%) in both proximal and distal resected cholangiocarcinoma.

The extent of lymphadenectomy has been an area of controversy, with some surgeons advocating for an extended nodal dissection. Prior studies have demonstrated

measurable 5-year actuarial survival in the presence of metastatic disease to distant lymph nodes in patients with hilar cholangiocarcinoma. However, an analysis of studies reporting 5-year survival suggests that distant nodal involvement is a marker of advanced/systemic disease and very few patients will benefit from an aggressive surgical approach.[117,118] With respect to the number of lymph nodes needed for accurate staging, the clinical implication of negative lymph nodes on histopathological analysis is likely dependent on the total number of lymph nodes sampled. A study from MSKCC reported that seven lymph nodes appear to be the target sampling number in order to accurately stage hilar cholangiocarcinoma.[119] This must be weighed against the reality that, in most series, the median number of nodes sampled from a porta hepatis lymphadenectomy is approximately three.

Lymphadenectomy is recommended for patients with cholangiocarcinoma, as it provides valuable staging information, with distant nodal disease portending poor 5-year survival. Furthermore, the therapeutic benefit and use of lymphadenectomy as a guide for adjuvant treatment has not been proven. Therefore, while a complete porta hepatis lymphadenectomy should be routinely performed at the time of resection, the authors do not advocate an extended lymph node dissection.

✔✔ Portal lymphadenectomy in patients with cholangiocarcinoma can provide important prognostic information.

## CAUDATE LOBECTOMY

En bloc resection of the caudate lobe should be performed for many patients undergoing hepatectomy for hilar cholangiocarcinoma, as it allows for complete resection of involved biliary radicals and is associated with improved postoperative outcomes. This is particularly true of tumours arising from the left hepatic duct since this is the primary source of caudate biliary drainage. A surgical approach that includes resection of the extrahepatic biliary tree along with hepatic resection including the caudate lobe should yield negative pathological margins in up to 80% of patients.[120]

Several studies have evaluated outcomes of hepatectomy including caudate lobectomy. In 171 patients with resected hilar cholangiocarcinoma, caudate lobectomy was associated with an increased incidence of curative resection ($P < 0.01$), without an increase in morbidity ($P = 0.39$) or mortality ($P = 0.67$) between groups.[121] In a study of 127 patients with resected hilar cholangiocarcinoma over 15 years, those who underwent caudate lobectomy ($n = 70$) had significantly improved OS compared with those who did not (64 vs 35 months, $P = 0.010$), and furthermore, multivariate analysis found caudate lobectomy to statistically improve disease-free survival ($P = 0.016$).[122] Additionally, caudate lobectomy was identified as an independent predictor of long-term survival ($> 5$ years; $P = 0.006$) in 243 patients with resected hilar cholangiocarcinoma.[123]

✔✔ Although initially controversial, resection of the caudate lobe en bloc for hilar cholangiocarcinoma is now widely accepted as standard in many patients, particularly tumours arising from the left hepatic duct.

## NO-TOUCH TECHNIQUE

The concept of the 'no-touch' technique was initially proposed by Neuhaus et al.[124] in 1999 for hilar cholangiocarcinoma arising from the right hepatic duct, and involves an extended right hepatectomy, caudate lobectomy and portal vein resection in order to avoid hilar dissection and possible microscopic dissemination of malignant cells. During this procedure, a vascular clamp is placed on the left portal vein branch within the umbilical fissure as well as on the main portal vein (directly above the head of the pancreas). These vessels are then divided without dissecting the portal vein within the hilar region.

A retrospective review of this technique found improved 5-year survival rates (58% vs 29%, $P = 0.02$) compared with those who underwent a conventional surgical approach.[125] Although the authors reported no increase in morbidity or mortality, the baseline mortality in both groups was high, and this technique may not be applicable to all surgeons or centres given the increased morbidity and mortality in less experienced hands. This surgical approach is likely best applied only to a highly selected population.

## PALLIATIVE SURGICAL INTERVENTION: INTRAHEPATIC BILIARY-ENTERIC BYPASS

Patients with unresectable hilar cholangiocarcinoma identified at operation may be candidates for intrahepatic biliary-enteric bypass. Decompression of one-third of the functioning hepatic parenchyma is usually sufficient to relieve jaundice and improve symptoms, and provided that the undrained lobe has not been percutaneously drained or otherwise contaminated, communication between the right and left hepatic ducts is not necessary.[126] The segment III duct is usually the most accessible and is the preferred approach of the authors, but the right anterior or posterior sectoral hepatic ducts can also be used.[127] A segment III bypass provides excellent biliary drainage and is less prone to occlusion since the anastomosis can be placed away from the tumour with 1-year patency rates of nearly 80%.[127] As discussed above for stenting, bypass to an atrophic lobe or a lobe heavily involved with tumour is generally not effective.

## LIVER TRANSPLANTATION

Orthotopic liver transplantation has been investigated for, and has become a well-established treatment, in highly selected patients with liver-only, unresectable hilar tumours, and rarely, ICC. In the USA, the use of liver transplantation is limited secondary to the number of available grafts, which has improved with the use of living liver donation and extended criteria grafts. Transplantation for hilar cholangiocarcinoma was first reported in 2000, and the use of liver transplantation has grown as it has been associated with good outcomes. The Mayo Clinic group has been the driving force behind this effort and has the largest experience worldwide.

Early studies evaluating liver transplantation for hilar cholangiocarcinoma were associated with high recurrence rates and poor OS,[128–130] but an improvement in outcomes were noted with the use of neoadjuvant therapy. The most widely used neoadjuvant regimen is external beam radiation plus brachytherapy with 5-flurouracil infusion, followed by capecitabine until transplantation. The use of liver transplantation for hilar cholangiocarcinoma has been shown to have positive outcomes,[131,132] with a 5-year RFS of 65% in a recent multicentre series.[133] In fact, data has demonstrated that patients who undergo neoadjuvant chemotherapy, radiation and liver transplantation have improved survival and lower recurrences than patients who undergo resection.[134] Patients with hilar cholangiocarcinoma and underlying PSC are recommended for neoadjuvant therapy and liver transplantation as this group of patients has specifically been shown to derive benefit from transplantation. Studies have demonstrated that patients with PSC who undergo liver transplantation for perihilar cholangiocarcinoma have better OS than their counterparts without PSC.[135]

Orthotopic liver transplantation has also been utilised in the management of some patients with ICC. While the treatment of choice is surgical resection, a subset of patients with locally unresectable, liver-only disease may be candidates for transplantation. It is recommended that patients with unresectable disease undergo neoadjuvant therapy, followed by transplantation in the setting of stable disease.[136,137] Furthermore, select patients with small tumours (< 2 cm) in the setting of cirrhosis can also be considered for liver transplant; early trials have demonstrated positive outcomes, yet it is recommended that this should be done in the setting of a clinical trial.[137]

## SYSTEMIC CHEMOTHERAPY

Systemic chemotherapy is the mainstay for locally advanced or metastatic disease, in patients in whom resection is not an option. There are a number of prior and ongoing trials that evaluate systemic therapy in the setting of advanced and metastatic disease, but details are beyond the scope of this chapter. The current first-line chemotherapy regimen is gemcitabine and cisplatin, as this regimen was associated with increased survival compared with gemcitabine alone in two trials.[143,144] Valle et al.[143] published the ABC-02 trial in 2010, a prospective randomised trial that included 410 patients with advanced biliary tract cancers. Results demonstrated that gemcitabine plus cisplatin was associated with a significant improvement in median OS (11.7 vs 8.1 months, $P < 0.001$) and median progression-free survival (8 vs 5 months, $P < 0.001$) compared with gemcitabine alone. Furthermore, the BT22 trial, which randomised 84 patients to gemcitabine and cisplatin or gemcitabine alone, demonstrated similar results with improved outcomes in the combination therapy arm.[144] Following the positive results of these trials, gemcitabine and cisplatin were used by some in the adjuvant setting.

✓✓ The combination of gemcitabine and cisplatin is the standard of care for patients with advanced biliary cancers, based on results from the ABC-02 and BT22 trials.[143,144]

## NEOADJUVANT THERAPY

There are no prospective randomised trials evaluating the use of neoadjuvant therapy in the treatment of ICC, ECC or hilar cholangiocarcinoma in patients with resectable disease. Theoretical benefits of neoadjuvant therapy include

**Table 14.3**    Prospective randomised trials evaluating adjuvant therapy in biliary tract cancers

| Trial | Number | Tumour types | Treatment | Overall survival (median) | Recurrence-free survival (median) |
|---|---|---|---|---|---|
| Takada et al. (2002)[146] | 508 | Cholangiocarcinoma Gallbladder Pancreatic Ampullary | Mitomicin/5-FU vs Observation | NS *gallbladder (5-yr OS) 26% vs 12%, $P = 0.0367$ | NS *gallbladder (5-yr RFS) 20% vs 12%, $P = 0.0210$ |
| BILCAP (2019)[149] | 447 | Intrahepatic CCA Hilar CCA Extrahepatic CCA Gallbladder | Capecitabine vs Surveillance | NS 51 vs 36 months HR: 0.81, 95% CI: 0.63–1.04, $P = 0.097$) *per protocol: 53 vs 36 months HR: 0.75, 95% CI 0.58–0.97, $P = 0.028$ | NS 24 vs 18 months HR: 1.48, 95% CI: 0.80–2.77, $P = 0.21$ |
| PRODIGE 12/ ACCORD 18 (2019)[147] | 196 | Intrahepatic CCA Extrahepatic CCA Gallbladder | Gemcitabine + oxaliplatin vs surveillance | NS 76 vs 51 months HR: 1.08, 95% CI: 0.70–1.66, $P = 0.74$ | NS 30 vs 19 months HR: 0.88, 95% CI: 0.62–1.25, $P = 0.48$ |
| BCAT (2018)[148] | 226 | Hilar CCA Extrahepatic CCA | Gemcitabine vs surveillance | NS 63 vs 64 months HR: 1.01, 95% CI: 0.70–1.45, $P = 0.964$ | NS 36 vs 40 months HR: 0.93, 95% CI: 0.66–1.32, $P = 0.693$ |
| ACTICCA-1 (2015)[213] | | Cholangiocarcinoma Gallbladder | Gemcitabine + cisplatin vs capecitabine | Ongoing | Ongoing |

downstaging locally advanced disease and increasing likelihood of R0 resection, and ultimately improving OS[138]; however, its utility remains unproven. There is limited retrospective data addressing this question, and instead there are primarily small case series and retrospective studies. However, there are several ongoing, prospective trials evaluating neoadjuvant chemotherapy in patients with cholangiocarcinoma.[139] The benefits of neoadjuvant therapy have been demonstrated with the use of successful liver transplantation for hilar cholangiocarcinoma, using the Mayo protocol as described previously.[140]

There are several small, retrospective studies evaluating the use of neoadjuvant therapy for ECC (hilar and distal), and show high rates of R0 resection.[139] One study included 40 patients who underwent resection for ECC. All patients who received neoadjuvant chemoradiotherapy had a margin-negative resection compared with 54% for the group who did not receive preoperative chemoradiotherapy ($P < 0.01$). Furthermore, a pathological complete response was observed in 3/9 (33%) patients.[141] Katayose et al.[142] published early results on a phase II trial evaluating gemcitabine and external beam radiation therapy (EBRT) for possibly resectable hilar and distal cholangiocarcinoma. Results demonstrated that R0 resection was 90% in patients who underwent resection, and treatment was well tolerated.

Neoadjuvant therapy has also been evaluated in patients with ICC in several retrospective studies. These series have looked at multimodality therapy in the locally unresectable setting, and a subset of patients have been downstaged and able to undergo resection.[139] A study by Le Roy et al. included a total of 186 patients; 74 patients with locally advanced ICC who underwent neoadjuvant therapy were compared with 96 with resectable disease who underwent upfront surgery. Results demonstrated similar morbidity and postoperative mortality between the groups; however, those who received neoadjuvant resection were less likely to have an R0 resection (31% vs 59%, $P = 0.004$). However, there was no difference in survival between groups (median OS, 24 months vs 26 months, $P = 0.391$).

## ADJUVANT CHEMOTHERAPY

There are several phase 3 randomised trials that evaluate the use of adjuvant therapy in patients with biliary malignancies (Table 14.3). All of these trials include multiple subtypes of biliary cancer, although do include subset analyses looking at adjuvant regimens in specific cohorts. A meta-analysis by Horgan et al.[145] demonstrated that the patients who derived the greatest benefit from adjuvant therapy included those with lymph node-positive disease (OR 0.49; $P = 0.004$) and those with positive margin disease (OR 0.36; $P = 0.002$). However, adjuvant therapy is not routinely used in these settings.

An early phase III trial investigating the use of mitomycin/5-fluorouracil (5-FU) included 508 patients with resected bile duct tumours ($n = 139$), gallbladder cancers ($n = 140$), pancreatic cancers ($n = 173$) and ampullary tumours ($n = 56$).[146] On subset analysis, there were no significant differences in OS or disease-free survival for bile duct tumours.

Following the ABC-02 and BT-22 trials which established gemcitabine and cisplatin as first-line standard of care therapy for advanced biliary tract cancers, the PRODIGE-12/ ACCORD-18 study evaluated gemcitabine plus oxaliplatin (GEMOX) compared with observation alone in the adjuvant setting.[147] This was a phase III randomised control trial that enrolled 196 patients with biliary cancers. Results demonstrated that there was no significant difference in OS (HR: 1.08, 95% CI: 0.70–1.66, $P = 0.74$) or RFS (HR: 0.88, 95% CI: 0.62–1.25, $P = 0.48$) between arms.[147]

The Bile Duct Cancer Adjuvant Trial (BCAT) randomised patients to gemcitabine versus observation following resection for hilar and distal cholangiocarcinoma.[148] A total of 226 patients were enrolled at 48 centres in Japan. Again, no significant difference was noted in overall OS (62 vs 64 months, $P = 0.96$) or RFS (36 vs 40 months, $P = 0.693$) between groups.[148]

Primrose et al.[149] reported results from the BILCAP trial, a phase III multi-institutional randomised trial, which randomised patients with biliary tract cancer to 6 months of adjuvant capecitabine ($n = 223$) versus observation ($n = 224$). Results demonstrated that there was no significant difference in median OS in the intention-to-treat analysis between the treatment and observation arms (51 vs 36 months, $P = 0.097$). However, in the per-protocol analysis, OS did reach statistical significance, with a median OS of 53 months in the treatment arm and 36 months in the observation arm ($P = 0.028$). Furthermore, patients who received adjuvant capecitabine had significantly longer RFS than those who underwent observation (25 vs 18 months, $P = 0.036$). Limitations of this trial include the heterogeneity of the patient population, as all sites of biliary tract cancers (ICC, hilar and distal cholangiocarcinoma, and gallbladder cancer), and both R0 and R1 resections were included. Although the grouping of all types of biliary tract cancer into a single trial can be criticised, it represents a clinical and practical reality given the rarity of these cancers and the feasibility of performing a clinical trial.

✓✓ Capecitabine is most commonly used in the adjuvant setting based on results of the BILCAP trial, which demonstrated improved OS on a per-protocol analysis in patients who received capecitabine compared with observation.[149]

## ADJUVANT RADIATION

There are currently no randomised trials evaluating the use of adjuvant radiotherapy in patients with biliary cancers, and no data supports its routine use. There are several small, single-centre studies that evaluate the use of adjuvant chemoradiotherapy in patients with hilar cholangiocarcinoma, especially in the setting of an R1 resection. Kamada et al.[150] suggested that radiation may improve survival in patients with histologically positive hepatic duct margins. Furthermore, in a study of 91 patients who underwent R1 resection for hilar cholangiocarcinoma, EBRT with or without intraluminal brachytherapy was associated with improved OS compared with those who did not receive radiation (24 vs 8 months, $P < 0.01$).[151] Lastly, a recent meta-analysis that included 6700 patients from 20 studies evaluating adjuvant therapy in biliary tract cancers demonstrated that patients receiving chemotherapy or chemoradiotherapy derived a greater survival benefit than radiotherapy alone (OR: 0.39, 0.61 and 0.98, $P = 0.02$).[145]

The SWOG S0809 study, a single-arm prospective phase II trial of adjuvant capecitabine/gemcitabine chemotherapy followed by concurrent capecitabine and radiotherapy in ECC and gallbladder cancer, assessed 79 patients to estimate 2-year survival and patterns of recurrence. The 2-year survival was 65% (95% CI: 53–74%) in all-comers and 67% and 60% in R0 and R1 patients, respectively. Disease-free survival was 52% at 2 years for all patients; there were 24 patients who developed distant recurrence and 14 patients with local recurrence, 9 of whom also recurred at a distant site.[152]

## TARGETED THERAPY AND IMMUNOTHERAPY

Over the last decade, improvements have been noted in targeted therapies and immunotherapy for cholangiocarcinoma as there has been an increased understanding of the genetic and molecular underpinnings of the disease. Studies have evaluated the use of targeted agents and immunotherapy in the treatment of biliary cancers, although most trials are in the advanced setting and therefore, are beyond the scope of this chapter.

Recently, there have been several trials that have evaluated targeted agents in the advanced setting in patients with cholangiocarcinoma. The ClarIDHy trial, a phase III randomised controlled trial evaluated the use of ivosidenib, an IDH1 inhibitor, in previously treated, *IDH1*-mutated ICC as compared to placebo. Patients who received ivosidenib had a significantly longer progression-free survival (median, 2.7 months vs 1.4 months, $P < 0.001$). Median OS was 10.3 months in the ivosidenib group and 7.5 months in the placebo group ($P = 0.09$); however, when adjusted for crossover, survival in the placebo group was 5.1 months ($P < 0.001$).[153] Furthermore, several targeted agents have shown promise in prospective phase II trials. For example, pemigatinib, FGFR1-3 inhibitor in cholangiocarcinoma, was evaluated in a single-arm, phase II trial including 146 patients, 107 of whom had an FGFR2 fusion or rearrangement. In this group, 38 patients (36%) had a complete or partial response, and median OS was 21 months.[154] There is an ongoing phase III trial, FIGHT-302, which is evaluating this agent compared with gemcitabine and cisplatin as a first-line agent in the locally advanced or metastatic setting.[155] Additionally, dabrafenib/trametinib has been evaluated in BRAFV600E mutated biliary tract cancers. Results of a single-arm, phase II trial evaluating dabrafenib and trametinib in BRAFV600E mutated biliary tract cancer in 43 patients (primarily ICC, $n = 39$) demonstrated a response rate in 22 (51%) patients, with a median OS of 14 months.[156]

There is little data regarding the use of immunotherapy in patients with biliary tract malignancies. The KEYNOTE-028 and KEYNOTE-158 trials evaluated the use of pembrolizumab in advanced biliary tract adenocarcinoma. KEYNOTE-028 was a phase 1b basket trial that included a subset ($n = 24$) of patients with biliary adenocarcinoma, while the KEYNOTE-158 trial enrolled 104 patients with advanced biliary adenocarcinoma.[157] Results demonstrated an objective response rate (ORR) of 13% (95% CI: 2.1–12.1%), median progression-free survival of 1.8 months (95% CI: 1.4–3.1 months) and median OS of 5.7 months (95% CI: 3.1–9.8) in KEYNOTE-028, and an ORR of 5.8%, median PFS of 2.0 months (95% CI: 1.9–2.1 months) and median OS of 7.4 months (95% CI: 5.5–9.6 months) in KEYNOTE-158.[158] Furthermore, Kim et al.[159] evaluated nivolumab in refractory, advanced biliary tract cancers. ORR was 22%, median PFS was 3.7 months (95% CI: 2.3–5.7 months) and median OS was 14.2 months (95% CI: 6 months to not reached). While early results demonstrate response in advanced disease, further studies are needed to elucidate the use of immunotherapy in cholangiocarcinoma. There are several ongoing phase I and II trials investigating the use of these agents in this population.

## REGIONAL TREATMENT MODALITIES

### HEPATIC ARTERIAL INFUSION

Hepatic arterial infusion (HAI) is most commonly used in the treatment of patients with unresectable colorectal liver metastases; however, several studies have evaluated its efficacy in ICC. Two early trials assessing the role of regional hepatic chemotherapy HAI with floxuridine (FUDR) with or without bevacizumab in unresectable ICC were performed at MSKCC.[160,161] Partial response was seen in 30–50% of patients and median survival was approximately 30 months in both trials. Of note, the addition of bevacizumab increased the incidence of biliary toxicity without any improvement in survival (31.1 vs 29.5 months; $P$ = NS). Furthermore, a retrospective study comparing systemic therapy plus HAI versus systemic therapy alone in 525 patients with ICC demonstrated that patients who received both systemic therapy and HAI had improved OS (31 vs 18 months, $P$ < 0.001).[162]

More recently, our group published a phase II study combining HAI of FUDR and systemic gemcitabine and oxaliplatin in patients with unresectable cholangiocarcinoma.[163] Of the 38 patients included, 22 (58%) achieved a partial radiographic response and 4 patients were converted to resectable. Median follow-up was 31 months, median progression-free survival was 11.8 months and median OS was 25 months.[163] HAI has demonstrated promising results for patients with unresectable cholangiocarcinoma, although additional studies are warranted prior to routine use.

### RADIOEMBOLISATION

Radioembolisation with yttrium-90 (Y-90) microspheres is another treatment modality for those with unresectable ICC. A systemic review and meta-analysis of 12 studies included 298 patients treated with Y-90 radioembolisation. Median OS was 15.5 months, with 28% of patients obtaining a partial response and 54% of patients with stable disease at 3 months. Seven patients responded sufficiently to undergo definitive resection.[164] Additionally, Ibrahim et al.[165] reported a median survival of 31.8 months in patients with unresectable ICC treated with Y-90 who had a performance status of ECOG 0; however, this effect was not seen in patients who underwent Y-90 embolisation but had a performance status of ECOG 1 or 2. Recently, a phase II study evaluated Y-90 selective internal radiotherapy (SIRT) combined with gemcitabine and cisplatin as first-line treatment for locally advanced ICC in 41 patients.[166] Results demonstrated a response rate of 40% and disease control rate of 98%, with a median OS of 22 months. Furthermore, 22% of patients were downstaged and able to undergo surgical resection.[166] In selected patients with locally advanced disease, radioembolisation may offer some benefit in terms of disease control and possibly converting a subset to resectability.

## POSTOPERATIVE OUTCOMES

The majority of patients with cholangiocarcinoma will develop a recurrence, and patients most often recur within the first 3 years of surgery. The liver is the most common site of recurrence for patients with ICC, hilar and distal cholangiocarcinoma. Of all resected patients, 50–65% of patients will develop a recurrence, and approximately 60% of recurrences will be in the liver.[100,167,168]

OS for cholangiocarcinoma is dependent on the stage at which it is diagnosed and the location of the primary tumour. Overall, 5-year survival ranges between 20–40% for ICC and 30–45% for perihilar cholangiocarcinoma, with 5-year survival rates reported to be approximately 50% for distal cholangiocarcinoma.[167–169]

## GALLBLADDER CANCER

The gallbladder is the most common site of biliary tract malignancy and the fifth most common GI malignancy overall. Historically, survival following a diagnosis of gallbladder cancer has been poor with a 5-year OS of less than 5%; however, a greater understanding of the disease and treatment has led to improved survival in selected patients. Currently, 5-year OS for all patients diagnosed is approximately 25%, and this is dependent on the stage at diagnosis.

## EPIDEMIOLOGY

Worldwide, the highest incidence of gallbladder cancer is found in South America and Asia.[170] In North America, the incidence is approximately 1.6 per 100 000 people, with a slightly decreasing incidence over the last several years.[171] It is more common in women than in men, and the highest incidence is among Native Americans.[170–172] Gallbladder cancer most commonly occurs in older adults, with a median age at diagnosis in the seventh decade.[171,173]

## RISK FACTORS

As with other biliary tract tumours, chronic inflammation leading to high cellular turnover is a common denominator of associated risk factors. The most common risk factor is cholelithiasis and approximately 85% of patients diagnosed with gallbladder cancer have associated gallstones. Other factors include gallbladder polyps, the presence of a cholecystoenteric fistula, typhoid bacillus infection and an anomalous pancreatico-biliary junction.[172]

Gallbladder polyps are noted in 3–6% of the population undergoing ultrasonography, although the vast majority are cholesterol polyps or adenomyomatosis, both of which are benign and have no malignant potential.[174] Approximately 1% of cholecystectomy specimens contain adenomatous polyps, which have malignant potential.[174] As with other GI malignancies, the adenoma to carcinoma sequence has been demonstrated within adenomatous polyps of the gallbladder. Conditions associated with an increased risk of malignancy in gallbladder polyps include size > 1 cm, patient age > 50 years, single polyps and sessile polyps.[174] Additionally, gallbladder polyps arising in the setting of PSC are more likely to be neoplastic, especially if greater than 0.8 cm in size. AGA guidelines recommend cholecystectomy if polyps are > 0.8 cm, while European guidelines recommend cholecystectomy in patients with PSC and polyps of > 0.6 cm.[175,176] Regarding management of gallbladder polyps, ultrasound surveillance is recommended for polyps < 1 cm, as polyps within this size range are associated with a decreased risk of malignancy compared with those > 1 cm.

A 'porcelain gallbladder', a gallbladder with a calcified wall, is also associated with an increased risk of malignancy. The risk of malignancy in a porcelain gallbladder previously was considered to be very high (10–50%), so routine prophylactic cholecystectomy was recommended. However, recent studies demonstrate a lower incidence of association with gallbladder cancer (< 10%) with stippled calcification actually carrying a higher risk than diffuse intramural calcification.[177–179] Therefore, now patients with a porcelain gallbladder can undergo surveillance, while resection is recommended in certain cases.

## CLINICAL PRESENTATION AND DIAGNOSIS

Many patients present late in the course of disease, and the majority of patients are unresectable at the time of diagnosis. Common symptoms include abdominal pain/biliary colic as seen in two-thirds of patients at presentation, while approximately one-third of patients will present with jaundice and 10% will have significant weight loss.

Jaundice in the setting of a newly diagnosed gallbladder cancer is an ominous finding, usually representing a sign of advanced disease. Except for the minority of patients with concomitant common bile duct stones, patients presenting with obstructive jaundice and a gallbladder malignancy will have tumour involvement of the porta hepatis by either direct extension of the tumour, diffuse invasion of the porta hepatis or extensive nodal disease. Prior studies have demonstrated that jaundice is an indicator of advanced malignancy and directly associated with poor OS. For example, in a study of 240 patients with gallbladder carcinoma, 34% of patients presented with obstructive jaundice.[180] Of this cohort, 67% underwent operative exploration; diagnostic laparoscopy was performed in 45% and peritoneal metastases precluding resection were found in 68% of this group. Ultimately, exploratory laparotomy was undertaken in 37 patients—distant peritoneal and liver metastases were found in 22% and locally unresectable disease in the porta hepatis was found in an additional 27% of patients. Ultimately, only 7% of all patients with jaundice underwent resection with curative intent.[180] Furthermore, patients with jaundiced were more likely to have advanced-stage disease (stage III/IV) at the time of presentation (96% vs 60%, $P <$ 0.001) and a lower median DSS (6 vs 16 months, $P < 0.0001$) than those without jaundice.[57] Although there is no proven correct approach to this patient population, a multidisciplinary discussion and consideration for systemic therapy prior to undertaking surgical exploration is warranted. As with cholangiocarcinoma, gemcitabine in combination with a platinum agent (cisplatin/oxaliplatin) remains the standard of care in the advanced setting.[143]

In a subset of patients with early-stage disease, gallbladder cancer is incidentally diagnosed on pathological examination of a cholecystectomy specimen resected for symptoms presumed to be benign biliary colic. Physicians should have an increased level of suspicion for a malignancy of the gallbladder in patients who present with a polyp > 1 cm, mass or irregularity of the gallbladder wall on radiological investigation.

## HISTOPATHOLOGY AND GENOMICS

The vast majority of gallbladder cancers are adenocarcinomas, of which there are multiple subtypes, the most common is the pancreato-biliary subtype. The papillary subtype is associated with a relatively better prognosis than others.[181] Certain histological subtypes, such as adenosquamous carcinoma or pure squamous cell carcinoma, are seen in the gallbladder more commonly than at any other site within the biliary tree.

Gallbladder cancer has a unique genomic profile. *TP53* is altered in approximately 50% of gallbladder cancers.[182] Furthermore, mutations in *ERBB2/3*, *EGFR* and *PTEN* alterations are common in gallbladder cancers, but less so in cholangiocarcinoma.[29] *IDH1* and *FGFR2* mutations are characteristic of ICC and are less common in gallbladder cancers.

## STAGING

The AJCC staging system is based on the standard TNM classification and was most recently updated in 2017 (8th edition).[183] The T-stage describes the depth of invasion in the gallbladder wall and has the greatest clinical impact on the extent of resection performed. The gallbladder wall consists of a mucosa and lamina propria, a thin muscular layer, perimuscular connective tissue and serosa. Of note, the gallbladder lacks a serosal covering along its border with the liver and the perimuscular connective tissue is continuous with the liver connective tissue. T1a tumours are limited to the lamina propria, which is important as a cholecystectomy can be curative in this subset of patient due to the limited invasion of the gallbladder wall. T1b tumours have invaded the muscle layer and T2 tumours have invaded through the muscle layer into the perimuscular connective tissue. T3 and T4 tumours are those that have penetrated the serosa and invade the liver or an extrahepatic organ (T3), or invade multiple extrahepatic organs or structures of the porta hepatis. In a study by Shindoh et al.,[184] the location of tumour on the gallbladder, specifically the peritoneal side versus the liver side, was associated with differences in recurrence and survival, but only for patients with T2 tumours.

In the 8th edition, N-stage is based on the number of lymph nodes that are positive; 1–3 positive lymph nodes constitute N1 disease, whereas four or more positive nodes represents N2. Metastatic disease (M1) refers to distant metastasis. Data has demonstrated that the AJCC 8th edition TNM staging system provides improved separation of survival by stage compared with the AJCC 7th edition.[185]

## RADIOLOGICAL ASSESSMENT

Many patients will present with an incidental finding of gallbladder cancer following cholecystectomy. In such cases, a

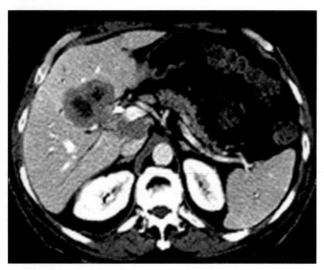

**Figure 14.5** Representative image of gallbladder cancer on CT.

post-cholecystectomy staging work-up should be completed. Many patients will undergo a right upper quadrant ultrasound as initial work-up, on which a polyp or mass may be noted. While ultrasound was able to detect the presence of a gallbladder mass in 85% of cases, its detection of advanced disease was only 37%.[186]

Complete staging work-up should involve assessment of the extent of local disease as well as the presence of any distant metastases using cross-sectional contrast-enhanced imaging (CT and/or MRCP)(Fig. 14.5) Multiphasic CT of the chest, abdomen and pelvis should include portal, venous and arterial phases, and is used to assess the extent of disease in the liver and porta hepatis while also evaluating for metastatic disease. In order to elucidate relationships between the tumour and porta hepatis structures, imaging should include thin cuts through the liver and porta hepatis. Similar to cholangiocarcinoma, initial imaging studies should be performed prior to biliary stenting (if it is to be performed) as stenting will cause local inflammation making assessment of tumour extent difficult.

With respect to the local assessment of disease, a study of 118 patients with gallbladder carcinoma found CT to be 79% accurate for differentiating T1 and T2 tumours, 93% accurate for differentiating T2 and T3 tumours and 100% accurate for differentiating T3 and T4 tumours.[48] Additionally, MRI with intravenous contrast and MRCP can contribute important diagnostic information during preoperative work-up to assess the extent of disease; prior studies evaluating MRI have shown sensitivities of 70–100% for hepatic invasion, 100% for vascular involvement and 75% for lymph node metastases.[187,188]

Similar to cholangiocarcinoma, FDG-PET imaging may help identify distant disease in patients with gallbladder cancer. A study of 61 patients with biliary tract malignancies found PET-CT to have a sensitivity of 100% compared with 25% for CT alone (P < 0.001) for the identification of distant metastases.[44] Furthermore, the use of PET-CT has been shown to change surgical management in 17–23% of cases.[44,51,189] Therefore, PET can be considered when evaluating patients with newly diagnosed gallbladder carcinoma, largely to evaluate for distant metastatic disease and to validate questionable findings on cross-sectional imaging.

## GENERAL OPERATIVE PRINCIPLES

The recommended surgical approach for gallbladder carcinoma greater than T1a utilises an extended cholecystectomy to include resection of segments IVb and V of the liver with a portal lymph node dissection, whereas patients with T1a disease can be treated with cholecystectomy alone. Contraindications to resection include distant metastases including multifocal liver involvement, tumour involvement of the hepatic vasculature or biliary tree that would preclude a complete resection, and presence of distant lymph node metastases. Although upfront resection is controversial in locally advanced disease, surgical intervention with negative margins remains the mainstay of definitive therapy for gallbladder cancer.

As in patients with suspected cholangiocarcinoma, a suspicious gallbladder mass does not require a preoperative tissue diagnosis. Biopsies can result in false-negative findings, and are associated with a risk of peritoneal seeding. Staging laparoscopy should be considered in patients with gallbladder cancer, especially with those associated with an increased risk of metastatic disease in an attempt to avoid non-therapeutic laparotomy, such as in those patients with an elevated CA 19-9 or T3 tumours.[93,190] The yield of staging laparoscopy has been demonstrated to be greatest in patients with gallbladder cancer compared with other biliary cancers.[91,92] Davidson et al.[93] demonstrated that in patients with extrahepatic biliary tumours, staging laparoscopy was associated with curative resection in gallbladder cancer (OR 2.41, 95% CI: 1.36–4.27).

### MARGIN-NEGATIVE RESECTION

Similar to cholangiocarcinoma, R0 resection is associated with improved outcomes in gallbladder cancer.[191–193] For example, in a study of 279 patients, 127 of whom had an R0 resection, a positive resection margin was associated with worse OS (HR: 2.29, 95% CI: 1.36–3.87, P = 0.002).[191]

Residual disease following cholecystectomy with an incidental gallbladder cancer was also associated with worse outcomes. In an analysis of 135 patients who underwent definitive resection following an incidentally diagnosed gallbladder carcinoma, the presence of residual disease at any site was associated with significantly worse median disease-free survival (11.2 vs 93.4 months, P < 0.0001) and DSS (25.2 months vs not reached, P < 0.0001). Furthermore, residual disease identified at any particular site predicted disease-free survival (HR: 3.3, 95% CI: 1.9–5.7, P = 0.0003) and DSS (HR: 2.4, 95% CI: 1.2–4.6, P = 0.01) and was independent of all other tumour-related variables.[194]

### PORTAL LYMPHADENECTOMY

Portal lymphadenectomy should be performed in patients undergoing extended resection for gallbladder carcinoma. Lymphadenectomy is needed for staging and does not have a therapeutic value. Specifically, with locally advanced lesions, it has been found that on progression of T-stage from T2 to T4, nodal and distant metastases increased from 16% to 79% and from 33% to 69%, respectively.[195]

Similar to cholangiocarcinoma, regional lymphadenectomy for gallbladder carcinoma should include removal of nodes in the porta hepatis, gastrohepatic ligament and retroduodenal space.[119,196] Prior data has suggested removal of at least six lymph nodes to improve staging.[119] Both the presence and location of nodal metastases have an association with survival. A study evaluating AJCC 8th edition staging using the NCDB demonstrates that the updated nodal staging system more accurately predicts OS.[185] Meng et al.[197] demonstrated that patients who have distant nodal metastases have a worse OS than those with disease in the portal nodes ($P = 0.007$). Early assessment of aortocaval, retropancreatic and/or celiac lymphadenopathy should be performed, and if suspicious for metastatic disease, intraoperative frozen section should be obtained as positive lymph nodes in these regions would be representative of distant metastatic disease and resection should be aborted.

✔✔ Positive distant lymph nodes are associated with worse OS than portal lymph nodes. If there is confirmed disease in distant lymph nodes at the time of resection, the operation should be aborted.

## T1 TUMOURS

T1a tumours, or those that are confined to the lamina propria, are most often discovered after, and adequately treated with, a simple cholecystectomy. This is because the potential for nodal involvement is minimal and cure rates approach 85–100% if negative margins are achieved.[198] Furthermore, a meta-analysis of T1 gallbladder cancers demonstrated that patients with T1a tumours who underwent radical resection had worse OS than cholecystectomy alone (RR: 0.82, 95% CI: 0.70–0.96, $P = 0.01$).[199]

It is recommended that patients with T1b or T2 gallbladder cancers undergo extended resection that includes a cholecystectomy, partial hepatectomy of segments IVb and V, and a portal lymphadenectomy. T1b tumours are those that have extended into, but not through, the muscle layer; a simple cholecystectomy can be curative in up to 85% of cases. While these tumours are relative early stage, nodal metastases have been found in up to 12% of patients with stage T1b cancers.[200]

## EXTENDED RESECTION

The goal of surgical resection for T1b and greater tumours is to obtain negative margins by performing a cholecystectomy, hepatectomy (segments IVb and V) and portal lymphadenectomy. In rare cases, a more extensive hepatectomy needs to be performed if there is tumour involvement of the right portal pedicle (i.e. major inflow vascular structures or right hepatic duct). Up to 50% of T2 tumours have associated lymph node metastases, and up to 25% of these patients can have liver involvement.[119,201] Studies have demonstrated that patients with T2/T3 tumours derive the greatest benefit from extended resections. Residual disease is associated with worse survival.[119,194,202] In a study of 135 patients who underwent re-exploration, residual disease was associated with worse disease-free survival (median, 11 vs 93 months, $P < 0.0001$) and worse DSS (25 months vs not reached, $P < 0.0001$).[194] Additionally, extended resections have been associated with improved survival. Goetze et al.[203] demonstrated that re-resection was associated with improved survival in patients with T2, but not T3, disease. A study evaluating 498 patients who underwent laparoscopic cholecystectomy

for gallbladder cancer demonstrated that improved OS was seen in patients with pathologic T2 or T3 tumours but not T1 or T4 tumours.[204]

In the setting of locally advanced disease (T3/T4), some cases will require additional resection and formal hepatectomy. This is true in tumours that involve the biliary confluence and/or right hepatic duct, with an extended right hepatectomy required for complete resection. In most cases, it is the involvement of major hepatic vascular and/or biliary structures rather than parenchyma involvement that dictates the extent of hepatic resection required. An analysis in 104 patients with gallbladder cancer determined that tumour biology and stage, rather than the extent of resection, is predictive of DSS. Major hepatic resections, including extended hepatectomy and common bile duct excision, were appropriate when necessary to achieve negative pathological margins and were associated with acceptable long-term survival.[205] Therefore, as in cholangiocarcinoma, the extent of resection should be dictated by what is necessary to achieve a negative margin.

The cystic duct margin should be evaluated to ensure an R0 resection, and frozen section should be obtained intraoperatively. Resection of the common bile duct should only be done if the cystic duct/common bile duct junction is grossly involved with tumour, as bile duct resection if it is not involved has not been shown to be associated with improved survival.[206]

## MALIGNANCY DIAGNOSED INTRAOPERATIVELY

If gallbladder carcinoma is suspected intraoperatively, an oncologic resection including a radical cholecystectomy, segment 4b/5 hepatectomy and lymphadenectomy should be performed. In select cases in which a diagnosis is uncertain, the gallbladder can be evaluated and suspicious lesions sent for frozen section. If a carcinoma is diagnosed, an appropriate oncologic resection should be performed. The authors prefer to perform an oncologically appropriate resection at the time the carcinoma discovered, unless there are extenuating circumstances that mandate otherwise. However, if the surgeon is not comfortable with performing a radical cholecystectomy/hepatic resection, the patient is best served by transferring the patient to a centre/surgeon with experience in performing the appropriate operation. A delayed radical and appropriate resection does not negatively influence the patient's outcome.[195]

## MALIGNANCY DIAGNOSED POST-CHOLECYSTECTOMY

When gallbladder cancer is diagnosed following a cholecystectomy on pathologic evaluation of the gallbladder, the need for a more radical resection is based on the pathologic T-stage of the tumour, as outlined above. Patients who are incidentally found to have T1a tumours do not require further intervention, but those with T2b or higher cancers are recommended for formal resection consisting of a segment 4b/5 hepatectomy and lymphadenectomy. Fong et al.[195] demonstrated an improved 5-year survival rate in patients undergoing a second operation compared with those who did not. Five-year survival rates of 61% were achieved in patients who were re-resected compared with 19% for patients who did not undergo a radical second operation. However, prior to undertaking a second operation, high-quality cross-sectional imaging (CT/MRI) should be obtained to appropriately stage the disease.

Resection of laparoscopic port site is no longer routinely recommended. Early data had demonstrated that port site recurrence was approximately 15%,[207] although this is now estimated to be lower. However, data has demonstrated that the presence of port site metastases is most likely reflective of underlying peritoneal disease,[208] and furthermore resection of port site metastases is not associated with improved survival.[209]

✓ In the past, routine resection of laparoscopic port sites was recommended in an effort to ensure clearance of microscopic disease that may have implanted during the laparoscopic procedure. However, there is little evidence to support the efficacy of routine resection of all port sites at reoperation. Recurrence at port sites is a harbinger of generalised peritoneal recurrence that will not be prevented with resection of these limited areas.

## ADJUVANT THERAPY

The large studies that evaluate adjuvant chemotherapy for biliary tract malignancies include gallbladder cancer (Table 14.3), and are described in detail above. Results of patients with gallbladder cancer included in these studies mirrored the larger study population. Takada et al.,[146] in an early phase III trial investigating the use of mitomycin/5-FU compared with observation alone in the adjuvant setting, included 508 patients with resected bile duct tumours ($n$ = 139), gallbladder cancers ($n$ = 140), pancreatic cancers ($n$ = 173) and ampullary tumours ($n$ = 56). Results demonstrated an improved 5-year OS (26% vs 14%, $P$ = 0.037) and disease-free survival (20% vs 12%, $P$ = 0.021) in patients with gallbladder cancer, but not the other subgroups.[146] While subsequent trials demonstrate no significant difference in survival outcomes, given the analysis of the BILCAP trial, the NCCN guidelines currently recommend adjuvant capecitabine for patients who undergo resection for gallbladder cancer.[112]

There are no randomised trials evaluating adjuvant radiation in gallbladder cancer. The SWOG S0809 study also included patients with gallbladder cancer, which was a single-arm, phase II trial evaluating the safety and efficacy of adjuvant gemcitabine and capecitabine with concurrent radiotherapy. Results demonstrated a 2-year OS of 65% (in all-comers, and 56% in patients with gallbladder cancer).[152] Other data is primarily retrospective, and some studies have demonstrated improved outcomes with the use of adjuvant radiotherapy. Kamarajah et al.[210] conducted a propensity score–matched analysis using data from the NCDB looking at patients who received adjuvant radiation compared with those who did not. Results demonstrated that the use of radiation was associated with improved survival, and on multivariable analysis demonstrated that this was regardless of margin status, nodal status or receipt of adjuvant chemotherapy. Given that there is limited data on the use of adjuvant radiation in gallbladder cancer, it is reasonable to consider in certain patients, and participation in clinical trial is encouraged.[112]

✓✓ Guidelines recommend the use of capecitabine in the adjuvant setting for patients with gallbladder cancer following the BILCAP trial.

## POSTOPERATIVE OUTCOMES

Prior data has demonstrated that most patients who undergo resection for gallbladder cancer will develop a recurrence. Jarnagin et al.[211] demonstrated that in patients with gallbladder cancers who underwent a potentially curative resection, 66% recurred within a median of 24 months, and median time to recurrence was 11.5 months. The majority of patients (85%) developed a recurrence at a distant site, whereas the remaining 15% developed a locoregional recurrence.

Overall 5-year survival for all patients diagnosed with gallbladder cancer is approximately 25%; however, overall outcome is dependent on the stage of disease.[185,212] Resectable disease is associated with significantly improved survival compared with patients who are unresectable secondary to locally advanced or metastatic disease, and T-stage is predictive of OS.[212] Furthermore, tumour size, T-stage and nodal status were all predictive of survival ($P < 0.001$).[212]

> **Key points**
>
> - Biliary tract cancers are a heterogenous group of malignancies that are associated with an overall poor prognosis. Surgical resection remains the mainstay of treatment and the only chance at cure.
> - Capecitabine is most commonly used for adjuvant systemic chemotherapy, and neoadjuvant chemotherapy is recommended in select cases of advanced disease.
> - The biological underpinnings of biliary tract cancers have been increasingly understood, and through the use of next-generation sequencing, certain targeted therapies have shown promise.
> - In hilar cholangiocarcinoma, complete resection necessitates a hepatectomy. Resectability is determined by the extent of bile duct involvement, portal vein involvement and to the presence or absence of hepatic atrophy.
> - In patients with a T1a gallbladder cancer, cholecystectomy is often curative. Those patients who have more advanced, but resectable disease require partial hepatectomy

🌐 References available at http://ebooks.health.elsevier.com/

## KEY REFERENCES

[6] Esnaola NF, Meyer JE, Karachristos A, et al. Evaluation and management of intrahepatic and extrahepatic cholangiocarcinoma. Cancer 2016;122:1349–69.
*This review focuses on the diagnosis and treatment of patients with cholangiocarcinoma and, in particular, on the role of endoscopy, surgery, transplantation, radiotherapy, systemic therapy and liver-directed therapies in the curative or palliative treatment of these individuals.*

[63] Bismuth H, Nakache R, Diamond T. Management strategies in resection for hilar cholangiocarcinoma. Ann Surg 1992;215:31–8.
*Seminal paper where results indicate that improved survival in hilar cholangiocarcinoma can be achieved by resection, with minimal morbidity and zero mortality rates, if histologically free resection margins are obtained.*

[65] Jarnagin WR, Fong Y, DeMatteo RP, et al. Staging, resectability, and outcome in 225 patients with hilar cholangiocarcinoma. Ann Surg 2001;234:507–17.
*Taking into account local tumor extent, the proposed staging system for hilar cholangiocarcinoma accurately predicts resectability, the likelihood of metastatic disease, and survival. Complete resection remains the only therapy that offers the possibility of long-term survival, and hepatic resection is a critical component of the surgical approach.*

[66] Matsuo K, Rocha FG, Ito K, et al. The Blumgart preoperative staging system for hilar cholangiocarcinoma: analysis of resectability and outcomes in 380 patients. J Am Coll Surg 2012;215:343–55.

*The preoperative clinical T-staging system of Blumgart, defined by the radial and longitudinal tumour extent, accurately predicts resectability of hilar cholangiocarcinoma.*

[79] Wiggers JK, Groot Koerkamp B, Cieslak KP, et al. Postoperative mortality after liver resection for perihilar cholangiocarcinoma: development of a risk score and importance of biliary drainage of the future liver remnant. J Am Coll Surg 2016;223:321–31.

*The mortality risk score for patients with resectable hilar cholangiocarcinoma identifies modifiable risk factors, including FLR volume, FLR drainage status, and preoperative cholangitis. The authors did not find evidence to support preoperative biliary drainage in patients with FLR volume >50%.*

[89] Ribero D, Abdalla EK, Madoff DC, et al. Portal vein embolization before major hepatectomy and its effects on regeneration, resectability and outcome. Br J Surg 2007;94:1386–94.

*This study evaluated the safety of portal vein embolisation (PVE), its impact on future liver remnant (FLR) volume and regeneration, and subsequent effects on outcome after liver resection.*

[121] Cheng Q-B, Yi B, Wang J-H, et al. Resection with total caudate lobectomy confers survival benefit in hilar cholangiocarcinoma of Bismuth type III and IV. Eur J Surg Oncol 2012;38:1197–203.

*This study identified prognostic predictors for overall survival in patients with hilar cholangiocarcinoma of Bismuth type III and IV, and evaluated survival benefit and safety of total caudate lobectomy. Resection with total caudate lobectomy is associated with high curative resectability rates and an acceptable safety profile.*

[124] Neuhaus P, Jonas S, Bechstein WO, et al. Extended resections for hilar cholangiocarcinoma. Ann Surg 1999;230:808–18.

*This is a retrospective study that evaluated the role of extended resections in hilar cholangiocarcinoma.*

[132] de Vreede I, Steers JL, Burch PA, et al. Prolonged disease-free survival after orthotopic liver transplantation plus adjuvant chemoirradiation for cholangiocarcinoma. Liver Transpl 2000;6:309–16.

*This paper demonstrates results from the initial experience at the Mayo Clinic using preoperative therapy followed by liver transplantation for unresectable cholangiocarcinoma.*

[137] Sapisochin G, Javle M, Lerut J, et al. Liver transplantation for cholangiocarcinoma and mixed hepatocellular cholangiocarcinoma: working group report from the ILTS Transplant oncology Consensus conference. Transplantation 2020:1125–30.

*Consensus paper approved by the International Liver Transplant Society that discusses the use of liver transplant for cholangiocarcinoma.*

[143] Valle J, Wasan H, Palmer DH, et al. Cisplatin plus gemcitabine versus gemcitabine for biliary tract cancer. N Engl J Med 2010;362:1273–81.

*Randomized controlled trial investigating gemcitabine plus cisplatin versus gemcitabine alone in patients with advanced biliary cancers. Results demonstrated that gemcitabine plus cisplatin was associated with improved OS and PFS as compared to gemcitabine alone.*

[147] Edeline J, Benabdelghani M, Bertaut A, et al. Gemcitabine and oxaliplatin chemotherapy or surveillance in resected biliary tract cancer (PRODIGE 12-ACCORD 18-UNICANCER GI): a randomized phase III study. J Clin Oncol 2019;37:658–67.

*Multicenter randomized controlled trial evaluating gemcitabine plus oxaliplatin versus surveillance after resection for localized biliary tract cancer did not demonstrate a difference in RFS between the two arms.*

[149] Primrose JN, Fox RP, Palmer DH, et al. Capecitabine compared with observation in resected biliary tract cancer (BILCAP): a randomised, controlled, multicentre, phase 3 study. Lancet Oncol 2019;20:663–73.

*Phase III trial comparing capecitabine versus observation in resected biliary tract cancer (BILCAP).*

[152] Ben-Josef E, Guthrie KA, El-Khoueiry AB, et al. Swog S0809: a phase II intergroup trial of adjuvant capecitabine and gemcitabine followed by radiotherapy and concurrent capecitabine in extrahepatic cholangiocarcinoma and gallbladder carcinoma. J Clin Oncol 2015;33:2617–22.

*Phase II trial evaluating the use of adjuvant capecitabine and gemcitabine followed by radiation in extrahepatic cholangiocarcinoma and gallbladder carcinoma.*

[163] Cercek A, Boerner T, Tan BR, et al. Assessment of hepatic arterial infusion of floxuridine in combination with systemic gemcitabine and oxaliplatin in patients with unresectable intrahepatic cholangiocarcinoma: a phase 2 clinical trial. JAMA Oncol 2020;6:60–7.

*Phase II trial evaluating the use of HAI floxuridine plus systemic gemcitabine and oxaliplatin in patients with unresectable intrahepatic cholangiocarcinoma.*

[205] D'Angelica M, Dalal KM, DeMatteo RP, et al. Analysis of the extent of resection for adenocarcinoma of the gallbladder. Ann Surg Oncol 2009;16:806–16.

*Tumour biology and stage, rather than extent of resection, predict outcome after resection for gallbladder cancer. Major hepatic resections, including bile duct excision, are appropriate when necessary to clear disease but are not mandatory in all cases.*

[211] Jarnagin WR, Ruo L, Little SA, et al. Patterns of initial disease recurrence after resection of gallbladder carcinoma and hilar cholangiocarcinoma: implications for adjuvant therapeutic strategies. Cancer 2003;98:1689–700.

*Retrospective study evaluating recurrence patterns in patients who undergo resection for gallbladder cancer and hilar cholangiocarcinoma.*

# 15 Complicated acute pancreatitis

C.L. van Veldhuisen | H.C. van Santvoort | C.H.J. van Eijck | M.G. Besselink

## INTRODUCTION

Acute pancreatitis is a common disease, characterised by painful inflammation of the pancreas. It is diagnosed if two of the following three criteria are present: abdominal pain, level of serum lipase (or amylase) three times the upper limit of normal serum levels, and characteristic finding on imaging (i.e., contrast-enhanced computed tomography [CECT]) (Fig. 15.1).[1-3] The clinical course and severity of acute pancreatitis varies widely. In most patients, acute pancreatitis is mild and self-limiting. With conservative therapy including adequate fluid resuscitation and analgesia, the vast majority of patients recover within days. However, approximately 20% of patients develop moderate or severe acute pancreatitis with local and/or systemic complications, such as necrosis of the (peri)pancreatic tissue and organ failure. Compared to mild acute pancreatitis, which has a mortality rate below 1%, complicated acute pancreatitis is associated with a high mortality of 10–30%, especially if necrosis becomes infected.[4-7]

The two most common causes of acute pancreatitis are biliary (e.g., gallstones or biliary sludge leading to temporary obstruction of the common bile duct and pancreatic duct) and alcohol.[8] Other causes include endoscopic retrograde cholangiography (ERCP), which although a minimally invasive procedure, is associated with a risk of post-ERCP pancreatitis in 6–15% of cases. Identifying the aetiology and early detection of complications following acute pancreatitis is key to offer accurate treatment. To date, the optimal timing and type of treatment required to manage the complications of acute pancreatitis remains challenging because of the heterogeneity of the disease and the complexity of clinical decision making.

## DEFINITIONS AND TERMINOLOGY

In 1993 the Atlanta Classification of acute pancreatitis categorised disease-related definitions and enabled specialists from different backgrounds to discuss various types of acute pancreatitis. It also introduced uniformity in the assessment of acute pancreatitis.[9]

Because of new and improved insights in the management of acute pancreatitis, the Atlanta Classification system was revised in 2012.[10] New definitions were added for different disease-phases, disease severity and local complications.

Based on the duration of disease-related symptoms, two phases of acute pancreatitis are now defined, that is, early and late, with a cut-off of less than or more than 4 weeks.

In addition, a third category was added to the severity of acute pancreatitis, resulting in mild, moderately severe or severe acute pancreatitis. The revised classification provided definitions for complications and categorised local fluid collections based on duration of symptoms, their content and whether they were sterile or infected. Several studies reported this revised classification system to be accurate and superior compared to the original Atlanta Classification.[11,12]

✓ Local complications of peripancreatic collections in acute pancreatitis are categorised based on duration of symptoms (with a cut-off of less than or more than 4 week) and whether this is sterile or infected.

## IMAGING IN ACUTE PANCREATITIS

### COMPUTED TOMOGRAPHY

CECT is the standard imaging modality in acute pancreatitis to establish the diagnosis, determine the severity and identify complications.[1,13] Computed tomography (CT) is best performed beyond 72 hours from disease onset to detect (peri)pancreatic necrosis, with a sensitivity rate close to 100%.[13] Therefore CECT on admission for acute pancreatitis is generally not recommended, except in patients with an uncertain diagnosis or with severe symptoms (e.g., organ failure). In these patients, a CT should be considered to exclude secondary peritonitis caused by perforation or mesenteric ischemia. Although concerns have been raised over the risk of post-contrast acute renal failure in severely ill patients, a recent meta-analysis showed no correlation.[14] Follow-up CT is indicated in patients with clinical deterioration or failure of continued clinical improvement.

### MAGNETIC RESONANCE IMAGING

Magnetic resonance imaging (MRI) in acute pancreatitis is recommended in patients with allergy to iodinated contrast, patients with renal impairment caused by the lack of renal nephrotoxicity and in young or pregnant patients to avoid radiation exposure. MRI might be superior in visualising necrosis within 'walled off necrosis' (WON) and can be useful in evaluating the pancreatic duct and the presence of a duct rupture resulting in a disconnected pancreatic duct syndrome.[15] MRI may also has a role in diagnosing acute pancreatitis and in assessing disease severity based on morphological changes and the (peri)pancreatic tissue.[16]

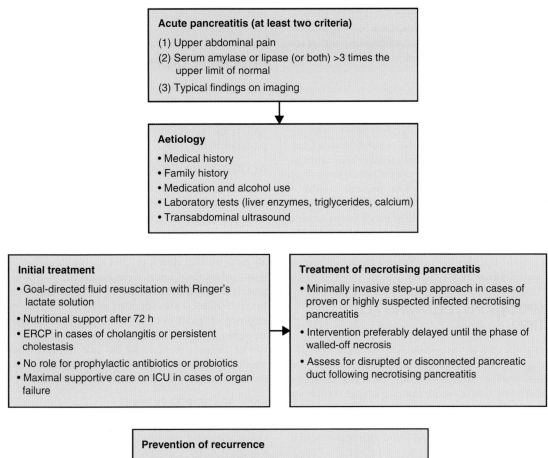

**Acute pancreatitis (at least two criteria)**

(1) Upper abdominal pain

(2) Serum amylase or lipase (or both) >3 times the upper limit of normal

(3) Typical findings on imaging

**Aetiology**

• Medical history
• Family history
• Medication and alcohol use
• Laboratory tests (liver enzymes, triglycerides, calcium)
• Transabdominal ultrasound

**Initial treatment**

• Goal-directed fluid resuscitation with Ringer's lactate solution
• Nutritional support after 72 h
• ERCP in cases of cholangitis or persistent cholestasis
• No role for prophylactic antibiotics or probiotics
• Maximal supportive care on ICU in cases of organ failure

**Treatment of necrotising pancreatitis**

• Minimally invasive step-up approach in cases of proven or highly suspected infected necrotising pancreatitis
• Intervention preferably delayed until the phase of walled-off necrosis
• Assess for disrupted or disconnected pancreatic duct following necrotising pancreatitis

**Prevention of recurrence**

• (Presumed) idiopathic pancreatitis:
  • Repeat abdominal ultrasound
  • Endoscopic ultrasound
• Mild biliary pancreatitis: cholecystectomy during admission
• Severe biliary pancreatitis: cholecystectomy after 6 weeks

**Figure 15.1** Algorithm for the management of acute pancreatitis. *ERCP*, Endoscopic retrograde cholangiopancreatography; *ICU*, intensive care unit.

## INITIAL GENERAL MANAGEMENT

Since the primary focus of this chapter is the management of complications of acute pancreatitis, the initial treatment of mild acute pancreatitis will not be addressed.

Antibiotic administration is not recommended for patients with mild pancreatitis, but should be reserved for severely ill patients, including those with systemic inflammatory response (SIRS), infected necrosis, multi-organ failure or extra-pancreatic infection. Early ERCP is not indicated in patients with mild biliary pancreatitis. In patients with predicted severe biliary pancreatitis without cholangitis, studies have shown that an early ERCP with sphincterotomy did not reduce the risk of major complications or mortality when compared to conservative management. However, ERCP should be considered in patients with cholangitis or persistent cholestasis associated with predicted severe acute biliary pancreatitis.[17]

In acute pancreatitis, a prolonged catabolic illness is often seen, especially in patients with more complex and severe disease. It is important to anticipate nutritional insufficiency and ensure optimal nutritional support. This will positively influence the maintenance of the intestinal barrier function, inhibiting bacterial translocation and reduce the systematic inflammatory response.[18] Multiple options for nutritional support are available. Bakker et al. found that early enteral tube feeding within 24 hours did not reduce risk of infection (25% vs. 25%) or mortality (11% vs. 7%).[19] However, enteral tube feeding should be considered if patients have insufficient intake after 72 hours, as commonly seen in the more severe cases. Nasogastric feeding, if tolerated, has been shown to be safe but nasojejunal feeding can be undertaken if required. Enteral feeding is preferred over parental feeding because of a lower risk on infectious complications, organ failure and mortality.[20,21]

## CLINICAL PATTERNS AND COMPLICATIONS

A wide variety of complications can occur in patients with acute pancreatitis and can be classified as local and/or systemic. The clinical course, disease manifestations, and prognosis of complications in acute pancreatitis is somewhat unpredictable and varies greatly between individuals. Timely diagnosis and accurate evaluation of severity are key for clinical management. Prediction of severity by surveillance of systematic inflammatory response or organ failure for a minimum of 48 hours after admission, and management by a multi-disciplinary team is therefore strongly recommended.[22]

## CLASSIFICATION OF SEVERITY

This chapter mainly focuses on moderately severe and severe acute pancreatitis as defined by the revised Atlanta Classification. Moderately severe acute pancreatitis is defined as local or systematic complications, without persistent organ failure. Organ failure can sometimes be present at admission but can improve within 48 hours after initial treatment. Persistent organ failure distinguishes moderately severe from severe acute pancreatitis, since severe acute pancreatitis is characterised by persistent organ failure, which generally requires urgent transfer for prolonged management in an intensive care setting (ICU).[10]

## LOCAL COMPLICATIONS FOLLOWING ACUTE PANCREATITIS

Acute pancreatitis can be accompanied by local complications of which (peri)pancreatic fluid collections are the most common. A clear distinction must be made between different collections based on location (peripancreatic or pancreatic area), the nature of the content (liquid, solid, gas) and the presence of a well-defined wall (Fig. 15.2).[3] Collections can be categorised as arising from either interstitial oedematous pancreatitis or collections deriving from necrotising pancreatitis.

## INTERSTITIAL OEDEMATOUS PANCREATITIS

In patients with interstitial oedematous pancreatitis, localised or diffuse enlargement of the pancreas is seen with homogeneous or slightly heterogeneous enhancement of the pancreatic parenchyma on CECT, without sings of (peri) pancreatic necrosis.

### ACUTE PERIPANCREATIC FLUIDS COLLECTION

One of the early complications associated with acute pancreatitis is the development of an acute peripancreatic fluid collection (APFC), defined as a non-encapsulated homogeneous peripancreatic collection that develops within the first 4 weeks after disease onset. Approximately 25% of all patients will develop APFC, which can be distinguished from other fluid collections based on morphological characteristics such as the absence of debris. APFCs are caused by (peri)pancreatic inflammation or as a consequence of rupture of small peripheral pancreatic side duct branches. In general, APFCs resolve spontaneously within a couple of weeks, remain sterile and do not require intervention. A small percentage of APFCs persist beyond 4 weeks and are then referred to as pancreatic pseudocysts.

### PANCREATIC PSEUDOCYST

Pancreatic pseudocysts are defined as encapsulated fluid collections and can be either asymptomatic or symptomatic,

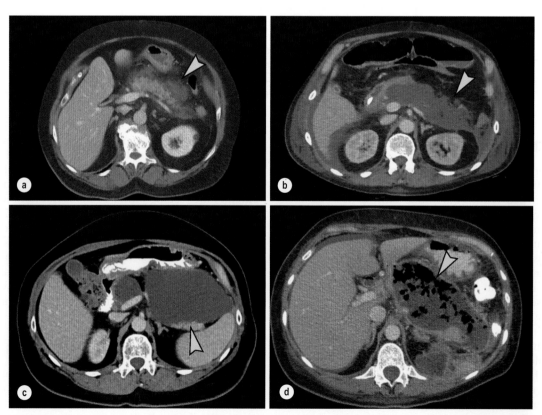

**Figure 15.2**    Local complications in acute pancreatitis, defined according to the Atlanta criteria. **(a)** Acute peripancreatic fluid collection (≤4 weeks). **(b)** Acute necrotic collection: necrotising pancreatitis (≤4 weeks). **(c)** Pancreatic pseudocyst (≥4 weeks). **(d)** Walled-off necrosis (≥4 weeks).

and may cause biliary or gastric outlet obstruction, bleeding or become secondarily infected (Fig. 15.3). Pancreatic pseudocysts are uncommon in patients with acute pancreatitis (approximately 10–20%), and are more frequently seen in patients with chronic pancreatitis.[23] Although the majority of pancreatic pseudocysts will resolve spontaneously and require no further intervention, treatment is needed in selected patients depending on the size and presence of clinical symptoms. Among the treatment options available, endoscopic transluminal drainage is the first choice and is preferably performed once the collection becomes encapsulated.[24] If there is communication with the main pancreatic duct, additional transpapillary drainage should be considered. Pancreatic pseudocysts rarely become infected and can be diagnosed on CECT by the presence of gas within the pseudocyst or by using fine-needle aspiration (FNA). Infected pseudocysts require antibiotics and either endoscopic or surgical drainage since complications of these pseudocysts include prolonged abdominal pain, sepsis, erosion into vessel leading to haemorrhage, obstruction and rupture leading to acute peritonitis.

## NECROTISING PANCREATITIS

Necrotising pancreatitis is present in approximately 5–10% of patients. Three different types of necrosis are defined in the revised Atlanta Classification, namely pancreatic parenchymal necrosis alone, peripancreatic necrosis alone or acute pancreatic parenchymal necrosis with peripancreatic necrosis. In most patients with necrotising pancreatitis (approximately 75–80%), the combined type is seen. Necrosis can be either sterile or infected, and infected necrotising pancreatitis typically requires 2 to 4 weeks to develop. Necrotic collections in the (peri)pancreatic area are divided into two groups (e.g., acute necrotic collection and walled-off necrosis), with an arbitrary cut-off of 4 weeks after onset of disease.[1]

### ACUTE NECROTIC COLLECTION

During the first 4 weeks, collections containing necrotic material are referred to as acute necrotic collections (ANC). ANCs can be distinguished from APFCs based on the presence of solid necrotic components, however, within the first week, it can be difficult to differentiate since both can manifest as homogeneous non-enhancing areas. On CECT,

necrosis usually involves both the pancreas and peripancreatic tissue and in approximately 50% of necrotic collections, it is located outside of the pancreas without interference of the pancreatic parenchyma.[25]

### WALLED-OFF NECROSIS

Over time, approximately after 4 weeks of persisting necrotising pancreatitis, ANCs become mature and encapsulated and are referred to as WON. In contrast to ANC, WON is surrounded by a fibrotic capsule. The size varies greatly, and these collections may or may not be infected. Multiple treatment options are available for the management of infected non-liquefied components (e.g., image-guided percutaneous drainage, laparoscopic or endoscopic procedures). Distinction between collections containing fluids only, such as pancreatic pseudocysts, are treated differently than collections containing fluid and non-liquefied material. In pancreatic pseudocysts, antibiotics or draining alone is effective in 30–50% of cases, in contrast to WON, which in general requires more invasive therapy.

## OTHER LOCAL COMPLICATIONS

### COLONIC ISCHEMIA

Colonic involvement is uncommon, however, potentially life-threatening in patient with severe acute pancreatitis. It is hypothesised that pancreatic enzymes spread through the retroperitoneum to the mesocolon could lead to colonic ischemia. Other theories include 'low flow state', thrombosis or compression of one of the mesenteric arteries causing ischemia. Colonic ischemia almost always requires surgical intervention and often requires the formation of a colostomy.

### GASTRIC OUTLET DYSFUNCTION

Delayed gastric emptying or gastric outlet obstruction should be suspected in patients with persistent vomiting or high-volume gastric aspirates from a nasogastric tube. It is seen in approximately 10% of all patients with severe acute pancreatitis and can occur as a consequence of ANCs, pancreatic pseudocysts or WON, causing a mechanical obstruction of the stomach. Treatment is indicated in those with persistent gastric dysfunction. According to the current guidelines, intervention is preferably performed when there is a well-defined wall, which is usually 4 to 8 weeks after onset of symptoms.

### GASTROINTESTINAL PERFORATION

An enteric perforation (e.g., duodenal or colon) is a rare complication following acute pancreatitis. It is more often seen in patients with necrotising pancreatitis, or in patients with post-ERCP pancreatitis. Depending on severity of the complication, additional antibiotics and or interventional treatment is recommended.

### ELEVATED INTRA-ABDOMINAL PRESSURE AND ACUTE COMPARTMENT SYNDROME

In patients with severe acute pancreatitis, an elevated intra-abdominal pressure (IAP) can lead to elevated IAP and intra-abdominal hypertension (IAH), which is present in 60–80%.[26] IAH is recognised to be a contributor to organ dysfunction involving the cardiovascular,

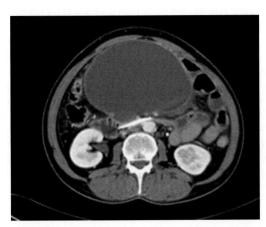

**Figure 15.3** Large pseudocyst causing gastric and extra-hepatic biliary obstruction with jaundice.

respiratory and/or renal systems. Eventually, IAH may lead to the abdominal compartment syndrome (ACS), characterised by multi-organ dysfunction syndrome.

Once IAH or ACS is suspected, regularly measurement of the urinary bladder pressure is recommended. With reference to the risk of clinical deterioration, surveillance of vital signs is indicated. Treatment is mainly focussed on non-surgical interventions, such as nasogastric decompression, short-term use of neuromuscular blockers and percutaneous drainage of fluid collections.[27] Before the 'last resort' including decompression surgery, deep sedation and paralysis can be needed if all non-operative options are insufficient. The role of decompression laparotomy is still debated. In critical medical conditions, decompression laparotomy is sometimes unavoidable, however, it should be a well-considered decision and caution should be applied because of high mortality rates.

## SYSTEMIC COMPLICATIONS FOLLOWING ACUTE PANCREATITIS

### ORGAN FAILURE

Despite better understanding of the underlying mechanism of severe acute pancreatitis and its complications, organ failure is commonly seen. Approximately 45% of patients with infected necrotising pancreatitis will develop organ failure, requiring invasive treatment strategies, prolonged support and treatment in the ICU.[5,10] Organ failure is defined as dysfunction of single or multiple organ systems and can be assessed using the modified Marshall scoring system.[28] Respiratory, cardiovascular and renal system failure are considered most important in acute pancreatitis. The early phase of severe acute pancreatitis is characterised by a SIRS with the release of inflammatory mediators (e.g., chemokines and cytokines) and an increased risk of organ failure. Since it is a dynamic process, organ failure is not limited to the first week and may develop at any stage. In moderately severe pancreatitis, organ failure can be present, however, it is transient (<48 h) and is associated with low mortality and complications. In severe pancreatitis, persistent organ failure is present and almost always requires management in a critical care facility. In patients with acute pancreatitis with organ failure, mortality rates are approximately 30%.[29] Interestingly, a study by Schepers et al. showed that in patients with organ failure, mortality rates were similar with or without infected necrosis.[4]

## MANAGEMENT OF COMPLICATION ASSOCIATED WITH ACUTE PANCREATITIS

The presence of secondary infection in a necrotic pancreatic collection is an important factor in predicting the clinical course and prognosis, and the need for medical, endoscopic or surgical intervention. Therefore clear distinction should be made between sterile and secondary infection of (peri) pancreatic necrosis because of the fact that treatment and prognosis are different.[30]

The vast majority of sterile fluid collections in acute pancreatitis are self-limiting and do not require intervention. Drainage of sterile infections can do harm by introducing iatrogenic infections and should therefore be reserved for a small subgroup with persistent symptoms.[31]

In patients with secondary infected (peri)pancreatic necrosis, invasive therapy is almost unavoidable. Clinical deterioration may be a warning symptom. Infected necrosis can be presumed when gas configurations are observed in peripancreatic collections on CECT. In case of diagnostic uncertainty, (additional) FNA for Gram stain should be considered.[32] The first step in the treatment of infected necrosis is the administration of broad-spectrum antibiotics, which may delay or even avoid intervention. Nevertheless, in the majority of patients, more invasive treatment strategies are required. Over the last two decades minimally invasive techniques have proven to be successful in management of pancreatic necrosis, including percutaneous, endoscopic and laparoscopic drainage procedures. The main goal in the treatment of necrotic collections has changed over the years; previously the main focus was on complete removal of the necrosis, however, this has been progressively challenged and now adequate sepsis control should be the primary focus, using a step-up strategy as detailed later if required.[33]

Infected necrotising pancreatitis is a complex disease and requires a multi-disciplinary team approach to management. The different procedures and techniques are discussed subsequently.

✅ An important factor in predicting the clinical course and need for intervention is the presence of secondary infection in a necrotic pancreatic collection.

## INTERVENTIONAL STRATEGIES

### SURGICAL AND ENDOSCOPIC STEP-UP APPROACH

In general, the first step of the step-up approach in patients with clinical deterioration and signs of infected necrotising pancreatitis after failure of antibiotic treatment is image-guided percutaneous or endoscopic drainage (Figs. 15.4 and 15.5).[34] Other indications include ongoing organ failure without radiological improvement of an infected necrotic collection and mechanical obstruction by large collections causing gastric outlet, biliary or intestinal obstruction. In later phases of the disease, interventional may be indicated in patients with on-going pain or discomfort.[35]

Preferably, intervention should be performed after 4 weeks when necrosis has become walled-off. This has been shown to allow safer and more effective interventions, and is associated with a lower risk of complications and less interventions.[36–38] To facilitate drainage of necrosis, percutaneous drainage of ascites may be required. If sepsis persists, drains should initially be upsized in diameter, with minimally invasive surgical necrosectomy only undertaken if clinically required.[1]

The endoscopy step-up approach is similar to the surgical step-up approach in terms of mortality and major morbidity but has been shown to be associated with lower rates of enteral- and pancreatico-cutaneous fistulae. Hospital stay following endoscopic management has also been shown to be shorter, compared to patients after surgical intervention.[39]

Percutaneous catheter drainage of infected necrotic collections can be first choice in specific patients, such as those with extended collections to the flank or pelvic region. Moreover, it may facilitate postponement of surgical intervention to a more favourable time or even enable patients to avoid surgery if there is complete resolution of the

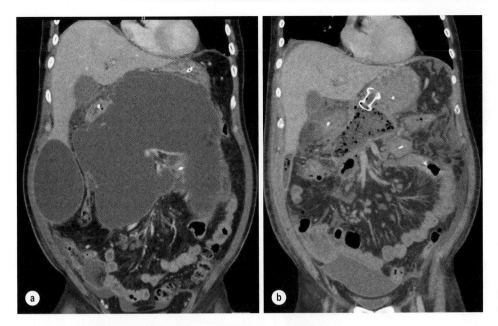

**Figure 15.4** Computed tomography **(a)** before and **(b)** after drainage.

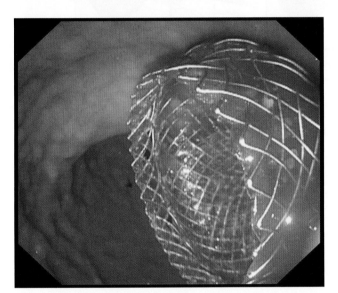

**Figure 15.5** Endoscopic transluminal drainage with a lumen-apposing self-expendable metal stent, placed via a transgastric approach.

infection. The preferred route for percutaneous catheter drainage is through the retroperitoneum, so this can be used as navigation in a later phase or if needed, for a minimally invasive retroperitoneal necrosectomy. Combined endoscopic transluminal and percutaneous catheter drainage in patients with large collections, spreading to the paracolic gutter and pelvic zone can also be considered.

✔ Intervention is more effective, safer and associated with lower risk of complications after 4 weeks when necrosis has become walled-off.

### MINIMALLY INVASIVE SURGERY

The benefit of video-assisted retroperitoneal debridement is in reducing the risk of an inflammatory response and local sepsis, compared to open necrosectomy as shown in the PANTER trial (Fig. 15.6).[33,40,41] Furthermore, high-risk

patients treated with minimally invasive surgery or endoscopic necrosectomy have a lower risk of mortality compared to open necrosectomy.[42] Minimally invasive surgery is indicated as a continuum in the step-up approach after unsuccessful percutaneous and/or endoscopic intervention. Other indications for surgical treatment are bleeding complication after unsuccessful attempts of endovascular approaches.

### OPEN LAPAROTOMY/DEBRIDEMENT

Over the past decade, the role for open surgery in infected necrosis has become much less and has been replaced by minimally invasive procedures. It is only indicated following failure of conservative treatment in patients with (the suspicion of) ACS and no other treatment options and in selected patients with sepsis/bleeding (Fig. 15.7).[43] With open decompression laparotomy, the retroperitoneal cavity should left intact, as well as the lesser omental sac, to lower the risk of infecting (peri)pancreatic necrosis.

### TIMING OF SURGICAL INTERVENTION

When considering mortality, it is important to note that a meta-analysis by Mowery et al. showed that late surgery resulted in a significant better survival compared to early surgery (e.g., 72 hours and 12 days). This seems to be related to lower bleeding risk and a more effective necrosectomy.[44] However, it is unknown how long surgery can be postponed and if patients do tolerate the delay of intervention. If possible, delaying surgical intervention for more than 4 weeks is recommended to minimise the mortality and bleeding risk and to optimise the efficiency of the necrosectomy.

✔ Open surgery has largely been replaced by endoscopic and minimally invasive techniques, however, is indicated in patients with (suspicion of) ACS if other available treatment options are unsuccessful, and in patients with signs of bowel ischaemia.

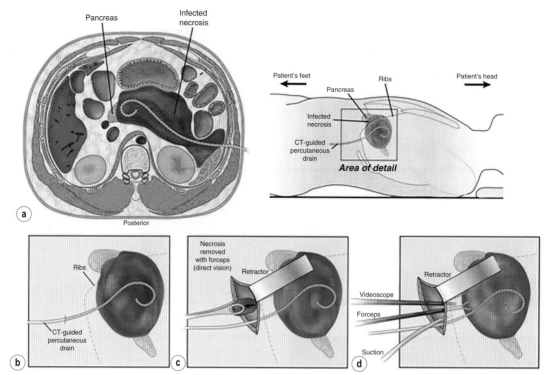

**Figure 15.6** Surgical step-up approach, including percutaneous catheter drainage and video-assisted retroperitoneal debridement (VARD). **(a)** Cross-sectional image and torso depicting an extra-pancreatic collection with fluid and necrosis. The preferred route is through the left retroperitoneal space between the left kidney, spleen and descending colon. **(b)** A percutaneous catheter drain is inserted in the collection to mitigate sepsis and postpone or even obviate necrosectomy. **(c)** A 5-cm subcostal incision is made and the previously placed percutaneous drain is followed into the retroperitoneum to enter the necrotic collection. Initially, necrosis is removed under direct vision using long grasping forceps. This is followed by further debridement under videoscopic assistance in **(d)**. (Reprinted from van Brunschot et al 2012, Elsevier.)

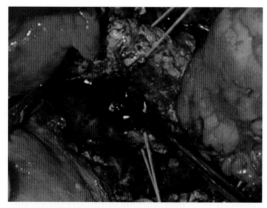

**Figure 15.7** Open necrosectomy following acute haemorrhage, managed by interventional radiological embolisation of a branch of the superior mesenteric artery, with loss of the head and uncinated process.

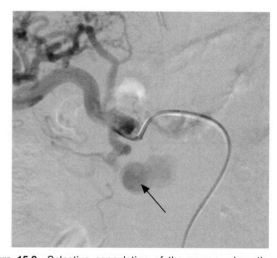

**Figure 15.8** Selective cannulation of the common hepatic artery showing filling of a pseudoaneurysm (marked with an *arrow*) arising from the gastroduodenal artery in a patient with haemorrhage into central pancreatic necrosis.

## MANAGEMENT OF ACUTE PHASE COMPLICATIONS

### HAEMORRHAGE

Haemorrhage in patients with severe acute pancreatitis is a fairly common complication. This may be explained by extravasation of exocrine proteolytic and lipolytic enzyme-rich fluid within areas of parenchymal necrosis. This may cause erosion of major vessels with or without pseudoaneurysm formation, which may rupture and result in significant haemorrhage. Splenic vein thrombosis, an underdiagnosed complication of severe acute pancreatitis, may cause left-sided portal hypertension, eventually leading to upper gastrointestinal variceal bleeding. If acute haemorrhage (e.g., blood in drain) is suspected, urgent CT angiography must be performed to identify the location of the bleeding. The first step in the treatment of (suspected) haemorrhage is embolisation with endovascular metal coils (Fig. 15.8). Some patients require more invasive strategies, for example, surgical interventions including suture ligation of the bleeding

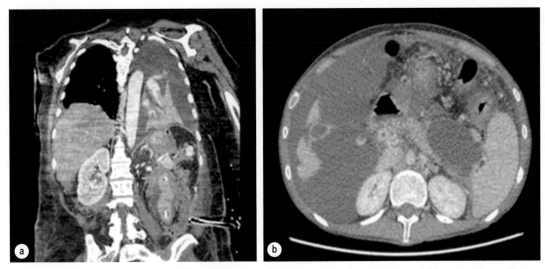

**Figure 15.9**  Post-acute pancreatitis complications. **(a)** Pancreatico-pleural fistula and **(b)** pancreatic ascites.

point. Gaining surgical access and achieving haemostasis in patients with active haemorrhage is challenging and is frequently accompanied with rapidly escalating organ dysfunction, coagulopathy and venous hypertension. Haemorrhage in patients with severe acute pancreatitis should therefore not be underestimated. The timing and type of surgical intervention are both important factors in preventing or aggravating the risk of bleeding in the course of the disease. An aggressive approach may lead to 'iatrogenic' injuries, whereas a hesitant approach could lead to death.

## VENOUS THROMBOSIS

In patients with severe acute pancreatitis, there is a relatively high risk of developing venous thromboembolic disease. Frequently affected areas are thromboses in the splenic vein and superior mesenteric or portal vein. CT may be useful to diagnose a venous thrombosis. The role of anticoagulation remains controversial and there are various opinions on whether prophylactic low molecular weight heparin should be administered or not, however, compression stockings are advised. Following venous thrombosis, regardless of active treatment, recanalization rarely occurs and collateralisation will ensue.

## LONG-TERM COMPLICATIONS

### PANCREATIC INSUFFICIENCY

In complicated acute pancreatitis, impaired exocrine and endocrine pancreatic function is a common consequence and development of pancreatic insufficiency is related to the severity of the pancreatitis. In severe pancreatitis, exocrine pancreatic insufficiency (EPI) is present in approximately 33% of patients compared to 19% of those with mild pancreatitis.[45] Most often a faecal elastase-1 test is used to diagnose EPI and clinical manifestations includes a variety of

symptoms, such as abdominal discomfort, steatorrhea and malnutrition. The treatment of EPI is focused on the administration of exogenous pancreatic enzymes. Endocrine insufficiency can be present after acute pancreatitis and is referred to as post-pancreatitis diabetes. Approximately a quarter of patients with severe acute pancreatitis patients develop endocrine insufficiency and several diagnostic tools are available such as fasting glucose and oral glucose tolerance testing.[46] Treatment can be either by lifestyle adjustments or medication (e.g., oral medication or insulin).

## PANCREATIC FISTULA

Pancreatic fistula is most commonly seen as a complication of previous intervention for fluid collections in patient with acute pancreatitis and is defined by persistent drainage of fluid with high amylase concentration. High amylase is defined as more than three times the upper limit of the institution's serum amylase. Closure of small leaks can often be managed by stepwise withdrawing of the drain once the patient's condition permits to do so. If a leak persists, endoscopic transpapillary stenting is recommended.[47] If a pseudocyst ruptures into the intra-peritoneal cavity, pancreatic ascites or a pleural effusion may occur if there is communication with the pleural cavity (Fig. 15.9). Some fistulas do not settle and if ductal stenting is unsuccessful, more invasive treatment is needed. Surgical resection (e.g., distal pancreatectomy with or without splenectomy) should be delayed until the patient has made a full recovery and their nutrition and physiology is optimised.

Pancreatic duct strictures can result from tissue damage and fibrotic repair after acute pancreatitis. This can be an isolated stricture or in association with duct disruption. Isolated pancreatic duct strictures can manifest with hyperamylasaemia and dilatation of the distal duct syndrome, typically presenting with recurrent bouts of abdominal pain. Treatment options are dilatation and temporary stenting, surgical drainage with a pancreato-jejunostomy or surgical resection of the stricture and distal pancreas.

## DISCONNECTED DUCT SYNDROME

Disconnected duct syndrome is a well-known complication of acute necrotising pancreatitis (ANP) and occurs in approximately 30% of patients with ANP. Predominantly, it affects the pancreatic neck and results in pancreatic juice leaking into the retroperitoneum, leading to either (peri)pancreatic necrosis or pseudocyst formation.[48] Surgical drainage procedures or resection are often needed to achieve resolution.

## Key points

- The majority of acute pancreatitis episodes are mild, however, approximately 20% of all patients develop severe acute pancreatitis, which is accompanied by local and/or systematic complications.
- The mortality rate of severe or complicated acute pancreatitis is 10–30%
- The Revised Atlanta Classification is used for the definition of acute pancreatitis. Local complications according to timing and presence of necrosis has been added to the original classification as well as a new category (moderately severe pancreatitis).
- Infected (peri)pancreatic necrosis is the most feared complication of acute pancreatitis.
- Interventional treatment of complications following acute pancreatitis should be delayed for as long as possible, preferably at least 4 weeks to allow maturation and encapsulation of collections.
- The key to successful treatment of infected (peri)pancreatic necrosis is adequate control of sepsis.
- Endoscopic and other minimally invasive techniques have mostly replaced open surgery because of the lower risks of complications and mortality.
- The key principle in management of complications following acute pancreatitis is 'Do as little as late as you can'.

References available at http://ebooks.health.elsevier.com/

# Chronic pancreatitis

# 16

Ajith K. Siriwardena

## SUMMARY

Chronic pancreatitis (CP) is an inflammatory disease of the pancreas characterised by inflammation and scarring resulting in irreversible damage to the gland, leading to variable loss of pancreatic exocrine and endocrine function.[1] The most common aetiological factor is long-term excessive consumption of alcohol.[2] There is also an association with cigarette smoking.[2,3] Chronic pancreatitis is associated with mutations in trypsin activation genes and mutations in cystic fibrosis genes.[4,5] Abdominal pain is typically the dominant symptom. Baseline assessment, in addition to careful clinical examination, must include cross-sectional imaging, typically by computed tomography (CT). Magnetic resonance (MR) scanning is also useful and endoscopic ultrasound (EUS) can be of value both in diagnosis and in treatment.

Treatment planning should ideally take place on a multidisciplinary basis. Interventions can be described as baseline treatments and more advanced interventions. Baseline treatment should be considered in all patients and includes assessment and management of pancreatic exocrine insufficiency and pain control. Analgesic prescription should follow the World Health Organisation (WHO)'s analgesic ladder originally developed for cancer pain.[6] Co-analgesics, such as gabapentin, may be used in conjunction with conventional analgesics.[7] Guidance on alcohol cessation and help on stopping smoking are important baseline interventions. More advanced interventions include endoscopic and surgical treatment. Endoscopic interventions are directed at improving pancreatic duct drainage, managing pancreatic duct disruption, treatment of extrahepatic biliary obstruction, and/or pain control through coeliac plexus nerve block.

Surgical treatments can be broadly categorised as main pancreatic duct drainage procedures, pancreatic resectional procedures and those which include a combination of main duct drainage and partial pancreatic resection.[8] To standardise the description and reporting of surgery for chronic pancreatitis, the International Study Group for Pancreas Surgery (ISGPS) has recently published a standardised nomenclature for surgical procedures.[8] This will be adopted in this chapter.

The long-term complications of chronic pancreatitis all relate to recurrent or persistent episodes of inflammation with subsequent healing with fibrosis. These include biliary stricture, duodenal stenosis, pseudocyst, false aneurysms of visceral vessels and portal or splenic vein occlusion leading to extrahepatic portal hypertension.[9] Important long-term risks of chronic pancreatitis to monitor for during follow-up include development of diabetes mellitus, malnutrition and in particular the increased risk for development of pancreatic cancer.[10]

## DEFINITION

✓✓ Chronic pancreatitis is defined as a benign inflammatory disease, characterised by chronic pancreatic inflammation and scarring, irreversibly damaging the pancreas and resulting in variable loss of exocrine and endocrine function.[1]

## CLASSIFICATIONS OF CHRONIC PANCREATITIS

Classifications of chronic pancreatitis have been based on the aetiology of the disease such as alcohol-related, genetic or idiopathic.[1] Alternatively, the disease can be classified according to morphology – large duct disease, small duct disease and minimal change pancreatitis.[11] Classifications incorporating the temporal changes along the time course of chronic pancreatitis have also been used (early stage, late stage disease).[12] The availability of better diagnostic tests such as endoscopic pancreatography were the stimulus for morphologically based categorisations and the Cambridge classification based on pancreatogram appearance is still used today.[11] Contrast-enhanced MR scanning has replaced diagnostic pancreatography.[13] Morphologically based classifications have the practical advantage that treatment can potentially be tailored to the disease variant. In addition to these systems of classification, there have since been several national classifications from (amongst others) Japan, Switzerland and the United States of America.[14–16] A widely used contemporary classification system is that described in the American Pancreatic Association's (APA) practice guideline on chronic pancreatitis in 2014.[16] The APA practice guideline provides criteria for the diagnosis of chronic pancreatitis based on CT, MR scanning and endoscopic ultrasonography.

## INCIDENCE

✓✓ Data from the North American National Pancreas Foundation suggests an incidence of about four new patients per 100 000 population per year in the USA.[17] As this is a chronic disease, the prevalence is 40–50 per 100 000 people.[17] There is substantial worldwide geographic variation in the clinical profile of the disease.[18]

## AETIOLOGY

The TIGAR-O risk factor list is a modern, comprehensive list of the aetiological causes of chronic pancreatitis (Table 16.1).[19] TIGAR-O considers toxic-metabolic causes, idiopathic, genetic, autoimmune, recurrent and obstructive factors. The M-ANNHEIM aetiology list is similar but adds the important option to consider multiple co-existent aetiological factors.[20] Excessive alcohol consumption is the single most common aetiologic factor.[19,20] Cigarette smoking is a common co-factor to alcohol, and as a modifiable risk factor, smoking cessation should be prioritised from the outset.[3] High caloric intake of protein and fat and deficiency of fat-soluble vitamins in the diet are associated with chronic pancreatitis but there is no proof of a causal link.[21,22]

There have been substantial important advances in understanding of the genetic basis of chronic pancreatitis.[4] Mutations in the cationic trypsinogen gene *PRSS1* lead to premature intra-acinar activation of trypsin.[4] Similarly, mutations in the pancreatic secretory trypsin inhibitor also termed *serine protease inhibitor Kazal Type 1 (SPINK1)* compromise intracellular inactivation of trypsin and are associated with chronic pancreatitis.[23] Cystic fibrosis gene mutations, especially the Δ508 mutation are associated with chronic pancreatitis and are thought to be caused by abnormalities in mucin production and secretion.[24] Alcohol susceptibility genes are also associated with alcohol-related chronic pancreatitis.[23]

### PATHOGENESIS OF PAIN IN CHRONIC PANCREATITIS

Pain in clinical chronic pancreatitis is complex and multifactorial. Logically, pain in chronic pancreatitis can be considered as having both a 'pancreatic' component and an 'extra-pancreatic' component. Pancreatic pain relates to inflammation of the gland and obstruction of the main pancreatic duct. Extra-pancreatic components relate to abnormal neural pathways and aberrant central nervous system perception of pain.[25,26] Objective evidence of the 'extra-pancreatic' component comes from studies, which show that the number and diameter of non-myelinated type C pain fibres are significantly increased in patients with chronic pancreatitis.[27,28] In addition, central nervous system processing of pain may be altered in longstanding chronic pancreatitis.[29] These 'extra-pancreatic' factors may account for some of the treatment failures of pancreas-directed surgery or endoscopy. It should also be remembered that there may be treatment-related side effects such as opiate-induced gut dysmotility. In practical terms, patients should be counselled before undergoing surgical or endoscopic intervention and should understand that no individual intervention is associated with an absolute guarantee of symptom relief in chronic pancreatitis.

✔✔ Pain in chronic pancreatitis is multi-factorial and can include a pancreatic parenchymal component, and an extra-pancreatic neural component and components caused by treatment-related side-effects such as opiate-induced gut dysmotility.

**Table 16.1    The TIGAR-O classification system of risk factors for chronic pancreatitis (modified from[19])**

| | |
|---|---|
| Toxic-metabolic | Alcohol, tobacco smoking, hypercalcaemia, hyperlipidaemia, chronic renal failure, medications, toxins |
| Idiopathic | Associated with early onset CP and also with late-onset CP, Tropical CP |
| Genetic mutations | *PRSS1, CFTR, SPINK 1*, others |
| Autoimmune | Isolated or as part of a syndrome |
| Recurrent and severe AP associated CP | Post-necrotic (severe AP), vascular disease/ischaemic, post-irradiation |
| Obstructive | pancreas divisum, sphincter of Oddi disorders, duct obstruction (e.g., tumour), post-traumatic pancreatic duct scars |

*AP*, Acute pancreatitis; *CP*, chronic pancreatitis.
The TIGAR-O classification is a comprehensive classification system of the risk factors for chronic pancreatitis.[19] It is worthwhile remembering that in clinical practice, there may be more than one co-existent aetiological factor.

## CLINICAL PRESENTATIONS

### ACUTE PRESENTATION OF CHRONIC PANCREATITIS

There is a substantial overlap between acute and chronic pancreatitis in their modes of presentation. To address this practically, if patients present with acute abdominal pain, hyperamylasaemia or meet the diagnostic criteria for acute pancreatitis defined in the Atlanta 2012 consensus[30] (see chapter on acute pancreatitis) they should be diagnosed as having acute pancreatitis and receive treatment according to the current International Association of Pancreatology/APA (IAP/APA) guidelines for the treatment of acute pancreatitis.[31] The practical importance of this is to ensure adequate initial resuscitation and also to detect and treat avoidable causes of recurrent pancreatitis. Principally, gallstones should be sought by trans-abdominal ultrasound and treated by cholecystectomy. The presence of parenchymal calcification on CT and/or a dilated main pancreatic duct are pointers toward an underlying diagnosis of chronic pancreatitis.

### CHRONIC PRESENTATION OF CHRONIC PANCREATITIS

The majority of admissions secondary to established chronic pancreatitis are as a result of abdominal pain with normal or marginally elevated pancreatic enzymes on blood testing. Unlike severe acute pancreatitis, these episodes usually require little more than a temporary escalation of analgesia and maintenance fluids, but to avoid recurrent admissions, an effective strategy is required. An important component of care is provision of counselling to help avoid continued alcohol overuse and there is good randomised trial evidence that professional counselling on the harms of alcohol consumption is associated with a reduction in future admissions with pancreatitis.[32,33] These patients may also be considered for endoscopic and/or surgical management (see later).

## INDEX PRESENTATION WITH COMPLICATIONS OF CHRONIC PANCREATITIS

Occasionally, the index presentation will be as a result of a complication of chronic pancreatitis such as a pseudocyst, bleed from a false aneurysm or biliary or duodenal obstruction from chronic fibrosis. The management of these is discussed in the section on complications.

## ASYMPTOMATIC INCIDENTAL FINDING

The widespread availability and use of CT occasionally results in the detection of patients with pancreatic parenchymal calcification without associated symptoms. In this setting, it is worthwhile assessing and excluding diabetes mellitus and malnutrition, but there is no role for intervention in the absence of symptoms.

## PRACTICAL DIFFERENTIAL DIAGNOSES IN CHRONIC PANCREATITIS

Three important differential diagnoses must be considered.

### PANCREATIC CANCER

Initial management of a patient presenting with a focal pancreatic mass, on a background of known or newly diagnosed chronic pancreatitis, should consider the possibility of pancreatic cancer in the differential diagnosis. Biomarkers such as carbohydrate antigen 19-9 (CA 19-9) are insufficiently accurate to allow for reliable distinction between chronic pancreatitis and cancer, especially in the setting of biliary obstruction.[34] Chronic pancreatitis is itself an independent risk factor for the development of pancreatic ductal adenocarcinoma.[35] Sonographic artifact from fibrosis and calcification compromises the accuracy of EUS, and whilst a diagnosis of cancer may be confirmed by EUS/fine-needle aspiration (FNA), it may not exclude neoplasia despite negative cytology and in patients in whom there is a suspicion of cancer, surgical resection should be considered.

### AUTOIMMUNE PANCREATITIS

Autoimmune pancreatitis (AIP) is a chronic inflammatory condition in which patients may present with a pancreatic mass, pain and jaundice and which can closely resemble chronic pancreatitis.[36,37] AIP is associated with stricture of the extra-pancreatic bile ducts and not typically with pancreatic calcification and these pointers may help differentiation from chronic pancreatitis.[38] AIP is also associated with elevation of the immunoglobulin IgG4 subtype.[39] The diffuse nature of the inflammatory process leads to a classical 'sausage-shaped' appearance of the swollen pancreas, which can be distinguished from chronic pancreatitis.[40] Ideally, a tissue diagnosis of AIP should be established, usually by pancreatic biopsy at EUS.

### MAIN-DUCT INTRADUCTAL PAPILLARY MUCINOUS NEOPLASM

Main-duct intraductal papillary mucinous neoplasm (IPMN) presents with dilatation of the main pancreatic duct and can closely resemble chronic pancreatitis.[41] Main-duct IPMN typically has intraductal mucin, which may be seen on side-viewing duodenoscopy to be extruding from the ampulla whereas the duct dilatation associated with chronic pancreatitis is associated with stricture formation and parenchymal calcification. It is important to distinguish between the two as main-duct IPMNs are regarded as pre-malignant lesions and if surgery is indicated, it should take the form of resection rather than drainage.[41]

✓ When establishing a diagnosis of chronic pancreatitis, the following conditions should be considered in the differential diagnosis:

- Pancreatic cancer
- Main-duct IPMN
- Autoimmune pancreatitis

## CLINICAL COURSE

Typically, the disease has a relapsing course characterised by intermittent abdominal pain.[42] At the onset, patients will have conserved exocrine and endocrine function, but both are compromised during the clinical course. Diabetes mellitus is more frequent in long-standing chronic pancreatitis.[43] Historical series proposed a 'burnout' hypothesis, suggesting pain may spontaneously decrease over time, coinciding with the occurrence of exocrine insufficiency.[44] However, two large prospective cohort studies[43,45] showed no association between the duration of chronic pancreatitis and resolution of pain.

## BASELINE ASSESSMENT OF A PATIENT WITH SUSPECTED CHRONIC PANCREATITIS

Clinical history is central to management and must focus on the nature and duration of symptoms, age of first onset of abdominal pain and associated factors such as jaundice and/or vomiting. An accurate history of alcohol consumption is important and must include information on type of alcohol, years of consumption and current intake in units. Smoking history and counselling on the significance of smoking on disease progression, and an accurate family history may identify hereditary kindreds. Clinical examination should record body mass index, abdominal examination findings and urinalysis.

Baseline laboratory tests include blood count, urea/electrolytes, biochemical liver function tests, blood glucose (and glycosylated haemoglobin), C-reactive protein and CA 19-9. Trans-abdominal ultrasonography will provide information on the presence or absence of gallstones and also on common co-existent liver diseases such as steatohepatitis. CT scan is the mainstay of detailed morphological assessment of the gland in chronic pancreatitis with additional or complementary information being provided by MR.[16]

The American Pancreatic Association (APA) Practice guidelines key points on the diagnosis of chronic pancreatitis:[16]

- Intraductal pancreatic calcifications are the most specific and reliable sonographic and CT signs of CP
- Compared with ultrasound and CT, MR is a more sensitive imaging tool for the diagnosis of CP
- Computed tomography is helpful for the diagnosis of complications of CP
- Computed tomography is helpful for diagnosis of other conditions that can mimic CP
- Endoscopic retrograde pancreatogram should not be used for diagnostic purposes
- The ideal threshold number of EUS criteria necessary to diagnose CP has not been firmly established, but the presence of five or more and two or less strongly suggests or refutes the diagnosis of CP, respectively. The relatively poor inter-observer agreement for EUS features of chronic pancreatitis limits the diagnostic accuracy and overall utility of EUS for diagnosis.[46]

CT features of chronic pancreatitis include dilatation of the main pancreatic duct, pancreatic calcification and parenchymal atrophy (Fig. 16.1). These features are usually present late in the course of the disease and thus may not be evident at an early stage. MR is reportedly more specific for the diagnosis of CP because ductal abnormalities are very reliably detected. The addition of intravenous secretin may improve the accuracy of MR and may provide indirect evidence of residual exocrine function.[47]

EUS complements cross-sectional imaging. EUS is more sensitive than CT in diagnosing the early stages of chronic pancreatitis and the Rosemont criteria[46] derived from a consensus conference combine the detection of parenchymal abnormalities with observations on pancreatic ductal irregularity or dilatation to produce a score for the prediction of chronic pancreatitis.

Although endoscopic retrograde cholangiopancreatography (ERCP) was a mainstay of diagnosis in the 1980s and was used in the Cambridge classification, purely diagnostic ERCP should no longer be undertaken as accurate information on ductal abnormalities can be obtained by cross-sectional imaging.

In addition to morphological assessment of the gland, functional assessment of the endocrine component of pancreatic function involves testing for diabetes mellitus. Baseline measurement of glycosylated haemoglobin (HbA1c) may be of value in non-diabetics at time of index presentation.

The exocrine component of pancreatic function can be assessed indirectly by measurement of faecal elastase, serum trypsinogen or chymotrypsin and does not require direct hormonal stimulation of the pancreas.[48] These tests are only of practical value in the late stages of the disease when clinical features such as steatorrhea are already present. Direct assessment of pancreatic exocrine function by intubation of the duodenum, provision of a secretory stimulus and collection of pancreatic juice is not widespread practice and seems to be most widely used in North America.[49] In many units, a clinical diagnosis of chronic pancreatitis serves as an indication for commencement of pancreatic exocrine replacement therapy given the high prevalence of subclinical malnutrition and vitamin deficiency in this disease.[48]

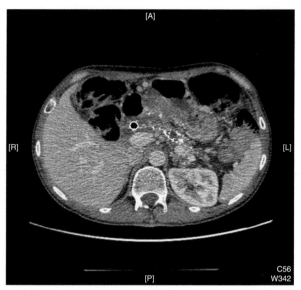

**Figure 16.1** Pancreatic parenchymal calcification. Venous contrast phase of a computed tomography showing typical pancreatic parenchymal calcification and segmental dilatation of the main pancreatic duct. An indwelling metallic endobiliary stent is also seen.

## MEDICAL MANAGEMENT OF CHRONIC PANCREATITIS

The treatment of chronic pancreatitis and its complications remains a major challenge. A holistic approach is based on accurate assessment of symptoms, nutritional status, pancreatic endocrine and exocrine function and morphological assessment of the integrity and patency of the duct and the nature of the pancreatic parenchyma.

### ANALGESIA

This is a key component of the non-operative treatment of chronic pancreatitis. Pain control should follow the WHO's analgesic ladder starting with a non-opioid, progressing to weak opioid and then a strong opiod.[6] Typically, patients will already be on regular analgesic medication by the time of referral to specialist care. Co-analgesics, such as gabapentin, may be used in conjunction with these medications.[7]

### ALCOHOL AVOIDANCE

There is good randomised trial evidence that professional alcohol avoidance counselling results in reduced hospital admission.[33] If alcohol consumption can be stopped at an early stage in the disease, progression may also be ameliorated.[32]

### SMOKING CESSATION

Formal guidance on cessation of smoking is useful. Cessation of smoking may modify disease progression.[3] If smoking cessation clinics are available, these should be used.

### EXOCRINE REPLACEMENT THERAPY

Exocrine replacement therapy should be considered in all patients with chronic pancreatitis. Treatment does not need to be dictated by complex pancreatic intubation tests or by measurement of faecal elastase but can be based on pragmatic clinical assessment.[48]

## MEDICATIONS OF UNPROVEN BENEFIT

The search for effective treatment in chronic pancreatitis has resulted in the assessment of a wide range of therapies of unproven benefit. Antioxidant therapy was evaluated on the assumption that orally administered cocktails of vitamin C, selenium and methionine would be absorbed into the pancreas in sufficient concentration to quench oxidative stress. Antioxidant therapy has been evaluated by two reasonably large and well-conducted randomised trials. The Indian trial from Delhi reported a reduction in 'painful days' but showed a substantial placebo response and treated a population with striking dietary deprivation.[50] The European ANTICIPATE trial randomised patients with painful chronic pancreatitis to a 6-month period of antioxidant therapy or placebo.[51] The principal findings were that there was no intervention-related reduction in pain or improvement in quality of life. Although there is one further study whose results are awaited, it is unlikely that antioxidant therapy is of any benefit in chronic pancreatitis. Medications of unproven benefit should be avoided in this population of vulnerable patients.

> ### KEY POINTS IN THE MEDICAL MANAGEMENT OF CHRONIC PANCREATITIS
>
> - Treatment decision making should be in a multidisciplinary forum.
> - Counselling on avoidance of alcohol consumption and cigarette smoking.
> - Treatment of malnutrition, pancreatic exocrine and endocrine insufficiency.
> - Analgesic use following the WHO ladder combined with co-analgesics such as gabapentin.
> - Antioxidant therapy has no role in the modern treatment of painful chronic pancreatitis.

## ENDOSCOPIC MANAGEMENT OF CHRONIC PANCREATITIS

Surgery and endoscopy should be seen as complementary rather than competitive treatments. Hence treatment planning is best undertaken on a multidisciplinary basis.

### ENDOSCOPIC DRAINAGE COMPARED TO SURGICAL DRAINAGE OF THE MAIN PANCREATIC DUCT

Two relatively small randomised trials compared surgical drainage of the main pancreatic duct to endoscopic therapy for painful chronic pancreatitis. The first in 2003 randomised 72 patients and reported the superiority of surgical resection or drainage over endoscopic duct stenting and/or clearance at 5 years in terms of pain relief and weight gain, with no difference in the rate of new onset diabetes.[52] In the second, a landmark study from Holland, endoscopic decompression (with prior pancreatic lithotripsy in 80%) was compared to open surgical duct drainage in 39 patients.[53] After 24 months follow-up, complete or partial pain relief was achieved in 32% assigned

to endoscopic intervention and 75% treated surgically ($P = 0.007$). Longer-term outcome in this cohort was reported in 2011 and demonstrated that the better outcomes in the surgically treated patients were maintained at 5 years.[54] Although rates of complications, length of hospital stay and changes in pancreatic function were similar between groups, endoscopically treated patients required more procedures than did patients in the surgery group (8 vs. 3; $P < 0.001$). The conclusion was that surgical drainage was more effective than endoscopic intervention. An important observation from the Dutch study was that whilst the response rate in terms of pain relief following endoscopy was inferior to surgery, those that did obtain relief did so within the first 3 months, suggesting persistence with endotherapy in the absence of a rapid response is unlikely to be beneficial. An important limitation of the Dutch study is that the findings apply only to patients with large duct disease without a pancreatic head mass as the surgical group was managed by longitudinal pancreatojejunostomy.[55]

More recently, the Dutch Pancreatitis Study Group reported the results of the ESCAPE randomised clinical trial comparing the effect of early surgery with an endoscopy-first approach in patients with painful, large-duct chronic pancreatitis.[56] Several lessons can be learnt from this important study. First, it is difficult to recruit patients to trials in chronic pancreatitis. ESCAPE recruited from 30 Dutch Hospitals between April 2011 and September 2016 and accrued 88 patients with chronic pancreatitis, a dilated main pancreatic duct and recent commencement of opiate analgesia (excluding patients on long-term opiate therapy). Second, the trial question was appropriate: patients were randomised to optimisation of analgesia followed by endoscopic intervention in the endoscopy arm and compared to patients undergoing surgery. Unlike previous trials surgery took the form of longitudinal pancreatojejunostomy for patients with a dilated duct and no mass and longitudinal pancreatojejunostomy with partial pancreatic head resection for those with a pancreatic head mass. The results showed that during 18 months of follow-up, patients in the early surgery group had lower pain scores than those randomised to receive the endoscopy-first approach (37 vs. 49; between-group difference, −12 points [95% confidence interval {CI}, −22 to −2]; $P=0.02$). Complete or partial pain relief at the end of follow-up was achieved in 23 of 40 patients (58%) in the early surgery compared to 16 of 41 (39%) in the endoscopy-first approach group ($P=0.10$). The total number of interventions was lower in the early surgery group (median 1 vs. 3; $P<0.001$). Treatment-related complications (27% vs. 25%), mortality (0% vs. 0%), hospital admissions, pancreatic function and quality of life were not significantly different between the early surgery group and those in the endoscopy-first arm.

The main conclusion was that in patients with chronic pancreatitis, early surgery compared with an endoscopy-first approach resulted in lower pain scores when followed over 18 months.

### ENDOSCOPIC DRAINAGE/STENTING OF THE MAIN PANCREATIC DUCT

Endoscopic drainage is best considered in patients with a dilated main pancreatic duct without a pancreatic head mass.

The principles of endoscopic drainage are to access the pancreatic duct, typically by pancreatic duct sphincterotomy, to remove intraductal stones and to leave either a single endobiliary stent or multiple stents in situ to facilitate prolonged drainage.[57–59]

More recently, fully covered self-expanding metallic stents have been used within the pancreas.[57] A variable proportion of patients will be definitively treated by endoscopic decompression. From a pathophysiological perspective, pancreatic ductal stones are different to common bile duct stones in that they may represent focal parenchymal calcifications with intraductal projections rather than being intra-luminal debris. Where large ductal calculi are evident on CT, extracorporeal shockwave lithotripsy can be used in combination with endoscopic attempts at clearance.[57,59]

### ENDOSCOPIC CELIAC PLEXUS BLOCK

Endoscopic ultrasonography allows for good visualisation of the celiac plexus around the celiac axis trifurcation. Injection of local anaesthesia at EUS can be used as a practical means of assessing for symptom relief.[60] In those patients who achieve an improvement in pain control after EUS-guided injection of local anaesthetic, destruction of the celiac plexus can be considered by injection of alcohol.

Some operators are reluctant to consider alcohol ablation of the coeliac plexus in benign conditions and in these, surgical ablation of the greater lesser and least splanchnic nerves in the thorax by the thoracoscopic route has been evaluated although unsatisfactory long-term outcomes have rendered this operation obsolete.[61,62]

### ENDOSCOPIC TREATMENT OF COMPLICATIONS OF CHRONIC PANCREATITIS

Endoscopic treatment can be considered for the treatment of distal bile duct stricture,[59] pancreatic pseudocyst (Fig. 16.2), and short-term duodenal stenting can be considered in patients with duodenal obstruction caused by inflammation. Long-term benign, symptomatic duodenal obstruction in chronic pancreatitis is better treated by gastrojejunostomy, which can be performed by the laparoscopic or open surgical routes.

## SURGICAL MANAGEMENT OF CHRONIC PANCREATITIS

### INDICATIONS FOR SURGERY

Surgery can be undertaken on an elective basis for pain control in patients with chronic pancreatitis. Surgery can also be indicated for management of the complications of chronic pancreatitis. Complications, which can be effectively managed by surgery include distal bile duct stricture in younger patients where long-term biliary stenting is not optimal; gastric outlet obstruction secondary to duodenal stricture and occasionally, patients with pseudocysts in the tail of the gland may require surgery.

### CASE SELECTION FOR SURGERY IN CHRONIC PANCREATITIS

In terms of elective surgery, there is evidence of substantial variation in the thresholds for intervention[63] and thus where possible, the decision to offer surgery should be taken in a multidisciplinary fashion. Pain is the typical symptom, which drives patients to seek treatment and for which surgery is considered. Although there is little evidence to support the view that patients who continue to drink alcohol must have a period of abstention (including avoidance of cigarette smoking), patients being selected for elective surgery for chronic pancreatitis should ideally have avoided alcohol consumption for at least the previous 6 months and preferably longer. The selection of the specific intervention is determined by the morphology of the gland, age and co-morbidity.

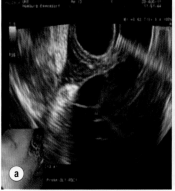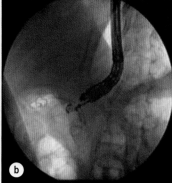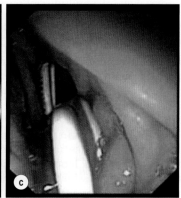

**Figure 16.2**   Endoscopic drainage of pancreatic pseudocyst. **(a)** Shows the pseudocyst on endoscopic ultrasound. **(b)** Shows the endoscopic approach to the pseudocyst and **(c)** shows a pigtail stent in situ protruding into the duodenal lumen.

## TIMING OF SURGERY

There is no clear consensus on the optimal timing of surgery. Earlier surgical intervention in the disease course of chronic pancreatitis may avoid long-term sequelae such as habituation to pain and opioids. However, earlier intervention may also result in patients having surgery when this could potentially have been avoided.

## WORKUP FOR SURGERY

Patients should have up-to-date cross-sectional imaging of the pancreas before surgery. The presence of extrahepatic portal hypertension caused by occlusion of the portal vein is a contra-indication to operation. Patients with long-standing chronic pancreatitis being considered for surgery are often on high-dose opiates, may be insulin-dependent diabetics and are likely to have varying degrees of malnutrition. Although cardiopulmonary exercise testing will provide a very reliable assessment of dynamic, functional reserve and modifiable risk factors and has been evaluated before elective pancreatic cancer surgery, it has not been formally evaluated as an assessment tool before surgery for chronic pancreatitis.[64] Dietitian and physiotherapy review before surgery should be considered and thought given to management of postoperative pain with either epidural or pain-controlled analgesia.

## PRACTICAL SURGICAL DECISION MAKING IN CHRONIC PANCREATITIS: SELECTION OF SURGICAL PROCEDURE

The current ISGPS terminology provides definitions of a range of elective operative procedures for chronic pancreatitis (Table 16.2).[8] It is not meant to be an exhaustive list of all reported surgical procedures. The terminology, which is based on an anatomical description of the procedure can be expanded to include other procedures.

## SELECTION OF SURGICAL PROCEDURE IN PATIENTS WITH A PANCREATIC HEAD MASS AND CONCERN ABOUT UNDERLYING CANCER

If there is a concern about underlying malignancy, which persists after assessment by EUS-FNA and/or [18]fluoro-deoxyglucose positron emission tomography, then pancreatoduodenectomy is an appropriate treatment.[65] Appropriate counselling is required to explain that major resection may be undertaken, with all its attendant risks, for a final diagnosis of benign disease.

## SELECTION OF SURGICAL PROCEDURE IN PATIENTS WITH A PANCREATIC HEAD MASS AND LOW INDEX OF CONCERN ABOUT UNDERLYING CANCER

In those patients with a pancreatic head mass but where pre-operative diagnostic tests have not shown features

**Table 16.2    Technical components of surgical procedures described in the ISGPS reporting standards[8]**

| ISGPS description | Duodenum | Pancreas Head | Pancreas Neck | Pancreas Body/Tail | Example of eponymous name |
|---|---|---|---|---|---|
| Longitudinal pancreatojejunostomy | Preserved | Preserved | Decompressed | Decompressed | Partington – Rochelle modification of Puestow |
| Longitudinal pancreatojejunostomy with partial pancreatic head resection | Preserved | Partial resection retaining parenchyma on duodenum and SMV/PV | Decompressed | Decompressed | Frey |
| Duodenum preserving subtotal pancreatic head resection with transection at neck of pancreas | Preserved | Subtotal resection retaining rim on duodenum | Transected | Not decompressed | Beger |
| Duodenum preserving subtotal pancreatic head resection without transection at neck of pancreas | Preserved | Resected, retaining rim on duodenum | Not transected | Not decompressed | Berne modification of Beger |
| Pylorus preserving pancreatoduodenectomy | Resected | Resected | Resected | Not decompressed | |
| Pancreatoduodenectomy | Resected | Resected | Resected | Not decompressed | Whipple |
| Distal pancreatectomy ± splenectomy | Preserved | Preserved | Resected | Resected | |
| Total pancreatectomy | Resected | Resected | Resected | Resected | |

*ISGPS,* International Study Group for Pancreas Surgery; *PV,* |portal vein; *SMV,* superior mesenteric vein.
Technical components of elective operations for chronic pancreatitis described using the current ISGPS terminology.[8]

of worry for malignancy, there are a range of possible treatment options. Main pancreatic duct drainage combined with partial pancreatic head resection (the Frey procedure) is one option with an alternative being the duodenum-preserving partial pancreatic head resection. It is important to emphasise that none of these drainage procedures are oncological operations. This is because they remove only part of the head of the pancreas and none of the lymph node drainage stations of the pancreatic head. Thus, careful pre-operative counselling is required. It is in this realm of drainage procedures where the proliferation of eponymously named variants has contributed to confusion and where the current ISGPS terminology standardises nomenclature.[8]

Both the duodenum-preserving pancreatic head resection (Beger procedure)[66,67] (Fig. 16.3) and the partial pancreatic head resection with longitudinal pancreatojejunostomy[68] (Frey procedure) (Fig. 16.4) are drainage procedures. There is ongoing debate in the published literature about the extent of pancreatic parenchyma removed from the head of the gland in each of these two procedures. Although the duodenum-preserving pancreatic head resection has proponents, a recent systematic review reported that worldwide, it is undertaken infrequently and has limited use outside Europe.[69] A global survey of elective surgery for chronic pancreatitis showed that there were 33 reports of duodenum-preserving pancreatic head resection of which 21 (64%) were from Germany.[69] Globally, the most widely practiced surgical procedure for patients with painful chronic pancreatitis, main duct dilatation and a pancreatic head mass is longitudinal pancreatojejunostomy with partial pancreatic head resection (the Frey procedure).[70]

It is important to appreciate that there are fundamental differences between the two. In the duodenum-preserving pancreatic head resection, the pancreas is divided at its neck.[66] This requires the establishment of a dissection plane behind the neck of the gland as in pancreatoduodenectomy. In the setting of chronic pancreatitis with post-inflammatory adhesions and a variable degree of compression of the portal vein leading to the development of a variceal collateral circulation, the attempt to create a tunnel behind the neck of the gland can be a highly risky step. In addition, the original description of the duodenum-preserving pancreatic head resection does not include a main duct drainage procedure.[66]

The combination of the risk inherent in the creation of a retropancreatic tunnel and the lack of main duct drainage along the length of the gland favour the longitudinal pancreatojejunostomy with partial pancreatic head resection (Frey procedure) over the duodenum-preserving pancreatic head resection (Beger). An unresolved debate remains about the extent of head resection required to achieve pain relief. However, in the original description of their procedure, Frey and Amikura describe resecting pancreatic parenchyma from the head of the gland to expose the duct towards the medial wall of the duodenum.[68]

In practice, when this is done, care must be taken to avoid injury to the superior pancreatoduodenal arcade and also the distal bile duct in the head of the pancreas.

One further option, which can be considered in settings where a duodenum-preserving head resection cannot be

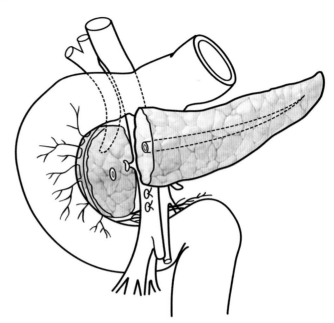

**Figure 16.3** Duodenum-preserving pancreatic head resection with subtotal pancreatic head resection (the Beger procedure). The pancreas is divided at its neck over the portal vein. The pancreatic head has been cored out and the bile duct is exposed within the head. Note that the duodenum has been preserved. Reconstruction is by a Roux pancreatojejunostomy.

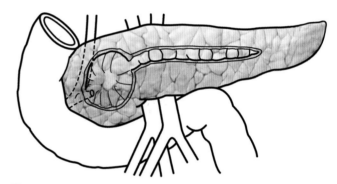

**Figure 16.4** Longitudinal pancreatojejunostomy with partial pancreatic head resection (the Frey procedure). Note the important similarities to and differences from the duodenum-preserving partial pancreatic head resection. Frey described a 'lateral' pancreaticojejunostomy, opening the main pancreatic duct out into the tail of the gland but making no attempt to undertake splenectomy. Current terminology would describe this as a longitudinal pancreatojejunostomy. Similarities to the duodenum-preserving pancreatic head resection are that pancreatic parenchyma from the head is removed. The key differences from duodenum-preserving pancreatic head resection are that the pancreas is not divided at its neck and that in the original description of the Frey procedure, the main pancreatic duct is opened along its length as in the illustration.

undertaken because of the difficulty in establishing a retropancreatic tunnel, is the duodenum-preserving pancreatic head resection without transection at the neck of the gland (the so-called *Berne modification of the Beger*).[71] This procedure has the advantage of closely following a recognised procedure but avoiding the risks inherent in creating a retropancreatic tunnel. Essentially, this procedure is a coring-out of parenchyma in the head of the pancreas and thus can be applied in settings where there is a degree of portal hypertension.

## SELECTION OF SURGICAL PROCEDURE IN PATIENTS WITHOUT A PANCREATIC HEAD MASS AND LARGE DUCT DISEASE

Duct drainage, either by longitudinal pancreatojejunostomy (Fig. 16.5) or by longitudinal pancreatojejunostomy with partial pancreatic head resection (see Fig. 16.4) are the surgical treatments of choice in this setting.[72,73]

### INDICATIONS FOR TOTAL PANCREATECTOMY FOR CHRONIC PANCREATITIS

In current practice, total pancreatectomy is not a widely used option in chronic pancreatitis. Total pancreatectomy with islet autotransplantation (TPIAT) does however have proponents.[74,75] In practical terms, this procedure can only be offered if there are facilities for islet isolation from the resected pancreas. Although tempting to consider TPI-AT as a salvage procedure after failed drainage or subtotal resection, prior surgical treatments reduce the possibility of achieving a successful islet yield. The Mayo clinic experience suggests that a tissue volume of 0.25 cc/kg be sought during islet manufacture and that intraportal infusion should be halted, at least temporarily, if the perfusion pressure exceeds 25 cm $H_2O$.[76] This procedure must be reserved for settings of established chronic pancreatitis with a low risk of cancer. In practice, the procedure is therefore optimal in younger patients with genetic chronic pancreatitis. It would be fair to say that as yet TPIAT for chronic pancreatitis is not a universally accepted procedure. The evidence supporting this procedure derives from cohort series, typically in younger patients with less advanced chronic pancreatitis and thus the question remains whether these patients truly required TPIAT. Although TPIAT has vocal proponents, questions remain about the validity of the procedure.

---

### KEY POINTS IN THE SURGICAL MANAGEMENT OF CHRONIC PANCREATITIS

- Large duct disease without a mass can be effectively treated by pancreatic duct drainage combined with 'coring-out' of parenchyma in the pancreatic head. The head and decompressed duct are then drained into a Roux loop by longitudinal pancreatojejunostomy.
- Globally, the most widely used operation for the surgical treatment of chronic pancreatitis with main duct dilatation and a pancreatic head mass is longitudinal pancreatojejunostomy with partial pancreatic head resection (the Frey procedure).
- Where there is a mass, consider pancreatoduodenectomy if there is a high index of suspicion of an underlying cancer.
- Duct drainage operations are not oncological procedures as they only remove part of the head of the gland and none of the lymph node drainage of the pancreatic head
- Total pancreatectomy with islet autotransplantation may be considered in young patients where there is a low risk of cancer. The procedure is not as yet widely accepted.
- Surgical bypass provides definitive treatment for biliary and/or duodenal strictures complicating chronic pancreatitis.

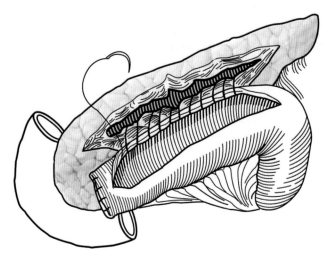

**Figure 16.5** Longitudinal pancreatojejunostomy. Longitudinal pancreatojejunostomy. The main pancreatic duct is opened longitudinally along its length and anastomosed to a Roux loop. This procedure is often incorrectly referred to as 'lateral pancreatojejunostomy'.

## COMPLICATIONS OF LONGSTANDING CHRONIC PANCREATITIS

Complications include distal bile duct stricture with jaundice,[77,78] gastric outlet obstruction secondary to duodenal stricture, pseudoaneurysm of one of the major peripancreatic visceral arteries,[79] duct disruption resulting in pseudocyst,[80] pancreatic ascites, fistula[81] or disconnected duct.[82]

### BILIARY STRICTURE

Long-term pancreatic and peripancreatic fibrosis can lead to distal bile duct stricture. Patients may present with jaundice or pain or following investigation of abnormal liver function tests.[77,78] Initial management will usually involve exclusion of neoplasia by combinations of cross-sectional imaging, EUS/FNA, and internal biliary drainage at ERCP whilst long-term options are evaluated. Jaundice secondary to extrahepatic biliary obstruction may be managed by multiple stents or self-expanding metal stents. However, in patients who are stent dependent and with minimal comorbidity, with persistent, symptomatic stricture, biliary bypass should be considered. Roux hepaticojejunostomy is the preferred intervention of choice. Choledochoduodenostomy is less widely practiced but may be a useful option in less fit patients and/or where there are contra-indications to the creation of a Roux loop.

### DUODENAL STENOSIS

Duodenal obstruction from fibrosis can be managed by short-term placement of a removable duodenal stent but gastrojejunostomy, ideally undertaken laparoscopically is the preferred treatment.

### PANCREATIC ASCITES

This is a rare complication. It is defined as a massive accumulation of pancreatic fluid in the peritoneal cavity.[81]

The amylase level in the ascitic fluid is typically elevated threefold above plasma levels although plasma amylase levels are usually also raised. Pancreatic fluid secondary to duct disruption may also track along tissue planes through the diaphragmatic hiatus to the mediastinum, occasionally reaching the pleura or bronchus. Initial management is usually by percutaneous drainage and nutritional support followed by ERCP to localise the site of leakage insertion and insertion of a trans-papillary pancreatic duct stent. Surgery is rarely required. Additional treatment with somatostatin or octreotide together with diuretics and repeated paracentesis may be beneficial for some patients.

## PSEUDOCYST COMPLICATING CHRONIC PANCREATITIS

The revised Atlanta Classification of acute pancreatitis retains the term *pseudocyst* when describing a persistent fluid collection lasting more than 4 wccks from an episode of acute pancreatitis but the definition also carries the cautionary advice that such a collection should contain little or no necrosis.[30] Features, which point to a pseudocyst complicating chronic pancreatitis include parenchymal calcification on CT, main pancreatic duct irregularity with segmental dilatation and absence of acute post-inflammatory changes in the peripancreatic fat. Pseudocysts complicating chronic pancreatitis are not liable to resolve spontaneously and usually require intervention. Endoscopic drainage is the preferred modality. Transpapillary stenting may be effective particularly where any duct stricture can be negotiated. EUS-guided transgastric drainage will often result in medium term resolution and stents are often left in situ to prevent closure of the endoscopic cystgastrostomy. Modern lumen-opposing stents can also be used in this setting. Once the pseudocyst has resolved, it is important to remove the stent. Disruption of the main pancreatic duct in its mid-body – typically a consequence of severe acute pancreatitis but also seen in chronic disease produces the 'disconnected duct syndrome' where the distal gland continues to secrete into the cavity around the middle of the gland.[83] Disconnected duct syndrome can be managed by endoscopic drainage but is one of the rare indications for distal pancreatectomy in chronic pancreatitis.[83]

## FALSE ANEURYSM OF VISCERAL VESSELS

Rarely, patients with chronic pancreatitis can present with gastrointestinal haemorrhage caused by false aneurysms of the visceral vessels (Fig. 16.6).[84] The splenic artery and gastroduodenal artery are the most frequently affected and optimal intervention is angiographic embolisation.[79]

## EXTRAHEPATIC PORTAL HYPERTENSION

Chronic peripancreatic inflammation and swelling involving the head of the gland can lead to portal vein occlusion resulting in the development of a collateral circulation and cavernous transformation (Fig. 16.7).[85] Often this is an asymptomatic late stage finding in chronic pancreatitis. Although there is some evidence favouring anticoagulation in acute portal vein thrombosis, the evidence in chronic

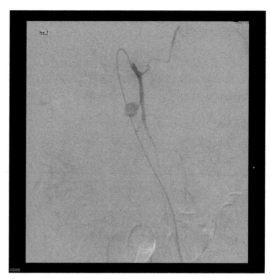

**Figure 16.6** False aneurysm in chronic pancreatitis. Selective mesenteric angiography with cannulation of the superior mesenteric artery (SMA) showing a 2-cm false aneurysm arising from the first jejunal branch.

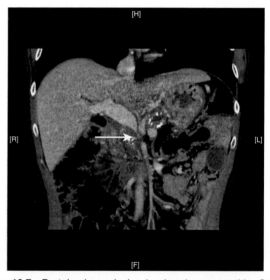

**Figure 16.7** Portal vein occlusion in chronic pancreatitis. Coronal view of a venous phase contrast computed tomography showing a smooth post-inflammatory stenosis of the main portal vein at the level of the spleno-portal confluence (highlighted by a *white arrow*). There is post-stenotic dilatation of the portal vein. Parenchymal calcification is also seen.

occlusion is less clear and the risks of anticoagulation are considerable. Occlusion of the splenic vein can lead to sinistral portal hypertension with a variceal collateral circulation running through the wall of the stomach.[86] It should be noted that transjugular portosystemic stent shunt is not effective in extrahepatic portal hypertension due to portal vein thrombosis as the procedure creates a shunt between the intra-hepatic portal circulation and the systemic circulation. Gastrointestinal bleeding is rare. Superior mesenteric vein/portal vein thrombosis with formation of venous collaterals is a contra-indication to elective surgery both because of the prohibitively high risk of major intra-operative haemorrhage but also because of the risk that disruption of the variceal collateral circulation compromises visceral venous return.

## PANCREATIC CANCER COMPLICATING CHRONIC PANCREATITIS

There is an increased lifetime risk of cancer arising in long-standing chronic pancreatitis. This must be borne in mind in older patients. There is a relative risk of 13.3 for developing pancreatic ductal adenocarcinoma in those with chronic pancreatitis, with a 10 to 20 year lag between the incidences of pancreatitis and pancreatic malignancy.[87]

---

### Key points

- Long-term alcohol overuse and cigarette smoking are the most common aetiological factors for chronic pancreatitis.
- Abdominal pain is the most frequent presenting symptom.
- Baseline assessment must include in addition to clinical history and physical examination, cross-sectional imaging (usually by CT) assessment of nutritional status, exocrine insufficiency and diabetes mellitus.
- Baseline intervention requires nutritional assessment, advice on alcohol and smoking cessation, pancreatic exocrine replacement and analgesic use following the WHO analgesic ladder.
- Advanced treatments include endoscopic and surgical approaches. These are complementary and treatment planning should be made in a multidisciplinary fashion.
- For patients with large duct disease, recent randomised trials favour surgery over endoscopic treatment.
- Selection of surgical treatment depends on the presence or absence of main pancreatic duct dilatation and the presence or absence of a pancreatic head mass.
- Operative procedures should be reported according to the current ISGPS terminology.
- In longstanding chronic pancreatitis, there is an increased risk of diabetes mellitus, malnutrition and pancreatic cancer.

---

 References available at http://ebooks.health.elsevier.com/

## KEY REFERENCES

[8] Siriwardena AK, Windsor J, Zyromski N, et al. Standards for reporting on surgery for chronic pancreatitis: a report from the International Study Group for Pancreatic Surgery (ISGPS). Surgery 2020;168:101–5.
 *This paper describes the current standardised international nomenclature for operations in chronic pancreatitis.*

[16] Conwell DL, Lee LS, Yadav D, et al. American Pancreatic Association Practice guidelines in chronic pancreatitis: evidence-based report on diagnostic guidelines. Pancreas 2014;43:1143–62.
 *This paper provides a concise but comprehensive overview of the diagnostic standards for chronic pancreatitis.*

[24] Aghdassi AA, Weiss FU, Mayerle J, et al. Genetic susceptibility factors for alcohol-induced chronic pancreatitis. Pancreatology 2015;15(Suppl):S23–31.
 *This paper provides a good overview of the genetic susceptibility factors for alcohol-induced chronic pancreatitis.*

[34] Nordback I, Pelli H, Lappalainen-Lehto R, et al. The recurrence of acute alcohol-associated pancreatitis can be reduced: a randomized controlled trial. Gastroenterology 2009;136:848–55.
 *This important randomised trial shows the effect of counselling in avoidance of repeat admission in alcohol-related pancreatitis.*

[54] Cahen DL, Gouma DJ, Nio Y, et al. Endoscopic versus surgical drainage of the pancreatic duct in chronic pancreatitis. N Engl J Med 2007;356:676–84.
 *This important randomised trial compares surgery to endoscopic therapy in patients with large-duct chronic pancreatitis.*

# 17 Pancreatic adenocarcinoma

Vikram Tewatia | Kevin C. Conlon

## INTRODUCTION

Pancreatic adenocarcinoma accounts for over 90% of tumours arising from exocrine pancreas.[1] Due to its late presentation at an advanced stage, it has a poor prognosis in the majority of patients. In the United States in 2020 there was estimated to be in excess of 47 000 deaths due to pancreatic cancer. The disease represents 3% of all new cancer cases and accounts for 8% of all cancer deaths in the United States.[2] The majority of cases are unresectable at the time of diagnosis and for the 15–20% who undergo resection, the 5-year survival is less than 20%.[3]

## EPIDEMIOLOGY

Globally, pancreatic adenocarcinoma is the seventh leading cause of cancer related mortality.[4] In 2020 there were 466 003 deaths reported worldwide.[5] The incidence varies with age, and worldwide 90% of new cases are diagnosed in those aged over 55 years. Males have an increased incidence compared to females and the incidence of pancreatic cancer is three times higher in Europe and North America compared to Africa and South Asia.[6] In the United Kingdom, the annual incidence is 16.9 per 100 000 population making it the 11th most common cancer.[7] The burden of disease is increased in the developed world and predicted to continue increasing and while the aetiology is not fully known, it is largely attributed to environmental factors.[8] Globally, the incidence and death caused by pancreatic cancer has more than doubled in last 30 years and is likely to continue as the population ages.[9,10]

✔ The incidence and mortality caused by pancreatic adenocarcinoma has more than doubled in the last 30 years and this trend is likely to continue.[8]

## RISK FACTORS (BOX 17.1)

### SMOKING

Tobacco smoking is a well-established lifestyle related modifiable risk factor in the development of pancreatic adenocarcinoma and smokers have a 75% increased risk compared to non-smokers. It has been suggested that up to 20% of cases are attributable to smoking and the risk has been shown to persist even following smoking cessation.[10,11] An Australian prospective pooled cohort study reported that the risk from current smoking is more pronounced for males (23.9% confidence interval [CI], 13.3–33.3% ) compared to females (7.2% CI, -0.4–14.2% $P = 0.007$).[12] There is also a negative impact on survival for smokers compared to ex or never smokers who develop the disease.[13] The mechanism of tobacco induced carcinogenesis is not fully understood but it is believed to be related to carcinogenic compounds from cigarette smoke inducing genetic mutation. In addition, cigarette smoke carcinogen 4-(methyln itrosamino)-1-(3-pyridyl)-1-butanone stimulates proliferation and inhibits cellular apoptosis in normal pancreatic ductal cells.[14]

## DIET AND ALCOHOL CONSUMPTION

Dietary factors are implicated in the development of many cancers including pancreatic cancer through several biological mechanisms.[15] A diet high in calories and fat over time leads to obesity, therefore having a negative impact on the pancreatic cancer risk, while meta-analyses have implicated red meat consumption as a factor in the development of pancreatic cancer.[16] Conversely, consumption of certain nutrients found in a diet rich in fruit, vegetables and grains may be protective.[17] Particular dietary nutrients associated with one carbon metabolism such as vitamin B6, B12, folate and methionine are thought to protect against cancer.[18] Alcohol consumption has also been associated with an increased risk of cancer. A pooled analysis of 14 cohort studies showed an increased risk of pancreatic cancer with an alcohol intake of more than 30 g/day.[19] A recent meta-analysis suggested that it is dose dependent, with high intake being more associated with an increased risk of pancreatic cancer in comparison to low to moderate intake.[20] Chronic alcohol intake causes structural and functional impairment in the pancreas and alcohol is a causative factor in the development of chronic pancreatitis, which is characterised by fibrosis. Pancreatic stellate cells are activated by alcohol and appear responsible for this fibrosis.[21]

## OCCUPATION

Occupational exposure to chlorinated hydrocarbons and polycyclic aromatic hydrocarbons through dry cleaning and metal related work is associated with a higher risk of developing pancreatic adenocarcinoma.[22]

## Box 17.1  Risk factors for pancreatic cancer

Age (above 60 years)
Smoking
Obesity
High fat diet
Alcohol abuse
Pancreatitis
   Chronic pancreatitis
   Hereditary pancreatitis
Diabetes mellitus
Family history of pancreatic cancer
Genetic predisposition
   Peutz–Jeghers' syndrome
   Li–Fraumeni's syndrome
   Fanconi's syndrome
   Familial adenomatous polyposis
   Lynch syndrome
   Gardner syndrome
   Multiple endocrine neoplasia
BRCA1
Von Hippel–Lindau's syndrome

## PAST MEDICAL HISTORY

There is an association between diabetes mellitus and pancreatic adenocarcinoma, particularly when diagnosed after the age of 50 years with an inverse relationship being described between the disease duration and the risk of adenocarcinoma.[10,23,24] The mechanism is not fully understood, however, reactive oxygen species are implicated as is the fibro-inflammatory process mediated through cytokines and pancreatic stellate cells, which induce pancreatic fibrogenesis, desmoplasia and thereby the promotion of pancreatic adenocarcinoma.[25]

✔ There is an association between diabetes mellitus and pancreatic cancer particularly when diagnosed after the age of 50 years.[10]

History of gallstone disease or prior cholecystectomy have also been shown to be independent risk factors for pancreatic carcinogenesis.[26,27]

Chronic pancreatitis is a fibro-inflammatory disease, which is characterised by irreversible glandular injury and current evidence strongly suggests that it increases the risk of pancreatic cancer.[28,29] However, only 4% of patients with chronic pancreatitis will develop pancreatic adenocarcinoma within 20 years. Many patients with pancreatic cancer may have associated pancreatitis, but whether this is implicated as a causative factor or represents a secondary feature remains controversial.[8]

A meta-analysis has shown that ABO blood group influences the risk of adenocarcinoma, with blood group A individuals having increased risk compared to other blood groups.[30]

## HEREDITARY PANCREATIC CANCER

Epidemiological evidence suggests that first-degree relatives with pancreatic cancer have at least a twofold increased risk of developing the disease.[31,32] Familial pancreatic cancer

shows a trend towards younger onset of age and ethnic deviation as compared to sporadic pancreatic cancer.[33] A meta-analysis of 6568 pancreatic cancer cases showed a significant increase in pancreatic cancer risk associated with having an affected relative, with an overall summary relative risk (RR) of 1.8 (95% CI, 1.48–2.12).[34] Patients with familial pancreatic cancer make up 8–10% of all cases of pancreatic cancer.[35,36]

✔ Compared to sporadic pancreas cancer, familial pancreas cancer has a younger age of onset. In addition, the lifetime risk for an individual in a familial pancreatic kindred increases with the decreasing age of onset of pancreatic cancer in family members.[33]

Although novel genes that predispose to familial pancreatic cancer remain to be fully elucidated, it is now well established that an increased risk is associated with familial conditions such as Peutz–Jeghers' syndrome and germline mutations in *BRCA1/BRCA2* (hereditary breast–ovarian cancer syndrome), *CDKN2A* (familial atypical mole and melanoma syndrome), *PALB2* (familial breast cancer syndrome),[37] *ATM* (familial breast cancer syndrome),[38] mismatch repair genes (hereditary non polyposis colorectal cancer or Lynch syndrome) and *PRSS1* and *SPINK1* of hereditary pancreatitis. Patient with hereditary breast and ovarian cancer syndrome are reported to have a 3.5–10-fold increased risk of developing pancreatic adenocarcinoma.[28] Mutations in the *CFTR* gene have been implicated in pancreatic cancer development.[39] Guidelines for family members at risk of hereditary pancreatic cancer are currently being developed, albeit based on expert opinion.[40]

## PRECURSOR LESIONS

Histologically, there are a number of distinct precursor lesions in regard to pancreatic carcinogenesis. Pre-neoplastic lesions are typically asymptomatic and small in size (<5 mm), therefore they are radiographically occult hence more commonly discovered at the time of resection. These lesions seem to follow a multi-step progression to invasive carcinoma, similar to that in colorectal carcinoma.[41] The precursor lesions include pancreatic intra-epithelial neoplasia (Pan-IN), intraductal papillary mucinous neoplasm (IPMN) and mucinous cystic neoplasm (MCN).[42] Pan-IN is the commonest of these, observed in approximately 82% of patients with pancreatic malignancy.[43] In terms of classification, following the Baltimore Consensus Meeting in 2015 for Neoplastic Pancreatic Precursor Lesions, a revised two-tier system was suggested. Therefore all precursor lesions are classified as either low-grade or high-grade dysplastic lesions.

At the time of resection, these lesions are observed adjacent to adenocarcinoma and exhibit highly similar genetic alterations to their invasive companions. Notably, the frequency of *p16* and K-*ras* mutations correlates directly with the severity of Pan-IN. This observation led primarily to the development of a pancreatic tumourigenesis model, which details a stepwise progression from Pan-IN to invasive carcinoma[44] and is characterised by diverse molecular changes (Fig. 17.1).

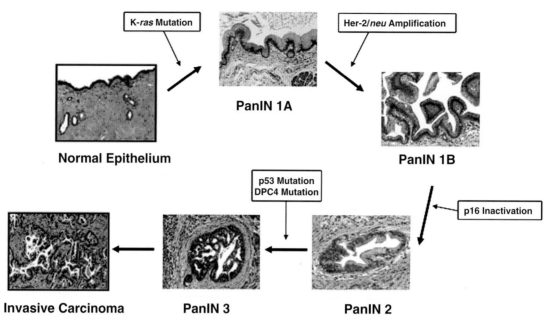

**Figure 17.1**    Diagrammatic representation of the multi-step progression to invasive carcinoma from low-grade to high-grade neoplasm. (Images courtesy of Dr Paul Crotty.)

Pancreatic adenocarcinoma exhibits approximately 63 genetic alterations, the majority of which are point mutations, which include genes such as *K-ras, p16/CDKN2A, TP53* and *SMAD4*.[45] K-ras is the most commonly observed mutation and is seen in >90% of pancreatic adenocarcinoma, in addition to about 45% of low-grade Pan-IN lesions.[46,47] K-ras is involved in a number of downstream signalling pathways hence mutations result in constitutive activation.[48]

*P16/CDKN2A* (cyclin-dependent kinase inhibitor 2A gene) is a tumour suppressor gene, which is inactivated in up to 90% of pancreatic adenocarcinoma.[49] The primary function is to regulate the cell cycle. In addition, *TP53* and *SMAD4* are tumour suppressor genes, which are inactivated in 75% and 55% of pancreatic cancer, respectively.[50,51] These changes are traditionally seen in late-stage precursor lesions, notably high-grade Pan-IN.[52] Wadell et al.[53] performed whole-genome analysis of 100 pancreatic adenocarcinomas thereby implicating several other genes, including *KDM6A, PREX2, ERBB, MET* etc. In addition, whole-genome sequencing of 456 pancreatic ductal adenocarcinomas identified 32 significantly mutated genes, which aggregated into 10 distinct molecular pathways.[14] Furthermore, work performed by the same group distinctly defined four pancreatic cancer subtypes; squamous, pancreatic progenitor, immunogenic and aberrantly differentiated endocrine exocrine. Each of these subtypes are characterised by different transcriptional networks, histopathological features and survival rates.

The development of this data offers important insight into the core mechanisms underlining pancreatic carcinogenesis and illuminating novel opportunities to target these molecular pathways.

## PRESENTATION

The manifestation of pancreatic cancer is often with non-specific symptoms such weight loss and anorexia (Box 17.2). As a result, the disease is usually at an advanced stage by the time a diagnosis is reached, and

**Box 17.2    Symptoms/signs suggestive of pancreatic neoplasm**

Early satiety
Obstructive jaundice (± pain)
Unexplained weight loss
Endoscopy-negative epigastric/back pain
Late-onset diabetes
Signs of malabsorption without defined cause

deemed surgically unresectable for approximately 80% of patients.[54] The most common symptoms for tumours in the head of the pancreas is asthenia, jaundice and abdominal pain. Tumours in the body and tail of the pancreas usually present later.[55] Less commonly, if the tumour invades surrounding structures such as the stomach or duodenum, melena and haematemesis may be reported.[56] In some cases, acute pancreatitis or new diagnosis of diabetes maybe the first sign of an underlying pancreatic neoplasm.[57] While widespread asymptomatic screening does not appear to be cost effective given the low incidence of the disease and the paucity of an affordable, sensitive and specific biomarker, there may be a role for surveillance in high-risk individuals. The relative inaccessibility of the pancreas and the inability to clearly define 'high risk' represents a major challenge in attempts to detect early cancers.[58] The classical Courvoisier's sign (palpable gallbladder with painless jaundice) occurs in less than 25% of patients. Jaundice may represent either primary disease causing biliary obstruction or external compression of the biliary system by metastatic nodal disease. Pain is a more common symptom than physicians typically appreciate, usually secondary to involvement of visceral afferent nerves or as a result of local pancreatitis. Pain on initial presentation is suggestive of unresectability. Weight loss is common, often associated with early satiety, nausea or vomiting. The latter may be caused by gastric outlet obstruction.

Virchow's node (left supraclavicular node associated with upper gastrointestinal malignancy), thrombophlebitis migrans (non-specific paraneoplastic sign named after Trousseau) and Sister Mary Joseph nodule (umbilical metastatic lesion via the falciform ligament) are well-recognised features of advanced disease. Hepatomegaly is seen in 65% of patients and may reflect hepatic metastases. Blumer's shelf (rectally palpable rectovesicle or rectovaginal mass) rarely occurs and is not usually sought as part of routine examination.

The most useful aid in making the diagnosis is a high index of suspicion. Vague epigastric symptoms and weight loss in the presence of normal endoscopy and preliminary radiology mandate further detailed investigation.

## INVESTIGATION

### SEROLOGY

Haematological and hepatic biochemical measurements are largely unhelpful in diagnosis. Many novel markers have been described over the past decade, however, none of these have yet been incorporated into routine clinical practice.[59] A mild normochromic anaemia may be present because of occult blood loss while thrombocytosis is also sometimes observed. Elevated serum bilirubin and alkaline phosphatase confirm obstructive jaundice; amylase and lipase may be elevated in those presenting with pancreatitis (5%). An elevated prothrombin time suggests hepatic dysfunction secondary to liver infiltration by metastases. Hyperglycaemia is non-specific and is seen in approximately 20% of patients and could be related to the fact that type 2 diabetes mellitus confers an increased risk of pancreatic cancer or may be the first presenting sign of the underlying cancer. Patients with malnutrition have hypoalbuminaemia and low cholesterol level.

### MARKERS

As of yet, there remains no effective tumour marker for pancreatic adenocarcinoma. The most widely used serum marker is sialylated Lewis blood group antigen on MUC-1 (Mucin 1, cell surface associated) carbohydrate antigen 19-9 (CA 19-9). It is a cell surface glycoprotein expressed by pancreatic neoplastic cells, as well as normal pancreatic and biliary duct cells, gastric, colonic, endometrial and salivary epithelia.[60] Systematic review reports that CA 19-9 has a diagnostic sensitivity ranging from 70–90% and specificity of 68–91%,[61] with 4–15% of the general population not expressing the antigen and hence do not have detectable serum CA 19-9 levels.[62] In addition, only 65% of patients with resectable pancreatic adenocarcinoma demonstrated an elevated CA 19-9, while the marker was increased in 40% of patients with chronic pancreatitis.[63] Because of these limitations, CA 19-9 is mostly used as a prognostic marker to assess response to therapy in patients already diagnosed with pancreatic cancer.[64]

Other potential markers include CA494,[65] CEACAM1 (carcinoembryonic antigen-related cell adhesion molecule 1),[66] PTHrP (parathyroid hormone-related protein),[67] TuM2-PK (tumour M2-pyruvate kinase)[68] and serum β-HCG (beta- human chorionic gonadotropin).[69] While many combinations of carbohydrate markers have been proposed to improve the specificity and sensitivity, there remains no single nor combination of antigens adopted in clinical practice, due to lack of standardisation and validation in larger cohorts.[70]

## DIAGNOSIS

### IMAGING STUDIES

Imaging studies play a crucial role in the diagnosis and staging of pancreatic cancer. Current protocol includes transabdominal ultrasound, computer tomography (CT) and magnetic resonance imaging (MRI), and is often complimented by endoscopic ultrasound (EUS), which offers the opportunity of tissue diagnosis. Transabdominal ultrasound (US) is the initial investigation in the jaundiced patient. It is superior to CT to detect cholelithiasis. Common bile duct dilatation (>7 mm, >10 mm in post-cholecystectomy patients) is an indirect sign, together with pancreatic duct dilatation (>2 mm). The primary pancreatic lesion is often visible together with hepatic metastases and ascites if present. For lesions >3 cm, US is approximately 95% sensitive; however, for lesions <1 cm sensitivity is approximately 50%.[71] Colour Doppler US has been suggested to assess vascular involvement (portal or superior mesenteric vein/ artery) by the tumour. While US remains a useful imaging modality for the initial workup of the jaundiced patient, additional imaging modalities are required to examine the pancreas and assess resectability status.

The diagnostic test of choice for suspected pancreatic lesions is multiphase multi-detector row CT with intravenous contrast. This modality is the most accurate in determining not only the primary tumour but also locoregional extension, vascular invasion, resectability and distant metastases.[72] Direct evidence of a tumour is often seen as a hypodense mass, with other subtle signs such as pancreatic atrophy, deformity of the glandular contour or double duct dilatation (common bile duct and pancreatic duct). Metastatic lesions can be detected as well as portal vein (PV) or superior mesenteric arterial involvement. For lesions >2 cm, the sensitivity is approximately 90%, decreasing to approximately 60% for smaller lesions.[73] Meta-analysis shows positive predictive value (PPV) of 81% for predicting the resectability of pancreatic cancer using contrast enhanced CT[74] (Figs. 17.2–17.6). However, despite these advances, CT-imaging is limited at detecting small liver or peritoneal metastatic deposits of occult disease.[75]

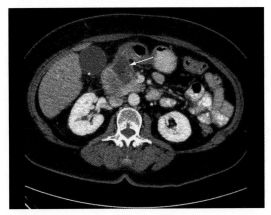

**Figure 17.2** Necrotic mass in the head of pancreas (*arrow*).

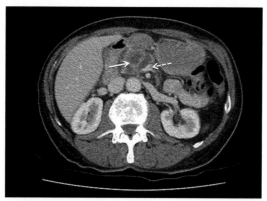

**Figure 17.3** Locally advanced borderline resectable tumour (*solid arrow*) with deformity of the superior mesenteric vein (*dashed arrow*).

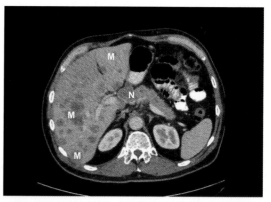

**Figure 17.5** Multiple hepatic metastases (M) from pancreatic neoplasm (N).

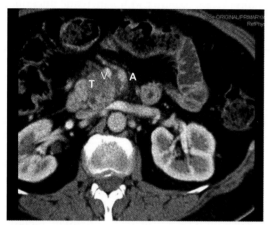

**Figure 17.4** Locally advanced unresectable tumour (T) with involvement of the superior mesenteric vein (V) and artery (A).

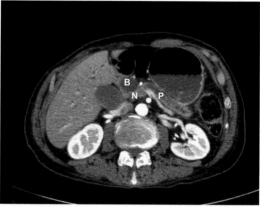

**Figure 17.6** Biliary duct (B) and pancreatic duct (P) obstruction by pancreatic neoplasm (N) denoting the double duct sign.

MRI is mainly used as an adjunct to CT for planning treatment options. The combination of T1/T2-weighted imaging and magnetic resonance cholangiopancreatography (MRCP) is useful to visualise the primary tumour and its relationship to the biliary and pancreatic ducts, as well as peripancreatic vasculature. MRI has 79% sensitivity in detecting invasive pancreatic cancer.[76]

Positron emission tomography (PET) shows accumulation of [18F]2-fluoro-2-deoxy-D-glucose (FDG) by tumour cells, and has the advantage of combining metabolic activity with imaging characteristics while imaging the whole body. Functional imaging is advantageous over CT and MRI in differentiating malignant from benign disease and detecting small lesions, as signal intensity is related to metabolic activity and uptake of the radiotracer rather than size of the lesion.[77] PET-CT scanners are able to detect small (up to 7 mm) pancreatic neoplasms and diagnose metastatic disease in about 40%.[78] PET is increasingly becoming a common method of assessing tumour response to treatment and may be prognostic. However, FDG-PET is not accurate in pancreatic disease due to its reliance on normal glucose homeostasis. The combination of PET-CT carries a sensitivity of 92%, and is superior to either modality alone.[79]

Endoscopic retrograde cholangiopancreatography (ERCP) is reserved mainly to assess obstructive intraductal lesions and to relieve biliary obstruction in selected cases. MRCP has replaced ERCP as a diagnostic modality of choice.

EUS detects lesions <2 cm with a sensitivity of 98%, however, it is costly, invasive and has substantial inter-operator variability. The sensitivity may be impaired in patients with concurrent pancreatitis.[71,80] It may help clarify benign conditions mimicking cancer, such as sclerosing pancreatitis or atypical choledocholithiasis. EUS also provides tissue diagnoses, in real time without contrast or radiation using fine-needle aspiration (FNA). There is a role for CT-guided percutaneous core needle biopsy for patients with indeterminate or inconclusive histology following EUS-guided FNA.[81]

## CYTOLOGY/HISTOLOGY

Multi-detector cross-sectional CT is the radiological modality of choice in the staging and diagnosis of pancreatic cancer. In selected cases, histological confirmation of malignancy may not be established before surgery. However, in patients selected for neoadjuvant therapy, histological confirmation is essential via FNA by EUS/ERCP or percutaneously by CT-guidance.

## ADVANCED STAGING TECHNIQUES

### LAPAROSCOPY

Despite advances in non-invasive imaging, laparoscopic staging and ultrasound have a role in selected cases. The routine use of diagnostic laparoscopy remains controversial and institution dependent. Contrast-enhanced CT accurately predicts resectability in approximately 75% of cases but for the remainder, occult metastatic diseases such as hepatic or peritoneal metastases, may not be evident. Laparoscopy is a minimally invasive modality for staging patients at high risk of unresectable disease, despite favourable CT imaging.[82] Laparoscopy can be performed immediately before conversion to laparotomy or as an interval staging measure. However, laparoscopic ultrasonography can potentially identify radiographically occult metastatic disease and hence obviate the need for non-curative laparotomies. It enables direct visualisation of intra-abdominal organs and can detect metastatic deposits <3 mm on peritoneal and hepatic structures, thereby offering more accurate disease staging (Figs. 17.7 and 17.8). Indeed despite the improvement of radiological staging investigations in recent years, current literature suggests that up to 30% of patients undergo a non-therapeutic laparotomy in the setting of advanced pancreatic cancer.[83]

A recent meta-analysis concluded that diagnostic laparoscopy with biopsy of suspected lesions before definitive laparotomy avoided non-curative laparotomies in 21% of cases, all of which were deemed resectable by CT imaging.[84] Detractors of laparoscopy argue that a significant proportion of patients require (open) surgical bypass and therefore laparoscopic staging should only be used if bypass would not be contemplated at open surgery.[85] Indications for staging laparoscopy include tumour size >3 cm, markedly elevated CA 19.9, indeterminate metastatic disease on imaging, and in the pre-operative staging of patients with borderline resectable pancreatic cancer.[86] Evidence from single-centre studies suggests that the need for subsequent operative palliation for established gastric outlet obstruction is less than 5%.[87] Moreover, less invasive options are now available for managing malignant gastric outlet obstruction such as endoscopic stenting and laparoscopic gastroenterostomy. A small randomised study of 24 patients comparing open versus laparoscopic gastroenterostomy concluded that the laparoscopic approach was associated with significantly less intra-operative blood loss, shorter time to oral solid food intake and less delayed gastric emptying.[88] Gurusamy et al. performed a meta-analysis to address the need for prophylactic gastrojejunostomy in patients with unresectable periampullary cancers (pancreatic cancer made up 92.1% of cases) and reported that prophylactic gastrojejunostomy was associated with a statistically significant lower risk of gastric outlet obstruction compared to controls.[89] However, there was no difference in quality of life between the two groups. The authors went on to recommend routine prophylactic gastroenterostomy in patients with unresectable disease (with or without hepatico-jejunostomy). However, it is important to mention that both trials included in this meta-analysis were associated with a high risk of bias and that all patients underwent exploratory laparotomy. Therefore, the results are not applicable to patients with unresectable disease diagnosed during staging laparoscopy.

General laparoscopy is performed with an angled (usually 30 degrees) lens looking for small-volume peritoneal and liver metastases. The liver is examined systematically and usually all but segment 7 can be viewed. Biopsy of

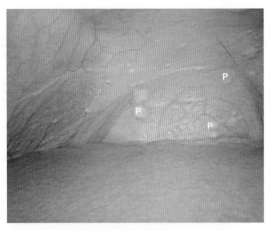

**Figure 17.7**  Staging laparoscopy demonstrating peritoneal metastases (P).

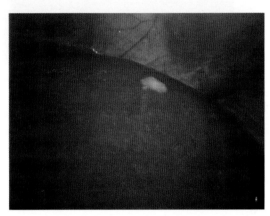

**Figure 17.8**  Staging laparoscopy demonstrating a liver metastasis.

hepatic or peritoneal deposits for frozen-section histology is taken, and the procedure is terminated if positive. If metastases are not seen, the hepatico-duodenal ligament is inspected for nodal disease. The lesser sac is opened by incising the gastrocolic omentum to inspect for tumour, and biopsies of the primary may be undertaken. This is achievable in 80% of cases. In certain institutions, the duodenum is mobilised, but this is unnecessary in the majority of cases. With more effective neoadjuvant regimens, it is important to use laparoscopic strategies to define patients who may be suitable for downstaging, similar to advanced rectal lesions.

Laparoscopic ultrasound has been advocated as an additional aid to detect intra-hepatic metastases, lymph node or vascular involvement to determine resectability (Fig. 17.9). A systematic review showed that staging laparoscopy with ultrasound correctly predicted resectablity in 79% of patients compared to 55% when using standard imaging, and prevented non-curative laparotomies in 33%.[90]

The role of peritoneal cytology taken during laparoscopic staging is less well defined, although it may improve staging accuracy. Recently, Oh et al. found that 14% of patients who would otherwise be classified as having potentially resectable disease had positive peritoneal cytology during routine staging laparoscopy and were subsequently upstaged to stage IV disease.[91] Moreover, most patients (86%) with positive cytology experienced disease progression after chemotherapy/chemoradiotherapy and their 5-year survival was zero.

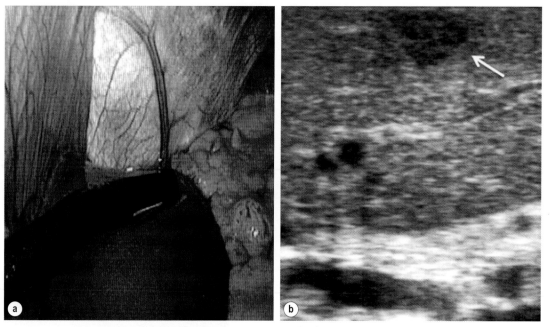

**Figure 17.9**  **(a)** Laparoscopic ultrasonography, and **(b)** liver metastasis (*white arrow*).

## PATHOLOGY

Ductal adenocarcinomas account for >85% of all pancreatic neoplasms. Other types of malignant tumours include the following:

- adenosquamous carcinoma
- mucinous non-cystic (colloid) carcinoma
- MCNs
- IPMN with an associated invasive carcinoma
- solid pseudopapillary neoplasm
- acinar cell carcinoma
- pancreatoblastoma
- serous cystadenocarcinoma
- undifferentiated (anaplastic) carcinoma
- signet-ring cell carcinoma
- giant cell carcinoma

## TREATMENT

Treatment strategies should be discussed at a multidisciplinary level, with emphasis on established guidelines. The American Joint Committee on Cancer TNM staging is outlined in Table 17.1.

Fig. 17.10 outlines the authors' current treatment algorithm for patients with pancreatic cancer.

Surgical treatment remains the only potential cure for pancreatic cancer, yet patient selection remains paramount.

In patients with obstructive jaundice and surgically resectable disease, the use of pre-operative biliary drainage is a topic of ongoing debate. Proponents of decompression argue that jaundiced patients undergoing surgery are at increased risk of peri-operative sepsis, pancreatic fistula and wound infections.[92] While detractors argue that routine biliary drainage is itself associated with an increased risk of procedure-specific complications such as cholangitis, pancreatitis and stent-related perforations.[93] A recent meta-analysis reported that patients who underwent internal pre-operative biliary drainage sustained statistically fewer major adverse events compared to those who had surgery only.[94] A recent retrospective cohort study showed increased risk of delayed gastric emptying post-pancreatoduodenectomy in patient who underwent pre-operative biliary drainage.[95] The authors' practice is not to decompress the bile duct pre-operatively unless symptoms and signs of cholangitis or secondary signs of hyperbilirubinaemia are present. If a neoadjuvant approach is being considered, biliary stenting is required before commencing chemo/radiotherapy. Coagulopathy, if present, is treated with vitamin K, before resection.

Patient selection is key, including cardiovascular and respiratory evaluation. Curative surgery is associated with a median survival of 11–23 months, with approximately 10–27% alive at 5 years.[96] Previously, pancreatic resections were associated with significant mortality; however, with advances in peri-operative supportive care, mortality rates are now <5% in high-volume centres.[97]

## PANCREATICO-DUODENECTOMY

Pancreatico-duodenectomy was first described by Kausch in 1912, and later popularised by Whipple in 1935. The classical Whipple procedure (two-stage) was an en bloc resection of the pancreatic head, duodenum, common bile duct, with the distal stomach and surrounding lymph nodes. Later being performed as a one-stage operation, it still remains the surgical therapy for tumours of the pancreatic head and neck.

The right colon is mobilised, exposing the third and fourth parts of the duodenum, and an extended Kocherisation is performed. This allows a tumour in the head of the pancreas to be palpated and exposes the left renal vein. The aortocaval and PV nodal packages are dissected, and the respective vessels are skeletonised. Resectability is finally assessed as extensive involvement of the confluence of the PV/superior mesenteric vein (SMV) may herald termination of the procedure. It is important to remember that short segments of the PV can be resected if necessary, and therefore an involved PV does not necessarily denote unresectability.

**Table 17.1    American Joint Committee on Cancer (AJCC) for pancreatic cancer, eighth edition**

| Primary tumour (T) | | Regional lymph nodes (N) | | Distant metastases (M) |
|---|---|---|---|---|
| T1 Maximum tumour diameter ≤2 cm | N0 | No regional lymph node metastasis | | M0 No distant metastasis |
| T2 Maximum tumour diameter >2 cm but ≤4 cm | N1 | Metastasis in 1-3 regional lymph nodes | | M1 Distant metastasis |
| T3 Maximum tumour diameter >4 cm | *N2* | Metastasis in ≥4 regional lymph nodes | | |
| T4 Tumour involves the celiac axis or the superior mesenteric artery (unresectable primary tumour) | | | | |
| Stage | | | | |
| Stage IA | T1 | N0 | M0 | |
| Stage IB | T2 | N0 | M0 | |
| Stage 2A | T3 | N0 | M0 | |
| Stage 2B | T1-T3 | N1 | M0 | |
| Stage 3 | Any T | N2 | M0 | |
| | T4 | Any N | | |
| Stage 4 | Any T | Any N | M1 | |

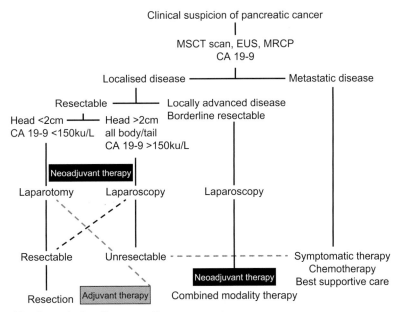

**Figure 17.10**    Treatment algorithm for patients with pancreatic cancer.

✔ The relationship of the tumour to the first jejunal branch of the SMV is often the critical determinant of resectability. If this is involved by tumour, the likelihood of successful reconstruction and R0 resection is low.

The remaining porta hepatis is dissected, and nodes are cleared. Cholecystectomy facilitates higher ligation of the bile duct, which is transected just proximal to the insertion of the cystic duct. It is the authors' practice to send a biliary aspirate for routine culture and sensitivity, as post-operative infective complications tend to involve enteric organisms.[98]

The common bile duct is mobilised distally and the hepatico-duodenal ligament is dissected along its length, taking care to identify and preserve the common hepatic artery and PV. The gastroduodenal artery is ligated while care is taken not to damage an aberrant right hepatic artery.

In a conventional Whipple, the distal stomach is resected. This is the authors' favoured approach as resection includes the nodes along the greater and lesser curves, reduces stomach-emptying dysfunction post-operatively, diminishes the density of parietal cells and theoretically reduces the risk of gastritis. The stomach is transected at the antrum along with the attached omentum. The proximal jejunum along with its mesentery is transected and the mobilised duodenum and jejunum is delivered back under the ligament of Treitz.

The pancreas is transected between four stay sutures (to facilitate haemostasis in the marginal arteries) after the uncinate process has been dissected from the superior mesenteric vessels. Retroperitoneal dissection allows the tumour and nodal package to be delivered en bloc. If any doubt exists regarding the adequacy of tumour clearance, the pancreatic resection margin should be sent for frozen section histology. Verbeke and Menon had shown that a discrepancy between margin status and clinical outcome is caused by frequent under-reporting of microscopic margin involvement.[99]

The lack of a standardised pathological examination, with confusing nomenclature and controversy regarding the definition of microscopic margin involvement, results in the wide variation of reported R1 rates (between 18% and 85%).[100] A recent meta-analysis showed that intra-operative margin clearance of the pancreatic neck was associated with improved overall survival for patients undergoing pancreatico-duodenectomy for pancreatic cancer. The survival benefit was even higher in patients with en bloc R0-resections compared to patients who either require intra-operative margin revisions or who have incomplete resections.[101]

Reconstruction is undertaken with the biliary anastomosis followed by the pancreatic and finally the gastric. Pancreatico-jejunostomy and pancreatico-gastrostomy are the most commonly used techniques for pancreatico-enteric reconstruction. A recent meta-analysis reported statistically significantly fewer rates of pancreatic fistula and intra-abdominal fluid collections after pancreatico-gastrostomy, with no significant differences in overall morbidity, mortality or length of hospital stay.

The nature of the pancreatic reconstruction is subject to individual variation. The authors favour a two-layered pancreatico-jejunal anastomosis with mucosa-to-mucosa reconstruction. Choledocho-jejunostomy is performed in a similar end-to-side manner, leaving the gastrojejunostomy until the end. Abdominal drains are not routinely placed.[102]

Morbidity following resection varies, with the majority of complications being minor. The most significant cause of morbidity is development of a pancreatic fistula, observed in 7–18% of cases.[103,104]

Most complications can be dealt with either conservatively or using drains placed by interventional radiology. A minority (<5%) of cases requires re-laparotomy.

## PYLORUS-PRESERVING PANCREATICO-DUODENECTOMY

Many centres recommend a pylorus-preserving pancreatico-duodenectomy (PPPDR) approach, first described by Watson in 1942. It is postulated to retain a functioning pylorus with an intact neurovascular supply, thereby ensuring good gastrointestinal function and diminishing nutritive, dumping and bile reflux sequelae.[105] A recent meta-analysis from Buchler's group showed no significant differences in overall survival, post-operative morbidity or mortality between PPPDR and a classical Whipple; however, the latter procedure was associated with significantly less delayed gastric emptying (DGE), whereas PPPDR resulted in significantly less operating time, intra-operative blood loss and red cell transfusions.[106] While pylorus preserving pancreatico-duodenectomy may offer modest advantages in the initial post-operative period, this did not translate in a long-term survival benefit or improved quality of life in comparison to standard pancreatico-duodenectomy.[107]

PPPDR dictates conventional mobilisation to the point where the stomach requires transection; the right gastric artery is preserved, and the duodenum is transected at least 2 cm distal to the pylorus. Reconstruction is usually accomplished by duodenojejunostomy or gastrojejunostomy.

Subtotal stomach-preserving pancreatico-duodenectomy (SSPPD) is a relatively novel technique developed in an attempt to decrease the incidence of DGE.[108] This is the authors' preferred technique. It involves division of the stomach 2–3cm proximal to the pyloric ring such that >90% of the stomach is preserved. In a meta-analysis comparing SSPPD and PPPDR, comprised of 650 patients, Huang et al. demonstrated that SSPPD was associated with a significantly lower rate of DGE but more intra-operative blood loss.[109] However, there were no differences in mortality, pancreatic fistula or intra-abdominal abscess rates between the two techniques. Nakamura et al. went one step further and compared rates of DGE between an antecolic side-to-side gastric greater curvature-to-jejunal anastomosis and a similar antecolic but end-to-side gastric stump-to-jejunal anastomosis in all patients undergoing SSPPD.[110] They showed that the former technique was associated with a significantly reduced rate of DGE, but similar overall morbidity compared to the end-to-side technique.

## EXTENDED LYMPH NODE AND VASCULAR DISSECTION

It is the authors' practice to perform extended dissection including aortocaval nodal clearance in the majority of cases. At presentation, most tumours have involvement of lymph nodes beyond the gland, and we believe that clearance of the left gastric and aortocaval nodes not only increases the specificity of staging and the resultant predicted prognosis but also the likelihood of a negative surgical margin. However, a recent meta-analysis examining previously published randomised trials failed to demonstrate improved overall survival with extended lymphadenectomy compared to standard dissection.[111] Moreover, extended dissection was associated with significantly worse post-operative morbidity. A recent meta-analysis showed no survival impact with extended lymph node dissection in comparison to standard lymph node dissection, however, it showed longer operating times with greater blood loss in the extended lymph node dissection group.[112]

✓ While an extended lymphadenectomy compared to a standard resection improves nodal yield, it is associated with increased operative time and blood loss without an impact on survival.[112]

The role of extensive vascular resection is very much an area of ongoing interest as the boundary of resectability for pancreatic cancer is continuously being pushed forward in an attempt to improve curability rates in patients who would otherwise be deemed unresectable. In a meta-analysis conducted by Zhou et al. comparing SMV/PV resection versus no resection in patients undergoing pancreatico-duodenectomy, there was no difference in post-operative morbidity or mortality between the two groups.[113] Furthermore, the 5-year overall survival rate was not significantly different between the two groups (12.3% in the vascular resection vs. 17% in the no resection group); translating into better outcomes compared to strict palliative therapy. On the other hand, arterial resections may be indicated in selected patients, despite being associated with increased peri-operative mortality compared to those without arterial resections.[114] A recent systematic review showed no statistically significant difference between the arterial resection and standard surgery group despite an overall increased mortality rate in group with arterial resection. This study also showed lower long-term survival rates in patients with arterial resection in comparison to standard resection. Patient selection and careful planning is paramount.[115]

## DISTAL PANCREATECTOMY

Distal pancreatectomy is the procedure of choice for tumours of the body and tail of the pancreas. The pancreatic neck is dissected from the PV and the splenic flexure of the colon is taken down. In the majority of ductal cancers, the spleen is also resected to achieve an en bloc clearance. Splenic preservation is generally limited to patients with benign or borderline neoplasms. Patients undergoing distal pancreatectomy and splenic resection are vaccinated prophylactically pre-operatively against encapsulated organisms such as *Haemophilus influenza* B, *Neisseria meningitidis* and *Streptococcus pneumoniae*.

## LAPAROSCOPIC PANCREATECTOMY

Laparoscopic pancreatectomy remains one of the most challenging minimally invasive abdominal operations to date. Accumulating evidence shows that laparoscopic pancreatico-duodenectomy is safe and feasible.[116] It has been shown to be associated with similar overall survival rates but significantly lower wound infection and pancreatic fistula rates, and reduced hospital stay, compared to the classic open approach.[117] Laparoscopic distal pancreatic resection is currently the most frequently performed minimally invasive pancreatic procedure, associated with decreased blood loss and reduced length of stay, as well as lower rates of wound infections and similar oncological outcomes.[118–120] The Memorial Sloan-Kettering Cancer Center group published their experience of distal pancreatectomy using open, laparoscopic or robotic approaches.[121] There were no significant differences in 90-day morbidity and mortality, or pancreatic fistula rates, or oncological outcomes between the three groups; however, the open group was associated with significantly more intra-operative blood loss. The LEOPARD randomised controlled trial showed that there was less intra-operative blood loss and a lower rate of delayed gastric emptying associated with laparoscopic distal pancreatectomy. However, longer operations were observed in minimally invasive distal pancreatectomy.[122] A recent review by Kocaay et al. concluded that laparoscopic pancreatic surgery remained a reasonable treatment modality for low-grade malignant tumours when performed by skilled surgeons in high-volume centres.[123] A recent meta-analysis suggested that laparoscopic pancreatico-duodenectomy is as safe and effective, both oncologically and surgically, as open pancreatico-duodenectomy.[124] A recent systematic review and meta-analysis of randomised controlled trials showed that there were no significant advantages of laparoscopic pancreatico-duodenectomy in comparison to open pancreatico-duodenectomy.[125] Further research into its oncological safety and long-term outcomes is needed before it can be firmly established as first-line treatment.

Robotic pancreatectomy is the most recent development in minimally invasive surgery and a recent meta-analysis suggested that it may be associated with reduced intra-operative bleeding, improved spleen preserving rate and an accelerated post-operative recovery, however, it is significantly more costly with no proven difference in oncological outcomes to date.[126]

## TOTAL PANCREATECTOMY

Some suggest that pancreatic cancer is a multicentric disease and therefore advocate total pancreatectomy. It was initially proposed to avoid the risk of pancreatico-enteric leaks and to remove potential undetected synchronous disease in other parts of the gland. Although total pancreatectomy can be carried out safely, the survival benefit is so dismal, it questions the indication for the operation.

## CENTRAL PANCREATECTOMY

The role of central pancreatectomy is rare and limited due to a narrow spectrum of indications. The procedure is historically reserved for patients with chronic pancreatitis and traumatic injuries. More recently, it has been advocated for use in lesions of the pancreatic neck. Opponents of this technique argue against higher rates of pancreatic anastomotic leakage whilst those in favour say it offers preserved functional elements (endocrine and exocrine) of the pancreas.[127]

## SURGICAL PALLIATION

### OBSTRUCTIVE JAUNDICE
In the majority of cases, biliary obstruction can be adequately relieved by endoscopic measures. However, in selected cases, surgical palliation may be required. Cholecysto-jejunostomy may be performed in cases where the cystic duct is patent and the tumour is not within 1 cm of the cystic duct. Alternatively, choledocho-jejunostomy may be used, which has equivalent outcomes.

## UPPER GASTROINTESTINAL TRACT OUTFLOW OBSTRUCTION

Gastric and duodenal outlet obstruction are said to occur in up to 20% of cases. Once jaundice has been addressed, persistent nausea and vomiting should raise the suspicion of underlying gastrointestinal obstruction. If biliary obstruction is being dealt with at open operation, prophylactic duodenal bypass should be considered. Laparoscopic gastro-jejunostomy has become the management of choice when warranted. Whilst endoluminal stenting is associated with more favourable short-term results, gastrojejunostomy may be a better treatment option in those with a predicted prolonged survival.

## ADJUVANT THERAPIES

Whilst surgical treatment is undertaken with curative intent, nonetheless the 5-year survival rate remains disappointingly low. There is evidence to support the use of chemotherapy as adjuvant therapy after curative resection for pancreatic adenocarcinoma. Randomised control trials such as ES-PAC-3[128] and CONKO-001[129] demonstrate improved survival compared with observation alone.

In terms of chemotherapy alone as an adjuvant therapy, the results of the European Study Group for Pancreatic Cancer 4 (ESPAC-4) showed promising results primarily in relation to gemcitabine plus capecitabine. Neoptolemos et al.[130] presented the results of the ESPAC-4 trial, which randomised 730 patients following surgery to either adjuvant gemcitabine ($n = 366$) or gemcitabine plus capecitabine ($n = 364$). The latter regimen resulted in a statistically significant increase in median overall survival (28.0 vs. 25.5 months, $P = 0.032$).

✓ Adjuvant therapy following resection with gemcitabine and capecitabine is associated with improved overall survival compared to gemcitabine monotherapy alone.[128]

More recently, there have been significant results established by the multicenter, randomised PRODIGE24/CCTGPA.6 French-Canadian trial comparing adjuvant modified FOLFIRINOX to gemcitabine monotherapy. Within the trial, 493 patients with macroscopically resected pancreatic ductal adenocarcinoma who were less than 80 years old were randomised to either modified FOLFIRINOX given every 2 weeks or gemcitabine monotherapy given every 4 weeks (days 1, 15 and 18) for a period of 24 weeks.[131] At a median follow-up of 33.6 months, the median disease-free survival was 21.6 months in the modified FOLFIRINOX group and 12.8 months in the gemcitabine group (stratified hazard ratio for cancer-related event, second cancer, or death, 0.58; 95% CI, 0.46–0.73; $P < 0.001$). The disease-free survival rate at 3 years was 39.7% in the modified FOLFIRINOX group and 21.4% in the gemcitabine group. The median overall survival was 54.4 months in the modified-FOLFIRINOX group and 35.0 months in the gemcitabine group (stratified hazard ratio for death, 0.64; 95% CI, 0.48–0.86; $P = 0.003$). The overall survival rate at 3 years was 63.4% in the modified FOLFIRINOX group and 48.6% in the gemcitabine group. Of note, grade 3/4 toxicities occurred in 75.9% of patients receiving modified FOLFIRINOX compared to 52.9% of those who received gemcitabine. These results were very promising, offering a new standard of care for pancreatic patients.

In comparison to chemotherapy, the role of adjuvant chemoradiotherapy is less clear with conflicting results from various trials. The Gastrointestinal Study Group (1) showed a survival benefit with 5-fluorouracyl and radiotherapy, albeit with a small sample size ($n = 43$) whilst the European Organisation of Research and Treatment of Cancer trial 116 failed to show a statistically significant survival benefit for those treated with adjuvant chemoradiation compared with an observation group. The mainstay of adjuvant treatment is chemotherapy.[132]

Adjuvant chemotherapy has played a pivotal role in improving outcomes, but overall survival rates remain far from optimal. More research is needed to discover the optimal therapeutic regime but recent developments and trials are promising.

## NEOADJUVANT THERAPY

The National Cancer Control Network guidelines list indications for neoadjuvant chemoradiotherapy, which include locally advanced or borderline resectable disease, in an attempt to downstage the disease and allow for subsequent resection. Theoretical advantages include delivery of chemotherapy and/or radiotherapy to well-oxygenated tissue, and hence early treatment of micrometastatic disease. Detractors of neoadjuvant therapy argue that the resultant delay in surgery may result in disease progression; however, this is difficult to prove. In a recent retrospective study consisting of 575 patients, Hackert et al. showed that neoadjuvant therapy with Folfirinox was associated with the highest resection rates (61%), compared to gemcitabine and radiation (46%) and other treatments (52%).[133]

✓ Neoadjuvant therapy for patients with borderline resectable disease improves the R0 resectability rate.[133]

Several studies have evaluated the use of neoadjuvant therapy in resectable pancreatic adenocarcinoma. In the retrospective study by Mirkin et al., comprising patients with resectable (clinical stages I–III) pancreatic cancer from the National Cancer Database, more than 1700 patients who underwent neoadjuvant therapy were compared to 6706 patients who were treated with surgical resection alone, and nearly 10 000 patients treated with surgery followed by adjuvant therapy.[134] Within the neoadjuvant cohort, 22% received chemotherapy only, 8.5% radiotherapy only and the rest received both treatment modalities. While neoadjuvant therapy was associated with similar median survival to adjuvant therapy in stage I disease, it resulted in significantly improved survival compared to both surgery and adjuvant therapy in stage III disease. These findings were corroborated by Mokdad et al., who showed that neoadjuvant treatment followed by surgery in early stage, resectable pancreatic cancer is associated with improved survival, compared to upfront surgery.[135] Moreover, patients who underwent surgery alone had significantly higher T stage, number of positive lymph nodes and positive resection margins. The Dutch Randomized Phase III PREOPANC trial demonstrated that pre-operative chemoradiotherapy for resectable or borderline resectable pancreatic cancer did not show a significant overall survival benefit.[136]

✓ In patients with resectable disease the use of neoadjuvant chemotherapy with or without radiation therapy appears to improve survival.[135]

## FUTURE AREAS OF INTEREST

Over the last decade, there has been significant improvement in the diagnosis and management of pancreatic adenocarcinoma due to advances in both imaging modalities and the widespread utilisation of minimally invasive surgery. However, overall mortality rates remain unsatisfactory. The need for earlier identification of patients most at risk of developing this disease and a better understanding of whole genomic sequencing, may contribute to earlier detection and survival outcomes. The role of nuclear medicine is expanding and its role in defining tumour characteristics at molecular level and also distinguishing neoplastic and inflammatory masses appears promising.

The role of neoadjuvant therapies in resectable pancreatic cancer has been limited to date, due to insufficient data to support its benefit. More recently, the survival benefit in both neoadjuvant and adjuvant settings has been accepted. Despite active research, there is not a unified approach and various regimens exist and vary according to institution. Further development of novel drug therapies and identification of optimal regimens may revolutionise the management of pancreatic adenocarcinoma going forward.

Minimally invasive surgery including laparoscopy and more recently robotic surgery have changed practice globally. Currently, robotic surgery is not yet accessible in all centres and there remains controversy about the learning curve, technical approaches, cost effectiveness and general feasibility. There are few high-quality comparative randomised control trials, however, as robotic surgery expands globally and further research emerges, the surgical management of pancreatic cancer may be transformed.

✅ Both robotic and laparoscopic distal pancreatectomy are safe and feasible. The robotic procedure has an improved splenic preservation rate but appears to be more costly.[126]

## Key Points

- Pancreatic adenocarcinoma is the seventh leading cause of cancer deaths globally
- Majority of cases are unresectable at the time of diagnosis
- Overall 5-year survival is less than 20%
- Screening is recommended for the following: patients from a familial pancreatic cancer kindred with ≥2 affected first-degree relatives, patients with Peutz–Jeghers' syndrome and p16, BRCA2 and HNPCC mutation carriers with ≥1 affected first-degree relative
- Multiphase multi-detector row CT with intravenous contrast is the radiological modality of choice
- Laparoscopic staging has a role in selected patients
- Neoadjuvant therapy followed by surgery is associated with improved survival compared to surgery
- Robotic surgery is an emerging field in pancreatic cancer surgery

 References available at http://ebooks.health.elsevier.com/

## KEY REFERENCE

[3] Bengtsson, A., Andersson, R., & Ansari, D. (2020). The actual 5-year survivors of pancreatic ductal adenocarcinoma based on real-world data. *Sci Rep*, *10*(1), 16425.
*This study indicates that actual 5 year survival is less than 5% despite an increase in survival for the subset of patient undergoing surgical resection.*

[8] Rawla, P., Sunkara, T., & Gaduputi, V. (2019). Epidemiology of pancreatic cancer: global trends, etiology and risk factors. *World J Oncol*, *10*(1), 10–27.
*This paper explores incidence, survival and risk factors.*

[44] Basturk, O., Hong, S. M., Wood, L. D., Adsay, N. V., Albores-Saavedra, J., Biankin, A. V., et al. (2015). A revised classification system and recommendations from the Baltimore consensus meeting for neoplastic precursor lesions in the pancreas. *Am J Surg Pathol*, *39*(12), 1730–1741.
*A two-tiered classification system (low versus high- grade dysplasia) was proposed for all pancreatic precursor lesions. Low-grade dysplastic lesions include PanIN-1 and PanIN-2, whereas high-grade lesions include PanIN-3 or carcinoma in situ.*

[34] Permuth-Wey, J., & Egan, K. M. (2009). Family history is a significant risk factor for pancreatic cancer: results from a systematic review and meta-analysis. *Fam Cancer*, *8*(2), 109–117.
*This paper explores family history as a significant risk factor for pancreatic cancer.*

[74] Somers, I., & Bipat, S. (2017). Contrast-enhanced CT in determining resectability in patients with pancreatic carcinoma: a meta-analysis of the positive predictive values of CT. *Eur Radiol*, *27*(8), 3408–3435.
*This meta-analysis describes use of CT in predicting resectability of pancreatic cancer.*

[83] Earley, H. S., Tewatia, V., & Conlon, K. C. (2021). The Role of Laparoscopic Staging in Pancreatic Cancer. In K. Søreide, & S. Stättner (Eds.), *Textbook of Pancreatic Cancer*. Cham: Springer. https://doi.org/10.1007/978-3-030-53786-9_52.
*This study determines the value of staging laparoscopy in potentially resectable disease.*

[94] Moole, H., Bechtold, M., & Puli, S. R. (2016). Efficacy of preoperative biliary drainage in malignant obstructive jaundice: a meta-analysis and systematic review. *World J Surg Oncol*, *14*(1), 182 PMID: 27400651.
*Preoperative biliary drainage was associated with fewer major adverse events compared to direct surgery, in patients with malignant obstructive jaundice undergoing surgery. No significant differences were observed in mortality or length of hospital stay between the two groups.*

[106] Huttner, F. J., Fitzmaurice, C., Schwarzer, G., et al. (2016). Pylorus-preserving pancreaticoduodenectomy (pp Whipple) versus pancreaticoduodenectomy (classic Whipple) for surgical treatment of periampullary and pancreatic carcinoma. *Cochrane Database Syst Rev*, 2, CD006053 PMID: 26905229.
*There were no significant differences in postoperative morbidity, mortality or overall survival between the two techniques. However, pylorus-preserving pancreatico-duodenectomy was associated with significantly less operative time, less blood loss and less red cell transfusion but higher incidences of delayed gastric emptying.*

[111] Dasari, B. V., Pasquali, S., Vohra, R. S., et al. (2015). Extended versus standard lymphadenectomy for pancreatic head cancer: meta-analysis of randomized controlled trials. *J Gastrointest Surg*, *19*(9), 1725–1732 PMID: 26055135.
*Extended lymphadenectomy was associated with significantly worse postoperative morbidity compared to standard lymph node harvest. There were no significant differences in 30-day mortality, length of hospital stay or overall survival between the two groups.*

[122] de Rooij, T., van Hilst, J., van Santvoort, H., Boerma, D., van den Boezem, P., Daams, F., et al. (2019). Minimally invasive versus open distal pancreatectomy (LEOPARD): a multicenter patient-blinded randomized controlled trial. *Ann Surg*, *269*(1), 2–9.
*While minimally invasive approach was associated with faster functional recovery, the overall rate of complications was not reduced when compared to open surgery.*

[132] Klaiber, U., Hackert, T., & Neoptolemos, J. P. (2019). Adjuvant treatment for pancreatic cancer. *Transl Gastroenterol Hepatol*, 4, 27.
*This paper reviews adjuvant therapy for pancreatic cancer. Poly-agent chemotherapy significantly prolongs overall survival after resection.*

[136] Versteijne, E., Suker, M., Groothuis, K., Akkermans-Vogelaar, J. M., Besselink, M. G., Bonsing, B. A., et al. (2020). Preoperative chemoradiotherapy versus immediate surgery for resectable and borderline resectable pancreatic cancer: results of the Dutch randomized phase III PREOPANC trial. *J Clin Oncol*, *38*(16), 1763–1773.
*The addition of Neoadjuvant chemoradiotherapy improves overall survival compare to those undergoing upfront surgery and adjuvant therapy.*

# 18 Cystic and neuroendocrine neoplasms of the pancreas

Andrew J. Healey | Ashley Clift | Andrea Frilling

## INTRODUCTION

Although pancreatic ductal adenocarcinoma accounts for the majority of pancreatic neoplasms, over the last three decades there has been increasing recognition of cystic and neuroendocrine pancreatic neoplasms.[1] The aim of this chapter is to examine these tumours in more detail, with particular emphasis on intraductal papillary mucinous neoplasms (IPMN) and pancreatic neuroendocrine neoplasms (PanNEN). Where possible, evidence-based recommendations for the investigation and management of these tumours will be provided.

## PANCREATIC CYSTIC NEOPLASMS

The prevalence of pancreatic cystic neoplasms (PCNs) in the general population ranges from 2.6–18% and 37% in those >80 years old.[2,3] PCNs represent different biological entities with variable potential for malignant transformation. The quality of modern cross-sectional imaging means that many are diagnosed incidentally (i.e., in asymptomatic patients). The reported prevalence of PCNs in computed tomography (CT) is 2.1–2.6%[4] and for magnetic resonance imaging (MRI) this is 13.5–45%.[5] Table 18.1 shows the World Health Organisation (WHO) Histological Classification of Pancreatic Cystic Tumours, (2010, revised 2020).[6]

The challenge facing all pancreatic specialists is in establishing the histological diagnosis of the cyst without exposing the patient to unnecessary surgical intervention, whilst ensuring close surveillance of correctly identified pre-malignant lesions and appropriate timing of treatment thereafter.

## DIAGNOSIS

### RADIOLOGY

The reporting accuracy for identifying specific types of PCNs is 40–95% for magnetic resonance cholangiopancreatography (MRCP)/MRI and 40–81% for CT.[7,8] Although CT and MR have comparable ability to characterise PCNs, MRI is superior in determining whether a cyst communicates with the pancreatic ductal system and internal structure: specifically the presence of nodularity and/or septations.[7,8] Furthermore, in patients who may require extensive surveillance, there is no associated ionising radiation exposure. CT is however, superior in patients in whom pancreatic parenchymal calcification is suspected, detailed vascular anatomy mapping is required, or in whom staging of suspected malignancy is required.

### ENDOSCOPY

Endoscopic ultrasound (EUS) is an important diagnostic adjunct to cross-sectional imaging in the assessment of PCNs. It is recommended in patients in whom imaging has identified worrisome features and surgical resection is being considered. Evidence for EUS-based differentiation between benign and malignant cysts remains mixed, but there is good evidence that the use of contrast-enhanced EUS helps identify hyper-enhancing mural nodules within cysts and that this is reproducible with increased inter-observer agreement.[9,10]

### CYST SAMPLING

Fine needle aspiration (FNA) of cyst fluid for carcinoembryonic antigen (CEA) can help in differentiating between mucinous and non-mucinous PCNs. Gillis et al. performed a meta-analysis demonstrating a 42% sensitivity but 99% specificity in differentiating between mucinous and non-mucinous cysts in 1115 patients.[11] These results have been replicated elsewhere using a cut off level of CEA level of >192 ng/L.[12] More specific cyst identification (i.e., mucinous cystic neoplasms [MCN] versus IPMN) has not yet been possible with fluid sampling alone for CEA,[13] but there are promising data regarding when fluid is assessed for *KRAS/GNAS* mutation analysis. In the same meta-analysis, Gillis et al. demonstrated that the combined sensitivity and specificity of cytology and *KRAS* was 0.71 and 0.88, respectively.[11]

## INTRADUCTAL PAPILLARY MUCINOUS NEOPLASMS

IPMN are defined as grossly visible, mucin-producing epithelial neoplasms of the pancreas. There are three types: main duct (MD-IPMN), branch duct (BD-IPMN) and mixed type. Main duct IPMN is characterised by segmental or diffuse dilation of the main pancreatic duct (MPD) of >5 mm without other causes of obstruction. BD-IPMN are pancreatic cysts >5 mm in diameter that communicate with the main duct. Mixed type meet the criteria for both, and a pancreatic pseudocyst is among the differential diagnoses for those patients with BD-IPMN in whom there is a history of pancreatitis. They are distinguished from MCNs by the absence of ovarian-type stroma.[14]

**Table 18.1   The WHO version 4 (2010) classification of pancreatic cystic neoplasms**

| Type | Histological classification |
|---|---|
| Benign | Acinar cell cystadenoma |
| | Serous cystadenoma |
| Premalignant | Intraductal papillary mucinous neoplasms (IPMN) |
| | Intraductal tubulopapillary neoplasms |
| | Mucinous cystic neoplasms (MCN) |
| Malignant | Acinar cell cystadenocarcinoma |
| | IPMN with an associated invasive carcinoma |
| | MCN with an associated invasive carcinoma |
| | Serous cystadenocarcinoma |
| | Solid pseudopapillary neoplasms |

The incidence is estimated at 2.04 (95% confidence interval [CI], 1.28–2.80) per 100 000 population; however, this increases significantly after the sixth decade of life.[15] The precise aetiology remains unknown, although an association with extra-pancreatic primary cancers (10%), most commonly colorectal, breast and prostate, has been reported, but this is not significantly different to that seen with primary pancreatic adenocarcinoma.[16] IPMN have also been shown to be a predictor of pancreatic cancer as compared to other intra-abdominal pathologies, with an odds ratio of 7.18.[17]

## CLINICAL PRESENTATION

IPMN most commonly present with symptoms related to pancreatic duct obstruction. The John Hopkins group reported their experience comparing the presentation and demographics to those patients presenting with pancreatic adenocarcinoma.[18,19] Although the mean age of presentation was similar to that of pancreatic adenocarcinoma (seventh decade), the clinical presentation was significantly different. Of the 60 patients with IPMN, 59% presented with abdominal pain but only 16% presented with obstructive jaundice, compared to 38% and 74% of patients with pancreatic adenocarcinoma, respectively.[18] This is in spite of the fact that only five of the 60 patients with IPMN had tumours within the body or tail.[18] In addition, those with IPMN were more likely to have been smokers and 14% had suffered previous attacks of acute pancreatitis (compared to 3% of those with pancreatic ductal adenocarcinoma).[18] Weight loss was a prominent factor reported in 29% of patients with IPMN.[19] Symptoms associated with invasive malignancy included the presence of jaundice, weight loss, vomiting[19] and diabetes.[20] Patients with invasive IPMN were a mean of 5 years older (68 vs. 63 years) compared to those with non-invasive IPMN.[19] This led the authors to conclude that IPMN are slow-growing tumours with a significant latency to develop invasive disease.[19] Increasingly, an important presentation is the incidental finding resulting from cross-sectional imaging for other medical indications. IPMN was the final diagnosis in 36% of pancreatic 'incidentalomas' that underwent pancreatico-duodenectomy.[21]

## INVESTIGATION

CT and MRI form the mainstay of non-invasive radiological imaging of suspected IPMN. The classical features of MD-IPMN are segmental or diffuse MPD dilatation greater than 5 mm as seen in Fig. 18.1, while branch-type IPMN can present with small cystic lesions (>5 mm) that may appear in a 'grape-like' configuration.[14] If both co-exist, they are classified as mixed type. Furthermore, BD-IPMN have been reported to be multifocal in distant regions of the pancreas in up to 30% of patients.[22] Although MRI and CT have been shown to accurately identify tumour location and communication with the pancreatic duct, the detection of invasive malignancy remains problematic.[23–25] Over the last 15 years, a number of guidelines have been developed based on earlier large series of resection pathology.[14,26–28]

At the time of the first consensus meeting on management of IPMN, the resection data assimilated by the International Association of Pancreatology (IAP) showed that the risk of malignancy was between 6% and 46%, with a mean of 25%, and a frequency of invasive cancer ranging between 0% and 31%.[13,14] For MD-IPMN, the frequency of malignancy (in situ and invasive) in eight series from Japan, Europe, and the USA ranged between 60% and 92%, with a mean of 70%. In 2006 the first widely applied management guidelines were published and have now been updated.[26]

These identify two subsets of cysts requiring careful management: worrisome features and high-risk stigmata, which may be defined by clinical and radiological features.[14] 'High-risk stigmata' include jaundice, the presence of an enhancing mural nodule (>5 mm) or a solid component, positive cytology or an MPD >10 mm. These are highly predictive of malignancy. Patients fit enough to undergo surgery should be investigated and worked up accordingly. 'Worrisome features' have been defined as cyst size >3 cm, cystic growth rate >5 mm/year, increased level of serum Ca19-9 (>37 U/mL), thickened enhanced walls, enhancing mural nodules <5 mm, MPD size 5–9.9 mm, abrupt change in MPD calibre with distal pancreatic atrophy, and lymphadenopathy.[26,29–32] A review of nine studies incorporating 1510 patients showed that an enhancing nodule, jaundice and PD >10 mm has a positive predictive value for malignancy of 56–89%.[27]

Differentiating IPMN from other cystic neoplasms (particularly branch-type IPMN from MCN or pseudocysts) can be difficult and the importance of considering the clinical picture cannot be underestimated, particularly the patient's age, gender, and history of pancreatitis or genetic syndromes. For example, in one series of SB-IPMN that had undergone surgery, the presence of a mural nodule >5 mm on EUS had a sensitivity of 73–85% and a specificity of 71–100% for the presence of high-grade dysplasia or cancer.[33–35]

Radiologically, localisation within the uncinate process, detection of non-gravity–dependent luminal filling defects (papillary projections) or grouped gravity-dependent luminal filling defects (mucin), and upstream dilatation of ducts (in MCN ducts are normal) all favour the diagnosis of branch-type IPMN.[36] Differentiating diffuse MD-IPMN from chronic obstructive pancreatitis can be challenging radiologically[36] – clinically, patients with IPMN tend to be (up to 20 years) older and lack a history of heavy alcohol use. On high-quality cross-sectional imaging, endoluminal filling defects (either mucin or papillary proliferations),

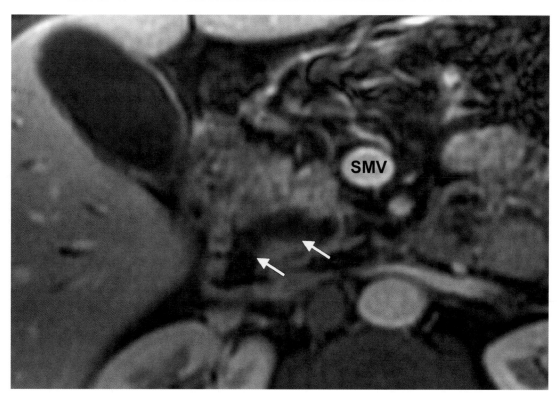

**Figure 18.1**   Magnetic resonance imaging (post-gadolinium, T1-weighted, fat-saturated) image of the pancreas. *White arrows* indicate a dilated pancreatic duct with a widely open ampulla consistent with a main duct intraductal papillary neoplasm. Histology is shown in Fig. 18.4. *SMV*, Superior mesenteric vein.

cystic dilatation of collateral branches (particularly within the uncinate process), communication of dilated ducts with normal ducts without evidence of an obstructing lesion or a widely open papilla (see Fig. 18.1) all favour IPMN.[36]

EUS has the advantage of being able to sample cystic fluid and biopsy solid lesions at the time of assessment.[37] Features seen at EUS suggestive of malignancy include main duct >10 mm (for MD-IPMN), while suspicious features for branch-type IPMN include tumour diameter >40 mm associated with thick irregular septa and mural nodules >10 mm,[38] (Fig. 18.2). In a systematic review and meta-analysis published in 2014, the sensitivity and specificity of EUS-FNA based cytology in detecting malignant IPMN was 65% and 91%, respectively.[39] Measuring tumour markers within cyst fluid has not proved to be accurate enough and as yet mutation analysis is not commonplace for EUS-obtained fluid aspirates but the low complication rate of EUS at 3.5% supports this in future studies. Confocal laser endomicroscopy represents an endoscopic modality for endoluminal pancreatic ductal and side branch tissue sampling to assess extent of cystic dilatation but procedure complications rates are almost three times that of EUS and FNA.[40] In the future, molecular analysis is likely to be more useful when combined with clinical presentation.[41] Although the absence of mucin does not exclude IPMN, the presence of necrosis is the only feature that is strongly suggestive of invasive carcinoma. Abundant background inflammation and parachromatin clearing are suspicious for carcinoma in situ.[42]

Endoscopic retrograde cholangiopancreatography (ERCP) can be used in the diagnosis of IPMN, although MRI (including the use of gadolinium-based contrast) is increasingly replacing it (see Fig. 18.1). The observation at ERCP of mucin protruding from a widely open papilla is diagnostic[43] (Fig 18.3). Biopsies and aspiration of ductal contents can be obtained; however, the yield is less than 50%.[43]

Although there are no tumour markers specific to IPMN, serum CA19-9, but not CEA, has been shown to be an independent predictor of malignancy.[20] Given the increasing frequency of diagnosis and relatively low rate of malignancy within BD-IPMN, clinico-radiological scoring systems have been proposed.[20,44] In a large study by Hwang et al., 237 patients with BD-IPMN who underwent resection were studied[44] with multivariate analysis used to identify independent predictors of either malignancy or invasiveness. However, the presence of a mural nodule, elevated serum CEA or cyst size >28 mm was sufficient to conclude that there was underlying malignant change or invasion and an indication for surgery.[44] An important point when considering the use of these scoring systems is that the radiological measurement varies by scan modality and may not correlate well with the final pathological measurement.[45]

✓ The European Study Group on Cystic Tumours of the Pancreas guidelines recommend use EUS-FNA in helping identify PCNs with features that should be considered for resection, for example, in helping differentiate mucinous versus non-mucinous PCNs and malignant versus benign PCNs, in cases where CT or MRI are unclear, (conditional recommendation, very low-quality evidence).[28]

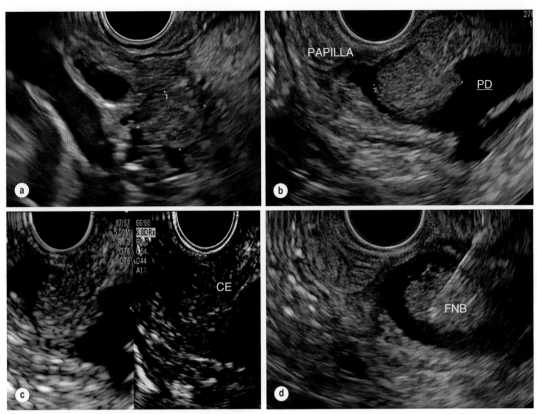

**Figure 18.2**    Contrast (Sonovue) enhanced assessment of pancreatic cystic neoplasm at endoscopic ultrasound. (a) Main duct intraductal papillary mucinous neoplasm (IPMN) with papillary projection; (b) Near papilla; (c) Contrast enhancement (CE) demonstrated uniformly in papillary projection. (d) Fine needle biopsy (FNB) confirms IPMN with low grade dysplasia *PD*, Pancreatic duct. (Image courtesy of I.D. Penman.)

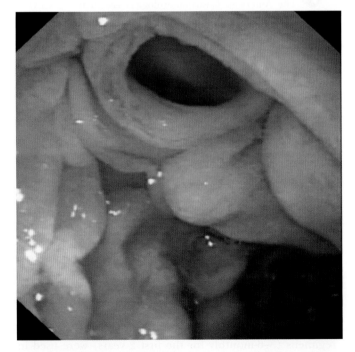

**Figure 18.3**    Endoscopic retrograde cholangiopancreatography view of mucin protruding from a widely open papilla in main duct intraductal papillary mucinous neoplasm , so called '*fishmouth*' appearances (Image courtesy of I.D. Penman).

## PATHOLOGY

The importance of assessment by experienced pathologists cannot be overemphasised. There are now pathological guidelines for reporting of IPMN[46] but discussion of these is beyond the scope of this chapter. IPMN involve the head of the gland in 70% of patients, while 5–10% are spread diffusely throughout the gland, and the rest are located within the body and tail.[47] On sectioning, the involvement can be diffuse or segmented, with projections of papillary epithelium (Fig. 18.4) and tenacious thick mucin within the involved dilated ducts. Branch-type neoplasms are

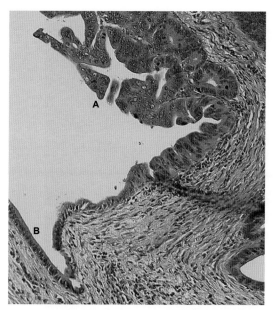

**Figure 18.4** Haematoxylin-and-eosin-stained section from the pancreatico-duodenectomy specimen of the patient in Fig. 18.1. Label A is in the lumen of the proximal pancreatic duct with adjacent proliferation of severely dysplastic glandular epithelium with intraluminal papillary growth, but no stromal invasion in this area. Elsewhere in the specimen, focal stromal invasion was identified. Label B indicates remnant low columnar non-neoplastic epithelium of the duct.

less likely to be associated with malignancy.[43] Surrounding pancreatic parenchyma may appear firm and hard because of scarring and atrophy from obstructive chronic pancreatitis secondary to the tumour. The presence of gelatinous or solid nodules should raise the suspicion of an invasive component. Microscopically, the most typical appearance is of mucin-secreting columnar epithelium with variable atypia (low-, moderate-, high-grade dysplasia or invasive carcinoma).[47] The growth pattern varies from flat ducts (ectasia) through to prominent papillae. The tumour tends to follow the pancreatic ducts and can be multifocal in 20–30% of patients.[47] IPMN can contain intestinal, gastric or, less commonly, pancreatico-biliary type differentiation. The gastric type are more often associated with branch-type IPMN and would seem to be associated with a different (lower) malignant potential, growth pattern and type of mucin production compared to the intestinal type.[48,49] Invasive carcinoma occurs focally and is thought to result from a stepwise progression through increasingly dysplastic lesions.[47] The invasive growth pattern can be muconodular (colloid) or a conventional ductal pattern and would appear to be related to the underlying cellular differentiation (intestinal vs. pancreatico-biliary, respectively).[47,49]

Pathologically, differentiating IPMN from other cystic neoplasms of the pancreas is important. The absence of ovarian stroma helps to separate IPMN from MCN.[14] For lesions between 0.5 and 1 cm, differentiating pancreatic intra-epithelial neoplasia (PanIN) from IPMN is difficult. IPMN tend to have taller and more complex papillae and are associated with abundant luminal mucin.[47] The presence of coarse and stippled chromatin with a smooth nuclear membrane will differentiate cystic pancreatic endocrine neoplasms from IPMN.[47]

## MANAGEMENT

In determining the most appropriate management of patients with IPMN, the following should be considered. Given the preponderance for these to present in older patients and the fact that the majority will be located within the head of the pancreas, it is important to assess for comorbidities and general fitness for major pancreatic surgery. If the patient is deemed not fit enough for surgery, then simple medical management of symptoms is appropriate. Equally, in the event of an incidental diagnosis, intensive follow-up regimens are not indicated if tumour progression would not lead to surgical intervention. Presuming the patient is a suitable candidate for surgery (if required), then appropriate staging to determine surgical resectability (criteria equivalent to those for pancreatic adenocarcinoma) should be performed.

Despite over 250 publications per year being dedicated to IPMN, the level of evidence available to make clinical recommendations remains poor. There are several published sets of guidelines with little concordance and few using an evidence-based approach.[14,26–28,50] Tanaka et al.'s 'Fukuoka Guidelines' dating back to 2006, but last updated in 2017, are perhaps the most established,[26] but the European Study Group for the Cystic Tumours of the Pancreas Guidelines in 2018, follow GRADE scoring on the basis of the evidence available.[27]

✔ A summary of the key findings as interpreted by the authors is shown in Table 18.2.[27,28]

✔ The American Gastroenterological Association (AGA) recommended that surgery was appropriate for asymptomatic patients with both a solid component and dilated pancreatic duct and/or concerning features on EUS and FNA (conditional recommendation, very low-quality evidence). Surgery should be performed in an expert centre (strong recommendation, very low-quality evidence).

Despite a robust methodological approach, it is important to recognise that these recommendations have not been met with universal acceptance and for those readers interested, the author recommends reading the accompanying published correspondence.[28]

Given that BD-IPMN would appear to be a pre-malignant lesion, albeit a slow-growing one, it is important to know the outcome from long-term follow-up if conservative management is to be successful. In two large prospective contemporary studies of BD-IPMN, in which indications for resection were based on IAP guidelines, patients were allocated to a surgical or intensive follow-up arm.[51,52] In both studies, 18% of patients met the criteria for surgery at initial presentation. Of these patients, the final histology was malignant (in situ or invasive disease) in three of 20 and eight of 34 patients. In those patients submitted to follow-up, intensive regimens (3–6-monthly for the first 2 years) were used in both studies, including combinations of CT, EUS and MRI. Between 5% and 12% of patients subsequently progressed to surgery during follow-up (median 12–18 months). Of these patients, 0 of five[51] and two of 18[52] had malignant disease. All remaining patients ($n = 84$[51] and $n = 132$[52]) that were followed remained alive during median follow-up periods of 30 months, with no deaths attributable to their disease.

**Table 18.2    Recommendation of management of IPMN as per current author's interpretation of current guidelines for pancreatic cystic neoplasms (Refs 27, 28 PMID)**

| Management strategy | Clinico-radiological feature |
|---|---|
| Conservative Management | Asymptomatic MCN <4 cm |
| | SB IPMN<3–4 cm without enhancing nodule |
| | Unfit for surgical intervention |
| Relative Indications for Surgical Resection | Main pancreatic duct dilatation (MD) 5–9.9 mm |
| | Cyst diameter >4 cm MCN |
| | Cyst diameter >3–4 cm SB IPMN |
| | Others to consider: |
| | Pancreatitis |
| | Abrupt cut-off of pancreatic duct (MD) with distal atrophy |
| | Thickened enhancing wall |
| | Lymphadenopathy |
| | *High-risk individual |
| Absolute Indications for Surgical Resection | Jaundice |
| | Enhancing mural nodule >5 mm |
| | Main pancreatic duct dilatation >10 mm |
| | Others to consider: |
| | Elevated serum Ca19-9 |
| | Cytological high-grade dysplasia (HGD) |

*High Risk Individual:
1: 2x First-degree relatives (FDR) diagnosed with pancreatic cancer
2: 1x FDR and a deleterious germline mutation (*BRCA1*, *PALB2*, *ATM* or *BRCA1*)
3: 1x FDR and a Peutz-Jeghers syndrome or Lynch syndrome
4: Diagnosis of hereditary pancreatitis or Familial Atypical Multiple Mole (FAMM) syndrome[50]
*MCN*, Mucinous cystic neoplasm; *SB IPMN*, side branch intraductal papillary mucinous neoplasms

The methodology of the follow-up regimen of both these studies raises further questions. Both used state-of-the-art imaging at a frequency that many health systems may struggle to provide. Both studies showed that although the current recommendations for BD-IPMN are very sensitive in detecting malignancy, the specificity remains low and hence many patients are followed intensively and subjected to surgery without clear benefit. Unique to the AGA guidelines, consideration is given to such issues as potential harm, adverse outcomes and cost from intensive follow-up or subsequent interventions.[28] Thus, the AGA recommendations with regard to follow-up are perhaps the most controversial. The more recent European Study Group Guidelines suggest that all patients without an indication for surgery should undergo a 6-monthly follow-up in the first year, (to assess cyst growth as a growth of >5 mm in 1 year confers a 20-fold higher risk of malignant progression), then annually thereafter until such point as there is a change in clinical symptoms to trigger further investigation. This was deemed a GRADE 1B recommendation. Similarly, in patients who have undergone pancreatic resection, the consensus of the European Group is that lifelong follow-up is still needed, that is, resection therefore does not negate the need for follow-up imaging.[53]

For those patients in whom surgery is indicated, the decision regarding the extent of pancreatic resection and nodal dissection needs to be decided. Falconi et al.[54] noted that there was lack of agreement amongst experts and some areas, such as use of duodenal sparing surgery, lacked evidence on which to make conclusive recommendations.

✔ Frozen section for margin assessment is currently recommended.[14,54] If there is high grade dysplasia or carcinoma then a further resection up to a total pancreatectomy is recommended. In contrast, lower grades of dysplasia at the resection margin do not require further resection. Given an IPMN-associated invasive carcinoma with no lymph node metastases has a better long-term outcome than pancreatic cancer-radical resection to negative/low-grade margins is warranted.[29]

Falconi et al. recommended frozen section with further resection until margins were without high-grade dysplasia or invasive malignancy.[54] Current recommendations from the IAP guidelines are that, in the presence of adenoma or borderline atypia, no further resection is required, but if in situ or invasive carcinoma is present, then further resection should be performed.[14] However, what has not yet been addressed in the literature is the effect of potentially spilling invasive carcinoma cells (i.e., cutting through invasive tumour) during surgery and the effect this has on long-term outcomes.

Fujino et al. reviewed the outcome in 57 patients who underwent surgical resection for IPMN.[55] Their approach was to perform a total pancreatectomy in patients with diffuse disease and a localised resection where pre-operative imaging revealed localised disease, using intra-operative ultrasound (IOUS) to determine the point of pancreatic transection. Frozen section was undertaken and for patients with invasive carcinoma, a radical resection was performed. Where non-invasive disease was detected, a tumour-free margin was sufficient. Of the 33 patients with MD-IPMN, 14 met the pre-resection criteria for total pancreatectomy. All 24 patients with BD tumours underwent partial resections, although two subsequently required completion pancreatectomy for complications. Correlating the IOUS findings with final pathological assessment indicated an accuracy of ductal spread of 74% for MD tumours and 96% for BD tumours. Frozen section was performed in 30 of the patients who underwent partial resection and in 29 patients, it correlated with the final result. Only one patient had invasive malignancy at the transected surface, while a further two patients who did not have frozen section assessment had invasive malignancy at the resection margin. In reviewing the final histology of the 16 patients undergoing total pancreatectomy, resection was found to be appropriate (frankly or potentially malignant tissue throughout all segments of the pancreas) in 12 patients. Importantly, six of these 16 patients had severe long-term problems with hypoglycaemia, two of whom died as a result of this complication. For those 41 patients undergoing partial pancreatectomy, five patients had an involved margin (three with invasive carcinoma, two with dysplasia). The three patients with invasive carcinoma all died from metastatic disease. Of the patients with clear margins, seven of 34 died from metastatic disease, while two developed metachronous pancreatic disease at 2 and 12 years. The authors of this study concluded that partial pancreatectomy should be performed if possible, and that the risk of severe long-term complications from total pancreatectomy outweighed the risk of patients developing recurrent malignancy in the remnant.

✅ For those undergoing resection, partial pancreatectomy is preferred to total pancreatectomy and intra-operative frozen section should be performed to ensure clear margins.[55]

## OUTCOME

The main determinant of survival following resection is the presence of invasive disease. The AGA review process identified 37 studies evaluating 3842 patients.[56] For those with non-invasive disease, 5-year survival was reported as between 80% and 100%, while for invasive disease, it was between 3% and 68%. Factors associated with poor survival in those with invasive disease include the presence of jaundice, tumour type (tubular worse than colloid), vascular invasion, perineural invasion, poorly differentiated tumours, percentage of tumour that was invasive and positive lymph node involvement, which has been reported in up to 41% of patients with invasive disease.[19,49,57–60] Invasive branch-type tumours have been shown to have similar survival to those with invasive MD disease.[57] Margin status has not been associated with worse long-term outcome.[19,57,58,60] In studies that have performed a multivariate analysis with adequate numbers of patients per variable, lymph node involvement,[58,60] invasive component >2 cm,[58] absence of weight loss,[58] morphological subtype[49] and tubular carcinoma[60] have been found to be independent predictors of poorer outcome. Invasive IPMN would still appear to have a better prognosis than pancreatic ductal adenocarcinoma,[59,60] although the tubular subtype may not.[60] The role of adjuvant therapy for those with invasive disease has not been addressed in formal trials. Outcomes from retrospective series have been analysed,[58,60] yet the role of either radiotherapy or chemotherapy remains unclear and currently cannot be recommended as the standard of care.

Recurrence following resection can be classified as disseminated, arising from invasive disease, or local (within the pancreatic remnant), which may or may not be invasive in nature. The AGA guidelines recommend that patients with invasive cancer or dysplasia in a cyst that has been surgically resected should undergo MRI surveillance of the remnant pancreas every 2 years (conditional recommendation, very low-quality evidence).[28] The authors acknowledge the lack of strong supporting evidence; however, the rationale is based on the concept that there may be a field change within the pancreatic remnant. Given the dismal survival for those with invasive disease and lack of subsequent curative therapies, it is questionable whether this type of follow-up should be limited to those with dysplasia or PanIN at the margin, or for patients with invasive disease >3 years from resection when the conditional survival is more favourable. In contrast, for those without high-grade dysplasia or malignancy at the margin, the AGA guidelines do not recommend ongoing surveillance (excluding mixed-type IPMN or family history of pancreatic cancer), again based on weak supporting evidence.[28]

✅ There is a lack of reliable evidence regarding recommended follow-up regimens. Both the IAP and AGA guidelines acknowledge this, but feel it is reasonable to perform cross-sectional imaging at a variable frequency (1–2 yearly).[14,28] The routine use of tumour markers is currently not supported.

Given that recurrence would seem to occur most commonly within the pancreatic remnant, Tomimaru et al. have proposed performing a pancreatico-gastrostomy to allow easy endoscopic follow-up of the duct.61 In addition, the association of IPMN with other gastrointestinal malignancies should alert physicians to investigate new gastrointestinal symptoms promptly.

# PANCREATIC NEUROENDOCRINE NEOPLASMS

PanNEN account for 1–2% of all pancreatic tumours.[62] In the past they were considered as rare tumours with a reported incidence of 0.2–0.4 per 100 000, although post-mortem studies have reported PanNEN in up to 10% of the population.[63] A steadily rising trend in their incidence has been documented in recent epidemiological studies.[64]

The majority of PanNEN (75–90%) are non-syndromic (i.e., non-functional/non-secreting). The rest comprise syndromic tumours,[65] of which serotonin secreting neoplasms ('carcinoids'), insulinoma and gastrinoma are the most common.[66] Some PanNEN secrete multiple hormones and may show secondary changes in the secreted hormone profiles during their clinical course. Their aetiology is poorly understood and although the majority of tumours are sporadic, there are associated with several hereditary syndromes, including Von Hippel–Lindau,[67] multiple endocrine neoplasia type 1 (MEN1),[68] neurofibromatosis type 1 and tuberous sclerosis.[69]

## PATHOLOGY, GENOMIC LANDSCAPE AND OUTCOME

Neuroendocrine tumour grading is based on the Ki67 index or number of mitoses per 10 high-powered fields (HPF).[70] Neuroendocrine neoplasms may be classified as neuroendocrine tumours (NET) or neuroendocrine carcinoma (NEC). Grade 1 (NET) have a Ki67 of <3% or <2 mitoses per 10 HPF. Grade 2 (NET) have a Ki67 index of between 3% and 20%, or between 2 and 20 mitoses per 10 HPF. Grade 3 NEN have a Ki67 index of >20%, or >20 mitoses per 10 HPF, and can be sub-classified into G3 NET and G3 NEC – this is on the basis of their differentiation: Grade 3 NET are well-differentiated, and G3 NEC are poorly differentiated.

Importantly, the diagnosis of functional tumours is not made histologically but clinically under consideration of hormonally induced symptoms and biochemical results. Immunohistochemical staining of specific hormones does not correlate with the clinical picture.[66] In 2010 the seventh edition of the American Joint Committee on Cancer (AJCC) published its first TNM staging classification for PanNEN.[71] Using this, Strosberg et al. retrospectively applied the staging system to a dataset of 425 patients with PanNEN.[72] Five-year overall survival for stages I–IV was 92%, 84%, 81% and 57%, respectively, thus indicating the proposed system is a useful adjunct for classifying PanNEN and assessing prognosis.[73] The WHO-AJCC classification grading systems demonstrated that in PanNEN patients grading is most probably the most powerful instrument for prediction of survival.[74]

Regarding the genomic landscape of PanNEN, comprehensive exome sequencing of sporadic tumours has demonstrated that 44% of cases harbour mutations in *MEN1*, with 43% showing mutations in *DAXX* or *ATRX*.[75] These and other 'omics'–based insights may have clinical relevance: the 5- and 10-year disease-specific survival were 40% and 50%, respectively, for *DAXX/ATRX*-negative PanNEN, compared to 96% and 89%, respectively, for *DAXX/ATRX* wild-type PanNEN.[76]

## CLINICAL PRESENTATION

The mode of presentation depends on the functional state of the tumour. Small non-functioning tumours are increasingly diagnosed incidentally,[77] whereas non-hormonal symptoms are usually related to mass effect or the presence of metastatic disease. For those tumours associated with a syndrome, this will be related to the specific hormone produced (Table 18.3).

## INVESTIGATIONS

The order of investigations also depends on presentation. The general principle for functional tumours is to confirm the diagnosis biochemically before localisation using imaging and endoscopic techniques.

### BIOCHEMICAL

Specific fasting gut hormones can be measured for functional tumours but testing is complex and subject to change, therefore it is recommended that tests are performed according to current guidelines in centres with significant experience.[78] The 72-h fast test is the gold standard for diagnosing insulinoma – it confirms autonomous insulin secretion and the failure of appropriate insulin suppression in the presence of hypoglycaemia. Elevated fasting gastrin in the presence of low gastric pH can be indicative for a gastrinoma.[79] In the majority of patients with PanNEN, including those with non-functional tumours, serum chromogranin A (an acid glycoprotein present in the secretory granules of most neuroendocrine cells) will be elevated.[66] Whilst chromogranin A is moderately sensitive, it is not highly specific and those interpreting the test must be aware of causes of false-positive results.[80]

Other investigations, such as calcium, parathyroid hormone and prolactin should also be considered, particularly if there is a history that suggests MEN 1.[66] For those in whom a hereditary component is suspected, referral to an appropriate genetic service for further investigation should be initiated. Assessment of 5-hydroxyindoleacetic acid (5-HIAA) in 24-h urine, a breakdown metabolite of serotonin, may be useful in PanNEN patients with carcinoid syndrome for diagnosis and monitoring of treatment.

**Table 18.3    Characteristics, diagnostic features and medical management of functional pancreatic neoplasm**

| Tumour type (secreted hormone) | Syndrome | Clinical features | Diagnosis | Medical options for initial symptom control |
|---|---|---|---|---|
| Insulinoma (insulin) | Whipple's triad | Fasting hypoglycaemia, neuroglycopaenic/autonomic symptoms relieved with eating | Insulin:glucose ratio >0.3 in presence of hypoglycaemia C-peptide suppression test | Overnight feeding Diazoxide titrated to symptom resolution Somatostatin analogue |
| Gastrinoma (gastrin) | Zollinger–Ellison | Treatment-resistant or complicated peptic ulceration (not related to NSAIDs or *H. pylori*), gastro-oesophageal reflux, chronic diarrhoea, abdominal pain | Serum fasting gastrin > 1000 pg/mL (if gastric pH <2.5) Secretin stimulation test | High-dose proton pump inhibition (may require up to 60 mg b.d.) |
| Glucagonoma (glucagon) | Glucagonoma syndrome | Necrolytic migratory erythema (characteristic rash), weight loss, new onset diabetes mellitus, stomatitis, diarrhoea, thromboembolism | Plasma glucagon > 1000 pg/mL | Somatostatin analogue, hyperalimentation, thrombosis prophylaxis |
| VIPoma (vasoactive intestinal peptide) | Verner–Morrison syndrome | Profuse watery diarrhoea with dehydration, hypokalaemia and achlorhydria | Plasma VIP >1000 pg/mL | Somatostatin analogue |
| Somatostatinoma (somatostatin) | | Gallstones, diabetes mellitus, weight loss, diarrhoea, steatorrhoea | Raised plasma somatostatin | Somatostatin analogue |
| Serotonin-producing PanNEN (serotonin) | Carcinoid syndrome | Abdominal pain, if metastases then flushing, palpitations, rhinorrhoea, diarrhoea, bronchospasm, pellagra | 24-hour urinary 5-HIAA | Somatostatin analogue |

*HIAA*, Hydroxyindoleacetic acid; *NSAIDs*, non-steroidal anti-inflammatory drugs; *PanNEN*, pancreatic neuroendocrine neoplasm; *VIP*, vasoactive intestinal peptide.

Novel circulating biomarkers (liquid biopsy) such as circulating tumour cells, cell-free deoxyribonucleic acid (DNA), circulating tumour DNA, messenger ribonucleic acid (mRNA), and microRNA have shown promising results in NEN and have the potential to change current clinical practice.[81,82]

## IMAGING AND ENDOSCOPIC LOCALISATION TECHNIQUES

For non-functioning tumours, where precise localisation of the primary tumour is often not problematic, a high-quality arterial and portal venous phase CT according to a pancreatic protocol is the gold standard imaging modality for primary tumour staging and direction of the therapy. It determines if surgery is indicated and technically feasible by ascertaining the vascular anatomy of the pancreas, identifying biliary and pancreatic duct abnormalities, as well as assessing for invasion of peripancreatic structures and nodal metastases. Features suggestive of a PanNEN on CT include the presence of a hypervascular or hyperdense lesion within the pancreas; however, they can also appear cystic or contain calcifications.[83] The presence of a large incidental mass within the pancreas, particularly without vascular encasement or desmoplastic reaction, should also alert the clinician to the possibility of a PanNEN.[83]

Although somatostatinomas, VIPomas (vasoactive intestinal polypeptide secreting) and glucagonomas tend to be large and easily identified and staged by contrast-enhanced CT, this is often not the case for insulinomas and gastrinomas, unless there is widespread metastatic disease. Most insulinomas are <2 cm in size and solitary. On CT, they tend to be hypervascular (Fig. 18.5) with either uniform or target enhancement; however, given that they are often non-contour–conforming, detection of the vascular blush is essential to localise them (the chance of detection can be maximised by timing the images 25 seconds after contrast injection).[83] MRI features include low signal intensity on T1-weighted images and they are particularly well seen on fat-suppressed (T1- and T2-weighted) images.[83] In contrast to insulinomas, which are located within the pancreas and only rarely seen as multifocal lesions within the MEN 1 syndrome, gastrinomas can be multiple and extra-pancreatic (located within the gastrinoma triangle; the junction between neck and body of the pancreas medially, the junction of the second and third parts of the duodenum inferiorly and the junction of the common bile duct and cystic duct superiorly).[84] On radiological examination, they tend to be less vascular than insulinomas[83] and they have a high rate (70–80%) of lymph node and hepatic metastases.[83] The sensitivity of CT in the detection of gastrinomas is related to size and can be as low as 30–50%.[84] Although slightly

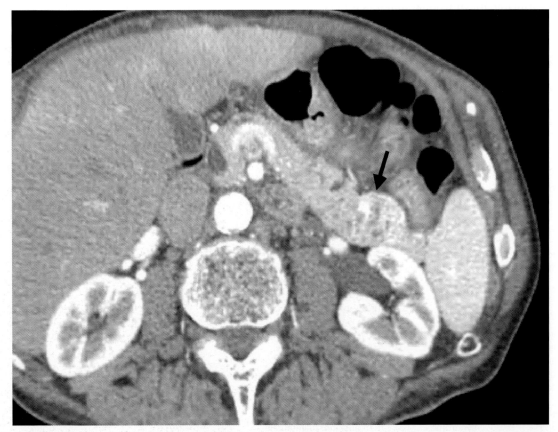

**Figure 18.5** A 78-year-old man presented with neuroglycaemic symptoms. Biochemical testing confirmed an insulinoma. Arterial phase computed tomography revealed a hypervascular lesion in the tail of the pancreas (*black arrow*). Laparoscopic spleen-preserving distal pancreatectomy was performed. Histology confirmed malignant, node-positive neuroendocrine tumour consistent with an insulinoma. After 4 years with no symptoms, the patient re-presented with symptoms of hypoglycaemia. Further investigation revealed an isolated nodal recurrence adjacent to the superior mesenteric artery. The patient underwent a completion radical antegrade modular distal pancreatico-splenectomy with resolution of hypoglycaemic symptoms.

better figures have been reported for insulinomas, this can be increased to 94% with the use of thin slice formats and, with the addition of EUS, sensitivities of 100% have been reported.[85]

EUS is particularly useful for imaging the duodenal wall, regional lymph nodes, the pancreatic head, and in MEN 1 patients in whom multifocal tumours can be expected.[86] A sensitivity of 79–100% is reported but is operator-dependent.[87,88] In combination with FNA (EUS-FNA), it can confirm the diagnosis and inform tumour grade.

Equally, the use of IOUS has also been shown to be useful, particularly in gastrinomas, by identifying occult multiple primaries or metastatic disease. The sensitivity for detecting small lesions in the pancreatic head is reported to be as high as 97%.[84] PanNEN hepatic metastases often appear as low-attenuation lesions on pre-contrast CT and hypervascular lesions on post-contrast imaging.[89] It is, however, important to perform a hepatic arterial phase as they can be isointense with normal parenchyma on portal venous imaging. MRI with hepatocyte-specific contrast agents (e.g., gadoxetic acid) is the imaging modality of choice for neuroendocrine liver metastases.[90,91] Their appearances are usually of low signal intensity lesions on T1- and high signal intensity on T2-weighted images. Qualitative features of MRI may help to discriminate liver metastases of PanNEN from those of small bowel NEN.[92] This might be of value particularly in patients presenting with neuroendocrine liver metastases and unknown primary tumour origin.

Somatostatin receptor based imaging within positron emission tomography (PET)/CT[93] or PET/MRI[94] techniques has evolved as the gold standard imaging modality for detection of metastatic disease and staging in patients with G1/G2 PanNEN (with the exception of insulinomas)[80]

(Fig. 18.6). It has replaced previously widely used [111]In-pentetreotide scintigraphy (Octreoscan). For patients with benign insulinomas, glucagon-like peptide 1-receptor (GL-1R) PET/CT may be useful, particularly in those with negative CT or MRI results.[95] Receptor-based functional imaging works by exploiting the observation that G1/G2 PanNEN express somatostatin receptors. The use of a somatostatin analogue labelled with a radioactive isotope (of which there are several; e.g., [68]Ga DOTATATE or [68]DOTATOC) allows a functional image to be obtained, guide surgical planning[96] and identify those patients who might be candidates for somatostatin receptor targeted therapy.[93]

[18]Fluorine-2-deoxyglucose ([18]F-FDG) PET/CT is used in pancreatic neuroendocrine carcinoma, G3 PanNEN and in G1/G2 PanNEN with mismatched lesions (seen on CT or MRI but not on [68]Ga DOTA-PET/CT).[97] Invasive investigations such as selective arterial calcium (insulinoma) and secretin (gastrinoma) stimulation with hepatic/portal venous sampling are not used routinely and are undertaken only if there is a high suspicion but non-invasive imaging has failed to localise the tumour.[80]

## TREATMENT

Once the diagnosis of a functioning tumour is established, control of the hormonal excess is the first priority in minimising symptoms and complications. Medications used for each individual tumour are shown in Table 18.3. Surgery offers the only chance of cure for those with localised disease.

Biochemically confirmed functional PanNEN, and those that are non-secreting but larger than 2 cm in size should be evaluated for surgery.[1] Approaches comprise typical resections (pancreato-duodenectomy [Whipple's procedure],

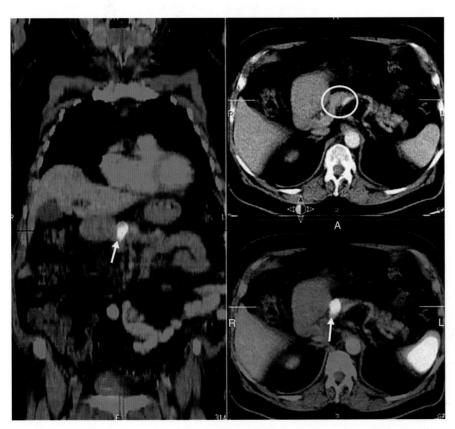

**Figure 18.6** 68Ga-DOTATATE positron emission tomography/computed tomography (CT) showing a 2-cm neuroendocrine neoplasm in the body of the pancreas (*arrow*). The uptake in the spleen is physiologic. On CT scan pancreas appears bulky in the corresponding area (*circle*).

distal and total pancreatectomy), or atypical, parenchyma-sparing techniques such as enucleation[98] and mesopancreatectomy. Atypical resections, whilst associated with a lower risk of endocrine and exocrine failure, may be associated with a higher incidence of pancreatic fistulae.[99] In locally advanced tumours, multivisceral resections might be required to achieve a R0 situation.[100]

MEN 1–associated non-functioning PanNEN ≤2 cm can be observed while larger lesions should be removed.[101] Functioning tumours should be resected if feasible and if the source of hormonal secretion within the pancreas can be regionalised.[102] Over 80% of sporadic insulinomas are solitary, benign and <2 cm in size, making them ideal for consideration of parenchyma-sparing procedures, preferably via a laparoscopic approach.[103] Enucleation is considered possible if the lesion can be clearly localised pre- or intra-operatively and if the relationship to the pancreatic duct has been reliably identified.[80] IOUS has been shown to be particularly valuable in helping to assess these factors.[80] Post-operatively, histological confirmation of the benign nature must be established.[66] Formal resection is required for tumours where malignancy is suspected (features of local infiltration, duct obstruction or lymph node involvement), if there is major vascular involvement, or the tumour is large.[104] Patients should be assessed for resection as for any pancreatic tumour. However, if a distal pancreatectomy is being performed, attempts to preserve the spleen should be made.[47] Blind pancreatic resection should be avoided.[98,104,105] Locally ablative therapies such as endoscopic transgastric radiofrequency ablation may also be appropriate in selected patients.[80]

✅✅ The majority of gastrinomas are malignant albeit small at diagnosis. For localised sporadic gastrinoma and for selected patients with resectable liver metastases, surgery has been shown to increase survival.[106]

Duodenotomy and IOUS combined with trans-illumination and palpation are the key to successful intra-operative localisation.[107] For duodenal gastrinomas, small tumours (<5 mm) can be enucleated from the submucosa while larger tumours require full-thickness excision.[107] For pancreatic gastrinomas, intra-operative assessment regarding the suitability for limited resection should be performed. However, if the tumour is not suitable, a formal pancreatic resection should be performed. It is now recommend that formal oncological lymph node dissection should be performed because of high rates of involvement, prognostic relevance and possible survival benefit it confers.[80]

Resection is the treatment of choice for sporadic non-functioning G1/G2 and selected G3 PanNEN.[1,108] A multi-centre analysis of 964 patients revealed an overall relative survival rate of 91.8%, and that 2019 WHO grade and European Neuroendocrine Tumour Society (ENETS) TNM stage were independent predictors of relative survival. The probabilities of a normal lifespan for patients with G1, G2, G3 PanNEN, and pancreatic NEC were 96.7%, 54.8%, 0%, and 0%, respectively. The probabilities of a normal lifespan were 99.8%, 99.3%, 79.8% and 46.8% for those with stage I, II, III and IV disease, respectively. The overall disease-rate was 73.6 % (95% CI, 65.2–79.5%), and 2019 WHO grade and ENETS TNM stage significantly influenced disease-free relative survival. The probabilities of disease-free survival were 93.2%, 84.9%, 45.2% and 6.8 % for patients with stage I, II, III and IV disease, and 91.9%, 45.2%, 9.4% and 0.7 % for those with G1, G2, G3 PanNEN, and pancreatic neuroendocrine carcinomas, respectively.[109]

Because of the long natural history of these tumours and given that many are symptomatic and difficult to palliate without resection (e.g., tumour bleeding), the criteria for what determines unresectable disease may not be the same as those for adenocarcinoma of the pancreas. The MD Anderson experience suggests that, in high-volume centres, major venous reconstruction can be performed safely, but only rarely should arterial reconstruction (isolated hepatic artery involvement) or upper abdominal exenteration be performed, because of the associated high long-term morbidity.[110] In addition, a recent report has also indicated that an incomplete resection (R2) is associated with a high peri-operative mortality and may in fact be detrimental to the patient's survival.[111] Continuous somatostatin analogue infusions are recommended peri-operatively for carcinoid tumours and/or patients with liver metastases to prevent intra-operative carcinoid crisis.[66]

There is controversial discussion regarding appropriate management of non-functioning ≤2 cm PanNEN, which are nowadays increasingly diagnosed incidentally on imaging for reasons not related to PanNEN. While some groups recommend watchful surveillance, others recommend resection despite small tumour size since lymph node metastases have been reported even in sub-centimetre PanNEN.[112,113] The risk of malignancy is related to size, and tumours between 1.5 cm and 2 cm can harbour malignant potential (Fig. 18.7).[110] Currently, patients should be assessed regarding fitness for surgery and an informed decision made with the patient regarding resection or observation under consideration of operative morbidity and mortality risks. Central pancreatectomy has also been shown to be feasible for selected smaller tumours and has the advantage of reducing the risk of post-operative diabetes.[114] A formal resection with lymphadenectomy should be performed for all potentially malignant tumours as lymph node metastases are common.[115]

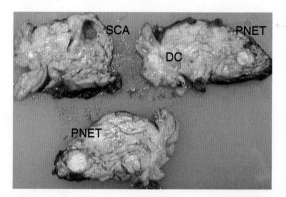

**Figure 18.7** A 30-year-old female with Von Hippel–Lindau disease underwent pancreatic screening. Radiological imaging revealed five neuroendocrine tumours within the pancreatic head. Pancreatico-duodenectomy was performed. Pathological sectioning of the pancreatic head revealed multiple neuroendocrine tumours (*PNET*), including at least one well-differentiated pancreatic endocrine carcinoma (node-positive) and a well-differentiated duodenal endocrine carcinoma (*DC*). All tumours were between 12 and 18 mm in diameter. An incidental serous cyst adenoma (*SCA*) was also identified.

## MANAGEMENT OF METASTATIC DISEASE

The liver is the commonest site of metastases from Pan-NEN.[116] Three classes of neuroendocrine liver metastases (NELM) exist, depending on lesion distribution and extent, and these inform amenability to surgery.[117] Because of the often bilobar distribution of NELM, only 20–30% of patients will be suitable for potentially curative resection. However, even after hepatectomy with curative intent, recurrence of NELM in general is high – up to 95% at 10-years.[118] Synchronous cholecystectomy may be considered to reduce complications from adjuvant therapy, such as increased risk of gallstones associated with somatostatin analogues.[119]

Palliative or 'debulking' surgery for NELM may be considered for patients with hormonal symptoms refractory to medical treatment. The impact of debulking on long-term prognosis of patients with PanNEN liver metastases remains debatable. In general, intra-hepatic disease progression within months will occur. Traditionally, the feasibility of resecting at least 90% of tumour bulk was used to select patients, but this cut-off was based on data from before the advent of modern treatments (such as somatostatin analogues), may be unnecessarily exclusive, and some centres report that a 70% debulking may not necessarily be associated with poorer prognosis compared to 90%.[120] However, the main consideration is caused by the development and availability of non-surgical techniques (see later), which may offer disease control without major surgery.

The other surgical approach is liver transplantation, usually as an isolated procedure, or within multi-visceral transplantation. Orthotopic liver transplantation according to stringent selection criteria such as the 'Milan NET' system may be associated with excellent long-term outcomes (up to 86.9% 10-year recurrence free survival), however, such data are from single-centre, non-randomised case series.[121,122]

Non-surgical therapeutic strategies for metastatic NEN have expanded in recent years beyond traditional cytotoxic chemotherapy and interferons.[123] Aside from recent trials of somatostatin analogues, molecularly targeted agents (sunitinib[124] and everolimus[125]) and peptide receptor radionuclide therapy,[126] there is increasing evidence supporting the use of interventional percutaneous and angiographic liver-directed therapies. Long-acting somatostatin analogues (SSAs) are cyclic peptides, are the cornerstone of NEN therapy, bind to the SSTR2 receptor often overexpressed on NEN, provide symptomatic relief and have an anti-proliferative effect that prolongs progression-free survival.[127] Peptide receptor radionuclide therapy comprises the administration of radiolabelled SSAs and by preferentially delivering radiotherapy to NEN, prolongs progression-free survival and offers significant symptom control benefits.[126] It has modest risks of myelo- and renal toxicity.[128]

Interventional liver-directed approaches comprise radioembolisation (also known as *selective internal radiotherapy*),[129] transarterial embolisation, and transarterial chemoembolization.[130] Meta-analyses of retrospective case series have clearly demonstrated favourable objective response and disease control rates.[129] Treatment with any liver-directed approach may lead to the 'post-embolisation syndrome' of fatigue, fever, deranged liver function and abdominal pain. Recent trials have evaluated the combination of peptide receptor radionuclide therapy with selective internal radiotherapy as one manifestation of an increasing focus on multimodal treatment concepts for NEN.[131]

Interferon alpha was in the past applied as a second-line anti-proliferative therapy for well-differentiated PanNEN. Due to its more florid side-effect and toxicity profile compared to SSAs, it is nowadays less frequently used.

✓✓ Sunitinib (tyrosine kinase inhibitor)[124] and everolimus (mTOR pathway inhibitor)[125] have both been shown to prolong progression-free survival in advanced, non-resectable NEN in randomised controlled trials. They are both first-line options for advanced PanNEN, or second line for progressive grade 1/2 tumours.

✓✓ A placebo-controlled trial of somatostatin analogue lanreotide in patients with enteropancreatic NEN has shown evidence of anti-proliferative activity.[127] The results of these three trials would suggest these treatments should represent the standard of care for non-resectable disease.

Systemic chemotherapy was traditionally centred on streptozocin for 5-fluorouracyl-based regimens, although oral temozolomide and capecitabine has emerged recently as a preferred regimen. Chemotherapy is usually first-line for advanced G3 NEN or advanced G1/G2NEN with large tumour burden, or second-line for G1/G2 NEN that have rapid substantial progression.[132]

The management of patients with PanNEN continues to evolve.[133] It is clear that decision-making is complex and dependent on tumour and patient factors. It is strongly recommended that management decisions for these patients are made under consideration of current guidelines in a multidisciplinary forum.[80,108,123]

## OTHER TUMOURS

The other two main types of cystic neoplasms are serous (SCA) and mucinous (MCN) cystic neoplasms. Because of the difference in malignant potential, the management of these two tumours differs, yet clinically and radiologically there is considerable overlap. It is therefore useful to compare and contrast them. The exact incidence of SCA and MCN is unknown; however, in a retrospective review of 24 039 patients undergoing radiological imaging, 0.7% had PCN. Of the 49 (0.2%) who underwent surgery, 10 and 16 patients had a final diagnosis of SCA and MCN, respectively.[5] A large multinational retrospective study reported on 2622 patients with SCA.[134] The median age at diagnosis was 58 years, with 74% occurring in women. Sixty-one percent of patients were asymptomatic. SCA were evenly distributed throughout the pancreas. In contrast, MCNs are almost exclusively found in women, with a peak incidence in the fifth decade, and are more likely to be located within the tail.[135] SCAs are also commonly associated with Von Hippel–Lindau syndrome[69] (see Fig. 18.7), and young patients presenting with multiple cystic lesions involving the pancreas and kidneys should be genetically assessed.[136]

On cross-sectional imaging, the four typical appearances of SCA were microcystic (45%, multiple <2 cm cysts, Fig. 18.8), macrocystic (32%, multiple >2 cm cysts), mixed type (18%, variable-sized cysts) and solid (5%, no cysts visible on cross-sectional imaging).[134] Central calcification (so-called '*sunburst calcification*') occurred in 15%. When the classic

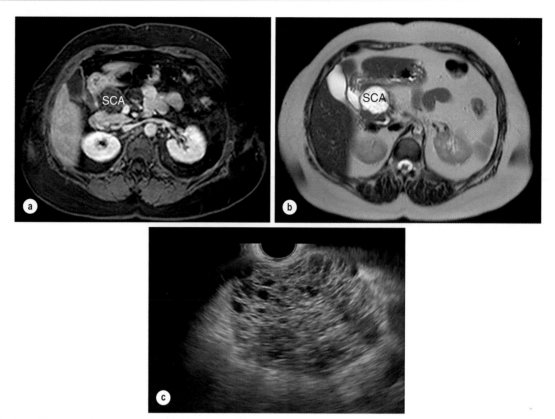

**Figure 18.8**   (a and b) Magnetic resonance imaging sequence of pancreatic microcystic serous cystadenoma (SCA). (c) Endoscopic ultrasound imaging characteristics of same lesion (Images courtesy of I.D. Penman).

features are present, differentiation from other tumours is not difficult; however, the presence of a uni- or oligo-locular macrocystic (>2 cm) lesion is more difficult to diagnose and a wide differential exists. Both SCAs (oligocystic type) and MCNs can fall into this group, although MCNs are less likely to be multilocular and, if calcification occurs, it does so peripherally and may be a marker of underlying malignancy.[137] The presence of solid components within a cystic lesion indicates the presence of, or high-risk of, malignancy and therefore surgical resection should be considered.[137] Included within this differential would be PanNEN, solid pseudopapillary neoplasm (young women) or mucinous cyst adenocarcinoma.[137] It is unusual for either SCAs or MCNs to communicate with the pancreatic duct, but it has been reported.[137]

The ability of non-interventional imaging to obtain an accurate diagnosis is limited. In a report of 100 SCAs from Bassi et al., the correct diagnosis was achieved in 53%, 54% and 76% by ultrasound (US), CT and MRI, respectively.[138] An incorrect diagnosis was made in 31%, 34% and 26%, and the investigation was non-diagnostic in 16%, 12% and 0% with US, CT and MRI, respectively.

In a study of solitary cystic (IPMN were excluded) neoplasms, 71 patients underwent EUS and fluid aspiration (for mucin, viscosity, amylase, lipase, CEA, CA19-9, cytology) followed by surgery to assess its accuracy.[139] The authors concluded that an accurate algorithm using measurement of viscosity, lipase and CEA can be used to determine the diagnosis of cystic lesions. A viscosity of ≥1.6 indicates an MCN and the patient should be offered resection. If it is <1.6 and the lipase is <6000 U/mL, this indicates an SCA. If the viscosity is <1.6

and lipase is >6000 U/mL, then a CEA measurement should be performed, and if this value is less than 480 U/mL the diagnosis is a pseudocyst. If it is >480 U/mL, a repeat EUS and FNA should be performed in 3–6 months. Using this algorithm, only two of 71 patients that underwent resection for suspected MCN had a final histology revealing a pseudocyst.

The management of SCAs and MCNs differs based on their malignant potential. SCAs rarely undergo malignant transformation and if asymptomatic, no intervention is required.[134] Patients with significant symptoms may be offered resection.[134] Until recently, it was recommended that all suspected MCNs undergo resection because of their malignant potential.[14] However, more recent series[140] have shown that it is safe to observe lesions less than 3 cm without mural nodules, thus aligning management with BD-IPMN.

Pathologically, SCAs demonstrate monomorphous cuboidal-shaped epithelium. The cells are glycogen-rich with cellular cytoplasm and small regular nuclei. There is a lack of mitotic activity. The cysts appear 'empty' on microscopy. In contrast, the cyst content of MCNs is turbid and tenacious,[136] and microscopically (unlike SCAs), the cyst lining can be highly variable. The cells are mucin-producing, which can be a single cell layer of flattened cuboidal epithelium or contain papillary tufting.[136] The tumours are classified as benign, borderline or malignant depending on the nuclear features of the cells.[136] It is important to examine the whole tumour as malignant invasion can occur without the presence of a mass.[136] The unique feature of MCNs, however, is the presence of ovarian stroma (highly cellular, densely packed, plump spindle cells). Current recommendations require the presence of this for a tumour to be classified as an MCN.[14] This is particularly important when the differential includes IPMN, in which this type of stroma is not seen.[14]

## Key points

- As the use of cross-sectional imaging has become more frequent, there has been an increase in the diagnosis of cystic neoplasms and small non-functioning neuroendocrine neoplasms within the pancreas.
- MD-IPMN should be resected because of the high incidence of underlying malignancy; however, a selective approach to intervention for side-branch IPMN should be taken (dependent on the presence of symptoms, tumour markers and tumour characteristics).
- Investigation and follow-up of cystic lesions of the pancreas requires a multimodal approach, of which EUS with biopsy is becoming an increasingly important component.
- While asymptomatic SCAs do not require intervention, some MCNs should be resected because of their underlying malignant potential.
- Somatostatin receptor-based PET/CT or PET/MRI techniques has evolved as the gold standard imaging modality for detection of metastatic disease and staging in patients with G1/G2 PanNEN (with the exception of insulinomas).
- The management of PanNEN will be dependent on the presence or absence of an underlying genetic syndrome, whether the tumour is hormonally active, and stage of disease.
- Biochemically confirmed functional PanNEN, and those that are non-secreting but larger than 2 cm in size should be evaluated for surgery.
- Neoadjuvant therapies have been shown to increase the resectability in patients with advanced PanNEN.
- Non-surgical therapeutic strategies for locally advanced and/or metastatic PanNEN encompass a panel of treatment options including traditional cytotoxic chemotherapy, interferons, somatostatin analogues, molecularly targeted agents, peptide receptor radionuclide therapy, and interventional percutaneous and angiographic liver-directed therapies.

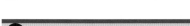 References available at http://ebooks.health.elsevier.com/

## ▶ RECOMMENDED VIDEOS

- Laparoscopic radical antegrade pancreatosplenectomy – https://tinyurl.com/yc3jgg9k (IHPBA members only)
- Laparoscopic pancreatico-jejunostomy during laparoscopic pancreatico-duodenectomy – https://tinyurl.com/y9gtsmwn
- University of Toronto video atlas of pancreatic techniques and procedures – https://tinyurl.com/ya96srgv
- Endoscopic ultrasound assessment of a pancreatic cystic neoplasm
- https://www.youtube.com/watch?v=jpzsSVLWors

## ACKNOWLEDGEMENT

We would like to acknowledge Saxon Connor who authored the previous version of this chapter.

## KEY REFERENCES

[1] Landoni L, Marchegiani G, Pollini T, et al. The evolution of surgical strategies for pancreatic neuroendocrine tumors (PanNENs): time-trend and outcome analysis from 587 consecutive resections at a high-volume institution. Ann Surg 2019;269(4):725–32. https://doi.org/10.1097/SLA.0000000000002594
*In this paper, development of surgical management of PanNEN over the last three decades is presented. The detection rate and the resectability have increased. Functioning and nodal status, tumour grade, and vascular invasion are of prognostic relevance.*

[14] Tanaka M, Fernandez-del Castillo C, Adsay V, et al. International consensus guidelines for management of intraductal papillary mucinous neoplasms and mucinous cystic neoplasms of the pancreas. Pancreatology 2012;12:183–97. PMID: 22687371
*This international guideline outlines a detailed management strategy for the IPMN and MCN of the pancreas.*

[28] Vege SS, Ziring B, Jain R, et al. Clinical guidelines committee. AGA Institute guideline on the diagnosis and management of asymptomatic neoplastic cysts. Gastroenterology 2015;148:819–22. PMID: 25805375.

[54] Falconi M, Crippa S, Chari S, et al. Quality and assessment of the guidelines on cystic neoplasms of the pancreas. Pancreatology 2015;15:463–9. PMID: 26100659
*This paper examines the quality of the published guidelines on pancreatic cystic neoplasms. It highlights the deficits of the current literature and tries to achieve expert consensus on clinically important questions.*

[106] Norton JA, Fraker DL, Alexander HR, et al. Surgery increases survival in patients with gastrinoma. Ann Surg 2006;244:410–9. PMID: 16926567
*In a study of 160 patients with gastrinomas, 35 patients (with similar staged localised disease) who did not undergo resection were compared to those who underwent resection. After 12 years' follow-up, 29% of those who did not undergo surgery had developed hepatic metastases compared to 5% in the resected group (P < 0.001).*

[124] Raymond E, Dahan L, Raoul JL, et al. Sunitinib malate for the treatment of pancreatic neuroendocrine tumors. N Engl J Med 2011;364:501–13. PMID: 21306237
*One hundred and seventy-one patients with advanced and progressive PNETs were randomised in double-blind fashion to placebo or sunitinib. The trial was stopped early because of increased complications and death in the placebo group. An improved progression-free survival (11.5 vs. 5.5 months, P < 0.001) and reduced risk of death (105 vs. 255, P = 0.02) were seen in the treatment group.*

[125] Yao JC, Shah MH, Ito T, et al. Everolimus for advanced pancreatic neuroendocrine tumours. N Engl J Med 2011;364:514–23. PMID: 21306238
*In a placebo-controlled randomised crossover design trial, 410 patients with advanced and progressive PNETs were enrolled to placebo or everolimus. In those patients who received everolimus, there was a 65% reduction in risk of progression (median progression-free survival was 11 months vs. 4.6 months) as compared to placebo. In addition, tolerance was high.*

[134] Jais B, Rebours V, Malleo G, et al. SCN of the pancreas: a multinational study of 2622 patients. Gut 2016;65:305–12. PMID: 26045140
*This large multinational study reported on 2622 patients with serous cystadenomas accumulated over three decades. The key points were: asymptomatic patients do not need resection and disease-specific mortality is extremely rare.*

# 19 Hepato-pancreato-biliary trauma

Michael Hughes | Kristoffer Lassen

## INTRODUCTION

Trauma care in general has been revolutionized by the increased availability and accuracy of cross-sectional imaging and interventional radiology. The 'trauma CT scan' is an integral part of most units' major trauma protocols and specialized trauma centres depend on 24-hour availability of endovascular embolisation. As a result, injuries are diagnosed quickly, often allowing detailed assessment of severity and direction of treatment strategy with traumatic haemorrhage frequently controlled without surgery.

As the diagnosis of hepatopancreaticobiliary (HPB) trauma has become faster and more accurate, the general surgeon will be obliged to manage and determine initial treatment strategies for a growing number of patients with, predominantly, liver trauma.

Accurate diagnosis of such trauma has led to an increased confidence in non-operative management (NOM) of isolated liver trauma, and this has become increasingly tolerated as experience has grown. Furthermore, interventional radiology is a crucial pillar of care for these patients and can augment non-operative as well as operative surgery and has become the platform for HPB trauma care.

Within this chapter the aims are to describe the presentation, assessment and treatment options as well as the outcomes related to these injuries and their treatment. Although some injuries such as liver trauma are common and there is good evidence available for scrutiny, some rarer aspects of HPB trauma are less well reported and the available evidence as well as the authors' experience are discussed.

## LIVER TRAUMA

### EPIDEMIOLOGY

The liver is a commonly injured abdominal organ.[1–3] With the increase in motor vehicle use and also the increased use of sensitive imaging modalities, both the occurrence and detection of liver injuries has greatly increased since the 1990s[4] and is reported at levels of up to 36% of all abdominal injuries.[5–8]

### MECHANISM OF INJURY

The mechanism of liver injury is dichotomised into blunt and penetrating injury and is critical when determining the treatment strategy. Blunt mechanisms of abdominal trauma most commonly include motor vehicle collisions, falls from height and assaults.[9] Blunt trauma in European centres is responsible for 85–90% of liver injuries and will be the focus of this chapter. In isolated liver injuries, the proportion of blunt liver injuries is less, reported in a major study as 64.5%.[10,11] Mortality rates of all liver injuries are reported between 14% and 16%. Due to the liver's size and position as well as its relatively fragile consistency, it is vulnerable to blunt abdominal trauma. The high vascular make-up of the liver makes injury a potentially catastrophic situation and must be carefully considered by an experienced trauma team, often in consultation with the HPB specialist team.

## LIVER INJURY GRADING

The American Association for the Surgery of Trauma Organ Injury Scale (AAST-OIS) grading classification of liver trauma is a validated and commonly used system to quantify liver injuries.[3]

In recognition of the increased reliance of computed tomography (CT) scanning to diagnose liver injury and also its significant influence on management, the AAST 2018 version update (Table 19.1) incorporates radiological findings and evidence of vascular injury into the grading system. This important inclusion therefore identifies and prioritises the presence of an identifiable vascular injury over more significant parenchymal compromise and any evidence of active bleeding detected on CT equates to at least a grade 3 injury. This is in recognition of ongoing bleeding as a predictor of failure of NOM, and mortality.[12]

The World Society of Emergency Surgery (WSES) guidelines for trauma management grades liver injury as follows: grades 1-2 are minor injuries, grade 3 is moderate and grades 4-5 are severe (with the caveat that haemodynamic instability of any grade is classified as severe).[13] This incorporates not only the anatomical and radiological findings but also the overall clinical stability of the patient and therefore the clinical context in which to determine a management strategy.

Minor hepatic injuries:

- **WSES grade I** includes AAST grade I-II hemodynamically stable either blunt or penetrating lesions.

Moderate hepatic injuries:

- **WSES grade II** includes AAST grade III hemodynamically stable either blunt or penetrating lesions.

Severe hepatic injuries:

- **WSES grade III** includes AAST grade IV-VI hemodynamically stable either blunt or penetrating lesions.
- **WSES grade IV** includes AAST grade I-VI hemodynamically unstable either blunt or penetrating lesions.

**Table 19.1    Liver injury scale—2018 revision**

| AAST grade | AIS severity | Imaging criteria (CT findings) | Operative criteria | Pathologic criteria |
|---|---|---|---|---|
| I | 1 | – Subcapsular hematoma < 10% surface area<br>– Parenchymal laceration < 1 cm in depth | – Subcapsular hematoma < 10% surface area<br>– Parenchymal laceration < 1 cm in depth<br>– Capsular tear | – Subcapsular hematoma < 10% surface area<br>– Parenchymal laceration < 1 cm<br>– Capsular tear |
| II | 2 | – Subcapsular hematoma 10–50% surface area; intraparenchymal hematoma<br>– ≤ 10 cm in diameter<br>– Laceration 1–3 cm in depth and ≤ 10 cm length | – Subcapsular hematoma 10–50% surface area; intraparenchymal hematoma < 10 cm in diameter<br>– Laceration 1–3 cm in depth and ≤ 10 cm length | – Subcapsular hematoma 10–50% surface area; intraparenchymal hematoma<br>– < 10 cm in diameter<br>– Laceration 1–3 cm depth and ≤ 10 cm length |
| III | 3 | – Subcapsular hematoma >5 0% surface area: ruptured subcapsular or parenchymal hematoma<br>– Intraparenchymal hematoma > 10 cm<br>– Laceration > 3 cm depth<br>– Any injury in the presence of a liver vascular injury or active bleeding contained within liver parenchyma | – Subcapsular hematoma > 50% surface area or expanding; ruptured subcapsular or parenchymal hematoma<br>– Intraparenchymal hematoma > 10 cm<br>– Laceration > 3 cm in depth | – Subcapsular hematoma > 50% surface area; ruptured subcapsular or intraparenchymal hematoma<br>– Intraparenchymal hematoma > 10 cm<br>– Laceration > 3 cm in depth |
| IV | 4 | – Parenchymal disruption involving 25–75% of a hepatic lobe<br>– Active bleeding extending beyond the liver parenchyma into the peritoneum | – Parenchymal disruption involving 25–75% of a hepatic lobe | – Parenchymal disruption involving 25–75% of a hepatic lobe |
| V | 5 | – Parenchymal disruption > 75% of hepatic lobe<br>– venous injury to include retrohepatic vena cava and central major hepatic veins | – Parenchymal disruption > 75% of hepatic lobe<br>– Juxtahepatic venous injury to include retrohepatic vena cava and central major hepatic veins | – Parenchymal disruption > 75% of hepatic lobe<br>– Juxtahepatic venous injury to include retrohepatic vena cava and central major hepatic veins |

Vascular injury is defined as a pseudoaneurysm or arteriovenous fistula and appeals as a focal collection of vascular contrast that decreases in attenuation with delayed imaging. Active bleeding from a vascular injury presents as vascular contrast, focal or diffuse that increases in size or attenuation in delayed phase. Vascular thrombosis can lead to organ infarction. Grade based on highest grade assessment is made on imaging, at operation or on pathologic specimen. More than one grade of liver injury may be present and should be classified by the higher grade of injury. Advance one grade for multiple injuries up to a grade III.

## ASSESSMENT OF LIVER INJURIES

Clinical assessment of liver trauma follows the same assessment protocol as for any trauma evaluation. Patients are evaluated as per the Advanced Trauma Life Support (ATLS) guidelines according to ABCDE approach. Clinical evaluation of circulatory status is carefully performed and response to fluid resuscitation is assessed.

Haemodynamic stability is a critical component of management of liver trauma as this is a crucial factor when determining the grade of liver injury and an appropriate management strategy. This is not a stand-alone measurement and involves serial assessment and evaluation in the context of clinical interventions and response to treatment. A recent review concluded that there is no universal consensus between care providers of the definition of haemodynamic instability.[14] Overall, the most common parameters quoted were systolic blood pressure, heart rate and response to fluid resuscitation, although the precise cut-off of these parameters at which a patient is deemed to be haemodynamically unstable was not universally defined.

This highlights the importance of recognition of difference in opinions regarding the classification of patients as haemodynamically unstable and if this has been achieved with or without intervention. As haemodynamic instability is a critical component of liver trauma assessment and care, what constitutes 'instability' needs to be defined, if not universally then between individuals' care providers. Changes in patient status and interventions performed to achieve stability must be recognized and managed accordingly in the appropriate locations.

## INVESTIGATION

Ultimately detailed imaging is required to fully examine the abdominal cavity if a liver injury is suspected. Focused Assessment with Sonography for Trauma (FAST) scanning can be performed in the emergency room, although the sensitivity of this to detect intracapsular bleeding, ongoing bleeding or small bleeds is compromised with reports of injury being picked up in less than 40% of liver injuries[15] compared with CT scanning.

The mainstay of imaging and investigation to diagnose and guide management of liver trauma has for around 20 years been CT scanning.[16,17] Importantly, CT scanning will provide a complete overview of injuries to other abdominal organs or in other compartments. With arterial and portovenous phases, one can identify the extent of injury as well as evidence of active haemorrhage from the liver. This provides the detail to determine if emergency interventional radiology is indicated. Furthermore, evidence of biliary complication can also be estimated from the initial CT pictures.[18] Timely CT scanning is therefore a requirement in order to safely assess and manage liver injuries.

Evidence of laceration and haematoma as well as evidence of active bleeding can all be detected by CT which, along with the clinical interpretation of haemodynamic stability contribute to assign a severity grading to liver injury.[19] Furthermore, injury to major hepatic veins and portal structures can also be identified which can aid surgical planning if appropriate.

CT scanning is reported as having 83.3% positive predictive value (PPV) for liver injuries with a negative predictive value (NPV) of 100%.[20] When compared with FAST scanning in a retrospective study looking at 226 trauma patients with liver or splenic injury, FAST scanning recorded a PPV and NPV overall of 99.5% and 83.3%, respectively. However, a 20% rate of missed injuries in FAST scans was reported compared with CT findings, with these cases having injuries or free fluid that was not detected by FAST. This was particularly evident in lower-grade solid organ injuries.[21] A negative FAST scan is therefore not reassuring in patients suffering major trauma.

Magnetic resonance imaging (MRI) scanning is not normally indicated in the acute stages but will be useful at a later evaluation of suspected biliary complications.

# MANAGEMENT

## EVOLUTION OF PRACTICE

The management of liver trauma has developed significantly over the past two decades. Major liver injury has historically been managed by exploratory laparotomy and surgical control of haemorrhage, but the development of selective non-operative management (SNOM) has completely changed the management approaches for these injuries.

A report of liver injuries over a 25-year period from 1975 to 1999 identified significant changes in the management of liver trauma over this time. There has been an evolution of practice away from surgical intervention for liver trauma in the 70s and 80s and increased use of NOM, packing and re-looking as part of damage control surgery and latterly, angiography and embolisation of bleeding vessels. This was also shown alongside a reduction in mortality rates associated with liver trauma overall and a general acceptance and favouring of NOM for the majority of cases.[11,22–24]

## SELECTIVE NON-OPERATIVE MANAGEMENT

The mainstay for the majority of blunt liver injury is SNOM. This requires the presence of a high-quality CT scan with quantification of the liver injury and confidence of absence of arterial bleeding that requires embolisation.[13] Additionally, SNOM should be undertaken in haemodynamically stable patients following initial resuscitation without suspicion of further abdominal injuries that require laparotomy A critical component of NOM is the use of embolisation of bleeding liver arterial vasculature. This is an established adjunct to conservative management. Patients undergoing SNOM should be monitored closely in a critical care environment

with on-site access to a surgeon experienced in managing liver trauma as well as access to on-site 24-hour interventional radiology capacity.

## DEFINITION OF NON-OPERATIVE MANAGEMENT

The precise NOM protocol will vary according to individual unit. The underlying premise is quantification of all underlying injuries to ensure no other indication for surgery has been missed. Once this has been established, close monitoring in a critical care environment is crucial.[13,25] Continuous observation of hemodynamic stability is required and also regular assessment of haemoglobin levels and liver function tests. This period of close monitoring will be variable but normally can be reduced after 48 hours if there are no signs of deterioration. The average length of stay of all liver injuries undergoing SNOM in a large trauma registry review of isolated blunt liver injuries was 2 days.[26] The recommendation being that patients with stable haemoglobin levels and normal abdominal examination can be discharged safely. Some units favour repeat imaging by way of further CT scan or contrast-enhanced ultrasound scan, but the benefits of this are uncertain. The critical component of NOM is the capacity to rapidly perform laparotomy if there is deterioration and for immediate access to interventional radiology and angiography with embolisation should active bleeding be encountered.

For patients with minor liver injuries, SNOM is the standard treatment recommendation. For patients with higher grade of injury 4-5, then particular consideration should be made to the potentially rapid deterioration from a secondary bleed. With this in mind, the logistical consideration of transport, availability of IR, operating theatres and the surgical team needs to be considered in case rapid intervention and change from conservative management is required. This will mean transfer of patients to tertiary HPB units for observation and readiness for rapid operative or IR intervention.

## OUTCOMES AND FAILURE OF SNOM

Failure of NOM is rare in low-grade isolated liver injuries.

The vast majority of such cases are managed with SNOM with studies reporting over 90% of cases of blunt low-grade trauma, without other indications for laparotomy, being managed non-operatively. Failure rates are reported as low as 3% in some series [27], although prospective data report failure of SNOM at up to 17% [28]. The reasons for failure are predominantly secondary bleeding, but biliary complications and missed injuries can manifest thus mandating laparotomy. SNOM demands close monitoring, and evidence of haemodynamic instability, haemoglobin drop or signs of infection suggests that repeat imaging is required and reconsideration of the continued appropriateness of NOM.

SNOM is more likely to be successful due to the de-selection of the majority of major hepatic vessel/retrohepatic caval injuries not surviving to reach a medical facility. The majority of survivable blunt injuries involves damage to the liver parenchymal vessels which will stop bleeding by tamponade and therefore are likely to be successfully managed with simple observation. [27-30]

## SNOM IN SEVERE LIVER INJURY

When looking at NOM in minor liver injuries, NOM is accepted as the first management option. When the extent of liver injury is severe, or classed as grades 3–5, then the evidence for SNOM is less well established.

Saqib[31] performed a systematic review of NOM in severe liver injury. No randomized trials were identified but of the included eight studies, five reported outcomes for SNOM in high-grade liver trauma. SNOM in these patients resulted in a success rate of 92.4% of 210 patients and a mortality rate of 3.3%. These figures were superior to the surgically treated patients with mortality figures of 15.8%. The author of this review raises the important issue of lack of randomisation and the inherent bias between the two groups in terms of haemodynamic instability, namely the definitions of haemodynamic stability, and also the almost exclusive inclusion of unstable patients in the surgically managed groups. Nevertheless, it does provide evidence that the extent of injury alone is not an immediate indication for surgery, rather, the overall stability and concern for other injuries. A further study from Italy reported a 100% success rate of SNOM with grade 1 patients and a 90% success rate in patients with grade 5 liver injuries, and of those requiring laparotomy, none of these was for bleeding[32] supporting the feasibility of this approach.

The use of transarterial embolisation (TAE) in NOM in severe hepatic injury is also less well established than for minor injuries. A systematic review by Virdis et al.[33] reported outcomes of 659 patients with severe liver injury undergoing TAE with a 6% failure rate, 28% morbidity rate and 5% mortality rate. Morbidity reported included bile leak (5.7%), abscess (6.8%), ischaemia (8.6%) and biloma (2.8%).

Melloul et al.[29] in 2015 conducted a systematic review of severe blunt hepatic injuries—namely grades 3–5 and identified just under 5000 patients from 12 studies. A success rate of 92% was reported in patients undergoing SNOM from eight studies, with up to 5% requiring TAE and 4% going on to record biliary complications and a 90-day mortality of 5%. This review also comments on a further group of patients with severe liver injury and active bleeding at the time of presentation. Five studies reported TAE performed initially in this group with a success rate of 94% in these patients. However, up to 30% of this group subsequently required laparotomy for abdominal compartment syndrome (ACS) or biliary complications, and the mortality rate was reported at up to 10%.

Similarly Gaski et al.[11] in 2018 addressed this issue with a SNOM protocol that included selective TAE in severe liver trauma with signs of active bleeding only, as opposed to a previous protocol of mandatory embolisation in the severe injury grade group. They reported a 0% failure rate in severely injured patients undergoing this approach, with 12% requiring TAE and a mortality rate of 15%. This was compared with a mortality rate of 46% for severe liver injuries requiring laparotomy. This protocol incorporated damage control resuscitation principles and the major haemorrhage protocol was only initiated in patients with a systolic blood pressure of less than 90 mmHg and when signs of ongoing active bleeding were present, and reported a liver-related death from haemorrhage of 4%.

These trials suggest that with the appropriate use of NOM and selection of patients with haemodynamic stability, as per DCR criteria, even in the most severely injured livers with signs of ongoing bleeding, the use of TAE can not only avoid laparotomy but this approach can also be associated with improved mortality rate and low failure rates of NOM. The caveat to this is that there are no randomised trials supporting this and there is always the risk of an operative comparative group selecting the sickest and most unstable patients with highest risk of death. Viewed together with the available data for SNOM, a randomised controlled trial is not likely to be possible in this population group.

Based on the current evidence, the WSES has published guidelines on the NOM of blunt hepatic injury[13] with findings as described above with the strongest evidence base supporting:

- Non-operative approach should not be undertaken for haemodynamically unstable patients, or those with diffuse peritonitis
- A laparotomy is not indicated if patient is haemodynamically stable without peritonitis
- A contrast CT scan is mandated to establish severity of liver injury
- The severity of hepatic injury is not an absolute contraindication to NOM
- TAE can be considered in actively bleeding but haemodynamically stable patients
- SNOM can only be trialled where there is capacity for close monitoring and emergency surgery.

## NON-OPERATIVE MANAGEMENT IN PENETRATING TRAUMA

Penetrating injury, less common in Western Europe than in USA, South Africa and other areas, mainly include gunshot wounds (GSWs) and stabbing incidents.[27,30] While SNOM is accepted initial management for the majority of blunt hepatic injuries, its role in the management of penetrating liver injuries is less well established. However, evidence is available to suggest that in selected patients NOM can provide satisfactory results and prevent non-therapeutic laparotomies.

The selection criteria for SNOM in penetrating liver injuries requires haemodynamic stability of patients at admission and also the absence of peritonitis due to hollow viscus perforation—more likely following penetrating trauma, and also the ability to perform serial accurate clinical examination without the masking effect of intoxication.

Data from the USA have reported that 33% of all penetrating liver injuries were selected for NOM; 28% of all penetrating liver injuries, including 23.5% of all severe injuries, were managed successfully non-operatively.[28] A recent study identified that 16.2% of all penetrating liver injuries were amenable to being managed successfully with SNOM. Only one patient selected for SNOM failed due to undetected hollow viscus injury.[34] Navsaria et al.[35] reported in 2015 a success rate of 91.4% for patients undergoing SNOM in liver GSWs from a large prospective trauma series from South Africa. More recently, the same group published outcomes of a larger series of liver GSWs, of which 71.7% of the cohort required emergency laparotomy. Of the 54 patients selected for SNOM, 3 patients required surgical intervention due to development of peritonitis and thus representing a 94.4% success rate for SNOM in carefully selected complex liver GSWs.[30]

These figures support the potential success for SNOM in penetrating trauma. However, caution must be exercised in this group as the data reveal high degrees of patient selection to achieve very low failure rates of SNOM in their population. The data are from high-volume trauma centres in the USA and South Africa, and a high level of experience in managing severe penetrating abdominal injuries is required to achieve good outcomes in this challenging group.[30]

## COMPLICATIONS OF LIVER TRAUMA

After the initial insult, mainly related to bleeding, has subsided, liver trauma carries with it the risk of further complications. The risk of morbidity increases with grade of injury and is also more common following surgically managed liver trauma. The most commonly reported morbidity following liver injury includes biliary complications, with bile leak or biloma encountered in 24% of patients in one case series, diagnosed on average 8 days from injury.[36]

A study by Kozar et al.[37] assessed 543 patients who had sustained high-grade blunt liver injury as part of a multicentre study. The overall morbidity rate of this group was 13%. The most common complications reported were bleeding (8%), biliary fistula (3.7%), infectious complication (3%) including abscess and ACS (1.1%). They reported that the morbidity rate increased with grade of injury and that bleeding and ACS were most likely to occur within 3 days of injury, but biliary and infectious complications occurred beyond this point. The authors of this study report that notwithstanding biliary peritonitis, biliary morbidity can be managed successfully with a combination of percutaneous drainage and endoscopic retrograde cholangiopancreatography (ERCP) stenting. Late bleeding was also managed by TAE for the majority of patients suffering this complication.

A further study looking specifically at bile leak post blunt liver trauma recorded a rate of 4.9%. Higher severity grade of injury, central injury and raised serum bilirubin levels were indicative of development of bile leak. Prompt diagnosis and treatment of bile leak in this study resulted in no mortality in this group. For patients with these risk factors as described, a high index of suspicion should be maintained.[38]

Green et al.[39] conducted a systematic review of outcomes following TAE for liver trauma; 998 patients were included from 11 studies, none of which were randomised trials and, of this group, 347 (34.8%) underwent TAE. The efficacy of this intervention was 93% and the overall mortality rate was reported as 9.6%. The study went on to report morbidity related to TAE and the most commonly reported complications were necrosis (14.9%), abscess (7.5%) with gallbladder infarction and bile leak recorded to a lesser degree.

Overall NOM is a favoured approach for almost all blunt liver injuries and a selected group of penetrating liver injuries. The adjuncts to NOM include TAE and also the modalities of treatment of the complications of liver injury. Percutaneous and endoscopic management of biliary complications will play a part in SNOM and the multidisciplinary approach to these complex patients will ensure optimum outcomes.

## OPERATIVE MANAGEMENT

Should NOM be contraindicated, the general emergency surgeon must be able to provide initial resuscitative operative management. Most commonly the indication for surgery is haemodynamic instability due to major, secondary or persistent haemorrhage whereby surgery is mandated.

The conventional approach to trauma damage control laparotomy is performed with the principles of achieving haemostasis and removal of contamination being the guiding principles.

## INITIAL LAPAROTOMY

A long midline incision is the standard approach. An extension of the midline incision can be made towards the subcostal margin, which will facilitate access to the right upper quadrant should this be required. The stomach, colon and small bowel can be retracted inferiorly and held in place with a large pack and further retractor to allow improved access to the liver and porta hepatis.

The first manoeuvre, once the field is exposed, is to establish and control the source of the bleeding that prompted the laparotomy. If the parenchyma of the liver has been fractured, then the fracture should initially be closed by direct manual pressure applied in the direction of the injury. It is advised to avoid packing or applying pressure directly into the injured area as this can open and push apart the injury and dislodge any clots aiding in haemostasis.

The next stage is packing. This is an active process that has been shown to be effective in not only smaller bleeds but also the most severe liver injuries. Packs should be able to sustainably reinforce the pushing manoeuvre. Rolled up packs are placed behind and in front of the right lobe as well as in a similar set up on the left side. Care must be taken to avoid 'over packing' as this can lead to pressure of the inferior vena cava (IVC), and also the renal veins, and can contribute to ACS.

If bleeding is not stopped by these measures, a Pringle manoeuvre can be performed with the fingers of the left hand or an atraumatic clamp to the porta hepatis. A tape can then be passed around the porta to perform the Pringle manoeuvre and have two hands free. Careful timing of the placement of the Pringle should be recorded. Consideration should be made of liver ischaemia and gut oedema secondary to Pringle placement and 15 minutes of Pringle should be sufficient to perform packing. This can be repeated after an interval of approximately 5 minutes.

## OPERATIVE INTERVENTIONS

Once these three steps have been performed, the expectation is that bleeding will be controlled. This will be true in the majority of cases. If this is not the case and bleeding continues, there is likely to be a bleed from juxtahepatic venous injury. This will be discussed later. However, in the case of significant haemorrhage that is controlled with the simple measures, the principles of damage control surgery should be followed to allow resuscitation, treatment of coagulopathy and rewarming of the patient.

The laparotomy should be completed, all contamination washed out and controlled and the patient should be transferred to the ICU where the lethal triad of acidosis, coagulopathy and hypothermia can be reversed. The patient can be returned to theatre, often between 24 and 48 hours later, for careful pack removal and inspection for any further bleeding or bile leak as well as other injuries not identified earlier and possible reconstruction or definitive repair of other injuries. Care must be taken on pack removal that re-bleeding does not occur and some surgeons advocate the placement of sterile sheets or even the omentum between the parenchyma and gauze packs to try and prevent re-bleeding at this point.

However, definitive techniques to stop bleeding are also possible and necessary. Techniques to stop small arterial bleeds include suture ligation, clips and energy device co-agulation. The use of hybrid theatres can facilitate the use of intraoperative or postoperative interventional arterial embolisation should the bleeding point not be visualised or readily accessible. Once the patient is stabilised by the use of packing and simple techniques, definitive embolisation can be performed in a controlled fashion with survival rates reported between 69% and 85%.[40–42]

In the case that the patient is stable and not coagulopathic, consideration can potentially be given to more definitive procedures to manage the injured liver. These techniques have been used preferentially in the past but are utilised less in modern practice. There may be circumstances where it is appropriate, but it is emphasised that the majority of liver injuries managed operatively are successfully managed by packing with or without prior or subsequent angiography and embolisation with subsequent debridement of devital-ised parenchyma following stabilisation if indicated.[13,43,44]

The use of selective hepatic artery ligation was historically the method of choice for treatment of significant hepatic vascular injury, along with selective vascular ligation following division of the liver parenchyma. In experienced hands successful results are reported, but their use in current practice is often not required due to the success of the methods described above.[22] These techniques have potential to cause further significant bleeding or necrosis and as such are not recommended. Similarly anatomical resection of injured lobes was performed extensively; however, results were often dire, likely reflecting the major extent of the underlying injury and its use is restricted to highly selected cases in centres with experience in these techniques.

## MAJOR LIVER VEIN INJURY

This is a high-risk situation that is rarely encountered and a major challenge for the experienced liver surgeon.

Damage to the main hepatic veins or the retrohepatic vena cava can result either in major bleed into the liver pa-renchyma or directly into the peritoneal cavity via the hepatic veins from their extra parenchymal portion. The shearing force of major trauma can avulse the veins from the cava or a direct force can rupture their relatively thin walls. The challenge for the trauma surgeon dealing with this injury is the relatively limited access to the hepatic veins and the limited options once the bleeding site has been identified.

Mobilisation of the liver to gain access to the hepatic veins as they enter the suprahepatic vena cava can have the detrimental effect of dislodging clot and leading to uncontrollable bleeding.

Total hepatic venous exclusion can be performed with clamping of the infra and supra hepatic vena cava, combined with Pringle manoeuvre. This has the benefit of stopping the bleeding, but it is often not tolerated in terms of reduced venous return to the heart. The use of venovenous bypass can potentially be used to mitigate this but is not reliably available on a 24-hour basis. Ligation or repair of the injured major vessel can be attempted although the mortality rates of such injuries are over 50%.[22] This strategy has historically been attempted in order to control the bleeding vessel and avoid late re-bleeding. This has been coupled with extensive mobilisation, total vascular hepatic exclusion with or without venovenous bypassing or

atriocaval shunting. The mortality rates have been reported as high as 90% with these techniques.[45,46] More modern thinking suggests that the appropriate strategy for this type of injury is packing with gauze or omentum and performing optimal damage control surgery combined with damage control resuscitation.[22,45,46]

## SUMMARY

Liver trauma is common and the vast majority of injuries are managed non-operatively. The use of TAE has extended the scope of NOM. Overall mortality has improved over the years and even the most severe injuries can be considered for SNOM. The critical issue is the availability of experienced surgical teams capable of rapidly shifting approach to surgical intervention when necessary. TAE can again augment surgical intervention with damage control surgery and packing being successful in the majority of cases. Following injury, managed operatively or not, the potential for biliary morbidity is high and should be closely observed for.

## EXTRAHEPATIC BILIARY TREE INJURIES

### INCIDENCE

Gallbladder and extrahepatic bile duct injuries (EHBTI) are rare and reported in 0.1% of abdominal trauma cases.[47] They are most commonly associated with additional injuries and isolated EHBTI are even rarer. Most frequently they are associated with liver injury, and this has been reported in over 80% of cases of EHBTI,[47,48] but associated injury to the duodenum and pancreas are also reported.

The mechanisms of injury most commonly reported for isolated EHBTI are penetrating injuries; however, blunt EHB-TI is the most common overall and results from compression of the biliary tree against the vertebrae, avulsion of the bile duct at its insertion into the pancreas (32%) or at its confluence at the hilum (23%).[49] These two areas represent the location where the bile duct is most vulnerable from shear forces as it goes to or from a fixed position. Gallbladder injury is most commonly a result of penetrating trauma at levels of up to 89% of all gallbladder trauma reported.[50]

### GRADE OF EXTRAHEPATIC BILIARY TREE INJURIES

EHBTI are graded according to the AAST grading system.[51] Grades 1–3 are considered mild, with grade 4 classified as moderate and grade 5 severe.

Grade 1 – Gallbladder contusion/portal triad contusion.
Grade 2 – Partial gallbladder avulsion from gallbladder bed, cystic duct intact/laceration or perforation of the gallbladder.
Grade 3 – Complete gallbladder avulsion from liver bed/cystic duct laceration.
Grade 4 – Partial or complete left/right hepatic duct laceration/partial < 50% common hepatic duct (CHD)/common bile duct (CBD) laceration.
Grade 5 – >50% transection of CHD/CBD/combined left and right hepatic duct laceration/intraduodenal/pancreatic CBD injury.

## PRESENTATION

The presentation of gallbladder injury and EHBTI may be subtle. In haemodynamically stable patients with liver injuries who undergo NOM, a high index of suspicion must be maintained, especially when a high grade of liver injury is sustained. EHBTI may present early in the non-operative course and may be detected as an acute abdomen, the development of sepsis or identified as free fluid on CT imaging. However, if these signs are not evident and the non-operative approach is successful in terms of the treatment of liver injury, then the diagnosis of EHBTI may be delayed. In a systematic review of EHBTI by Pereira et al.,[52] of the 66 patients with EHBTI, 23 were haemodynamically stable and managed non-operatively. The mean time to diagnosis of biliary tract injury in this group of patients was 11 days.

MRCP and CT are useful if NOM is being undertaken or after the initial damage control surgery. Moreover, percutaneous transhepatic cholangiography and/or ERCP can be diagnostic and therapeutic.

Furthermore, unless there is a high index of suspicion, patients undergoing laparotomy for liver trauma or a damage control laparotomy for abdominal trauma, can have injuries missed unless specifically searched for. Operative findings suggestive of EHTBI include major liver laceration, retroperitoneal bile staining, or portal haematoma. There may also be evidence of free bile and biliary peritonitis. High-risk injuries to the porta hepatis will also include vascular injury and this can lead to significant blood loss, liver ischaemia and portal haematoma.

## TREATMENT

In patients who are diagnosed with EHPTI while undergoing NOM, the EHBTI may be managed with percutaneous drainage of biloma should this be appropriate. Ongoing bile leak may benefit from ERCP and stent with preferential drainage via the ampulla. Stenting can be performed across partial defects in the extrahepatic biliary tree.[51] MRCP is beneficial in investigating ongoing biliary leak in patients percutaneously drained. This combination of biliary stent and percutaneous drain can be successful in cases where limited biliary leak is evident in a haemodynamically stable patient.[52]

However, surgical management is often required.[47,52] In unstable patients undergoing damage control laparotomy, EHBTI can be missed as priority is often rapid control of life-threatening haemorrhage. However, decontamination of the surgical field is a critical component of damage control surgery and this should include bile drainage.

Injury to the gallbladder can be identified preoperatively and also at laparotomy. Signs of gallbladder injury include haematoma or perforation with subsequent leakage of bile. The management of this is cholecystectomy and its presence should alert the surgeon to the possibility to EHBTI.

Large-bore drainage can be performed as a temporizing measure to control sepsis while the patient's physiology improves. Ongoing high-volume bile leak can also be treated with ERCP and stenting when there is clinical stability. This will successfully treat the majority of partial ductal injuries[47] and can be performed in the delayed setting once clinical condition is stable. If high-grade injury is suspected or confirmed, then definitive management will be required at a later stage.

Extensive EHBTI found upon a trauma laparotomy can be drained externally for weeks or months until the patient is amenable to definitive repair. Such definitive treatment will most likely involve biliary enteric anastomosis. The overriding principles of reconstruction are similar to iatrogenic bile duct injuries. Definitive reconstruction is most likely to be successful once the patient is haemodynamically and nutritionally stable and infection is controlled. Hepaticojejunostomy is the most commonly performed biliary reconstruction. This is most commonly indicated for complete transection of the duct, corresponding to the most severe grade of injury. This reconstruction should be performed by the specialist HPB team.

Less severe injuries involving less than 50% of the duct can potentially be managed surgically with T-tube insertion with subsequent delayed removal, or direct primary repair. Long-term morbidity in this group is common and a small case series examining seven traumatic bile duct injuries repaired with either T-tube/primary repair or biliary enteric anastomosis observed that five of the seven cases were complicated by either leak or stricture during the follow-up period.[53] Again, management of these injuries beyond drainage should be performed in specialist HPB units.

## SUMMARY

Isolated EHBTI are rare and the evidence assessing these injuries is limited. In general terms, a high index of suspicion is required if there is evidence of biliary morbidity and no liver injury. Management of major ductal disruption will require reconstruction, but this will likely be more successful away from the initial damage control period. Drainage and endoscopic stenting remain appropriate adjuncts to management in non-operative treatment or following surgical identification of partial ductal injury.

# PANCREATIC TRAUMA

## INCIDENCE

Pancreatic trauma is a less commonly encountered injury with rates of injury reported between 3% and 5% of cases abdominal trauma.[54-56]

It is a potentially dangerous situation, not only because of the underlying pancreas injury itself but also because of its proximity to major vascular structures, a high association with other abdominal organ injuries and also the potential for late complications resulting in a prolonged clinical course.

Mortality rates associated with pancreas trauma are reported at up to 15%,[49,57] and the mortality is complex and bimodal. The early deaths are related to exsanguination following major retroperitoneal vascular injury. The later deaths are related to multiorgan failure and sepsis with the impact of the individual pancreas injury not clearly established.[57] A retrospective analysis of 432 patients with pancreatic injuries from South Africa reported that the head was injured in 32% and the majority of injuries involved the body and tail, and 22% had an associated major vascular injury.[49] An overall morbidity rate of 64% was reported and this included intra-abdominal morbidity (27%) as well as pancreas-specific morbidity (21%), namely pancreatic pseudocysts and pancreatic fistulae. This distribution is likely also biased by patients who have penetrating injuries to the head of the pancreas with associated portal and caval injuries who are unlikely to make it to hospital at all.

## GRADE OF INJURY

When determining management for pancreatic injuries, mortality rate has been shown to be associated with pancreas trauma grade and this is reflected by the validated AAST grading system.

Grade 1 – Minor injury – no duct disruption.
Grade 2 – Major injury – no duct disruption.
Grade 3 – Distal duct disruption.
Grade 4 – Proximal duct disruption.
Grade 5 – Complete destruction of head of pancreas.

A study by Heuer et al.[56] from Germany showed that in their cohort of 284 patients with pancreatic injury following severe abdominal trauma, the AAST grading was associated with early and late mortality rates in this group of patients. Grade 2 injuries had an 8.9% total mortality rate, whereas the mortality rates for grades 3–5 injuries were 27.8%, 30% and 33%, respectively. This pattern was observed when looking at mortality rates in the first 24 hours also.

## PRESENTATION

Pancreatic injures are most often associated with additional injuries rather than in isolation, with multiorgan injury being commonly reported.[54,58] Isolated injuries are more common in children and associated with handlebar injuries and also penetrating trauma in slim adults.

Identification of pancreatic injury is challenging and a high index of suspicion must be maintained. CT scan imaging may identify major injuries with obvious parenchymal transection, but the presence of free fluid is non-specific. Sensitivity and specificity for CT detection of main ductal injury has been reported at 78.7% and 61.6%, respectively.[59] This is an improvement from earlier[60] data as a result of more detailed CT imaging but still reflects a challenge when diagnosing ductal injury radiologically. A low threshold for MRI/MRCP should be exercised when ductal disruption is suspected. MRCP is useful to identify pancreatic ductal disruption[61] but may not be appropriate in the acute situation.

Pancreas injuries are often not diagnosed until laparotomy indicated for haemodynamic instability or concern of GI contamination from small bowel injury.

Serial examination, interval imaging and a high index of suspicion in the non-improving patient with no other injuries is required with repeat CT and/or MRCP imaging. Serum amylase levels are not always raised in the early stages following pancreatic fistula and not related to the degree of severity of injury. Normal amylase levels should not reassure the clinician, although a raised level can alert to the need for prompt repeat cross-sectional imaging.

Delayed presentation of missed pancreatic injury may present later, up to 6 months reported by one study, most likely with pancreatic fistula, pseudocyst or pancreatitis.[62]

## MANAGEMENT

Management is based on the grade of injury, overall clinical condition, the timing of presentation and also the presence of other abdominal injuries. Most often, an indication for emergency laparotomy in a trauma setting will be dictated by injury to another organ than the pancreas, and this will dictate the degree of urgency.

The majority of pancreatic injuries are grades 1 and 2 where there is no disruption to the main pancreatic duct.[54,59,63,64] Isolated pancreatic injuries without duct disruption in haemodynamically stable patients can potentially be managed non-operatively or with percutaneous drainage along with close observation.[65] Further assessment can be obtained with MRCP, with ERCP and pancreatic duct stent if drainage volume does not come down following these non-operative measures,[66] with laparotomy, washout and drainage reserved for inability to control the injury.[54,64] Non-operative approach to these injuries has been reported at 59.1% of cases from a large US data registry study with a mortality rate of 8.6%.[67]

Major surgical intervention is associated with a high morbidity and mortality burden. Overall mortality rates of between 7% and 12% per cent are reported following surgical intervention for pancreas injury.[63,64,68,69] Morbidity rates are also reported as high as 75%[68], with pancreatic fistula, abscess and pseudocyst being responsible for the majority of morbidity with fistula rates reported in up to 40% of patients.[67,69]

If surgery is unavoidable, either because of a mandatory laparotomy to control other injuries or because of significant duct disruption being diagnosed, the approach depends on the grade and position of ductal injury.

The majority of grade 3 injuries managed operatively are managed by distal pancreatectomy. Grade 4 injuries are more frequently managed with drainage.[64,69] Mortality rates are reported to be lower in grade 3 injuries managed by distal pancreatectomy compared with drainage[64] (6% compared with 16% mortality rate for those with grade 3 injury managed without resection), and pseudocyst formation is also reported to be reduced in grade 3 patients managed with distal pancreatectomy.[70] Higher grade of pancreatic fistula is also reported in patients with grade 3 injuries undergoing drainage.[67]

Major ductal disruption represents a dangerous condition with often a long complex hospital stay requiring multimodal management and treatment of complications. Despite the lack of high-quality evidence, postoperative pancreas-specific morbidity emerges from the evidence available as higher in a non-resection group following major duct disruption. The recommendation is therefore resection for this type of injury when laparotomy is indicated (for whatever reason) and distal duct transection is evident[64] and surgical drainage of more proximal, grade 4 injuries.

The subsequent treatment of pancreas-related morbidity either post-surgical or after a non-operative approach, namely fistula, can be effectively managed by percutaneous drainage with or without ERCP and pancreatic duct stenting,[71,72] and endoscopic drainage of pseudocyst.[49]

Finally surgical management of the most severe pancreatic injuries remains challenging but is also very rare. Significant destruction of the pancreatic head is almost always involving the duodenum also. Consideration in this case has to be given to performing pancreatoduodenectomy. Again, feasibility of this is often compromised in the unstable patient, but consideration to staged resection and reconstruction can be given in selected cases. This major procedure is rarely performed and drainage of significant injuries to the pancreatic head is almost always attempted initially.

# DUODENAL TRAUMA AND INJURIES OF THE PANCREATODUODENAL COMPLEX

## INCIDENCE

Isolated duodenal trauma is rare. Hollow viscus injuries make up approximately 1% of all blunt trauma admissions, and a large retrospective cohort analysis showed that duodenal injuries represented 12% of these injuries.[73] Isolated traumatic devascularization with necrosis of the second part of the duodenum (D2) but sparing of the avulsed papilla, especially in children, has been reported by several authors.[74,75] This is a further rare injury of the duodenal/papillary complex but a recognised pattern of injury.

However, due to the proximity of the duodenum to pancreas, liver as well as major vascular structures including the IVC, aorta and mesenteric vessels, duodenal trauma is often associated with other life-threatening injuries.[68] It was reported that patients suffered on average five associated injuries, most commonly liver and colon, and with each additional injury the odds of mortality increased by 27.4%. Associated vascular injury was reported in 30.7% of these patients with penetrating duodenal injuries, and this was associated with a mortality rate of 32.2%.[68]

Penetrating injuries to the duodenum associated with pancreatic injury were reported to represent 36% of duodenal injuries.[70] A multicentre retrospective analysis of duodenal injuries reported outcomes on 372 patients suffering duodenal injuries, of which 79% were penetrating and 68% had associated injuries. Of these, 29% were associated with pancreatic injuries, 6% with liver injuries and 9% with IVC injuries. Overall mortality rate was 24% and injury to the pancreas was an independent predictor of mortality.[69] This injury presents a significant challenge to the HPB surgeon.

## GRADES OF DUODENAL INJURIES

Duodenal injuries are classified according to the AAST-OIS (Table 19.2) ranging from minor serosal haematoma to complete avulsion and devascularisation. This scale is used commonly and has been validated by Phillips et al.[68] in a large registry study assessing penetrating duodenal injuries where mortality was associated with OIS grade.

## DIAGNOSIS

Clinical evaluation can be challenging in patients with injuries of the pancreatic duodenal complex. Clinical signs may be minimal without evidence of overt peritonitis and most patients will require detailed cross-sectional imaging with high-resolution CT scanning. However, CT may not always provide hard evidence to mandate a laparotomy. In this group of patients, signs suggestive of duodenal injury such as small-volume periduodenal fluid or duodenal haematoma may be present but have been reported to have a PPV of duodenal injury requiring surgical repair of only 21%.[76]

Appropriate diagnosis of duodenal injury is critical to avoid prolonged morbidity following major abdominal trauma. Identification of duodenal injury requires an index of suspicion and will often require laparotomy and kocherisation of the duodenum to fully visualise the posterior aspect.

## TREATMENT

Treatment remains a challenge, especially in the rapid laparotomy as part of damage control surgery.

Due to the rarity of duodenal injuries, a large evidence base to guide management is lacking. The original descriptions of surgical repair of large duodenal injuries describe techniques to protect the duodenal repair, should a primary repair be deemed appropriate.

One of the largest retrospective analyses of duodenal trauma identified a high proportion (80%) of primary repairs being performed in patients with all grades of duodenal injuries, with good outcomes achieved.[69] The leak and re-laparotomy rates were lower in the primary repair group. A small proportion underwent additional procedures to protect the primary repair including pyloric exclusion, diverting procedures and gastroenterostomy. Additional procedures beyond primary repair alone were not predictive of mortality, and the significant factor associated with poor outcome was the presence of significant bleeding related to injury to surrounding major vasculature.

A considerable challenge arises when the duodenum and the pancreas are both significantly injured. Primary repair of the duodenum and drainage of the head of pancreas are potential treatment strategies but on rare occasions the destruction and devitalisation of the pancreatic-duodenal complex is such that major resection in the form of a pancreatoduodenectomy is indicated. This injury is most often secondary to penetrating trauma (80%) with mortality rates reported at up to 30%.[77] The largest registry study reporting outcomes following trauma pancreatoduodenectomy reported 39 cases and a mortality rate of 33%, with the authors concluding that such a procedure may not be of benefit[78] (van der wilden), although can be attempted in highly selected cases.

### Table 19.2  AAST organ injury scale for duodenal injuries

**Duodenum injury scale**

| Grade* | Type of injury | Description of injury |
|---|---|---|
| I | Hematoma | Involving single portion of duodenum |
|   | Laceration | Partial thickness, no perforation |
| II | Hematoma | Involving more than one portion |
|   | Laceration | Disruption < 50% of circumference |
| III | Laceration | Disruption 50–75% of circumference of D2 Disruption 50–100% of circumference of D1.D3.D |
| IV | Laceration | Disruption > 75% of circumference of D2 |
|   |   | Involving ampulla or distal common bile duct |
| V | Laceration | Massive disruption of duodenopancreatic complex |
|   | Vascular | Devascularization of duodenum |

*Advance one grade for multiple injuries up to grade III. D1, first portion of duodenum; D2, second portion of duodenum; D3, third portion of duodenum; D4, fourth portion of duodenum.

## SUMMARY

HPB trauma represents a complex and challenging facet of surgery. Liver trauma is common and the vast majority can be managed non-operatively by the general surgeon, with interventional radiology and only occasionally operative intervention indicated. Other areas of HPB trauma are rare and may not be part of many surgeons' experience. The evidence guiding treatment strategies is generally of low quality, retrospective and low in numbers. Rapid damage control surgery, often for other injuries, will form a key treatment, so too are close observation, endoscopic and percutaneous interventions as well as late reconstructive procedures by a specialist HPB surgeon. The multidisciplinary team plays a significant part in the management of hepatobiliary trauma and will continue to do so.

---

### Key points

#### Liver

- Majority of cases can be managed with non-operative management if haemodynamically stable.
- Transarterial embolisation can be an adjunct to non-operative management.
- Majority of unstable cases can be managed with packing at damage control surgery.
- The main complications of liver trauma are biliary morbidity which can be treated with percutaneous drainage and stenting at a later stage.

#### Extrahepatic bile duct injuries

- These are rare injuries.
- Diagnosis may be missed unless searched for.
- Operative management includes drainage in the early stage.
- Reconstruction of major biliary injuries can be performed in a delayed fashion when conditions are optimum.

#### Pancreas

- Pancreatic trauma is challenging to diagnose and associated with high mortality and morbidity.
- Low-grade injuries can be managed non-operatively.
- Severe injuries with ductal disruption are often managed operatively with distal pancreatectomy indicated for distal duct disruption and drainage for proximal disruption.
- High levels of postoperative morbidity are encountered, but the majority can be managed endoscopically/percutaneously.

#### Duodenum

- Challenging to diagnose both radiologically and at operation.
- Primary repair treatment of choice.
- Can be associated with major pancreaticobiliary injuries in rare cases.

---

 References available at http://ebooks.health.elsevier.com/

## KEY REFERENCES

[4] Malhotra AK, et al. Blunt hepatic injury: a paradigm shift from operative to nonoperative management in the 1990s. Ann Surg 2000;231(6):804–13.

*An important recognition of the major changes in management of liver injuries that has influenced trauma care significantly.*

[31] Saqib Y. A systematic review of the safety and efficacy of nonoperative management in patients with high grade liver injury. Surgeon 2020;18(3):165–77.

*Important finding supporting the concept of selective non operative management not only in minor liver injuries.*

[64] Ho VP, et al. Management of adult pancreatic injuries: a practice management guideline from the eastern association for the surgery of trauma. J Trauma Acute Care Surg 2017;82(1):185–99.

*Large review identifying benefits of pancreatic resection in grade 3/4 injuries.*

[78] van der Wilden G., et al. Trauma Whipple: Do or don't after severe pancreaticoduodenal injuries? An analysis of the national trauma data bank (NTDB). World J Surg 2014;38:335–340.

*Limited series but identifies no major benefit in performing trauma Whipple in this group.*

# INDEX